Functional and Bioactive Foods in Promoting Health

Functional and Bioactive Foods in Promoting Health

Edited by Teresa Clarke

SYRAWOOD
PUBLISHING HOUSE
New York

Published by Syrawood Publishing House,
750 Third Avenue, 9th Floor,
New York, NY 10017, USA
www.syrawoodpublishinghouse.com

Functional and Bioactive Foods in Promoting Health
Edited by Teresa Clarke

International Standard Book Number: 978-1-64740-371-3 (Hardback)

Cataloging-in-publication Data

Functional and bioactive foods in promoting health / edited by Teresa Clarke.
p. cm.
Includes bibliographical references and index.
ISBN 978-1-64740-371-3
1. Functional foods. 2. Bioactive compounds--Health aspects. 3. Food. 4. Nutrition. 5. Health. I. Clarke, Teresa.
QP144.F85 F86 2023
613.2--dc23

TABLE OF CONTENTS

PREFACE

Every book is initially just a concept; it takes months of research and hard work to give it the final shape in which the readers receive it. In its early stages, this book also went through rigorous reviewing. The notable contributions made by experts from across the globe were first molded into patterned chapters and then arranged in a sensibly sequential manner to bring out the best results.

Functional foods are highly nutritious food items. Their consumption provides a number of health benefits such as protection against disease, promotion of proper growth and development, and prevention of nutrient deficiencies. The health benefits of functional foods extend beyond their nutritional value. They are also called as nutraceuticals. Bioactive foods are food items that contain certain non-essential biomolecules, which owing to their bioactive properties can affect one or more metabolic processes. These bioactive compounds have beneficial effects on the body that result in the promotion of better health. Bioactive food components are studied for their beneficial effects with respect to the prevention of cancer, heart disease, and other diseases. Lycopene, resveratrol, lignan, tannins, and indoles are some of the examples of bioactive compounds. This book outlines the role of functional and bioactive foods in promoting health in detail. Scientists and students actively engaged in the field of food science will find it full of crucial and unexplored concepts.

It has been my immense pleasure to be a part of this project and to contribute my years of learning in such a meaningful form. I would like to take this opportunity to thank all the people who have been associated with the completion of this book at any step.

Editor

1

Assessment of Tryptophan, Tryptophan Ethylester and Melatonin Derivatives in Red Wine by SPE-HPLC-FL and SPE-HPLC-MS Methods

Daniela Fracassetti [1,*], Ileana Vigentini [1], Alfredo Fabrizio Francesco Lo Faro [2], Patrizia De Nisi [3], Roberto Foschino [1], Antonio Tirelli [1], Marica Orioli [2] and Marcello Iriti [3]

1 Department of Food, Environmental and Nutritional Sciences, Università degli Studi di Milano, Via G. Celoria 2, 20133 Milan, Italy; ileana.vigentini@unimi.it (I.V.); roberto.foschino@unimi.it (R.F.); antonio.tirelli@unimi.it (A.T.)

2 Department of Biomedical, Surgical and Dental Sciences, Università degli Studi di Milano, Via Mangiagalli 37, 20133 Milan, Italy; fabriziolofaro09@gmail.com (A.F.F.L.F.); marica.orioli@unimi.it (M.O.)

3 Department of Agricultural and Environmental Sciences - Production, Landscape, Agroenergy, Università degli Studi di Milano, Via G. Celoria 2, 20133 Milan, Italy; patrizia.denisi@unimi.it (P.D.N.); marcello.iriti@unimi.it (M.I.)

* Correspondence: daniela.fracassetti@unimi.it

Abstract: Melatonin (MEL) is an indoleamine produced mainly by the pineal gland in vertebrates. It plays a significant role in the regulation of circadian rhythms, mitigation of sleeping disorders, and jet lag. This compound is synthetized from tryptophan (TRP) and it has been found in seeds, fruits, and fermented beverages, including wine. Wine is also a source of other tryptophan derivatives, the tryptophan ethylester (TEE) and MEL isomers (MISs), for which the biological properties need to be elucidated. An analytical method for the simultaneous quantification of TRP, TEE, and MEL was developed by a Solid Phase Extraction (SPE) of a preconcentration of wine followed by high performance liquid chromatography (HPLC) analysis either with fluorescence or mass spectrometer detectors. The analytical method showed a relative standard deviation (RSD) lower than 8%, except for TRP (RSD 10.5% in wine). The recovery was higher than 76%. The versatility of SPE preconcentrations allowed for the adequate preconcentration of wine sample as well as detection of low concentrations, an important aspect especially for MEL (detection limit 0.0023 μg/L). The proposed method proved to be suitable for assessing the investigated compounds in some red wine samples, where 74.4–256.2 μg/L and 0.038–0.063 μg/L of TEE and MEL were detected, respectively. Five MISs were also found in wine samples in concentrations up to 1.97 μg/L.

Keywords: indoleamines; grapevine; liquid chromatography; UHPLC/ESI-QTRAP; wine

---

1. Introduction

Melatonin (*N*-acetyl-5-methoxytryptamine; MEL) is an indoleamine produced mainly by the pineal gland in vertebrates [1] and its synthesis also occurs in other tissues, such as the gastrointestinal tract, bone marrow, and lymphocytes [2–4]. It is synthetized from L-tryptophan metabolism via serotonin [5,6]. In animals, MEL modulates the circadian and circannual rhythms, reproductive functions, bone metabolism, and turnover via cell-receptor-mediated mechanisms. It also shows a powerful antioxidant activity by directly scavenging free radical species (both reactive oxygen and nitrogen species) and stimulating the activity of antioxidant enzymes [7]. MEL has been found in edible plants [8–10] as a phytohormone protecting against oxidative stress and regulating growth [11,12]. Consequently, MEL is also present in plant foods, including seeds, fruits, and fermented beverages [11,13,14]. Several authors evidenced the presence of MEL in wines [15–18]. The circulating levels of MEL in mammals are very low (about 200 pg/mL at the maximum night peak and lower than 10 pg/mL during the day) [19] compared to MEL in grape products (about 1000 pg/g in berry skin and 500 pg/mL in wine) and, therefore, the intake of grape products represents a relevant topic [16,20]. The content of MEL increases during the fermentation step of the winemaking and other fermented beverages, meaning the yeast plays a significant role in its biosynthesis [14,21–23]. Besides MEL, its isomers (MISs) were also detected, and one of them was recently identified as tryptophan-ethyl ester (TEE) [24,25]. This compound was the most abundant tryptophan derivative, and its concentration was higher than that of MEL [26,27].

The analytical methods described for the detection of MEL in wine were based on liquid chromatography separation coupled with fluorescence [15,28,29] and mass spectrometry detectors [21,26,27]. Recently, Muñiz-Calvo and coauthors [30] proposed voltammetric techniques for the determination of MEL, TRP, and other TRP derivatives (TEE excluded). However, the authors evidenced the high performance liquid chromatography (HPLC) analysis had high discriminating capability and unambiguous identification and quantification. Due to the fact that wine is a complex matrix and MEL and its derivatives are present in low concentrations, the use of a solid phase extraction (SPE) technique is beneficial to use due to its removal of interferences, isolation, and concentration capabilities.

This study aimed to develop an HPLC method for the simultaneous determination of TRP, MEL, and TEE. In this respect, we developed a sample preparation protocol by means of SPE preconcentration allowing the detection of the three compounds by fluorescence and mass spectrometry detectors. The proposed method was used to determine the content of TRP, MEL, MISs, and TEE in red wine samples.

2. Materials and Methods

2.1. Chemicals and Materials

Melatonin (MEL), tryptophan-ethyl ester (TEE), methanol, and formic acid were purchased from Sigma-Aldrich (St. Louis, MO, USA). All the chemicals were of analytical grade. HPLC grade water was obtained by a Milli-Q system (Millipore Corp., Bedford, MA, USA).

MEL and TEE stock solutions were prepared in an ethanol:water ratio of 80:20 at 100 mg/L, while TRP was dissolved in water at 1000 mg/L. The stock solutions were stored covered with aluminum foil in order to protect the compounds against the light at −20 °C and they were thawed once.

Synthetic wine solution (SWS) contained 5.0 g/L tartaric acid and 12% ethanol (*v*/*v*) at a pH of 3.2, adjusted with sodium hydroxide (Merck, Darmstadt, Germany).

Eight red wine samples were analyzed. The wines were produced from *Vitis vinifera* cv. Nebbiolo in vintage 2015 in the Valtellina area (Lombardia, Italy), and they were collected at the market.

2.2. Sample Preparation

The preconcentration of red wine was developed by means of a solid phase extraction (SPE) technique. The SPE cartridges tested were Strata C18-T 500 mg/3 mL and Strata X-Polymeric Reversed Phase 200 mg/3 mL (Phenomenex, Torrance, CA, USA).

The final SPE protocol was set with Strata X-Polymeric Reversed Phase 200 mg/3 mL. After the SPE activation with methanol (4 mL) and conditioning with 0.1% formic acid (*v*/*v*) (8 mL), 5 mL of sample was loaded and the eluate was recovered (fraction A). The cartridge was firstly washed with 5 mL 0.1% formic acid in water (*v*/*v*) (fraction B) and then with 5 mL of 40% methanol (*v*/*v*) (fraction C). The elution was carried out with 5 mL of 100% methanol (fraction D), which was evaporated under vacuum (Rotavapor R 110, Büchi). The sample was re-suspended in 500 μL of 10% methanol acidified with 0.1% formic acid (*v*/*v*) corresponding to a concentration fold of 10. Each fraction was analyzed after filtration through a 0.22 μm polyvinilidene fluoride (PVDF) filter (Millipore). Samples were protected from the light during the preparation.

The setting of the SPE procedure was carried out on both spiked SWS and red wine at two concentration levels: 1 mg/L TRP, 50 μg/L TEE, and 50 μg/L MEL (level 1); and 2 mg/L TRP, 500 μg/L TEE, and 500 μg/L MEL (level 2). A higher concentration of TRP was chosen because its average content has been reported to be 3 mg/L [31]. The SPE procedure setup included differences in (i) volume of sample loaded (5 mL and 10 mL); (ii) volume of washing with 0.1% formic acid (*v*/*v*) (5 mL and 10 mL); (iii) volume and composition of washing with methanolic solution (5 mL and 10 mL; methanol 40%, 50%, 60%, and 70% (*v*/*v*)); (iv) recovery of fraction D with a different methanolic solution (methanol 50% (*v*/*v*), methanol 50% (*v*/*v*) acidified with 0.1% formic acid (*v*/*v*), 10% methanol (*v*/*v*), and 10% methanol (*v*/*v*)acidified with 0.1% formic acid (*v*/*v*)).

2.3. Chromatographic and Quantification Conditions

The HPLC system consisted of an Agilent 1260 Infinity Quaternary LC equipped with an Agilent G1321B Fluorescence Detector and an Agilent LC/MS 6130 Quadrupole (Agilent, Santa Clara, CA, USA) operating in multimode source (simultaneous electrospray (ESI) and atmospheric pressure chemical ionization (APCI)). The MS operative conditions included a spray voltage of +3.5 kV, vaporizer temperature of 250 °C, gas temperature of 350 °C, drying gas at 12 mL/min, and a nebulizer pressure of 55 psig. The fluorescence detector was set at 280 nm and 350 nm for excitation and emission, respectively. The column used for the separation was an Accucore C18 (100 × 3 mm, 2.7 μm particle size, Thermo Scientific, San Jose, CA, USA) set at 40 °C. The elution solvents were: (A) 0.1% formic acid (*v*/*v*), and (B) methanol acidified with 0.1% formic acid (*v*/*v*), and the flow rate was 0.5 mL/min. Elution conditions were as follows: 5% B for 1 min, from 5% to 40% B in 15 min followed by the column washing with 100% B and re-equilibration for a total of 25 min for each run. Injection volumes were 5 μL and 20 μL for HPLC-MS and HPLC-FL methods, respectively.

Chromatographic data were processed using Agilent OpenLab ChemStation software (Agilent). For the MS detector, data acquisition was performed in a single ion monitoring (SIM) setting [m/z]+ 205 for TRP and 233 [m/z]+ for MEL and TEE. MEL, TEE, and TRP were quantified using the external standard method. Six-level calibration curves were obtained with standard solutions containing the analytes at the respective concentrations spanning the expected ranges in wine.

The UHPLC/ESI-QTRAP analysis was carried out to identify MEL, MISs, and TEE eluting in the chromatograms of the wine samples. A UHPLC model HP 1290 (Agilent) coupled with a Mass Spectrometer Detector 5500 TRIPLE QTrap model 1024945-AX (ABSCIEX, Framingham, MA, USA) equipped with an HESI-II probe for electrospray ionization and a collision cell (HCD) was used. Data were acquired in a multiple reaction monitoring (MRM) mode. The operative conditions were: spray voltage +2.2 kV, sheath gas flow-rate 50, auxiliary gas flow-rate 55, capillary temperature 360 °C, capillary +95 V, tube lens +170 V, Skimmer +38 V, and heater temperature 500 °C. The chromatographic separation was carried out on a BEH C18 column (100 × 2.1 mm, 1.7 μm particle size, Waters, Milford, MA, USA). The column was maintained at 30 °C and the injection volume was 0.3 μL. The elution solvents were (A) 0.1% formic acid (*v*/*v*), and (B) acetonitrile. The elution conditions were as follows: 10% B for 0.30 min, from 10% to 30% B in 5 min, from 30% to 85% in 0.5 min followed by column washing with 90% B and re-equilibration for a total of 10.5 min for each run. The flow rate was set at 0.55 mL/min. The MS data were processed using MultiQuant software (AB Sciex). The peak identity was ascertained by evaluation of both the accurate mass and the fragments obtained in the collision cell. MEL, TEE, and TRP were quantified using the external standard method with the respective standards; MISs were quantified with the calibration curve obtained for MEL.

2.4. Method Validation

The in-house validation of the method was carried out in terms of selectivity, linearity, limit of detection (LOD), limit of quantification (LOQ), repeatability, and recovery [32].

The selectivity of the method was evaluated by analyzing TRP, TEE, and MEL both in the absence and presence of possible interferences originating from the wine matrix. With this aim, the separations of a SWS at the concentrations 2 mg/L TRP, 50 μg/L TEE, and 50 μg/L MEL analyzed with both FL and MS detectors were compared with those of a purified SWS and a red wine sample spiked with the three analytes at the same concentrations.

Linearity was tested on six concentration levels within the intervals reported in Tables 1 and 2. The SWS samples were purified and analyzed in triplicate as well as spiked red wine samples at the same concentration levels. The equations of the calibration curves and the correlation coefficients (r) were obtained by linear regression analysis.

The values of limit of detection (LOD) and limit of quantification (LOQ) were calculated as the lowest concentration of analyte in a sample that resulted in a signal-to-noise ratio of 3 and 10 for LOD and LOQ, respectively. Values were measured in three independent replicates.

The recovery (%) in purified SWSs and spiked wine samples was calculated using the SWSs added with the same concentrations of the analytes. The spiking concentrations were 5.3 μg/L, 10.6 μg/L, 21.2 μg/L, 53.0 μg/L, 106.0 μg/L, and 212 μg/L for TEE and MEL, and 110 μg/L, 220 μg/L, 550 μg/L, 1100 μg/L, 2200 μg/L, and 5500 μg/L for TRP. SWSs and spiked red wine samples were purified and analyzed in triplicate. Triplicate analyses of unpurified SWSs spiked with the same concentrations of the analytes were also carried out. The accuracy was evaluated by means of recovery assay of replicate preconcentrations of both SWS and spiked red wine samples at levels of 10.6 μg/L and 106.0 μg/L for TEE and MEL, and 220 μg/L and 2200 μg/L for TRP. Duplicate preconcentrations were carried out in two different days for SWSs (n = 4) and for three different days for spiked red wine samples (n = 6).

Precision was expressed as relative standard deviation (RSD) of the analytical response. Both the SWSs and red wine samples spiked at the three levels of concentration were analyzed (10.6 μg/L, 53.0 μg/L, and 106.0 μg/L for TEE and MEL, and 220 μg/L 1100 μg/L, and 2200 μg/L for TRP). Three independent replicates were carried out on three different days (n = 9). For the repeatability of the SPE procedure and instrumental repeatability, duplicate injections were carried out from the same vial at the two concentration levels on three different days (n = 12). The repeatability of the retention times was also evaluated over a total of 54 injections carried out on three different days.

2.5. Statistical Analysis

Statistical analysis was carried out with SPSS Win 12.0 program (SPSS Inc., Chicago, IL, USA). The equations of the calibration curves were assessed by the linear regression analysis. Differences between the calibration curve slopes obtained in aqueous solution and white wine were evaluated by the F-test ($p < 0.05$).

3. Results and Discussion

3.1. Analytical Method Development

The chromatographic conditions by means of both FL and MS detectors were firstly optimized using the SWS at the concentration 2 mg/L TRP, 50 μg/L TEE, and 50 μg/L MEL. While the analytical response (area) was similar for MEL and TEE using MS detector, it resulted lower in fluorescence for TEE analyzed at the same concentration (Figure 1).

A standard water solution with the same levels of analytes was analyzed, and no differences were observed in comparison to SWS. The SPE preconcentration allowed both the removal of compounds potentially interfering in the HPLC separation from the wine matrix and the concentration of the analytes of interest, making their detection possible because of their presence in low amounts in wine [33]. Although other authors applied the SPE preconcentration for MEL detection from wine and other food matrices [15,27,29,34], the SPE approach presented in this study allowed the simultaneous elution of TRP, TEE, and MEL. For the development of the SPE preconcentration, several assays were carried out using the SWS containing concentrations of 2 mg/L TRP, 50 μg/L TEE, and 50 μg/L MEL. The setup method by using a blank matrix added with the compounds of interest is considered acceptable [35] since a Certified Reference Material for wine containing TRP, TEE, and MEL does not exist. First, preconcentrations by using two different SPE cartridges were compared by loading 10 mL of spiked SWS and washing with methanol 40% methanol (*v*/*v*). Higher recovery (>15%) was observed by the preconcentration with Strata X-Polymeric Reversed Phase 200 mg, in accordance to El-Moussaoui and Bendriss [29]. These SPE cartridges were used for the development of the analytical method. Trials loading 5 mL and 10 mL of spiked SWS at two concentration levels (see Paragraph 2.2), and washing with 5 mL and 10 mL 0.1% formic acid (*v*/*v*), and 5 mL 40% methanol (*v*/*v*), led to comparable recovery values. The lower amounts were chosen in order to reduce the solvent amounts needed for the SPE, which were 5 mL of 0.1% formic acid and 5 mL of methanol in total for the four steps of preconcentration. The analyses of all these fractions were carried out. TRP was detected in the sample loading (fraction A) and in the washing with 40% methanol (fraction C), TEE was revealed in fraction C and in the methanolic solution (fraction D), while MEL was only found in fraction D. The major interferences of red wine are represented by phenols, compounds completely soluble in methanol. In order to reduce the possible interferences in fraction D, different concentrations of methanol (40–70% (*v*/*v*)) were assayed. However, the increase of methanol in the washing step led to a loss of MEL in fraction D, even when the washing was carried out with 50% methanol (*v*/*v*). The recovery of fraction D, after methanol evaporation under vacuum, was carried out with different methanol amounts (500 μL and 1 mL) and concentrations (10% and 50% (*v*/*v*)), with and without acidification with 0.1% formic acid (*v*/*v*). The best chromatographic separation in terms of peak shape was obtained with methanol 10% acidified with 0.1% formic acid (*v*/*v*). Formic acid 0.1% (*v*/*v*) was the solvent for the HPLC separation and no change of sample pH was generated through the analysis.

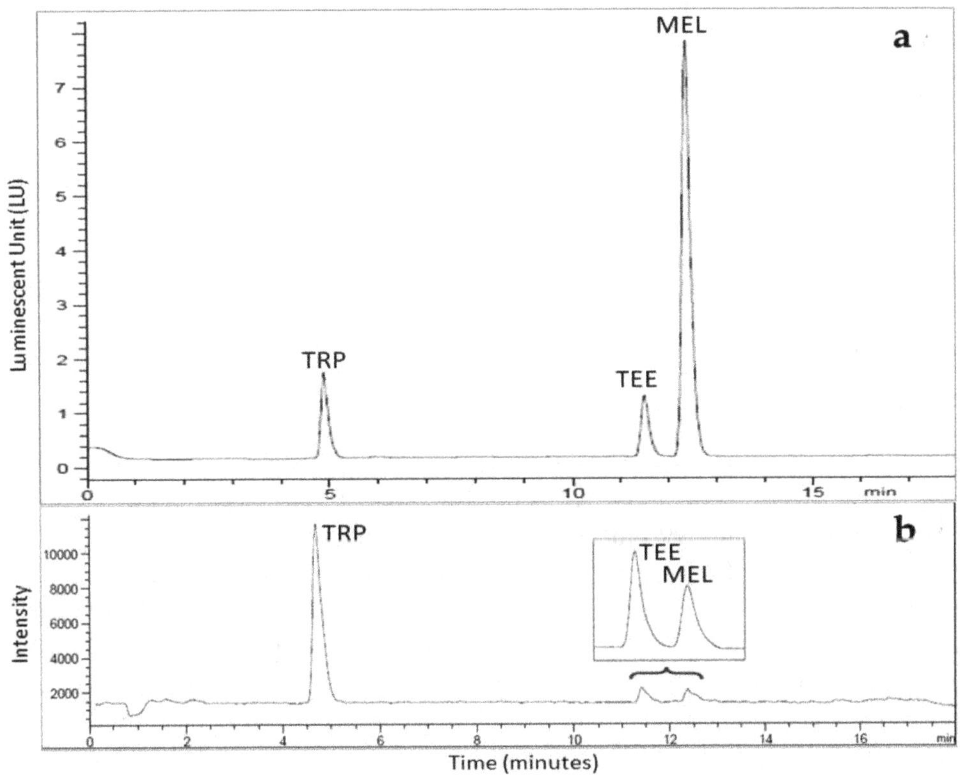

Figure 1. (**a**) HPLC-FL and (**b**) HPLC-MS chromatograms of tryptophan (TRP) (1 mg/L), tryptophan ethyl ester (TEE) (50 μg/L), and melatonin (MEL) (50 μg/L) in standard synthetic wine solution.

Based on the results obtained for the spiked SWS, the SPE procedure was carried out by loading 5 mL of spiked SWS and spiked wine sample recovering the eluate (fraction A). The cartridge was firstly washed with 5 mL of 0.1% formic acid (*v*/*v*) (fraction B) and then with 5 mL of 40% methanol (*v*/*v*) (fraction C). The elution was carried out with methanol 100% (fraction D) which was evaporated under vacuum. The fraction D was re-suspended in 500 μL of 10% methanol acidified with 0.1% formic acid (*v*/*v*), meaning a 10-fold concentration of wine sample.

Before proceeding to method validation, spiked red wine samples at two concentration levels (see Paragraph 2.2) were SPE preconcentrated in order exclude any possible interferences arising from the HPLC separation of red wine, especially for the concentrated fraction D. As shown in Figure 2, the HPLC separation was interference-free, not only for fraction D, but also for fractions A and C.

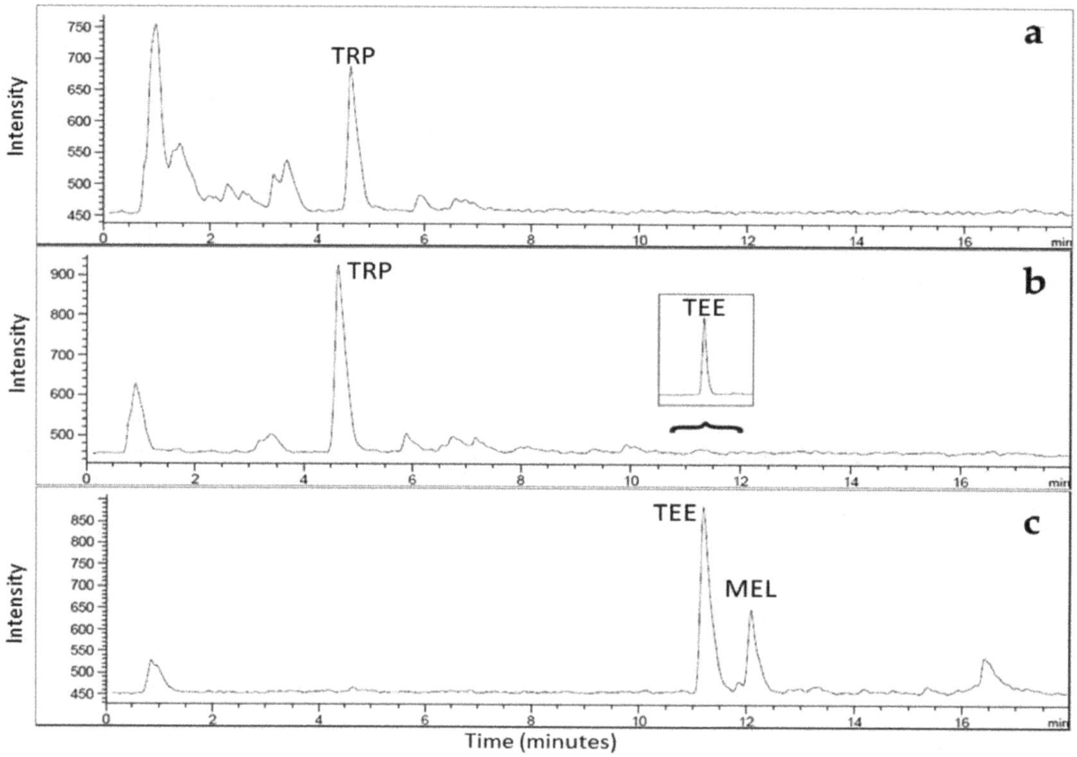

Figure 2. HPLC-MS chromatograms of (**a**) fraction A, (**b**) fraction C, and (**c**) fraction D obtained for solid phase extraction (SPE)-preconcentrated red wine sample spiked with TRP (1 mg/L), TEE (50 μg/L), and MEL (50 μg/L). Peak identity: TRP, tryptophan; TEE, tryptophan ethyl ester; MEL, melatonin.

3.2. Validation of the Analytical Method

The linearity was firstly assessed for TRP, TEE, and MEL added to SWS by calculating six-point calibration curves without SPE preconcentrations. Both the FL and MS detectors showed correlation coefficient (r) values higher than 0.99 (Table 1). A linear response was also found for TRP, TEE, and MEL determined in spiked SWSs after SPE preconcentration and analyzed by the FL detector ($y = 39.03 \times x + 0.07$ for TRP, $y = 0.51 \times x + 58.46$ for TEE, and $y = 1.19 \times x - 9.00$ for MEL) with r values that corresponded to 1, 0.991, and 0.998 for TRP, TEE, and MEL, respectively. The LOD and LOQ were assessed for the three compounds and they resulted in lower than the average concentrations found in wine [21,28,33,36] for both TRP (5.16 μg/L and 17.18 μg/L for LOD and LOQ, respectively) and 22 MEL (0.12 μg/L and 0.41 μg/L for LOD and LOQ, respectively). Higher LOD and LOQ were found for TEE (1.17 μg/L and 3.91 μg/L, respectively) making the analytical method proposed less sensitive for TEE quantification in comparison to MEL. However, Vigentini et al. [26] and Fernández-Cruz et al. [27] reported concentrations of TEE higher than the LOQ value; the mentioned authors found TEE amounts in most cases higher than 5 μg/L and up to 1126 μg/L.

A linear response was observed for both spiked SWSs and red wine samples analyzed by the MS detector, and no significant difference was found between the two matrices. The r values were higher than 0.99 for all the compounds investigated, and no significant differences were found in the calibration curve slopes calculated in spiked SWSs and red wine samples purified with SPE (Table 2).

As expected, both LOD and LOQ values were lower when the detection was carried out by the MS detector (Table 2), which is more sensitive than FL detector. The LOD values we found were on the same order of magnitude as other analytical methods previously proposed for TEE, while the results were lower in the case of MEL, indicating a high sensitivity of the analytical method proposed [26–28,37]. In addition, the chromatographic separation was interference-free (Figure 2), facilitating the identification and quantification.

Table 1. Linearity obtained with standard synthetic wine solutions by fluorescence (FLD) and mass spectrometry (MSD) detectors.

	FLD			MSD		
Compound	Concentration Range (μg/L)	Linearity		Concentration Range (μg/L)	Linearity	
		Equation	*r*		Equation	*r*
TRP	110–5500	$39.03 \times x - 0.08$	0.996	110–5500	$3389.30 \times x + 49.99$	1
TEE	50–2000	$0.064 \times x + 7.308$	0.998	5–200	$23.40 \times x + 111.85$	0.999
MEL	20–500	$0.15 \times x + 0.41$	1	1–200	$15.04 \times x + 109.10$	0.998

The equations and the correlation coefficients (*r*) were calculated by means of linear regression. *x*, concentration; TRP, tryptophan; TEE, tryptophan ethyl ester; MEL, melatonin.

The recovery of the SPE preconcentration was evaluated for both spiked SWSs and red wine samples at six concentration levels (see Paragraph 2.4). The average values of percent recovery were all higher than 75% (Table 2). Only negligible differences were obtained by analyzing the spiked SWSs and red wine samples, thus a matrix effect could be excluded (Table 2).

The repeatability of the method was calculated as the relative standard deviation (RSD) of the analytical response (peak area) obtained by analyzing both spiked SWSs and red wine samples (n = 9). The average RSD values obtained for the TRP, TEE, and MEL in spiked SWSs ranged between 4.6% and 9.1%, whereas values obtained for spiked red wine samples were between 5.4% and 10.5% (Table 2). The repeatability of the SPE preconcentration was also evaluated for two concentration levels in both spiked SWS (n = 4) and red wine (n = 6). The average values determined for spiked SWS were 5.4%, 7.4%, and 4.0%for TRP, TEE, and MEL, respectively, and the values for spiked red wine samples were 4.2%, 5.2%, and 5.2% for TRP, TEE, and MEL, respectively. The intra-day precision (n = 12) corresponded to 3.8%, 2.6%, and 3.1% for TRP, TEE, and MEL, respectively. The repeatability of retention times (n = 54), estimated on three different days, was negligible (<2%). Overall, these data confirm the reliability of the analytical method here proposed.

The last step of the developed sample preparation method was the evaporation of methanol under vacuum and the re-suspension of samples in 500 μL of 10% methanol acidified with 0.1% formic acid (*v*/*v*), meaning a 10-fold concentration of wine sample. Assays were carried out by concentrating the wine samples up to 25-fold, and results were in accordance to those found for 10-fold concentrated samples (data not shown). These findings indicated the high versatility of the developed SPE preconcentration, making possible the detection of the investigated compounds, MEL and TEE in particular, even when they are present in very low concentrations (<0.02 μg/L).

3.3. Analysis of Red Wine Samples

In order to evaluate the suitability of the analytical method proposed, the determinations of TRP, TEE, and MEL were carried out in eight red wine samples produced from *Vitis vinifera* cv. Nebbiolo in vintage 2015. The wine samples were also analyzed by UHPLC/ESI-QTRAP in order to confirm the presence of MEL and TEE. Besides the latter two compounds, five MISs were detected, and fragmentation is reported in Table 3. This is an improvement of the existing methods since one MIs [38,39] to three MISs [26,33] were previously detected in wine.

Table 2. Linearity, limits of detection (LOD) and quantification (LOQ), recovery (%), and repeatability (as relative standard deviation, %RSD) for the analytical method developed in HPLC-MS.

Compound	Concentration Range Added (μg/L)	SWS		Spiked Red Wine		LOD (μg/L) ($n = 3$)	LOQ (μg/L) ($n = 3$)	Recovery (%) ($n = 6$)		Repeatability (%RSD) ($n = 9$)	
		Equation	r	Equation	r			SWS	Spiked Red Wine	SWS	Spiked Red Wine
TRP	110–5500	$3284.2 \times x + 328.3$	0.999	$3257.4 \times x + 3132.1$	0.995	0.75	1.25	89	84	9.1	10.5
TEE	5–250	$659.2 \times x - 440.4$	0.997	$677.4 \times x + 3861.0$	0.999	0.038	0.12	88	76	6.5	7.9
MEL	0.05–250	$242.2 \times x + 2748.6$	0.996	$269.5 \times x + 840.1$	0.997	0.0023	0.018	86	79	4.6	5.4

The equations and the correlation coefficients (r) were calculated by means of linear regression. Recovery and repeatability values were determined at two and three different concentration levels, respectively. SWS, synthetic wine solution; x, concentration; TRP, tryptophan; TEE, tryptophan ethyl ester; MEL, melatonin.

Table 3. Identification of MEL (melatonin), TEE (tryptophan ethyl ester), and MISs (MEL isomers) by HUPLC/ESI-QTRAP.

Compound	Exact Mass	MS/MS Fragmentation	
	$[M + H]^+$	MS/MS Fragments	Collision Energy (μV)
MEL	233.1	188.1 216.1 174.1	30 30 30
TEE	233.1	174.1 159.0 130.1 178.1	20 36 55 29
MIS 1	233.1	141.0 216.0 174.1	20 20 20
MIS 2	233.1	141.1 196.0	20 20
MIS 3	233.1	130.0	50
MIS 4	233.1	141.0 216.0 174.1	20 20 20
MIS 5	233.1	141.0 159.0	35 35

The concentration of TRP varied from 0.44 ± 0.05 mg/L to 4.39 ± 0.46 mg/L (Table 4); the concentration of free amino acids can be quite variable in wine, depending on the initial content in grapes and cellular lysis occurrence of wine-related microorganisms [31]. The revealed TEE was variable among wine samples, ranging from 74.4 ± 5.9 μg/L to 256.2 ± 20.2 μg/L (Table 4). These amounts were higher in comparison to the values reported by Vigentini et al. [26] and Fernández-Cruz et al. [27] who monitored the TEE content in laboratory-scale fermentations in real must and in synthetic must, respectively. Maybe winemaking at an industrial-scale or the unknown fermenting yeast could affect the level of TEE. MEL was detected in the analyzed red wine samples, ranging from 0.038 ± 0.001 μg/L to 0.063 ± 0.004 μg/L (Table 4), on the same order of magnitude as the concentration reported by Vitalini and co-authors [33] who detected MEL in red wines at 0.05–0.62 μg/L. These amounts could be of physiological interest since the MEL detected in wine was higher than its circulating levels in humans during the day (10 pg/mL) [19].

Table 4. Levels of TRP (tryptophan), TEE (tryptophan ethyl ester), MEL (melatonin), and MEL isomers (MISs) in red wine samples. Data are expressed as mean ± standard deviation.

Sample Code	TRP	TEE	MEL	MIS 1	MIS 2	MIS 3	MIS 4	MIS 5
	mg/L	μg/L	μg/L	μg/L	μg/L	μg/L	μg/L	μg/L
Red wine 1	3.85 ± 0.40	172.2 ± 13.6	0.057 ± 0.003	1.64 ± 0.09	<LOQ	<LOQ	0.0043 ± 0.0002	<LOQ
Red wine 2	4.39 ± 0.46	212.0 ± 16.8	0.062 ± 0.003	1.97 ± 0.11	<LOQ	<LOQ	0.0041 ± 0.0002	<LOQ
Red wine 3	1.56 ± 0.16	256.2 ± 20.2	0.063 ± 0.004	0.74 ± 0.04	<LOQ	<LOQ	<LOQ	<LOQ
Red wine 4	1.02 ± 0.11	223.2 ± 17.6	0.038 ± 0.002	0.67 ± 0.04	<LOQ	<LOQ	<LOQ	<LOQ
Red wine 5	0.98 ± 0.10	113.0 ± 8.9	0.046 ± 0.003	0.58 ± 0.03	<LOQ	<LOQ	<LOQ	<LOQ
Red wine 6	0.84 ± 0.09	92.9 ± 7.3	0.054 ± 0.003	0.86 ± 0.05	<LOQ	<LOQ	<LOQ	<LOQ
Red wine 7	0.44 ± 0.05	71.7 ± 5.7	0.063 ± 0.004	0.91 ± 0.04	<LOQ	<LOQ	<LOQ	<LOQ
Red wine 8	0.57 ± 0.06	74.4 ± 5.9	0.038 ± 0.001	0.80 ± 0.04	<LOQ	<LOQ	<LOQ	<LOQ

Several factors can affect the concentration of MEL in red wine, including agrochemicals (i.e., plant activators, treatment with copper) and winemaking practices (i.e., barrel-aging, content of sulphur dioxide, and the use of fining agents), fermenting microorganisms (different strains of both *Saccharomyces cerevisiae* and non-*Saccharomyces* yeasts), and maybe even the grape/wine composition (i.e., phenol content, antioxidant capacity) [18,26]. However, further investigations will be carried out in order to elucidate the effects of both winemaking and grape/wine composition. Most of the MISs were detected at trace levels except for MIS 1, for which the concentrations ranged from 0.58 ± 0.03 μg/L to 1.97 ± 0.11 μg/L (Table 4), more than one order of magnitude higher in comparison to MEL. MIS biosynthesis is still not clear, and their antioxidant and cytoprotective activities are dependent on the position of two side chains in the indole ring [40].

4. Conclusions

The proposed analytical method allowed the detection and reliable quantification of TRP, TEE, and MEL simultaneously. In general, this protocol may represent a useful tool for monitoring the release of MEL and TEE, even when their concentration is very low (<0.02 μg/L), and their fate throughout the wine production and storage. Moreover, the sample preparation method and chromatographic conditions presented in this study allowed the detection of five MISs, for which the molecular structure, in particular the position of two side chains in the indole ring, will be evaluated.

The obtained results suggested the amounts of MEL detected in the wine samples may be of biological importance, as MEL was higher than its circulating levels in humans during the day; bioavailability studies are necessary to confirm this hypothesis. TEE is more highly concentrated than MEL (over one thousand times) in Nebbiolo wine samples, as well as MIS 1, confirming the outcome of previous works [24,26], even though the origin and the putative nutritional role of this molecule have not been elucidated yet. Since chromatographic analysis does not allow getting information about the chemical structure of MISs, further investigations will be carried out in order to clarify the position of two side chains in the indole ring for the MISs detected. We can suppose that the proper choice of the winemaking procedures could lead to higher levels of MEL, TEE, and MISs, and this needs further investigation.

Author Contributions: Conceptualization, D.F., M.I. and I.V.; Methodology, D.F.; Validation, D.F., A.F.F.L.F., P.D.N.; Data Curation, D.F.; Resources, R.F., M.I., M.O. and A.T.; Writing—Original Draft Preparation, D.F. and I.V.; Writing—Review & Editing, P.D.N., Roberto Foschino, M.I., A.F.F.L.F., M.O. and A.T.

Acknowledgments: We are grateful to Sonia Moiola and Alice Boletti for their technical support.

References

1. Reiter, R.J. The pineal and its hormones in the control of reproduction in mammals. *Endocr. Rev.* **1980**, *1*, 109–131. [CrossRef] [PubMed]
2. Huether, G.; Poeggeler, B.; Reimer, A.; George, A. Effect of tryptophan administration on circulating melatonin levels in chicks and rats: Evidence for stimulation of melatonin synthesis and release in the gastrointestinal tract. *Life Sci.* **1992**, *51*, 945–953. [CrossRef]
3. Huether, G. The contribution of extrapineal sites of melatonin synthesis to circulating melatonin levels in higher vertebrates. *Experientia* **1993**, *49*, 665–670. [CrossRef] [PubMed]
4. Tan, D.X.; Manchester, L.C.; Terron, M.P.; Flores, L.J.; Reiter, R.J. One molecule, many derivatives: A never-ending interaction of melatonin with reactive oxygen and nitrogen species? *J. Pineal Res.* **2007**, *42*, 28–42. [CrossRef] [PubMed]
5. Reiter, R.J. Pineal melatonin—Cell biology of its synthesis and of its physiological interactions. *Endocr. Rev.* **1991**, *12*, 151–180. [CrossRef]
6. Chattoraj, A.; Liu, T.; Zhang, L.S.; Huang, Z.; Borjigin, J. Melatonin formation in mammals: In vivo perspectives. *Rev. Endocr. Metab. Disord.* **2009**, *10*, 37–243. [CrossRef]
7. Reiter, R.J.; Paredes, S.D.; Manchester, L.C.; Tan, D.X. Reducing oxidative/nitrosative stress: A newly-discovered genre for melatonin. *Crit. Rev. Biochem. Mol. Biol.* **2009**, *44*, 175–200. [CrossRef]
8. Dubbels, R.; Reiter, R.J.; Klenke, E.; Goebel, A.; Schnakenberg, E.; Ehlers, C.; Schiwara, H.W.; Schloot, W. Melatonin in edible plants identified by radioimmunoassay and by high performance liquid chromatography-mass spectrometry. *J. Pineal Res.* **1995**, *18*, 28–31. [CrossRef]
9. Hattori, A.; Migitaka, H.; Iigo, M.; Itoh, M.; Yamamoto, K.; Ohtani-Kaneko, R.; Hara, M.; Suzuki, T.; Reiter, R.J. Identification of melatonin in plants and its effects on plasma melatonin levels and binding to melatonin receptors in vertebrates. *Biochem. Mol. Biol. Intern.* **1995**, *35*, 627–634.
10. Paredes, S.D.; Korkmaz, A.; Manchester, L.C.; Tan, D.X.; Reiter, R.J. Phytomelatonin: A review. *J. Exp. Bot.* **2009**, *60*, 57–69. [CrossRef]
11. Manchester, L.C.; Tan, D.X.; Reiter, R.J.; Park, W.; Monis, K.; Qi, W. High levels of melatonin in the seeds of edible plants: Possible function in germ tissue protection. *Life Sci.* **2000**, *67*, 3023–3029. [CrossRef]
12. Tan, D.X.; Hardeland, R.; Manchester, L.C.; Korkmaz, A.; Ma, S.; Rosales-Corral, S.; Reiter, R.J. Functional roles of melatonin in plants, and perspectives in nutritional and agricultural sciences. *J. Exp. Bot.* **2012**, *63*, 577–597. [CrossRef]
13. Sturtz, M.; Cerezo, A.B.; Cantos-Villar, E.; Garcia-Parrilla, M.C. Determination of the melatonin content of different varieties of tomatoes (*Lycopersicon esculentum*) and strawberries (*Fragaria ananassa*). *Food Chem.* **2011**, *127*, 1329–1334. [CrossRef] [PubMed]
14. Garcia-Moreno, H.; Calvo, J.R.; Maldonado, M.D. High levels of melatonin generated during the brewing process. *J. Pineal Res.* **2012**, *55*, 26–30. [CrossRef] [PubMed]
15. Mercolini, L.; Saracino, M.A.; Bugamelli, F.; Ferranti, A.; Malaguti, M.; Hrelia, S.; Raggi, M.A. HPLC-F analysis of melatonin and resveratrol isomers in wine using an SPE procedure. *J. Sep. Sci.* **2008**, *31*, 1007–1014. [CrossRef]
16. Iriti, M.; Varoni, E.M.; Vitalini, S. Melatonin in traditional mediterranean diets. *J. Pineal Res.* **2010**, *49*, 101–105. [CrossRef] [PubMed]

17. Stege, P.W.; Sombra, L.L.; Messina, G.; Martinez, L.D.; Silva, M.D. Determination of melatonin in wine and plant extracts by capillary electrochromatography with immobilized carboxylic multi-walled carbon nanotubes as stationary phase. *Electrophoresis* **2010**, *31*, 2242–2248. [CrossRef]
18. Vitalini, S.; Gardana, C.; Zanzotto, A.; Fico, G.; Faoro, F.; Simonetti, P.; Iriti, M. From vineyard to glass: Agrochemicals enhance the melatonin and total polyphenol contents and antiradical activity of red wines. *J. Pineal Res.* **2011**, *51*, 278–285. [CrossRef]
19. Bonnefont-Rousselot, D.; Collin, F. Melatonin: Action as antioxidant and potential applications in human disease and aging. *Toxicol* **2010**, *278*, 55–67. [CrossRef] [PubMed]
20. Iriti, M.; Vitalini, S. Health-promoting effects of traditional mediterranean diets—A review. *Pol. J. Food Nutr. Sci.* **2012**, *62*, 71–76. [CrossRef]
21. Rodriguez-Naranjo, M.I.; Gil-Izquierdo, A.; Troncoso, A.M.; Cantos-Villar, E.; Garcia-Parrilla, M.C. Melatonin is synthesised by yeast during alcoholic fermentation in wines. *Food Chem.* **2011**, *126*, 1608–1613. [CrossRef] [PubMed]
22. Mena, P.; Gil-Izquirdo, A.; Moreno, D.A.; Martí, N.; García-Viguera, C. Melatonin is detected in pomegranate wines. Influence of variety and winemaking stage. *LWT-Food Sci. Technol.* **2012**, *47*, 13–18. [CrossRef]
23. Fernandez-Pachon, M.S.; Medina, S.; Herrero-Martin, G.; Cerrillo, I.; Berna, G.; Escudero-Lopez, B.; Ferreres, F.; Martin, F.; Garcia-Parrilla, M.C.; Gil-Izquierdo, A. Alcoholic fermentation induces melatonin synthesis in orange juice. *J. Pineal Res.* **2014**, *56*, 31–38. [CrossRef] [PubMed]
24. Gardana, C.; Iriti, M.; Stuknyte, M.; De Noni, I.; Simonetti, P. "Melatonin isomer" in wine is not an isomer of the melatonin but tryptophan-ethylester. *J. Pineal Res* **2014**, *57*, 435–441. [CrossRef] [PubMed]
25. Iriti, M.; Vigentini, I. Tryptophan-ethylester, the false (unveiled) melatonin isomer in red wine. *Int. J. Tryptophan Res.* **2015**, *8*, 1–3. [CrossRef] [PubMed]
26. Vigentini, I.; Gardana, C.; Fracassetti, D.; Gabrielli, M.; Foschino, R.; Simonetti, P.; Tirelli, A.; Iriti, M. Yeast contribution to melatonin, melatonin isomers and tryptophan ethyl ester during alcoholic fermentation of grape musts. *J. Pineal Res.* **2015**, *58*, 388–396. [CrossRef] [PubMed]
27. Fernández-Cruz, E.; Álvarez-Fernández, M.A.; Valero, E.; Troncoso, A.M.; García-Parrilla, M.C. Melatonin and derived L-tryptophan metabolites produced during alcoholic fermentation by different wine yeast strains. *Food Chem.* **2017**, *217*, 431–437. [CrossRef]
28. Mercolini, L.; Mandrioli, R.; Raggi, M.A. Content of melatonin and other antioxidants in grape-related foodstuff: Measurement using MEPS-HPLC-F method. *J. Pineal Res.* **2012**, *53*, 21–28. [CrossRef]
29. El Moussaoui, N.; Bendriss, A. Analysis of melatonin by high performance liquid chromatography after Solid-Phase Extraction (SPE/HPLC-FD). *Int. J. Eng. Res. Technol.* **2015**, *4*, 988–993.
30. Muñiz-Calvo, S.; Guillamón, J.M.; Domínguez, I.; Doménech-Carbó, A. Detecting and monitoring the production of melatonin and other related indole compounds in different *Saccharomyces* strain by solid-state electrochemical techniques. *Food Anal. Methods* **2017**, *10*, 1408–1418. [CrossRef]
31. Ribéreau-Gayon, P.; Dubourdieu, D.; Donèche, B.; Lonvaud-Funel, A. The microbiology of wine and vinifications. In *Handbook of Enology*; Ribéreau-Gayon, P., Ed.; Wiley: Hoboken, NJ, USA, 2006.
32. Magnusson, B.; Örnemark, U. Eurachem Guide: The Fitness for Purpose of Analytical Methods—A Laboratory Guide to Method Validation and Related Topics. Available online: https://www.eurachem.org/images/stories/Guides/pdf/MV_guide_2nd_ed_EN.pdf (accessed on 14 March 2018).
33. Vitalini, S.; Gardana, C.; Simonetti, P.; Fico, G.; Iriti, M. Melatonin, melatonin isomers and stilbenes in Italian traditional grape products and their antioxidant capacity. *J. Pineal Res.* **2013**, *54*, 322–333. [CrossRef] [PubMed]
34. Ramakrishna, A.; Giridhar, O.; Sankar, K.U.; Ravishankar, G.A. Melatonin and serotonin profiles in beans of Coffea species. *J. Pineal Res.* **2012**, *52*, 470–476. [CrossRef] [PubMed]
35. 2002/657/EC: Commission Decision. Official Journal of the European Communities L221, 17.8.2002. Available online: https://eur-lex.europa.eu/legal-content/EN/TXT/PDF/?uri=OJ:L:2002:221:FULL&from=HR (accessed on 14 March 2019).
36. Amerin, M.A.; Ough, C.S. *Alcohols, in Methods for Wine and Must Analysis*; Amerine, M.A., Ough, C.S., Eds.; John Wiley and Sons: New York, NY, USA, 1980.
37. Huang, X.; Mazza, G. Simultaneous analysis of serotonin, melatonin, piceid and resveratrol in fruits using liquid chromatography tandem mass spectrometry. *J. Chromatogr. A* **2011**, *1218*, 3890–3899. [CrossRef] [PubMed]

38. Gomez, F.J.V.; Raba, J.; Cerutti, S.; Silva, M.F. Monitoring melatonin and its isomer in *Vitis vinifera* cv. Malbec by UHPLC-MS/MS from grape to bottle. *J. Pineal Res.* **2012**, *52*, 349–355. [CrossRef] [PubMed]
39. Kocadağli, T.; Yılmaz, C.; Gökmen, V. Determination of melatonin and its isomer in foods by liquid chromatography tandem mass spectrometry. *Food Chem.* **2014**, *153*, 151–156. [CrossRef]
40. Spadoni, G.; Diamantini, G.; Bedini, A.; Tarzia, G.; Vacondio, F.; Silva, C.; Rivara, M.; Mor, M.; Plazzi, P.V.; Zusso, M.; et al. Synthesis, antioxidant activity and structure-activity relationships for a new series of 2-(acylaminoethyl) indoles with melatonin-like cytoprotective activity. *J. Pineal Res.* **2006**, *40*, 259–269. [CrossRef]

2

How Safe is Ginger Rhizome for Decreasing Nausea and Vomiting in Women during Early Pregnancy?

Julien Stanisiere, Pierre-Yves Mousset and Sophie Lafay *

GYNOV SAS, 5 rue Salneuve, 75017 Paris, France; j.stanisiere@gynov.com (J.S.); py.mousset@jenwin.fr (P.-Y.M.)
* Correspondence: s.lafay@gynov.com

Abstract: Ginger, *Zingiber officinale* Roscoe, is increasingly consumed as a food or in food supplements. It is also recognized as a popular nonpharmacological treatment for nausea and vomiting of pregnancy (NVP). However, its consumption is not recommended by all countries for pregnant women. Study results are heterogeneous and conclusions are not persuasive enough to permit heath care professionals to recommend ginger safely. Some drugs are also contraindicated, leaving pregnant women with NVP with few solutions. We conducted a review to assess effectiveness and safety of ginger consumption during early pregnancy. Systematic literature searches were conducted on Medline (via Pubmed) until the end of December 2017. For the evaluation of efficacy, only double-blind, randomized, controlled trials were included. For the evaluation of the safety, controlled, uncontrolled, and pre-clinical studies were included in the review. Concerning toxicity, none can be extrapolated to humans from in vitro results. In vivo studies do not identify any major toxicities. Concerning efficacy and safety, a total of 15 studies and 3 prospective clinical studies have been studied. For 1 g of fresh ginger root per day for four days, results show a significant decrease in nausea and vomiting and no risk for the mother or her future baby. The available evidence suggests that ginger is a safe and effective treatment for NVP. However, beyond the ginger quantity needed to be effective, ginger quality is important from the perspective of safety.

Keywords: pregnancy; *Zingiber officinale* R; ginger; NVP; toxicity; safety; adverse effects; food supplement; CAM

---

1. Introduction

According to the World Health Organization, the growth and expansion of traditional and complementary medicine (T&CM) products is worldwide phenomenon. These days, this sector plays a significant role in the economic development of number of countries [1]. The growing mistrust of the side effects of pharmaceuticals products coupled with the desire for more traditional medicines perceived as natural and safe by consumers, may partially explain the increase in the use of herbal remedies.

In Europe, many herbal remedies are sold as food supplements and meet Directive 2002/46/EC [2]. Regarding botanicals, particularly, the European Food Safety Authority (EFSA) published, in 2012, a compendium of botanicals and associated substances of concern. The objective is to have a guideline for the evaluation of specific ingredients in food supplements, identifying the compound(s) to monitor [3]. In parallel, positive and/or negative lists of botanicals are published by authorities in different European countries [4–7] to control and guarantee the quality and traceability of used botanical ingredients in food supplements. These regulatory approaches aim to protect consumer health by ensuring that Complementary and Alternative Medicine (CAM) are safe and of high quality.

More than 100 million Europeans use regularly CAM, and the prevalence varied from 5.9 to 48.3% [8]. However, women in the middle-age, tertiary educated are typical consumers. In France [9], women consume more food supplements than men. This is also true in Belgium [10], Australia, and the USA [11]. Despite higher consumption by women in Europe, there are variations by country [12]. The differences in consumption by country and gender are summarized in Table 1.

Table 1. Comparison of food supplement consumption between men and women by country [12].

Country	Men (%)	Women (%)
France	17–21.6	26.3–28.5
Belgium	11–14	22.5–30
Australia	34.9	50.3
USA	45	58
Greece	2	6.7
Spain	5.9	12.1
Italy	6.8	12.6
Germany	20.7	27
The Netherlands	16	32.1
UK	36.3	47.5
Denmark	51	65.8
Sweden	30.5	42.4

Not only women, but also pregnant women, consume food supplements. In the United States, 36.7% of pregnant women from the ages of 19 to 49 reported using CAM in the last year compared to 40.7% of non-pregnant women [13]. In the UK and Australia, 57.8% and 52% of pregnant women, respectively, had used an herbal remedy during pregnancy [14,15].

Some studies showed that the women had a positive opinion on the safety of herbal remedies during pregnancy [16,17]. Moreover, a minimum of one-third of the healthcare professionals are willing to recommend the use of CAM to pregnant women [18,19], and the majority (69.2%) agreed that there was some value in CAM use during pregnancy [20]. Nevertheless, the safety of CAM was also a key concern. Despite this, documentation on the safety and efficacy of many herbs used during pregnancy is limited. Whereas most Member States update and regularly implement regulations relative to herbal substances/products according to the most recent scientific evaluations, few toxicological data coming from studies on pregnant women are available.

A multinational, cross-sectional study [18] identified 126 specific herbal medicines used by 2379 women. They were classified on three categories: safe, caution, and contraindicated, and their consumption was observed. Women used herbal medicine mainly classified as safe for pregnancy use. However, a difference between regions was observed (Figure 1). This study shows that there is still work to be done in informing pregnant women. Information confirmed by Pallivalappila et al. [19], 61% (n = 127) of dietary supplement users during pregnancy and 44% (n = 54) of non-users responded that CAM should be available through the NHS (the publicly-funded healthcare system in Scotland).

One of the most popular botanical remedies during pregnancy is ginger (*Zingiber officinale* Roscoe) [14,18,21]. Ginger is an Asian native plant. Its aromatic rhizome is used as a spice, but also in traditional medicine since ancestral times. Ginger belongs to the official pharmacopoeias of different countries, including Austria, China, Egypt, India, United Kingdom, Japan, Switzerland, and the Netherlands.

For around 10 years, ginger imports in Europe have increased significantly [22], and many foods and food supplements have appeared on the market. Most of these food supplements are dedicated to pregnant women (Table 2).

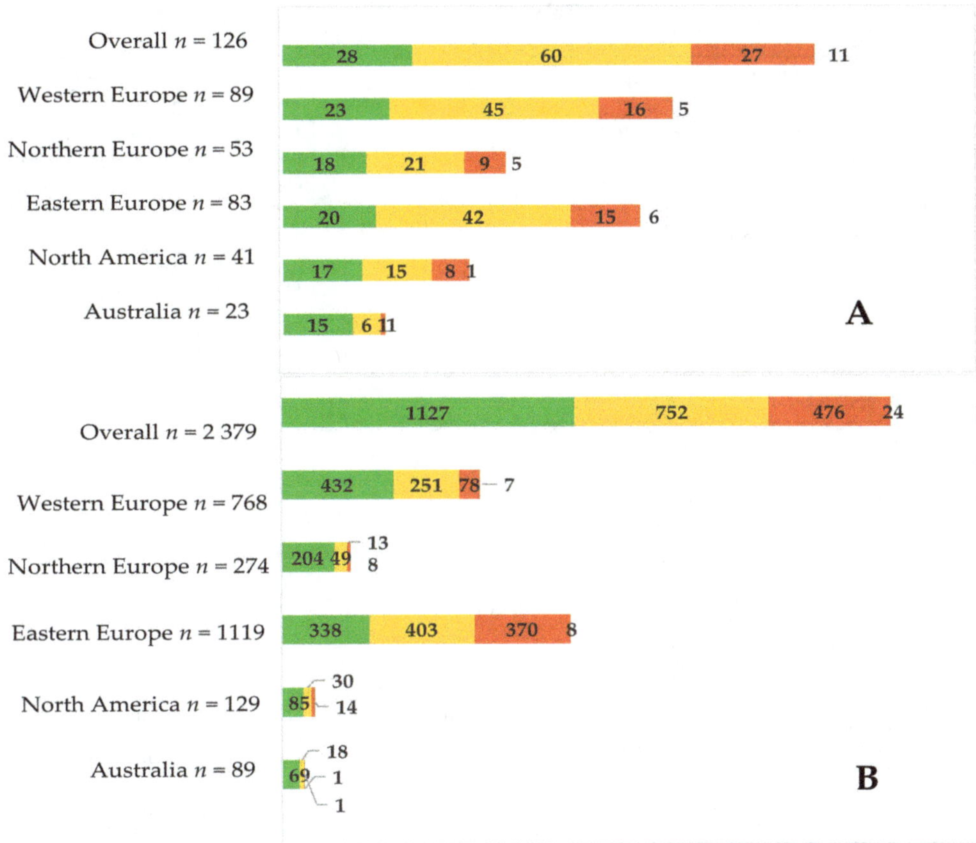

Figure 1. Herbal medicine used (**A**) and number of women who used them (**B**) by safety classification (green = safe; orange = caution; red = contraindicated; white = unknown). From Kennedy et al. [18].

Table 2. Sample of food supplements with ginger sold around the world; composition and claims.

Country	Composition	Daily Dose	Claims
Belgium	Cellulose; standardized ginger extract 50 mg with 10% gingerols (equal to 500 mg of powder); calcium phosphate; silicon dioxide, magnesium stearate; hypromellose, titanium dioxide; talc; glycerol	2/day for pregnant women	Helps you regain optimal digestive balance in the following situations: - in case of overeating - in case of unusual diets - when agitated or on trips - too much stress Can be used in pregnant women who wish to return to digestive well-being during pregnancy
	Ginger bio extract (6 × concentrated) 200 mg	1/day	Digestive comfort
	500 mg of ginger rhizome powder and 5 mg of ginger rhizome extract per caps	1/day	Sexual fatigue; nausea in pregnant women; travel sickness
	Ginger rhizome extract: 67 mg, eq. to 1 g of ginger rhizome, magnesium carbonate, vitamin B6	1/day	Ginger contributes to the normal functioning of the stomach in case of early pregnancy (Claim under consideration (EFSA)) Magnesium contributes to a reduction of tiredness and fatigue Vitamin B6 contributes to the regulation of hormonal activity

Table 2. *Cont.*

Country	Composition	Daily Dose	Claims
France	Organic ginger rhizome powder: 250 mg	4/day	Nausea in pregnant women
	Ginger rhizome powder (*Zingiber officinale* R): 365 mg/hard caps	4/day	Lower bowel contractions and digestive acids; prevent motion-induced nausea and vomiting
	Organic ginger rhizome extract (*Zingiber officinale* R): 200 mg	2/day	Ginger contributes to the normal functioning of the stomach in case of early pregnancy
	Organic ginger rhizome extract (*Zingiber officinale* R): 200 mg	5/day	Travel sickness
	Zingiber officinalis R (roots): 230 mg.	6/day	Helps to support the digestion/contributes to the normal function of intestinal tract Travel sickness Joint mobility Libido in men
	Sorbitol, rhizome ginger extract (*Zingiber officinale* R), natural orange flavor, sodium starch glycolate, microcrystalline cellulose, natural lemon flavor, magnesium stearate, silica, sucralose.	2/day	-
	Ginger, lemon, B6, magnesium, iron, B9	5 biscuits/day	-
	B6, folates, cocoa, strawberry pulp, ginger	1/day	-
	Ginger (*Zingiber officinale* Roscoe), cinnamon (*Cinnamomum verum* J. Presl), fennel (*Foeniculum vulgare* Mill.), lemon (*Citrus limon* (L.) Burm f.), Tumeric (*Curcuma longa* L.), hibiscus (*Hibiscus sabdariffa* L.), liquorice (*Glycyrrhiza glabra* L), natural lemon flavor and natural vanilla flavor	1–3 sachets /day	-
	Cellulose, silicon dioxide, magnesium stearate, standardized ginger extract (*Zingiber officinale* R) 50 mg; HPMC, titanium dioxide, talc, copper complexes of chlorophyllins	Pregnant women: 2/day Children from 6 to 11 years old: 1 to 4/day Adults and Children >12 years old: 2 to 8/day	Nausea in pregnant women; travel sickness Ginger contributes to the normal functioning of the stomach (Claim under consideration (EFSA))
	Cellulose, standardized ginger extract (10% of gingerols) 50 mg eq. to 500 mg of ginger powder; calcium phosphate; silicon dioxide; magnesium stearate; HMPC; titanium dioxide, talc, glycerol.	2/day for pregnant women	Helps to support the digestion/contributes to the normal function of intestinal tract/contributes to the normal functioning of the stomach in case of early pregnancy or travel sickness For adults and children aged 12 years and above
	Microcrystalline cellulose, standardized ginger extract 50 mg, eq. to 500 mg of rhizome powder, silicon dioxide, fatty acid magnesium salts, hypromellose, titanium dioxide, talc, glycerol	2 hard caps 3 times per day	Helps to support the digestion Contributes to decrease discomforts in case of travel nausea, pregnant women nausea, or chemotherapy
	Bach flowers, essential oils, and plant extracts	5 sprays if nauseous	Quick-acting oral spray against discomfort, apprehension and transport.
	Ginger root extract (160 mg of extract, 16 mg of gingerols); lemon balm extract (100 mg)	4/day	Stomach; antiemetic; pregnant women
Italy	Standardized root extract: 300 mg (5% gingerols) Whole root pulverized: 1500 mg	2/day	Regulate the gastro-intestinal motility and gas elimination of in case of nausea Promotes joint function and counteracts the localized states of tension Counter menstrual cycle disorders
	Hydro-alcoholic standardized ginger extract (5% of gingerols)	2/day	Reducing nausea, gas, bloating and intestinal spasms
Poland	Ginger rhizome extract 75 mg (eq. to 300 mg of powder); Vitamin B6: 0.5 mg	3/day	Adults and children poorly tolerating travel by vehicles and craft: cars, buses, trains, ships, planes
UK	Ginger extract 55 mg eq. to 1.1 g of root powder	1/day	Helps calm a queasy stomach; an excellent stomach soother; excellent travel companion
	Ginger extract 120 mg eq. to 14 g of root powder (24 mg of gingerols) (120:1 extract)	1/day	Do not take if pregnant or breastfeeding
	Ginger extract 138 mg eq. to 550 mg	2/day	-
	Ginger root 500 mg	2/day	-
	Ginger root extract (*Zingiber officinale* R) 500 mg, vitamin B6 25 mg, vitamin D 200 IU, calcium (carbonate and lactate) 240 mg, red raspberry leaf 25 mg, mint leaf 25 mg *Citrus aurantifolia* 10 mg Contains no artificial colors or flavors.	2/day	-
US	Ginger root powder	2/day	-
	Ginger root powder	2/day	May soothe an upset stomach and support digestion Promotes a healthy inflammation response May help reduce nausea, vomiting and dizziness
	Ginger root powder	2/day	Helps calm a queasy tummy an excellent stomach soother Excellent travel companion

Whereas ginger rhizome consumption is described for Nausea and Vomiting of Pregnancy (NVP) in different monographs [23–25], it is not recommended in others as a precautionary measure [26]. In the same way, ginger rhizome consumption by pregnant women is tolerated or authorized in several countries (France, Belgium) or forbidden in others (Finland, Russia). Without scientific evidence established in the concerned population, clear recommendations, and harmonized regulations, it is difficult for healthcare professionals to provide safe advice.

This review focuses on the efficacy for NVP of ginger and the safety of its use in pregnant women. The main goal is to have an objective treatment of safety, so non-clinical and clinical data were analyzed to present and discuss factual information to healthcare professionals.

2. Generality

2.1. *Zingiber Officinale Roscoe*

Ginger, *Zingiber officinale* Roscoe is originated from Asia. It is a plant of the genus *Zingiber* and of the family Zingiberaceae, whose rhizome is used worldwide in cooking and traditional medicine. It is considered as premium spices, like cardamom and turmeric. Ginger was first cultivated in the Asian subcontinent, probably in South East Asia [27]. It migrated to Europe by Greek and Roman times and was used as digestive aids wrapped in bread. Ginger was then incorporated into bread and confections. In the 1600s, the Spanish established ginger plantations in Jamaica and in the 19th century some physicians used it to induce sweating, to improve the appetite or decrease the nausea [28].

Ginger is cultivated in the tropical regions from both hemispheres and India is the largest producer (32.75% of the world's production), followed by China (21.41%) and Nigeria (12.54%) [23,29].

2.2. *Nutritional Composition and Chemical Composition*

The main ginger constituents are starch (up to 50%), lipids (6 to 8%), proteins, and inorganic compounds [25,30]. When referring to the USDA National Nutrient Database for Standard Reference and DTU Fødevaredatabanken, raw ginger root is a source of potassium (415 mg/100 g). When referring to the ANSES Table Ciqual 2017 [31], data are very different: ginger powder is a source of phosphorus (168 mg/100 g) and is rich in magnesium (214 mg/100 g), potassium (1320 mg/100 g), manganese (33.3 mg/100 g), zinc (3.64 mg/100 g), iron (19.8 mg/100 g), and niacin (9.62 mg/100 g) (Table 3). These differences between nutrient databases showed high quantitative variations that could be explained by the plant variability itself but also by used analytical methods which can differ from database to another.

Table 3. Nutritional composition of ginger root (USDA, ANSES, DTU).

	USDA (National Nutrient Database for Standard Reference)	**ANSES (Table Ciqual 2016 Composition Nutritionnelle des Aliments)**	**DTU (Fødevaredatabanken Version 7.01)**
Ginger type	**Ginger Root, Raw**	**Ginger, Powder**	**Ginger Root, Raw**
Phosphorus (mg/100 g)	34	168	34
Magnesium (mg/100 g)	43	214	43
Potassium (mg/100 g)	415	1 320	415
Manganese (mg/100 g)	-	33.3	0.229
Zinc (mg/100 g)	0.34	3.64	0.34
Iron (mg/100 g)	0.60	19.8	0.60
Calcium (mg/100 g)	16	114	16
Niacin (mg/100 g)	0.750	9.62	0.950
Folate (µg/100 g)	11	13	11

The non-volatile pungent principles responsible of spicy aroma are the gingerols, shogaols, paradols, and zingerone. They represent 4 to 7.5% [27,29] (Figure 2). The principal compound of these is 6-gingerol. In dried ginger, the concentrations of gingerols are reduced whereas the concentrations of shogaols are more abundant, coming from gingerol dehydration [27,32–35].

Volatile oils represent 1–4%. More than 100 compounds are identified. Most of them are terpenoids, mainly sesquiterpenoids (α-zingiberene, zingiberol, β-sesquiphellandrene ...) and smaller amounts of monoterpenoids (camphene, cineole, geraniol ...) [34,35].

All the *Z. officinale* samples coming from different origins are genetically indistinguishable. However, their metabolic profiling showed quantitative variation [27] function of the type, the variety but also the agronomic conditions, harvest, drying methods, and storage conditions [35,36].

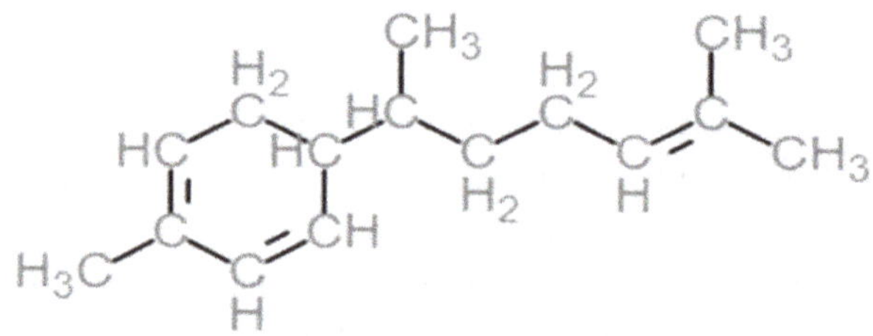

Zingiberene

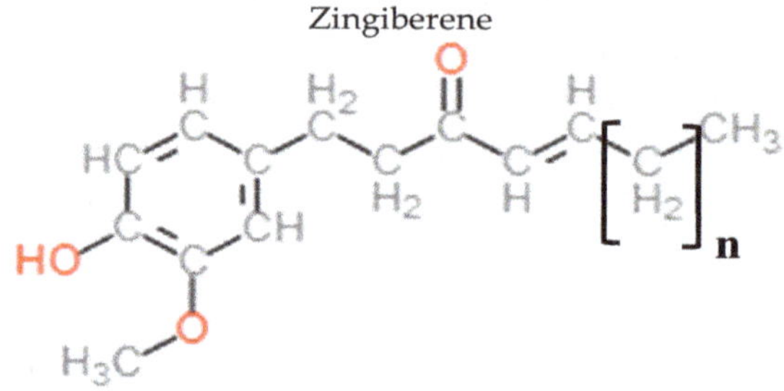

Shogaols (n = 4, 5, 7, 9, 10)

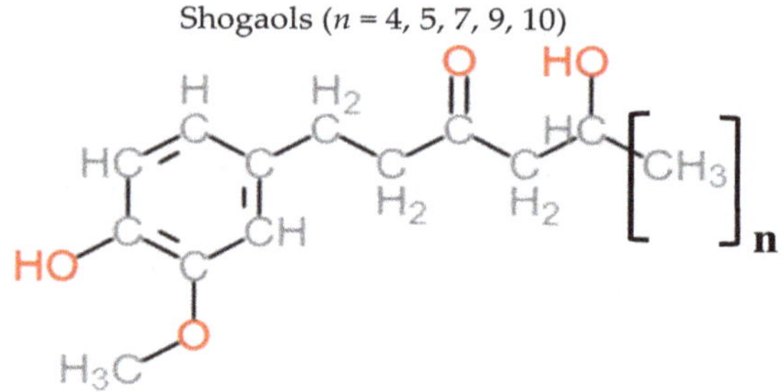

Gingerols (n = 2, 3, 4, 5, 7, 9)

Figure 2. Chemical structures of active constituents: zingiberene, shogaols, and gingerols.

2.3. Ginger Consumption

In EU countries, the apparent consumption (henceforth referred to simply as 'consumption') of ginger amounted to 58,000 tons in 2014 [22]. A large part of the consumption (around 70–80% of demand) comes from the food processing industry. Dried ginger is especially used in significant amounts in bakery (e.g., gingerbread, cookies) and Asian food products, as well as various drinks (e.g., ginger ale and ginger beer) [22].

Western EU countries accounted for 77% of EU consumption in 2014. The UK (32% of consumed volume), Germany (20%), and the Netherlands (13%) were the largest EU consumers. Concerning the UK, its large ethnic community is an important driver of the national consumption. The volume of consumed ginger in the EU increased by an average of 11% per year between 2010 and 2014, despite the economic crisis. This increase was greatest (over 20% per year) in the Eastern and Northern EU countries [22].

2.4. *Women's Perception of Ginger*

In a multinational survey (Europe, North America, and Australia) including 9113 pregnant women and new mothers, Petersen et al. [37] determined their perception of risks related to medicines, foods or herbal substances, alcohol, tobacco, and thalidomide.

The least harmful products were cranberries and ginger, whereas antidepressants, alcohol, smoking, and thalidomide were rated as the most harmful. Mean risk perception scores for ginger is 1.5 on a 10-point scale (n = 8318, Table 4)

Table 4. Mean risk perception scores for 13 individual items by geographical region (dark green = 0–2; pale green = 2–4; yellow = 4–6; orange = 6–8; red = 8–10). From Petersen et al. [37].

	Australia	Eastern Europe	Eastern Europe	Western Europe	North America
Cranberries	dark green	dark green		dark green	
Ginger	dark green	dark green	dark green		dark green
Eggs	pale green	dark green	dark green	pale green	dark green
Paracetamol	dark green	pale green	pale green	pale green	pale green
OTC (against nausea)	pale green	yellow	pale green	pale green	yellow
Antibiotics	pale green	orange	yellow	yellow	yellow
Swine flu vaccine	yellow	orange	yellow	yellow	yellow
Blue-veined cheese	orange	yellow	orange	orange	
Dental X-ray	orange	red	yellow	orange	orange
Antidepressants	yellow	red	orange	orange	orange
Alcohol (1st trimester)	orange	red		red	red
Smoking	red	red		red	red
Thalidomide	red	red			red

3. Non-Clinical Data

3.1. *Cytotoxicity*

The cytotoxic potential of ginger has been studied for many decades. Various cell lines or in-tissue culture cells were used. Results appeared very different from one study to another (Table 5).

Table 5. In vitro cytotoxicity of ginger extracts and main related compounds.

Ginger, Ginger Extracts, or Related Compounds	Cell Line	IC50	Reference
Ethanol extract of ginger	CL-6–Calcein assay	10.95 μg/mL	Plengsuriyakarn et al., 2012 [38]
Ethanol extract of ginger	CL-6–Hoechst 33342 assay	53.13 μg/mL	Plengsuriyakarn et al., 2012 [38]
Ethanol extract of ginger	HepG2–Calcein assay	71.89 μg/mL	Plengsuriyakarn et al., 2012 [38]
Ethanol extract of ginger	HepG2–Hoechst 33342 assay	92.88 μg/mL	Plengsuriyakarn et al., 2012 [38]
Ethanol extract of ginger	HepG2	358.71 μg/mL	Harliansyah et al., 2007 [39]
Ethanol extract of ginger	HRE–Calcein assay	198.15 μg/mL	Plengsuriyakarn et al., 2012 [38]
Ethanol extract of ginger	HRE–Hoechst 33342 assay	245.91 μg/mL	Plengsuriyakarn et al., 2012 [38]
Ethanol extract of ginger	Hamster ovary	245 μg/mL	Unnikrishnan et al., 1988 [40]
Ethanol extract of ginger	Vero cells	120 μg/mL	Unnikrishnan et al., 1988 [40]
Ethanol extract of ginger	Dalton's Lymphoma Ascites	200 μg/mL	Unnikrishnan et al., 1988 [40]
Aqueous extract of ginger	Dalton's Lymphoma Ascites	420 μg/mL	Unnikrishnan et al., 1988 [40]
Aqueous extract of ginger	NRK-52E Cells (MTT test)	No cytotoxicity	Abudayyak et al., 2015 [41]
Chloroform extract of ginger	NRK-52E Cells (MTT test)	9.08 mg/mL	Abudayyak et al., 2015 [41]
Methanol ginger extract	MCF7 (Breast)	75 μg/mL	Zaeoung et al., 2005 [42]
Methanol ginger extract	LS174T (Colon)	80 μg/mL	Zaeoung et al., 2005 [42]
Volatile oil of ginger	MCF7 (Breast)	14.2 μg/mL	Zaeoung et al., 2005 [42]
Volatile oil of ginger	LS174T (Colon)	15.9 μg/mL	Zaeoung et al., 2005 [42]
Related compounds			
Diarylheptanoids and gingerol-related compounds	HL-60	<50 μmol/L	Wei et al., 2005 [43]
6-gingerol	HepG2	431.7 μg/mL	Harliansyah et al., 2007 [39]
6-gingerol	MCF7 (Breast)	31.6 μg/mL	Zaeoung et al., 2005 [42]
6-gingerol	LS174T (Colon)	30.6 μg/mL	Zaeoung et al., 2005 [42]
6-gingerol	HepG2	89.58 μg/mL	Yang et al., 2010 [44]
6-shogaol	MCF7 (Breast)	6 μg/mL	Zaeoung et al., 2005 [42]
6-shogaol	LS174T (Colon)	4.2 μg/mL	Zaeoung et al., 2005 [42]

Wei et al. [43] indicated that diarylheptanoids and gingerol-related compounds were cytotoxic against human promyelocytic leukemia (HL-60) cells (IC50 < 50 μM), while Zaeoung et al. [42] reported that the IC50 of ginger was higher than 39.2 μg/mL against breast (MCF7) and colon (LS174T) cell lines.

In 2008, Kim et al. [45] investigated the cytotoxicity of five compounds of ginger (4-, 6-, 8-, 10-gingerols, and 6-shogaol) on four human tumor cell lines. 6-shogaol showed the most potent cytotoxicity against the four tumor cell lines (IC50 from 1.05 to 1.76 μg/mL) while the others showed moderate activity [45]. Peng et al., for their part, isolated 13 compounds from fresh ginger and studied their cytotoxicity against nine human tumor cell lines. Three of them were identified to be cytotoxic in cell lines tested: 6-shogaol, 10-gingerol, and an enone-diarylheptanoid analog of curcumin [46].

When comparing the IC50 of different chemical constituents to their maximum plasma concentration (see Section 4.1: Pharmacokinetic Data) after an intake of 1.5 or 2 g of ginger, the IC50 value corresponds to concentrations that are not achievable in the human body. IC50 values represent from 7 to ca. 692 times the maximum concentration reached in the plasma (Table 6).

Table 6. IC50 values and plasma concentration comparison.

Ginger Related-Compounds	IC50 (μg/mL)	Plasma Concentration after 1.5 or 2 g of Ginger (μg/mL)	Ratio IC50/Concentration	References
6-gingerol	15.72 to 431.7	1.69	9.3 to 255.4	Zaeoung et al., 2005 [42]; Harliansyah et al., 2007 [39]; Kim et al., 2008 [45]; Zick et al., 2008 [47]
6-shogaol	1.05 to 6	0.0136 to 0.15	7 to 441.2	Zaeoung et al., 2005 [42]; Kim et al., 2008 [45]; Zick et al., 2008 [47]; Yu et al., 2011 [48]
8-gingerol	8.85 to 12.57	0.23	38.5 to 54.7	Kim et al., 2008 [45]; Zick et al., 2008 [47]
10-gingerol	4.2 to 6.57	0.0095 to 0.53	7.9 to 691.6	Kim et al., 2008 [45]; Zick et al., 2008 [47]; Yu et al., 2011 [48]

Moreover, according to pharmacokinetics data [48] no free 6-, 8-, and 10-gingerols and 6-shogaol were detected in the plasma of all the volunteers 24 h after ginger consumption. Only glucuronide and sulfate metabolites were observed at very low concentration [48]. It is difficult to conclude that ginger is toxic in humans on the basis of these results. The studies presented here cannot be generalized to ginger activity in the body. The potential cytotoxic effects of ginger have to be studied, taking account of the whole plant and its absorption metabolites.

3.2. Genotoxicity/Mutagenicity

Ginger showed some mutagenicity in TA 100, TA 1535 [49,50], and T 98 strains [41]. However, ginger's mutagenicity was much lower than established mutagens, such as sodium azide or MNNG [49]. This mutagenicity could be linked to gingerols and shogaols [44,50]. However, in the presence of zingerone, mutagenic activity of gingerols and shogaols was suppressed in a dose-dependent manner (Table 7).

Thus, the observed mutagenic activity of ginger extracts in vitro is the result of the combined action of pro and antimutagenic compounds present in the ginger [50]. However, as for cytotoxic assays, studies presented here cannot be extrapolated to in vivo mutagenicity because of the tested compounds and their concentrations, which are not representative to absorption metabolites and their blood concentration.

Others in vitro and in vivo studies showed antimutagenic properties of ginger or ginger extracts [38,49,51]. When rats fed diets containing 0.5, 1, and 5% of powdered ginger for one month and are exposed to benzopyrene, the mutagenicity in vitro test realized with urine samples showed a reduced number of TA 98 and TA 100 revertants exposed to treated urine at all ginger concentrations compared to control urine [51]. On the basis of ingested dry matter, the ingested daily dose is approximately 0.1, 0.2, and 1 g of ginger by rats, which corresponds to 2.5, 5, and 25 g of ingested powdered ginger in humans, respectively.

Plengsuriyakarn et al., using a crude ethanol extract of ginger, concluded there was an absence of any toxicity at maximum dose of 5 g/kg body weight (BW) using a hamster model [38].

In the in vitro microbial test system, ginger root has mutagenic and antimutagenic properties. In vivo, it appears to be antimutagenic when it is consumed at the human dose.

3.3. *Acute/Subacute Toxicity (Repeated Dose Toxicity)*

Many acute (oral administration of a single dose of a substance in rodents within 24 h) or subacute (oral administration of a test substance in rodents for 28 days) toxicity studies were realized with different rhizome ginger extracts or related compounds. Five studies with ginger powder or ginger extracts (freeze-dried or ethanol extracts) [38,52–55], and one with related compound [56] showed no treatment-related signs of toxicity or mortality in any animals at tested doses. One of them was realized on pregnant rats and showed neither embryotoxic nor teratogenic effects of the tested ginger [55]. The No Observable Adverse Effect Level (NOAEL) was 5000 mg/kg per day whatever the used extract (freeze dried or Ethanol extract) [38,53] whereas the NOAEL of ginger oil is up to 500 mg/kg per day [57]. In four studies [54,58–60], the oral LD50 is far above the highest dose used for human food, dietary supplements or drugs (Table 8).

Table 7. Genotoxicity/mutagenicity of ginger and related compounds.

	Test Object	Concentration	Results	References
		In Vitro		
		Ginger		
Ames assay	*Salmonella typhimurium* strains TA 100, TA 98, TA 1535, and TA 1538 with and without activation	5 to 200 µg/plate	Mutagenic on metabolic activation in strains TA 100 and TA 1535	Nagabhushan et al., 1987 [50]
Ames assay	*S. typhimurium* TA 100 and TA 1535, with and without activation	25 and 50 mg/mL	Mutagenic in both TA, at both concentrations	Soudamini et al., 1995 [49]
Ames assay	*S. typhimurium* TA 100 and TA 98, with and without activation	0.78 to 25 mg/mL	Mutagenic on TA 98 activated cells from 3.13 mg/mL	Abudayyak et al., 2015 [41]
		6-gingerol		
Comet assay	HepG2	0 to 80 µmol/L	DNA strand breaks from 5.89 mg/mL (20 µmol/L)	Yang et al., 2010 [44]
Ames assay	*Salmonella typhimurium* strains TA 100, TA 98, TA 1535, and TA 1538 with and without activation	5 to 200 µg/plate	Mutagenic on metabolic activation in strains TA 100 and TA 1535	Nagabhushan et al., 1987 [50]
		Shogaol		
Ames assay	*Salmonella typhimurium* strains TA 100, TA 98, TA 1535, and TA 1538 with and without activation	5 to 200 µg/plate	Mutagenic on metabolic activation in strains TA 100 and TA 1535	Nagabhushan et al., 1987 [50]
		Zingerone		
Ames assay	*Salmonella typhimurium* strains TA 100, TA 98, TA 1535, and TA 1538 with and without activation	5 to 200 µg/plate	No mutagenic effect	Nagabhushan et al., 1987 [50]

Table 8. Acute/subacute toxicity of ginger extracts and the main related compounds.

	Administration	Species	Oral LD50	References
	Ginger dried rhizome powder			
Ginger powder	per os	Rats	No mortality	Rong et al., 2009 [52]
	Ginger dried rhizomes extracts			
Ginger dried rhizomes ethanol extract	intraperitoneal	Mice	1551 ± 75 mg/kg	Ojewole et al., 2006 [58]
Ginger dried rhizomes ethanol extract	per os	Hamsters	No mortality	Plengsuriyakarn et al., 2012 [38]
Patented standardized ethanol extract of dried rhizomes of ginger (EV.EXT 33)	per os	Pregnant rats	No mortality	Weidner et al., 2001 [55]
Freeze-dried ginger powder	per os	Rats	No mortality	Malik et al., 2011 [53]
Dry ginger decoction	per os	Rats: Gastric ulcer models	250 g/kg	Wu et al., 1990 [60]
Roasted ginger decoction	per os	Rats: Gastric ulcer models	170.6 g/kg	Wu et al., 1990 [60]
Ginger dried rhizomes ethanol extract		Mice	No mortality at 2.5 g/kg	Anonymous, 2003 [54]
Ginger oil	per os	Rabbits	5 g/kg	Anonymous, 2003 [54]
Ginger oil	per os	Rats	No mortality	Jeena et al., 2011 [57]
	Related compounds			
	(E)-8 beta,17-epoxylabd-12-ene-15,16-dial (ZT)			
(E)-8 beta,17-epoxylabd-12-ene-15,16-dial (ZT) from ginger	per os (25 mg/kg)	Mice	No mortality	Tanabe et al., 1993 [56]
(E)-8 beta,17-epoxylabd-12-ene-15,16-dial (ZT) from ginger	Intra-abdominal (25 mg/kg)	Mice	No mortality	Tanabe et al., 1993 [56]
	6-shogaol			
6-shogaol	intravenous	Mice	50.9 mg/kg	Suekawa et al., 1984 [59]
6-shogaol	intraperitoneal	Mice	109.2 mg/kg	Suekawa et al., 1984 [59]
6-shogaol	per os	Mice	687 mg/kg	Suekawa et al., 1984 [59]
	6-gingerol			
6-gingerol	intravenous	Mice	25.5 mg/kg	Suekawa et al., 1984 [59]
6-gingerol	intraperitoneal	Mice	58.1 mg/kg	Suekawa et al., 1984 [59]
6-gingerol	per os	Mice	250 mg/kg	Suekawa et al., 1984 [59]

3.4. Reproductive Toxicity

One in vivo study was made with a patented ginger extract [55]. Three groups of 22 pregnant female rats from days 6 to 15 of gestation received by gastric intubation of the extract in concentrations of 100, 333, and 1000 mg/kg and were killed on day 21 of gestation. A fourth group received sesame oil as control. Body weight, food, and water intakes were recorded during the study. Standard parameters of reproduction and performance were analyzed. Signs of teratogenic and fetuse toxic effects were determined. No adverse effects or deaths were observed and ginger supplementation was well tolerated. Neither embryotoxic nor teratogenic effects were showed by analysis of fetuses and the authors concluded that the ginger extract administered to pregnant rats during the organogenesis period caused neither maternal nor developmental toxicity at doses of up to 1 g/kg body weight per day [55].

By contrast, some ginger adverse events have been reported on pregnant rats [61]. Pregnant Sprague–Dawley rats received ginger tea (15, 20, or 50 g/L) on day 6 of gestation onwards until day 15 of gestation. They were sacrificed at day 20. No maternal toxicity was observed, but embryonic loss was increased in the treatment group compared to control. No gross morphologic malformations were seen but fetuses exposed to ginger tea were significantly heavier than control and had more advanced skeletal development. This effect was greater in female fetuses and not correlated with increased placental size. Thus, results of this study suggest that in utero exposure to ginger tea leads to an increased early embryo loss with increased growth in surviving fetuses [61].

In 2009, Sukandar et al. studied the effect of ethanol extracts of ginger and noni fruit in pregnant rats. The blend was administered per os at three different doses on days 6–15 of gestation (50 and 50, 500 and 500, 1000 and 1000 mg/kg BW). Sacrifices were realized on day 19 of gestation to observe live fetus, resorption, and growfail fetus. No malformation was found. The combination, did not cause any fetus resorption, growth failure, malformation in organs nor in the skeleton, whatever the dose. The highest dose (500 and 500 and 1000 and 1000 mg/kg BW) caused liver color change of 7.3% and 8.3% of rat fetuses, respectively [62].

In a double-blind randomized cross-over clinical trial, ginger per os, 250 mg, four times daily did not generate teratogenic aberrations in newborns and Apgar scores of these babies were 9 to 10 after five minutes [63].

Reproductive and developmental toxicity has been investigated in three studies in rats [55,61,62] and one double-blind randomized cross-over clinical trial [63]. All these studies showed no teratogenic aberrations. Extensive data do not suggest any major concerns with respect to reproductive and developmental safety of ginger root.

4. General Population Safety Data

Many reviews have been published on ginger effects and few minor adverse events have been reported with the use of ginger in humans [34,64–67].

A systematic review by Betz et al. [65] including 15 randomized studies with safety data showed that, among the 777 patients included, 3.3% reported slight side effects that did not require treatments like mild gastrointestinal symptoms and sleepiness.

In a clinical trial involving 12 healthy volunteers who consumed 400 mg of ginger three times per day for two weeks, one subject reported mild diarrhea during the first two days of treatment. Authors explained that ginger could cause heartburn and as a gastric irritant with doses higher than 6 g. Moreover, its inhalation could produce an IGE-mediated allergy [64].

An assessment report on *Zingiber officinale* Roscoe made by the Committee on Herbal Medicinal Products (HMPC) in 2012 summarized the published clinical studies with safety data indexed by PubMed through June 2010 [30].

Adverse effects resulting from the intake of ginger root observed in clinical studies occur with low frequency, low intensity, and are mainly gastrointestinal. No severe events have been reported. An interaction between ginger and warfarin has been showed in some case reports however the latter are unconvincing. Moreover, one randomized study in healthy volunteers failed to demonstrate any warfarin interaction. No sufficient evidence are available to suggest induction or inhibition of CYP-enzymes by ginger or its constituents [30]. Consequently, the committee concluded that the benefit/risk balance is in favor of the oral use of ginger extract and complies with the criteria for well-established use in the prevention of nausea and vomiting in motion sickness [30]. However, ginger's effect on platelet aggregation cannot be confidently dismissed and future clinical trials are needed to further investigate this area, particularly in risk population [68].

More recently, Wang et al. [69] assessed daily ginger consumption in adults, explored its correlation with chronic diseases and analyzed further how different levels of ginger intake may affect the prevalence of chronic diseases. A total of 4628 participants (1823 men and 2805 women), aged from 18 to 77 years old, completed face-to-face dietary and health questionnaires. Daily ginger consumption was associated with a decreased risk for hypertension ((OR), 0.92; 95% confidence interval (CI), 0.86–0.98) and chronic heart disease (CHD) (OR, 0.87; 95% CI, 0.78–0.96) in adults ≥18 years old. Differences were also observed in adults ≥40 years old: hypertension (OR, 0.92; 95% CI, 0.87–0.99), CHD (OR, 0.87; 95% CI, 0.78–0.97). However, after 60 years old, no association was seen for hypertension, but there was still a difference regarding CHD (OR, 0.84; 95% CI, 0.73–0.96). Again, the probability of illness (hypertension or CHD) decreased when the dosage of daily ginger intake increased. No adverse events were reported [69].

4.1. Pharmacokinetic Data

In 2008, Zick et al. [47] realized a single dose pharmacokinetic escalation study of the ginger constituents 6-gingerol, 8-gingerol, 10-gingerol, and 6-shogaol. 27 healthy volunteers were recruited, three participants per dose except for the highest doses for which 6 and 9 participants were included. Administrated doses of ginger extract were 100 mg, 250 mg, 500 mg, 1.0 g, 1.5 g, and 2.0 g. The dry extract of ginger root used in the study was standardized to 6% of gingerols. A dose of 250 mg correspond to 15 mg of total gingerols, with 5.38 mg 6-gingerol, 1.28 mg 8-gingerol, 4.19 mg 10-gingerol, and 0.92 mg 6-shogaol. Blood was sampled at different times after ginger intake and analysis showed that no free 6-gingerol, 8-gingerol, 10-gingerol, or 6-shogaol was detected and no conjugate metabolite were detected below the 1 g ginger extract dose, except for 6-gingerol. However, as of this dose, all metabolites were quickly absorbed and detected as glucuronide and sulfate conjugates. Conjugate metabolite appeared 30 min after 2 g dose intake, with their T_{max} between 45 and 120 min and their elimination half-lives between 75 to 120 min. The maximum concentrations were 1.69 μg/mL for 6-gingerol, 0.23 μg/mL for 8-gingerol, 0.53 μg/mL for 10-gingerol, and 0.15 μg/mL for 6-shogaol at either the 1.5 g or 2.0 g dose. No pharmacokinetic model was able to be constructed due to the low levels of ginger constituent absorption, and the pharmacokinetic parameters were based on a non-compartment analysis with an elimination half-life only presented for the 2.0 g dose [47].

Another study made by Yu [48] in 2011 with 12 volunteers receiving 2 g of ginger extract per os for 24 days showed that no 6-, 8-, and 10-gingerols, and 6-shogaol under free form were detected in the plasma of all the participants 24 h after the last dosing. Concentrations of 6-gingerol glucuronide (from 5.43 to 13.6 ng/mL), 6-gingerol sulfate (from 6.19 to 7.29 ng/mL), and 10-gingerol glucuronide (from 6.96 to 9.33 ng/mL) were low whereas levels of other conjugate metabolites were not detectable in all the volunteers. Maximum concentrations determined for 10-gingerol and 6-shogaol were 9.5 ± 2.2 ng/mL (0.027 ± 0.006 μM) and 13.6 ± 6.9 ng/mL (0.049 ± 0.025 μM), whereas the IC50s of 10-gingerol and 6-shogaol were 12 and 8 μM, or 4.2 and 2.2 mg/mL, respectively. The half-lives of all metabolites are between 1 and 3h [48].

Table 6 reviews the pharmacokinetic data and IC50 values of some ginger metabolites absorbed and detected in plasma, such as 6-, 8-, 10- gingerols, and 6-shogaol. As mentioned before, IC50 values represents between 7 to 692 times the maximum concentrations detected in plasma.

5. Pregnant Women Data

5.1. Safety Data

We analyzed 14 randomized clinical studies from 1991 [63] to 2017 [70] and three prospective studies [71–73]. In randomized clinical studies, a total of 1 331 pregnant women have been studied, including 617 who consumed ginger (Tables 9 and 10). Paritakul et al. studied 63 postpartum women (33 for the placebo group and 30 for ginger group). Studies included pregnant women at less than 20 weeks of gestation and only for one greater than or equal to 37 weeks of gestation [74].

Different types of ginger were used, like fresh ginger, ginger powder, ginger extract, or ginger essence. The ginger dose ranges studied were from 500 mg/d to 2.5 g/d. The recommended daily doses were: 3 × 650 mg, 4 × 250 mg, 2 × 500 mg, 4 × 125 mg, 3 × 350 mg, 3 × 250 mg, and five biscuits. The majority of the studies were conducted over four days, but three studies chose seven days [75–77], one study was conducted for two weeks [78], and one study was conducted for three weeks [79]. Clinical studies were realized in Asia (Thailand), Europe (Denmark), Oceania (Australia), and the Middle East (Iran). The majority of studies (12/14) lasted between four and seven days, which is consistent with the symptomatology of pregnant women with regard to nausea and vomiting. Ten studies, all randomized versus placebo or positive control (vitamin B6 or dimenhydrinate), have highlighted various side effects.

Table 9. Randomized double-blind trials investigating the effectiveness and safety of ginger for pregnancy.

Objective	Population	Number	Treatment	Ginger Definition	Duration	Results	Adverse Events	Reference
To determine the effectiveness of ginger for the treatment of NVP	Women NVP < 17 weeks of gestation	$n = 67$ 35 placebo 32 ginger	1000 mg/day (4×250 mg) of ginger (powder capsules) vs. placebo	Fresh ginger root	4 days + follow-up visit 7 days later	Significant decrease of nausea in the ginger group vs. placebo group ($p = 0.014$) Significant decrease of vomiting in the ginger group vs. placebo group ($p < 0.001$) Follow-up visits:Significant symptom improvement in the ginger group vs. placebo group ($p < 0.001$)	Headache: - 5 in the placebo group - 6 in the ginger group. Ginger group: - 1 abdominal discomfort - 1 heartburn - 1 diarrhoea for one day **Side effects reported as minor.** Spontaneous abortions: - 3 in the placebo group - 1 in the ginger group Term delivery: - 91.4% in the placebo group - 96.9% in the ginger group Cesarean deliveries: - 4 in the placebo group - 6 in the ginger group **No infants had any congenital anomalies recognized.** **No significant adverse effect of ginger on pregnancy outcome was reported.**	Vutyavanich et al., 2001 [80]
To compare the effectiveness of ginger and vitamin B6 for treatment of NVP	Women NVP < 16 weeks of gestation	$n = 123$ 62 vit. B6 61 ginger	1950 mg/day of ginger (3×650 mg) or 75 mg/day of vitamin B6 (3×25 mg)	Fresh ginger root	4 days	Nausea/vomiting: Improvement of nausea vomiting scores in both group from baseline The average score change in the ginger group was better than that of vitamin B6 group ($p < 0.05$)	Side effects: - 16 in ginger group - 15 in B6 group (NS) Heartburn: - 8 in ginger group - 2 in B6 group Sedation: - 7 in ginger group - 11 in B6 group Arrhythmia: - 1 in ginger group Headache: - 2 in B6 group **Side effects were reported to be minor**	Chittumma et al., 2007 [81]
To determine the effectiveness of ginger for the treatment of NVP	Women NVP < 20 weeks of gestation	$n = 67$ 35 placebo 32 ginger	1000 mg/day (4×250 mg) of ginger (powder capsules)	Ginger root powder (Zintoma, Goldaroo Company, Tehran, Iran)	4 days	Nausea: Significant improvement in 84% of ginger users vs. 56% in the control group ($p < 0.05$) Vomiting: Significant improvement in the treated group vs. the control group ($p < 0.05$)	No complication during the treatment period was reported **Reported as a safe remedy to improve the nausea and vomiting of pregnancy.**	Ozgoli et al., 2009 [82]

Table 9. *Cont.*

Objective	Population	Number	Treatment	Ginger Definition	Duration	Results	Adverse Events	Reference
To compare the effectiveness of ginger and vitamin B6 for the treatment of NVP	Women with nausea with or without vomiting < 17 weeks of gestation	$n = 69$ 34 vit. B6 35 ginger	1000 mg/day (2 × 500 mg) of ginger (powder capsules) or 40 mg/day of vitamin B6 (2 × 20 mg)	Fresh ginger root	4 days + follow-up visit 7 days later	Nausea score: Better score in the ginger group vs. the vitamin group ($p = 0.024$) Vomiting episodes: No significant difference between the groups Follow-up visits: 82.8% reported an improvement in the ginger group vs. 67.6% in the vitamin group ($p = 0.52$)	Spontaneous abortions: - 2 in the ginger group - 1 in the B6 group ($p > 0.05$) Term birth: - 82.9% in the ginger group - 82.4% in the B6 group Caesarean deliveries: - 4 in the ginger group - 6 in the B6 group ($p > 0.05$) **No babies had any congenital anomalies All were discharged in good condition** **No adverse effects of ginger on pregnancy outcome were reported**	Ensiyeh et al., 2009 [83]
To compare the effects of ginger on nausea and vomiting caused by pregnancy and compares it with metoclopramide medicine	Women NVP < 20 weeks of gestation	$n = 102$ 34 placebo 34 metoclopramide 34 ginger	600 mg/day (3 × 200 mg) ginger;30 mg/day (3 × 10 mg) metoclopramide;600 mg/day (3 × 200 mg) placebo	Ginger essence	5 days	Intensity of nausea: Significant difference in the two supplemented groups (ginger or metoclopramide) vs. placebo ($p < 0.05$) Not statistically significant between treated groups	-	Mohammadbeigi et al., 2011 [84]
To determine if ginger syrup mixed in water is an effective remedy for the relief of NVP	Women with nausea with or without vomiting first trimester	$n = 23$ 10 placebo 13 ginger	1 g/day (4 × 250 mg) ginger (tablespoon) vs placebo	Ginger including 1 mg pungent compounds from ginger rhizome juice, 1 mg of 20% pungent compounds and 5% zingiberene coming from CO_2 supercritical extract of ginger rhizome	2 weeks	Nausea: 77% improvement in ginger group vs. 20% in placebo group Vomiting: 67% in ginger group stop vomiting at day 6 vs 20% in placebo group	Delivered viable infant at term without major complications **Safe option in the treatment of NVP**	Keating et al., 2002 [78]

Table 9. *Cont.*

Objective	Population	Number	Treatment	Ginger Definition	Duration	Results	Adverse Events	Reference
To investigate the effect of a ginger extract (EV.EXT35) on the symptoms of morning sickness.	Women with morning sickness < 20 weeks of gestation	$n = 9951$ placebo48 ginger	500 mg/day (4 × 125 mg) eq. 6 g/day ginger vs. placebo	EV.EXT35: ginger extract (125 mg eq to 1.5 g of dried ginger)	4 days	Nausea experience score: - except for day 3, the difference parameter for each day post-baseline, was significantly less than zero Vomiting: - no significant difference between the groups	Spontaneous abortion: - 3 in the ginger group - 1 in the placebo group Intolerance of the treatment: - 4 in the ginger group Worsening of treatment requiring further medical assistance: - 1 in the ginger group - 2 in the placebo group Allergic reaction to treatment: - 1 ginger group **No apparent increased risk of fetal abnormalities or low birth weight.**	Willetts et al., 2003 [85]
To estimate whether the use of ginger to treat nausea or vomiting in pregnancy is equivalent to pyridoxine hydrochloride (vitamin B6)	Women NVP Between 8 and 16 weeks of gestation	$n = 235$ 115 vit. B6 120 ginger	1.05 g/day ginger (3 × 350 mg) vs. 75 mg/day vitamin B6 (3 × 25 mg)	-	3 weeks	53% reported an improvement taking ginger, and 55% reported an improvement with vitamin B6 Ginger was equivalent to vitamin B6 for improving nausea, dry retching, and vomiting	Belching: - ginger (9%) vs. B6 (0%) ($p < 0.05$) Dry retching after swallowing: - ginger (52%) vs. B6 (56%) Vomiting after ingestion: - ginger (2%) vs. B6 (1%) Burning sensation: - ginger (2%) vs. B6 (2%) Pregnancy outcome: - 272 (93%) gave birth to 278 infants - 12 women with spontaneous abortion (first or second trimester) - 3 women with stillbirth - No differences were found between study groups - 9 babies born with congenital abnormality (3 ginger, 6 B6) (NS) - 6 cases of urogenital disorders - 2 cases of minor gastrointestinal abnormalities -1 case of a minor congenital heart defect	Smith et al., 2004 [79]

Table 9. *Cont.*

Objective	Population	Number	Treatment	Ginger Definition	Duration	Results	Adverse Events	Reference
To examine the evidence for the safety and effectiveness of ginger for NVP	Women NVP Between 7 and 17 weeks of gestation	$n = 62$ 30 placebo 32 ginger	5 biscuits/day (2.5 g of ginger) vs. placebo	-	4 days + follow-up visit 7 days later	Nausea scores: - significantly greater in the ginger group vs. in placebo group ($p = 0.01$) Vomiting episodes: - no significant difference ($p = 0.243$) No vomiting after 4 days: - 34% in ginger group vs. 18% in placebo group Follow-up visits: - 87.5% ginger group reported improvement vs. 70% in placebo group ($p = 0.043$)	In ginger group: - 1 dizziness - 1 heartburn **The side effects reported as minor.** **No abnormal pregnancy and delivery outcome occurred. No infants had any congenital abnormalities recognized.** **All discharged in good condition**	Basirat et al., 2009 [86]
To compare the breast milk volume during the early postpartum period between women receiving dried ginger capsules with those receiving placebo	Women ≥ 37 weeks gestation	$n = 63$ 33 placebo 30 ginger	1 g of ginger (500 mg × 2) vs. placebo	Dried ginger powder	7 days	Breast milk volume: - day 3 ginger group has higher milk volume than the placebo group ($p < 0.01$) - day 7, the ginger group does not differ from the placebo group Prolactin levels is similar in both groups	No notable side effects	Paritakul et al., 2016 [74]
To study the efficacy of ginger and dimenhydrinate in the treatment of NVP	Women NVP < 16 weeks of gestation	$n = 170$ 85 dimenhydrinate 85 ginger	1 g (500 mg × 2) of ginger vs. 100 mg (50 mg × 2) of dimenhydrinate	-	1 week	Nausea: - the mean score in day 1-7 decreased in both groups - daily mean scores between both groups were not statistically different Vomiting: - frequency of vomiting times in day 1-7 decreased in both groups - daily mean vomiting times in the dimenhydrinate group in day 1-2 were less than the ginger group ($p < 0.05$) - after day 3–7 post treatment, the daily mean vomiting times in both groups were not statistically different	Drowsiness: - 5/85 in the ginger group vs. 66/85 in dimenhydrinate group ($p < 0.01$) Heart burn: - 13/85 in the ginger group vs. 9/85 in dimenhydrinate group ($p = 0.403$) **No other adverse effect was reported in both groups**	Pongrojpaw et al., 2007 [75]

Table 9. *Cont.*

Objective	Population	Number	Treatment	Ginger Definition	Duration	Results	Adverse Events	Reference
To study the efficacy of ginger and placebo in hyperemesis gravidarum.	Women hyperemesis gravidarum < 20 weeks of gestation	$n = 27$ 13 lactose 14 ginger	1 g (250 mg × 4) of ginger vs. placebo	Powdered root	2 × 4 days 2 days washout	The preference: - ginger treatment period was statistically significant ($p = 0.003$) Relief of the hyperemesis symptoms: - significantly greater in ginger group vs. placebo ($p = 0.035$)	One spontaneous abortion, which was not a suspicious high rate of fetal wastage in early pregnancy No side effects were observed All infants were without deformities and discharged in good condition.	Fischer-Rasmussen et al., 1991 [63]
To compare the effectiveness of ginger and acupressure in the treatment of NVP	Women NVP < 16 weeks of gestation	$n = 143$ 45 control 48 acupressure	750 mg (250 mg × 3) of ginger vs. acupressure	-	7 days - 3 with no intervention - 4 with treatment	Rhodes index scores: - better in the ginger group vs. acupressure and control ($p < 0.001$) - reduced 49% in ginger group and 29% in acupressure group. - increased up to 0.06% in control group Post hoc test showed significant differences in vomiting, nausea, retching, and total scores between the groups except for vomiting score between acupressure and control groups and for retching score between acupressure and ginger groups	1 case of heartburn with ginger capsules	Saberi et al., 2013 [76]
To determine the effect of ginger to relieve NVP	Women NVP < 16 weeks of gestation	$n = 106$ 36 placebo 33 control 37 ginger	750 mg (250 mg × 3) of ginger vs. acupressure	-	7 days - 3 with no intervention - 4 with treatment	Rhodes index scores: - greater in the ginger group vs. placebo and control ($p < 0.001$) - reduced 48% in ginger group,13% in placebo group and -10% in control group Post hoc test showed significant difference between the groups in reduction of vomiting, nausea, retching and total Rhodes Index scores ($p < 0.001$)	1 case of heartburn with ginger capsules	Saberi et al., 2014 [77]
To compare the effects of ginger, pyridoxine (vitamin B6), and placebo for the treatment of NVP	Women between 6 and 16 weeks of pregnancy; mild and moderate NVP	$n = 77$ 23 placebo 26 vit. B6 28 ginger	1 g (500 mg × 2) ginger capsules 80 mg (40 mg × 2) Vit. B6 capsules	-	4 days	Rhodes index scores: - ginger > placebo ($p = 0.039$) - Vit. B6 > placebo ($p = 0.007$) - ginger = Vit. B6 ($p = 0.128$) Ginger was more effective for - nausea intensity - nausea distress - distress of vomiting	Ginger is effective and safe	Sharifzadeh et al., 2017 [70]

Table 10. Prospective studies investigating the effectiveness and safety of ginger for pregnancy.

Study Type	Objective	Population	Number	Treatment	Ginger Definition	Duration	Results	Adverse Events	Reference
Prospective cohort study (Korean Motherisk Program)	To determine if ginger exposure during pregnancy would increase the risk of adverse fetal and neonatal outcomes	Women Cough and cold preparations (49.7%) Functional gastrointestinal disorders (37.7%) 3 days to 20.7 weeks	159 306 (control group)	Median dose: 470 mg/day Maximum dose: 7.2 g/day	Dried ginger	Median length: 2 days		Spontaneous abortion: - 7 in the ginger group vs. 17 in the control group (NS) Stillbirths: - 2.7% in the ginger group vs. 0.3% in the control group (NS) NICU admission: - 4.7% in the ginger group vs. 1.7% in the control group (NS) The admission rate was marginally different between cases and controls however, no difference was observed when admission rate was compared with that reported in 2012 at the hospital. **They concluded that dried ginger is not a major human teratogen**	Choi et al., 2014 [73]
The Norwegian Mother and Child Cohort study	To evaluate the safety of ginger use during pregnancy on congenital malformations	Women NVP first trimester	*n* = 68 522 - 1020 (use ginger) - 466 (use ginger during 1st trimester)					Not increase the risk of malformations No significant associations between ginger use risk of: - Stillbirth - Perinatal death - Low birth weight - Preterm birth - Low Apgar score	Heitmann et al., 2013 [72]
Prospective cohort study (The Motherisk Program)	The primary objective: - to examine the safety The secondary objective: - to examine the effectiveness of ginger for NVP	Women first trimester	187 (ginger group) 187 (comparison group)	Various types of ginger: - Capsules (49%) - Ginger tea - Fresh ginger - Pickled ginger - Ginger cookies - Ginger candy - Inhaled powdered ginger - Ginger crystals - Sugared ginger		Minimum 3 days	Ginger effectiveness scores (overall) on 66 women - 3.6 ± 2.4 (SD) Scale range of effectiveness: - 0 => 29 (43.9%) - 2–4 => 19 (28.8%) - 5–7 => 13 (19.7%) - 8–10 => 6 (7.6%) 0 = No effect; 1–4 = mild effect; 5–7 = moderate effect; 8–10 = best effect.	- 3 spontaneous abortions - 2 stillbirths - 1 therapeutic abortion (Down syndrome) 3 major malformations in the ginger group: - ventricular septal defect - lung abnormality - kidney abnormality (pelviectasis) - 1 idiopathic central precocious puberty at 2 years old No significant differences between the groups in terms of live births, spontaneous abortions, stillbirths, therapeutic abortions, birth weight, or gestational age. Eight sets of twins in the ginger group. More babies < 2.5 Kg in the control group	Portnoi et al., 2003 [71]

The various adverse effects founded in RCTs are listed in Table 11. There are no common side effects from one study to another with the exception of heartburn and spontaneous abortion, which are quoted six and five times, respectively.

Table 11. List of adverse effects identified in the different clinical studies.

Adverse Effects Identified (No Significance)	References
Headache, abdominal discomfort, diarrhea, heartburn, spontaneous abortion	Vutyavanich et al., 2001 [80]
Sedation, arrhythmia, heartburn	Chitumma et al., 2007 [81]
Intolerance, allergic reaction, medical assistance, spontaneous abortion	Willets et al., 2003 [85]
Dry retching, vomiting, burning sensation, belching, spontaneous abortion	Smith et al., 2004 [79]
Dizziness, heartburn	Basirat et al., 2009 [86]
Drowsiness, heartburn	Pongrojpaw et al., 2007 [75]
Spontaneous abortion	Ensiyehh et al., 2009 [83]
Spontaneous abortion	Fisher Rasmussen et al., 1991 [63]
Heartburn	Saberie et al., 2013 [76]
Heartburn	Saberie et al., 2014 [77]

This diversity of side effects can be explained by changes in several parameters depending on the studies. The most important point is that ginger quality is never specified and there are many variations on the type of ginger, recommended daily doses, and the duration of treatment.

According to Boltman-Binkowski [87], ginger does not increase spontaneous abortion compared to the control group (relative risk with 95% CI = 0.80 (0.21, 2.99)) and does not increase the rate of stillbirth (relative risk with 95% CI = 0.64 (0.03, 13.59)) and congenital abnormalities (relative risk with 95% CI = 2.11 (0.07, 65.87)) compared to the general population.

In Saberi's studies made in 2013 and 2014 [76,77], a total of 249 women participated to RCTs, 87 of whom are treated with ginger, and only two cases of heartburn were detected. Babies whose mothers were exposed to ginger during Saberi's study did not appear to be at an increased risk of fetal abnormalities or low birth weight. All these side effects were reported by subjects as minor and did not preclude them from taking their prescribed medication [76,77].

Three prospective studies [71–73] focus on the exposure of pregnant women to ginger and the possible side effects that would result from it. In 69 361 women, 812 pregnant women were studied because they took ginger during first trimester. Choi et al. [73] noted seven cases of spontaneous abortions in the ginger group and 17 cases in the control group (OR: 0.8; 95% CI: 0.3–1.9; $p = 0.59$). At first reading, rates of stillbirths and babies that required attention at the neonatal intensive care unit (NICU) were marginally superior in the ginger group vs. the control group. However, no difference was observed when the NICU admission rate was compared with what was reported from the hospital and Women's Healthcare Center in 2012.

Heitmann et al. [72] found that ginger use during pregnancy at any time did not increase the risk of malformations (4.7% in the no exposure to ginger group vs. 4,1% in those exposed to ginger during the first trimester group, adjusted OR (95 % CI) 0.8 (0.5–1.4)). Moreover, ginger use during pregnancy is not significantly associated to the risk of stillbirth/perinatal death, low birth weight, preterm birth, or low Apgar score. Equivalent results were found by Portnoi et al. [71], with no differences between the groups in terms of live births, spontaneous abortions, stillbirths, therapeutic abortions, birth weight, or gestational age. One exception: there were more infants who weighed less than 2500 g in the control group. Unfortunately, Heitmann et al. [72] specified neither the duration, nor the dose, nor the type of ginger used. Several types of ginger were consumed by women in Portnoi's study [71] and Choi et al. [73] did not give any details except that it is a dried ginger.

Three studies [70,78,82], used ginger in syrup and powder form, respectively, on 14, 28, and 32 pregnant women during two weeks or four days. None of them had safety outcomes, but they concluded that ginger is a safe option in early pregnancy.

Term birth parameter is mentioned in three others studies [79,80,83]. In two of them, there was no significant difference between ginger groups vs. other groups (placebo or B6) [80,83]. Conversely,

Smith, et al., showed that term birth in the ginger group was significantly better than placebo (93% vs. 98% for placebo and of ginger groups, respectively, $p = 0.03$) [79].

A randomized, double-blind controlled trial was conducted by Paritakul et al. [74] in 2016 on women for seven days postpartum. Sixty-three women (30 ginger group, 33 placebo group) received 500 mg of dried ginger powder in capsules twice a day and no notable side effects are mentioned.

The 14 randomized and three prospective clinical studies have observed more than 70,000 pregnant women, including more than 1500 who have consumed ginger during their pregnancy. Studies ran through over more than 25 years. Doses, durations, types of ginger, and countries vary from one study to another, thus addressing the different possibilities of current consumption. The use of ginger during pregnancy do not present a risk for the mother or her future baby. All studies conclude the safety of ginger. We can, however, note a side effect inherent to the composition of ginger—heartburn—which must be monitored in sensitive persons.

According to McLay [88], ginger could potentially cause interactions with concurrent prescription medicines: one major interaction with nifedipine, and three moderate interactions with metformin, insulin, and aspirin. In France, these drugs—except insulin—are not recommended for use or are contraindicated in pregnant women.

5.2. *Efficacy*

The mechanisms of action underlying ginger's efficiency in reducing NVP has been investigated [89], dual antiemetic action have been highlighted: (i) gingerols and shogaols act as antagonists of cholinergic M3 and serotonin 5-HT3 receptors of the central nervous system; (ii) ginger's constituents improve the gastric tonus, motility, and emptying due to peripheral anticholinenergic and antiserotonergic actions. However, these data need further investigations to elucidate and confirm those preliminary findings.

Concerning the efficacy of ginger on pregnant women, Mohammadbeigi's study is added to the previous studies mentioned in Section 5.1 [84]. The total number of pregnant women studied in randomized clinical studies was 1433, with 651 pregnant women who consumed ginger. The doses used and the duration of treatment vary according to the studies.

To determine the effectiveness of ginger on NVP, its effect was compared to control [77] or placebo [77,78,80,84–86] groups, but also vitamin B6 [70,79,81,83], drugs like dimenhydrinate [75], metoclopramide [84], or acupuncture [76].

A minimum of 1 g of fresh ginger root per day during at least four days significantly decreased nausea and vomiting and improved significantly symptoms vs. placebo or vitamin B6 [79–81,83].

Willets, et al., [85] investigated in a randomized double-blind placebo-controlled study, the effect of a ginger extract (EV.EXT35) on morning sickness symptoms in 120 pregnant women. 125 mg of ginger extract was equivalent to 1.5 g of dried ginger. After four days, the nausea experience score was significantly less than zero (except for day 3). Concerning vomiting symptoms, there was no significant difference between ginger extract and placebo groups

Keating et al. [78] demonstrated that 1 g/d (4×250 mg) of ginger syrup for a two-week period revealed that 67% of women in the ginger group stopped vomiting at day 6 vs. 20% in the placebo group. Additionally, 77% of women in the ginger group had a four-point improvement on the nausea scale at day 9 vs. 20% in the placebo group.

Mohammadbeigi et al. [84] used 600 mg/d (3×200 mg) of ginger essence for five days vs. 30 mg/d (3×10 mg) of metoclopramide and 600 mg/d (3×200 mg) of placebo. Significant decreases in the severity of nausea and vomiting, as well as the Rhodes Index for ginger and metoclopramide groups vs. the placebo group, was shown. There was also no difference between both groups.

Basirat et al. [86] realized a randomized double-blind clinical trial on 62 pregnant women. Thirty-two women took five biscuits daily for four days. Each biscuit contained 0.5 g of ginger. The average change in nausea scores in the ginger group was significantly better ($p = 0.01$) than that in the placebo group. The average change in the number of vomiting episodes was not significantly different between the ginger group and the placebo group. However, after four days of treatment, the proportion of women who had no vomiting in the ginger group (11/32 patients) was greater than that in the placebo group (6/30).

Regardless of the dose, duration, or type of ginger, there is a significant impact on nausea and there are no safety concerns. In 4/15 studies either ginger had no effect on vomiting or there was no significant difference with placebo or vitamin B6.

According to Ding et al. [90], all various forms of ginger studied were a safe and effective treatment for NVP when compared to placebo and vitamin B6. Two meta-analyses made in 2014 [67,91] concluded also that ginger could be considered as an effective and harmless alternative option for women suffering from the symptoms of NVP and that 1 g/day for a duration of at least four days is better than placebo in improving NVP.

6. Conclusions

NVP affect 7 in 10 pregnant women and have a deep impact on the quality of life. Recently, increasing concerns have been pointed out regarding the safety of traditional antiemetic drugs (metoclopramide, domperidone, etc.). Thus, considering natural options, such as ginger, with a favorable risk/benefit ratio and a good level of evidence, is now part of several practice guidelines [92].

Many food supplements with ginger powder or ginger extracts are used to decrease symptoms of nausea and vomiting associated with pregnancy. This effect is supported by a European claim (ID 2172) that it "*Helps to support the digestion/contributes to the normal function of intestinal tract/contributes to physical well-being/contributes to the normal functioning of the stomach in case of early pregnancy*" provided the product contains the equivalent of 0.5 to 2 g of root per day.

Beyond the quantity of ginger needed to be effective, the quality of the ginger is important for the safety aspect. For example, in France, it is mandatory to monitor the concentration of methyleugenol because of its potential toxicity [5]. It is important to focus special attention on pungent components of ginger powder, including the main components, 6-gingerol, 8-gingerol, and 10-gingerol [89]. It is also important to highlight the wide variability in 6-gingerol, 6-shogaol, 8-gingerol, and 10-gingerol composition from one food supplement to another. The 6-gingerol concentration ranged from 0.0 to 9.43 mg/g, 6-shogaol ranged from 0.16 to 2.18 mg/g, 8-gingerol ranged from 0.0 to 1.1 mg/g, and 10-gingerol ranged from 0.0 to 1.40 mg/g [93]. Variations could be due to sourcing, method and period of harvest, storage, and processing methods [93]. The main critical control points to assure safety and quality of ginger used are chemical constituents (actives like gingerols, or potentially toxics like methyleugenol), contaminants (microbiology, pesticides, heavy metals, residual solvents), and adulteration risks. In view of the sensitivity of this raw material, control and qualification procedures appear mandatory: supply chain transparency, traceability, management of material safety, and quality standards are keys to assure consumer safety. Processes have to be in place to approve the suppliers' production sites and the relationship between buyer and supplier is critical to support any adulteration prevention effort.

With regard to toxicity associated with ginger chemical constituents, such as gingerols, cytotoxic or mutagenic in vitro studies already performed are not representative and difficult to extrapolate to humans. Potential toxic effect of ginger have to be studied taking account of the whole plant and its absorption metabolites in humans (glucuronides and sulfates of gingerols, for example), not plant metabolites. Recently, one in vitro study showed that free forms are more cytotoxic compared to the glucuronide conjugates [94].

All the in vivo results do not suggest any major concerns with respect to reproductive and developmental safety of ginger root. At least, no associations were found between the use of ginger and malformations in humans. This finding is reassuring and supports previous findings. Moreover, according to the data, the use of ginger during pregnancy does not increase the risk for any of the following pregnancy outcomes: stillbirth/perinatal death, low birth weight, preterm birth, and low Apgar score [72].

It is interesting to note that one member of the Committee on Herbal Medicinal Products (HMPC) did not agree with HMPC's opinion on *Zingiber officinale* Roscoe rhizome [30,95]. He reported that ginger is used in food without any restrictions. Additionally, there are results of tests on reproductive toxicity and results of clinical trials including pregnant women published which support safe use during pregnancy. Therefore, the restriction for use during pregnancy is not justified. Moreover the results of the clinical trials for pregnancy-induced vomiting are such a quality that well-established use could be established for ginger rhizomes [92].

Finally, a recent consensus [96] was published on a list of benefits and potential harms of ginger use for the management of NVP. The authors suggest that this guideline should be addressed during the clinical consultation for NVP and should help to take a decision to use ginger or not. They reported that even if no conclusive evidence of adverse events of ginger on fetus was shown nowadays, the potential anti-coagulant effect of ginger is still equivocal and have to take account by clinicians before ginger recommendation.

Can we safely give ginger rhizome to decrease nausea and vomiting in women during early pregnancy?

First, medical supervision is mandatory. Ginger recommendation has to be done on a case-by-case basis after evaluation of patient medical history. Then, the quality of the finish product containing ginger and the quality of ginger itself, the quality of its transformation process (powder, extract, oils, etc.), and its relative standardization have to be mastered to assure consumer safety. If all the prerogatives are met, doctors could recommend ginger for NVP in early pregnancy.

At the least, further clinical studies are still needed to highlight the effect of ginger on platelet aggregation, particularly in pregnant women population.

Acknowledgments: The author(s) received no specific funding for this work.

Author Contributions: J.S., P.-Y.M. and S.L. made literature searches. S.L. analyzed the data and all authors discussed them. J.S. & S.L. wrote the manuscript, P.-Y.M. reviewed it.

Abbreviations

T&CM	traditional & complementary medicine
CAM	complementary and alternative medicine
USDA	United States Department of Agriculture
INCA	Étude individuelle nationale des consommations alimentaires
ANSES	Agence nationale de sécurité sanitaire de l'alimentation, de l'environnement et du travail (France)
UK	United Kingdom
EU	European Union
USA	United States of America
RCT	randomized clinical trial
EC	European Commission
EFSA	European Food Safety Authority
NVP	nausea and vomiting of pregnancy
BW	Body Weight
ca.	circa
HMPC	Committee on Herbal Medicinal Products

References

1. Organisation mondiale de la santé (OMS). *Stratégie de L'oms Pour la Médecine Traditionnelle Pour 2014–2023*; Organisation mondiale de la santé: Genève, Suisse, 2013.
2. Parlement Européen et Conseil de l'Europe. Directive 2002/46/ce du Parlement Européen et du

Conseil du 10 Juin 2002 Relative au Rapprochement des Législations des Etats Membres Concernant les Compléments Alimentaires. 2002. Available online: https://www.legifrance.gouv.fr/affichTexte.do?cidTexte=JORFTEXT000000337464&dateTexte=20090923 (accessed on 27 November 2017).

3. European Food Safety Authority (EFSA). Scientific report of EFSA—Compendium of botanicals reported to contain naturally occuring substances of possible concern for human health when used in food and food supplements. *EFSA J.* **2012**, *10*, 2663.
4. Ministère Croate [MINISTARSTVO ZDRAVLJA]. Liste positive vitamines, minéraux, plantes, substances à but physiologiques [pravilnik o tvarima koje se mogu dodavati hrani i koristiti u proizvodnji hrane te tvarima čije je korištenje u hrani zabranjeno ili ograničeno]. *Off. J.* **2013**, *160*, 13.
5. Etat Français. Arrêté du 24 Juin 2014 Etablissant la Liste des Plantes, Autres que les Champignons, Autorisées dans les Compléments Alimentaires et les Conditions de Leur Emploi. 2014. Available online: https://www.legifrance.gouv.fr/affichTexte.do?cidTexte=JORFTEXT000029254516&categorieLien=id (accessed on 27 November 2017).
6. Etat Belge; Etat Français; Etat Italien. Liste Belfrit—Harmonisation de L'emploi des Plantes dans les Compléments Alimentaires au sein D'un Espace Européen: Belgique, France, Italie. 2014. Available online: https://www.economie.gouv.fr/dgccrf/projet-belfrit-cooperation-reussie-au-sein-lunion-europeenne (accessed on 27 November 2017).
7. Etat Hongrois. Az oéti Szakértői Testülete Altal Etrend-Kiegészítőkben Alkalmazásra nem Javasolt Növények [Plantes Pour une Utilisation Dans les Compléments Alimentaires ne sont pas Recommandés par L'oéti Body Expert]. 2013. Available online: https://anzdoc.com/az-oeti-szakerti-testlete-altal-etrend-kiegeszitkben-alkalma.html (accessed on 27 November 2017).
8. Eardley, S.; Bishop, F.L.; Prescott, P.; Cardini, F.; Brinkhaus, B.; Santos-Rey, K.; Vas, J.; von Ammon, K.; Hegyi, G.; Dragan, S.; et al. A systematic literature review of complementary and alternative medicine prevalence in eu. *Forsch. Komplementmed.* **2012**, *19* (Suppl. 2), 18–28. [CrossRef] [PubMed]
9. Agence Nationale de Sécurité Sanitaire Alimentation, de L'alimentation, de L'environnement et du Travail (ANSES). Étude Individuelle Nationale des Consommations Alimentaires 3 (inca 3). 2017. Available online: https://www.anses.fr/fr/content/etude-inca-3-pr%C3%A9sentation (accessed on 29 November 2017).
10. De Ridder, K.; Bel, S.; Brocatus, L.; Lebacq, T.; Ost, C.; Teppers, E. *Enquête de consommation alimentaire 2014-2015*; Numéro de dépôt: D/2016/2505/51 Référence Interne: PHS Report 2016-042; Institut Scientifique de Santé Publique: Bruxelles, Belgique, 2016.
11. O'Brien, O.A.; Lindsay, K.L.; McCarthy, M.; McGloin, A.F.; Kennelly, M.; Scully, H.A.; McAuliffe, F.M. Influences on the food choices and physical activity behaviours of overweight and obese pregnant women: A qualitative study. *Midwifery* **2017**, *47*, 28–35. [CrossRef] [PubMed]
12. Skeie, G.; Braaten, T.; Hjartaker, A.; Lentjes, M.; Amiano, P.; Jakszyn, P.; Pala, V.; Palanca, A.; Niekerk, E.M.; Verhagen, H.; et al. Use of dietary supplements in the european prospective investigation into cancer and nutrition calibration study. *Eur J. Clin. Nutr.* **2009**, *63* (Suppl. 4), S226–S238. [CrossRef] [PubMed]
13. Birdee, G.S.; Kemper, K.J.; Rothman, R.; Gardiner, P. Use of complementary and alternative medicine during pregnancy and the postpartum period: An analysis of the national health interview survey. *J. Womens Health (Larchmt)* **2014**, *23*, 824–829. [CrossRef] [PubMed]
14. Holst, L.; Wright, D.; Haavik, S.; Nordeng, H. Safety and efficacy of herbal remedies in obstetrics–review and clinical implications. *Midwifery* **2011**, *27*, 80–86. [CrossRef] [PubMed]
15. Frawley, J.; Adams, J.; Sibbritt, D.; Steel, A.; Broom, A.; Gallois, C. Prevalence and determinants of complementary and alternative medicine use during pregnancy: Results from a nationally representative sample of australian pregnant women. *Aust. N. Z. J. Obstet. Gynaecol.* **2013**, *53*, 347–352. [CrossRef] [PubMed]
16. Hastings-Tolsma, M.; Vincent, D. Decision-making for use of complementary and alternative therapies by pregnant women and nurse midwives during pregnancy: An exploratory qualitative study. *Int. J. Nurs. Midwifery* **2013**, *5*, 76–89. [CrossRef]
17. Olowokere, A.; Olajide, O. Women's perception of safety and utilization of herbal remedies during pregnancy in a local government area in nigeria. *Clin. Nurs. Stud.* **2013**, *1*. [CrossRef]
18. Kennedy, D.A.; Lupattelli, A.; Koren, G.; Nordeng, H. Safety classification of herbal medicines used in pregnancy in a multinational study. *BMC Complement. Altern. Med.* **2016**, *16*, 102. [CrossRef] [PubMed]
19. Pallivalappila, A.R.; Stewart, D.; Shetty, A.; Pande, B.; Singh, R.; McLay, J.S. Complementary and alternative

medicine use during early pregnancy. *Eur. J. Obstet. Gynecol. Reprod. Biol.* **2014**, *181*, 251–255. [CrossRef] [PubMed]

20. Stewart, D.; Pallivalappila, A.R.; Shetty, A.; Pande, B.; McLay, J.S. Healthcare professional views and experiences of complementary and alternative therapies in obstetric practice in north east scotland: A prospective questionnaire survey. *BJOG* **2014**, *121*, 1015–1019. [CrossRef] [PubMed]
21. Ahmed, M.; Hwang, J.H.; Choi, S.; Han, D. Safety classification of herbal medicines used among pregnant women in asian countries: A systematic review. *BMC Complement. Altern. Med.* **2017**, *17*, 489. [CrossRef] [PubMed]
22. CBI Market Intelligence; The Ministry of Foreign Affairs. CBI Product Factsheet: Dried Ginger in Europe. Available online: www.cbi.eu/market-information (accessed on 3 November 2017).
23. World Health Organization (WHO). *Who Monographs on Selected Medicinal Plants Volume 1*; World Health Organization (WHO): Geneva, Switzerland, 1999.
24. Bradley, P. British Herbal Compendium. In *A Handbook of Scientific Information on Widely Used Plant Drugs*; British Herbal Medicine Association: Bournemouth, UK, 1992; Volume 1.
25. European Scientific Cooperative on Phytotherapy (ESCOP). *Escop Monographs: The Scientific Foundation for Herbal Medicinal Products*, 2nd ed.; European Scientific Cooperative on Phytotherapy: Stuttgart, Germany, 2009; ISBN 9783131294210.
26. European Medicines Agency (EMA); Committee on Herbal Medicinal Products (HMPC). *Community Herbal Monograph on Zingiber Officinale Roscoe, Rhizoma*; European Medicines Agency: London, UK, 2012.
27. Khan, S.; Pandotra, P.; Qazi, A.; Lone, S.; Muzafar, M.; Gupta, A.; Gupta, S. Medicinal and nutritional qualities of zingiber officinale. In *Fruits, Vegetables, and Herbs*; Watson, R.R., Preedy, V.R., Eds.; Academic Press: Oxford, UK, 2016; pp. 525–550.
28. Kemper, K. Ginger (*zingiber officinale*); Longwood Herbal Task Force and the Center for Holistic Pediatric Education and Research. Longwood Herbal Task Force. 1999. Available online: http://www.mcp.edu/herbal/default.htm (accessed on 15 November 2017).
29. Dhanik, J.; Arya, N.; Nand, V. A review on zingiber officinale. *J. Pharmacogn. Phytochem.* **2017**, *6*, 174–184.
30. European Medicines Agency (EMA); Committee on Herbal Medicinal Products (HMPC). *Assessment Report on Zingiber Officinale Roscoe, Rhizome*; European Medicines Agency: London, UK, 2012.
31. Agence Nationale de Sécurité Sanitaire Alimentation, de L'alimentation, de L'environnement et du Travail (ANSES). Ciqual, Table de Composition Nutritionnelle des Aliments. Available online: https://ciqual.anses.fr/#/aliments/11006/gingembre-poudre (accessed on 6 November 2017).
32. Jolad, S.D.; Lantz, R.C.; Solyom, A.M.; Chen, G.J.; Bates, R.B.; Timmermann, B.N. Fresh organically grown ginger (*zingiber officinale*): Composition and effects on lps-induced pge2 production. *Phytochemistry* **2004**, *65*, 1937–1954. [CrossRef] [PubMed]
33. Jolad, S.D.; Lantz, R.C.; Chen, G.J.; Bates, R.B.; Timmermann, B.N. Commercially processed dry ginger (*zingiber officinale*): Composition and effects on lps-stimulated pge2 production. *Phytochemistry* **2005**, *66*, 1614–1635. [CrossRef] [PubMed]
34. Ali, B.H.; Blunden, G.; Tanira, M.O.; Nemmar, A. Some phytochemical, pharmacological and toxicological properties of ginger (*zingiber officinale* roscoe): A review of recent research. *Food Chem. Toxicol.* **2008**, *46*, 409–420. [CrossRef] [PubMed]
35. Sharifi-Rad, M.; Varoni, E.M.; Salehi, B.; Sharifi-Rad, J.; Matthews, K.R.; Ayatollahi, S.A.; Kobarfard, F.; Ibrahim, S.A.; Mnayer, D.; Zakaria, Z.A.; et al. Plants of the genus zingiber as a source of bioactive phytochemicals: From tradition to pharmacy. *Molecules* **2017**, *22*. [CrossRef] [PubMed]
36. Agrahari, P.; Panda, P.; Verma, N.; Khan, W.; Darbari, S. A brief study on zingiber officinale-a review. *J. Drug Discov. Ther.* **2015**, *3*, 20–27.
37. Petersen, I.; McCrea, R.L.; Lupattelli, A.; Nordeng, H. Women's perception of risks of adverse fetal pregnancy outcomes: A large-scale multinational survey. *BMJ Open* **2015**, *5*, e007390. [CrossRef] [PubMed]
38. Plengsuriyakarn, T.; Viyanant, V.; Eursitthichai, V.; Tesana, S.; Chaijaroenkul, W.; Itharat, A.; Na-Bangchang, K. Cytotoxicity, toxicity, and anticancer activity of zingiber officinale roscoe against cholangiocarcinoma. *Asian J. Cancer Prev.* **2012**, *13*, 4597–4606. [CrossRef]
39. Harliansyah; Murad, N.; Ngah, W.; Yusof, A. Antiproliferative, antixoidant and apoptosis effects of zingiber officinale and 6-gingerol on hepg2 cells. *Asian J. Biochem.* **2007**, *6*, 421–426.
40. Unnikrishnan, M.C.; Kuttan, R. Cytotoxicity of extracts of spices to cultured cells. *Nutr. Cancer* **1988**, *11*,

251–257. [CrossRef] [PubMed]

41. Abudayyak, M.; Ozdemir Nath, E.; Ozhan, G. Toxic potentials of ten herbs commonly used for aphrodisiac effect in turkey. *Turk. J. Med. Sci.* **2015**, *45*, 496–506. [CrossRef] [PubMed]
42. Zaeoung, S.; Plubrukarn, A.; Keawpradub, N. Cytotoxic and free radical scavenging activities of zingiberaceous rhizomes. *Songklanakarin J. Sci. Technol.* **2005**, *27*, 799–812.
43. Wei, Q.; Ma, J.; Cai, Y.; Yang, L.; Liu, Z. Cytotoxic and apoptotic activities of diarylheptanoids and gingerol-related compounds from the rhizome of chinese ginger. *J. Ethnopharmacol.* **2005**, *102*, 177–184. [CrossRef] [PubMed]
44. Yang, G.; Zhong, L.; Jiang, L.; Geng, C.; Cao, J.; Sun, X.; Ma, Y. Genotoxic effect of 6-gingerol on human hepatoma g2 cells. *Chem. Biol. Interact.* **2010**, *185*, 12–17. [CrossRef] [PubMed]
45. Kim, J.; Lee, S.; Park, H.; Yang, J.; Shin, T.; Kim, Y.; Baek, N.; Kim, S.; Choi, S.; Kwon, B.; et al. Cytotoxic components from the dried rhizomes of zingiber officinale roscoe. *Arch. Pharm. Res.* **2008**, *31*, 415–418. [CrossRef] [PubMed]
46. Peng, F.; Tao, Q.; Wu, X.; Dou, H.; Spencer, S.; Mang, C.; Xu, L.; Sun, L.; Zhao, Y.; Li, H.; et al. Cytotoxic, cytoprotective and antioxidant effects of isolated phenolic compounds from fresh ginger. *Fitoterapia* **2012**, *83*, 568–585. [CrossRef] [PubMed]
47. Zick, S.M.; Djuric, Z.; Ruffin, M.T.; Litzinger, A.J.; Normolle, D.P.; Alrawi, S.; Feng, M.R.; Brenner, D.E. Pharmacokinetics of 6-gingerol, 8-gingerol, 10-gingerol, and 6-shogaol and conjugate metabolites in healthy human subjects. *Cancer Epidemiol. Biomark. Prev.* **2008**, *17*, 1930–1936. [CrossRef] [PubMed]
48. Yu, Y.; Zick, S.; Li, X.; Zou, P.; Wright, B.; Sun, D. Examination of the pharmacokinetics of active ingredients of ginger in humans. *AAPS J.* **2011**, *13*, 417–426. [CrossRef] [PubMed]
49. Soudamini, K.K.; Unnikrishnan, M.C.; Sukumaran, K.; Kuttan, R. Mutagenicity and anti-mutagenicity of selected spices. *Indian J. Physiol. Pharmacol.* **1995**, *39*, 347–353. [PubMed]
50. Nagabhushan, M.; Amonkar, A.J.; Bhide, S.V. Mutagenicity of gingerol and shogaol and antimutagenicity of zingerone in salmonella/microsome assay. *Cancer Lett.* **1987**, *36*, 221–233. [CrossRef]
51. NIrmala, K.; Prasanna Krishna, T.; Polasa, K. In vivo antimutagenic potential of ginger on formation and excretion of urinary mutagens in rats. *Int. J. Cancer Res.* **2007**, *3*, 134–142.
52. Rong, X.; Peng, G.; Suzuki, T.; Yang, Q.; Yamahara, J.; Li, Y. A 35-day gavage safety assessment of ginger in rats. *Regul. Toxicol. Pharmacol.* **2009**, *54*, 118–123. [CrossRef] [PubMed]
53. Malik, Z.; Sharmaa, P. Attenuation of high-fat diet induced body weight gain, adiposity and biochemical anomalies after chronic administration of ginger (*zingiber officinale*) in wistar rats. *Int. J. Pharmacol.* **2011**, *7*, 801–812. [CrossRef]
54. Anonymous. Zingiberis rhizome. In *Escop Monographs*; Stuttgart, T.P., Ed.; European Scientific Cooperative on Phytotherapy: New York, NY, USA, 2003; pp. 547–553.
55. Weidner, M.; Sigwart, K. Investigation of the teratogenic potential of a zingiber officinale extract in the rat. *Reprod. Toxicol.* **2001**, *15*, 75–80. [CrossRef]
56. Tanabe, M.; Chen, Y.D.; Saito, K.; Kano, Y. Cholesterol biosynthesis inhibitory component from zingiber officinale roscoe. *Chem. Pharm. Bull. (Tokyo)* **1993**, *41*, 710–713. [CrossRef] [PubMed]
57. Jeena, K.; Liju, V.B.; Kuttan, R. A preliminary 13-week oral toxicity study of ginger oil in male and female wistar rats. *Int. J. Toxicol.* **2011**, *30*, 662–670. [CrossRef] [PubMed]
58. Ojewole, J.A. Analgesic, antiinflammatory and hypoglycaemic effects of ethanol extract of zingiber officinale (roscoe) rhizomes (zingiberaceae) in mice and rats. *Phytother. Res.* **2006**, *20*, 764–772. [CrossRef] [PubMed]
59. Suekawa, M.; Ishige, A.; Yuasa, K.; Sudo, K.; Aburada, M.; Hosoya, E. Pharmacological studies on ginger. I. Pharmacological actions of pungent constitutents, (6)-gingerol and (6)-shogaol. *J. Pharmacobiodyn.* **1984**, *7*, 836–848. [CrossRef] [PubMed]
60. Wu, H.; Ye, D.; Bai, Y.; Zhao, Y. Effect of dry ginger and roasted ginger on experimental gastric ulcers in rats. *China J. Chin. Mater. Medica* **1990**, *15*, 278–280, 317–318.
61. Wilkinson, J.M. Effect of ginger tea on the fetal development of sprague-dawley rats. *Reprod. Toxicol.* **2000**, *14*, 507–512. [CrossRef]
62. Sukandar, E.; Qowiyah, A.; Purnamasari, R. Teratogenicity study of combination of ginger rhizome extract and noni fruit extract in wistar rat. *Indones. J. Pharm.* **2009**, *20*, 48–54.
63. Fischer-Rasmussen, W.; Kjaer, S.K.; Dahl, C.; Asping, U. Ginger treatment of hyperemesis gravidarum. *Eur. J. Obstet. Gynecol. Reprod. Biol.* **1991** *38*, 19–24. [CrossRef]

64. Chrubasik, S.; Pittler, M.H.; Roufogalis, B.D. Zingiberis rhizoma: A comprehensive review on the ginger effect and efficacy profiles. *Phytomedicine* **2005**, *12*, 684–701. [CrossRef] [PubMed]
65. Betz, O.; Kranke, P.; Geldner, G.; Wulf, H.; Eberhart, L.H. Is ginger a clinically relevant antiemetic? A systematic review of randomized controlled trials. *Res. Complement. Nat. Class. Med.* **2005**, *12*, 14–23. [CrossRef] [PubMed]
66. Haniadka, R.; Saldanha, E.; Sunita, V.; Palatty, P.L.; Fayad, R.; Baliga, M.S. A review of the gastroprotective effects of ginger (*zingiber officinale* roscoe). *Food Funct.* **2013**, *4*, 845–855. [CrossRef] [PubMed]
67. Viljoen, E.; Visser, J.; Koen, N.; Musekiwa, A. A systematic review and meta-analysis of the effect and safety of ginger in the treatment of pregnancy-associated nausea and vomiting. *Nutr. J.* **2014**, *13*, 20. [CrossRef] [PubMed]
68. Marx, W.; McKavanagh, D.; McCarthy, A.L.; Bird, R.; Ried, K.; Chan, A.; Isenring, L. The effect of ginger (*zingiber officinale*) on platelet aggregation: A systematic literature review. *PLoS ONE* **2015**, *10*, e0141119.
69. Wang, Y.; Yu, H.; Zhang, X.; Feng, Q.; Guo, X.; Li, S.; Li, R.; Chu, D.; Ma, Y. Evaluation of daily ginger consumption for the prevention of chronic diseases in adults: A cross-sectional study. *Nutrition* **2017**, *36*, 79–84. [CrossRef] [PubMed]
70. Sharifzadeh, F.; Kashanian, M.; Koohpayehzadeh, J.; Rezaian, F.; Sheikhansari, N.; Eshraghi, N. A comparison between the effects of ginger, pyridoxine (vitamin b6) and placebo for the treatment of the first trimester nausea and vomiting of pregnancy (nvp). *J. Matern. Fetal Neonatal Med.* **2017**, 1–6. [CrossRef] [PubMed]
71. Portnoi, G.; Chng, L.A.; Karimi-Tabesh, L.; Koren, G.; Tan, M.P.; Einarson, A. Prospective comparative study of the safety and effectiveness of ginger for the treatment of nausea and vomiting in pregnancy. *Am. J. Obstet. Gynecol.* **2003**, *189*, 1374–1377. [CrossRef]
72. Heitmann, K.; Nordeng, H.; Holst, L. Safety of ginger use in pregnancy: Results from a large population-based cohort study. *Eur J. Clin. Pharmacol.* **2013**, *69*, 269–277. [CrossRef] [PubMed]
73. Choi, J.S.; Han, J.Y.; Ahn, H.K.; Lee, S.W.; Koong, M.K.; Velazquez-Armenta, E.Y.; Nava-Ocampo, A.A. Assessment of fetal and neonatal outcomes in the offspring of women who had been treated with dried ginger (*zingiberis rhizoma* siccus) for a variety of illnesses during pregnancy. *J. Obstet. Gynaecol.* **2015**, *35*, 125–130. [CrossRef] [PubMed]
74. Paritakul, P.; Ruangrongmorakot, K.; Laosooksathit, W.; Suksamarnwong, M.; Puapornpong, P. The effect of ginger on breast milk volume in the early postpartum period: A randomized, double-blind controlled trial. *Breastfeed. Med.* **2016**, *11*, 361–365. [CrossRef] [PubMed]
75. Pongrojpaw, D.; Somprasit, C.; Chanthasenanont, A. A randomized comparison of ginger and dimenhydrinate in the treatment of nausea and vomiting in pregnancy. *J. Med. Assoc. Thai* **2007**, *90*, 1703–1709. [PubMed]
76. Saberi, F.; Sadat, Z.; Abedzadeh-Kalahroudi, M.; Taebi, M. Acupressure and ginger to relieve nausea and vomiting in pregnancy: A randomized study. *Iran. Red Crescent Med. J.* **2013**, *15*, 854–861. [CrossRef] [PubMed]
77. Saberi, F.; Sadat, Z.; Abedzadeh-Kalahroudi, M.; Taebi, M. Effect of ginger on relieving nausea and vomiting in pregnancy: A randomized, placebo-controlled trial. *Nurs. Midwifery Stud.* **2014**, *3*, e11841. [CrossRef] [PubMed]
78. Keating, A.; Chez, R.A. Ginger syrup as an antiemetic in early pregnancy. *Altern. Ther. Health Med.* **2002**, *8*, 89–91. [PubMed]
79. Smith, C.; Crowther, C.; Willson, K.; Hotham, N.; McMillian, V. A randomized controlled trial of ginger to treat nausea and vomiting in pregnancy. *Obstet. Gynecol.* **2004**, *103*, 639–645. [CrossRef] [PubMed]
80. Vutyavanich, T.; Kraisarin, T.; Ruangsri, R. Ginger for nausea and vomiting in pregnancy: Randomized, double-masked, placebo-controlled trial. *Obstet. Gynecol.* **2001**, *97*, 577–582. [CrossRef] [PubMed]
81. Chittumma, P.; Kaewkiattikun, K.; Wiriyasiriwach, B. Comparison of the effectiveness of ginger and vitamin b6 for treatment of nausea and vomiting in early pregnancy: A randomized double-blind controlled trial. *J. Med. Assoc. Thai.* **2007**, *90*, 15–20. [PubMed]
82. Ozgoli, G.; Goli, M.; Simbar, M. Effects of ginger capsules on pregnancy, nausea, and vomiting. *J. Altern. Complement. Med.* **2009**, *15*, 243–246. [CrossRef] [PubMed]
83. Ensiyeh, J.; Sakineh, M.A. Comparing ginger and vitamin b6 for the treatment of nausea and vomiting in pregnancy: A randomised controlled trial. *Midwifery* **2009**, *25*, 649–653. [CrossRef] [PubMed]
84. Mohammadbeigi, R.; Shahgeibi, S.; Soufizadeh, N.; Rezaiie, M.; Farhadifar, F. Comparing the effects of ginger

and metoclopramide on the treatment of pregnancy nausea. *Pak. J. Biol. Sci.* **2011**, *14*, 817–820. [PubMed]
85. Willetts, K.E.; Ekangaki, A.; Eden, J.A. Effect of a ginger extract on pregnancy-induced nausea: A randomised controlled trial. *Aust. N. Z. J. Obstet. Gynaecol.* **2003**, *43*, 139–144. [CrossRef] [PubMed]
86. Basirat, Z.; Moghadamnia, A.; Kashifard, M.; Sharifi-Ravazi, A. The effect of ginger biscuit on nausea and vomiting in early pregnancy. *Acta Medica Iran.* **2009**, *47*, 51–56.
87. Boltman-Binkowski, H. A systematic review: Are herbal and homeopathic remedies used during pregnancy safe? *Curationis* **2016**, *39*, 1514. [CrossRef] [PubMed]
88. McLay, J.S.; Izzati, N.; Pallivalapila, A.R.; Shetty, A.; Pande, B.; Rore, C.; Al Hail, M.; Stewart, D. Pregnancy, prescription medicines and the potential risk of herb-drug interactions: A cross-sectional survey. *BMC Complement. Altern. Med.* **2017**, *17*, 543. [CrossRef] [PubMed]
89. Lete, I.; Allue, J. The effectiveness of ginger in the prevention of nausea and vomiting during pregnancy and chemotherapy. *Integr. Med. Insights* **2016**, *11*, 11–17. [CrossRef] [PubMed]
90. Ding, M.; Leach, M.; Bradley, H. The effectiveness and safety of ginger for pregnancy-induced nausea and vomiting: A systematic review. *Women Birth* **2013**, *26*, e26–e30. [CrossRef] [PubMed]
91. Thomson, M.; Corbin, R.; Leung, L. Effects of ginger for nausea and vomiting in early pregnancy: A meta-analysis. *J. Am. Board Fam. Med.* **2014**, *27*, 115–122. [CrossRef] [PubMed]
92. Campbell, K.; Rowe, H.; Azzam, H.; Lane, C.A. The management of nausea and vomiting of pregnancy. *J. Obstet. Gynaecol. Can.* **2016**, *38*, 1127–1137. [CrossRef] [PubMed]
93. Schwertner, H.A.; Rios, D.C.; Pascoe, J.E. Variation in concentration and labeling of ginger root 39 dietary supplements. *Obstet. Gynecol.* **2006**, *107*, 1337–1343. [CrossRef] [PubMed]
94. Mukkavilli, R.; Yang, C.; Tanwar, R.S.; Saxena, R.; Gundala, S.R.; Zhang, Y.; Ghareeb, A.; Floyd, S.D.; Vangala, S.; Kuo, W.W.; et al. Pharmacokinetic-pharmacodynamic correlations in the development of ginger extract as an anticancer agent. *Sci. Rep.* **2018**, *8*, 3056. [CrossRef] [PubMed]
95. European Medicines Agency (EMA); Committee on herbal medicinal products (HMPC). *Opinion of the HPMC on a Community Herbal Monograph on Zingiber Officinale Roscoe, Rhizome*; EMA/HPMC/216956/2012; European Medicines Agency (EMA): London, UK, 2012.
96. Shawahna, R.; Taha, A. Which potential harms and benefits of using ginger in the management of nausea and vomiting of pregnancy should be addressed? A consensual study among pregnant women and gynecologists. *BMC Complement. Altern. Med.* **2017**, *17*, 204. [CrossRef] [PubMed]

3

Enrichment of Biscuits with Matcha Green Tea Powder: Its Impact on Consumer Acceptability and Acute Metabolic Response

Benjapor Phongnarisorn [1,2], Caroline Orfila [1,*], Melvin Holmes [1] and Lisa J. Marshall [1,*]

[1] School of Food Science and Nutrition, University of Leeds, Leeds LS2 9JT, UK; nbjp459@hotmail.com (B.P.); prcmjh@leeds.ac.uk (M.H.)

[2] Faculty of Agricultural Technology, Phuket Rajabhat University, Phuket 83000, Thailand

[*] Correspondence: c.orfila@leeds.ac.uk (C.O.); L.J.Marshall@leeds.ac.uk (L.J.M.)

Abstract: Matcha green tea powder (MGTP) is made with finely ground green tea leaves that are rich in phytochemicals, most particularly catechins. Shortbread biscuits were enriched with MGTP and evaluated for consumer acceptability and potential functional health properties. Baking decreased the content of total catechins by 19% compared to dough, although epimerization increased the amount of (+)-gallocatechin gallate at the expense of other catechins such as (−)-epigallocatechin gallate. Consumer acceptability tests using a 9-point hedonic scale showed that consumers preferred enriched biscuits with low content of MGTP (2 g of MGTP 100 g^{-1} of flour), and an increase of sugar content did not significantly improve the acceptability of MGTP-enriched biscuits. Overall, enrichment of biscuits with MGTP did not significantly affect the postprandial glucose or triglyceride response (area under curve) compared to non-enriched biscuits consumed with water or MGTP drink. Enriching biscuits with Matcha green tea is acceptable to consumers, but may not bring significant postprandial effects.

Keywords: Matcha green tea powder; catechin stability; consumer acceptability; acute metabolic response; functional food

---

1. Introduction

Catechins are the main polyphenols found in green tea. As shown in Figure 1, catechins have a common carbon backbone with variations in the substitutes at the C-3 and C-5′ positions [1]. The four major catechins found in green tea are (−)-epigallocatechin (EGC), (−)-epicatechin (EC), (−)-epigallocatechin gallate (EGCG), and (−)-epicatechin gallate (ECG). Their trans epimer forms, namely (+)-catechin, (+)-gallocatechin gallate (GCG), (+)-gallocatechin (GC), and (+)-catechin gallate (CG), are found in minor amounts. The epimerization from cis to trans is reversible and can occur when cis catechins are exposed to high temperatures [2]. EGCG is the most abundant catechin in green tea leaves and contributes to 50% of total catechins in tea leaves. Hence, it is been used as a quality indicator in green tea products [3]. It is also found at low levels in a range of foods including apples, red berries, nuts, and legumes.

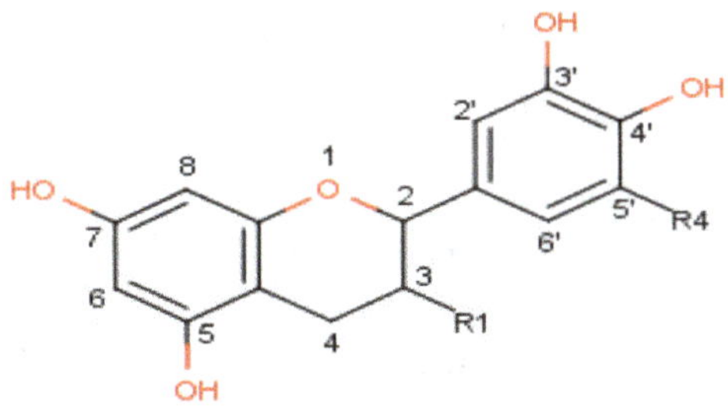

	R1	R4
Catechin	OH	H
Epicatechin (EC)	OH	H
Epigallocatechin (EGC)	OH	OH
Epicatechin gallate (ECG)	Gallate	H
Epigallocatechin gallate (EGCG)	Gallate	OH

Figure 1. Structure of the main catechins found in green tea.

Consumer research has suggested that even though green tea is unfamiliar to most non-Asian consumers, their desire to drink green tea is enhanced due to its perceived health benefits [4,5]. Moreover, there are also the demands for convenience products (i.e., biscuits) with value-added components [6,7]. Incorporating green tea powder into bakery products may mask the bitterness or astringency of green tea perceived by consumers. A few studies have incorporated green tea into bakery products and have shown effects on the physicochemical, colour, textural, and shelf life properties [8–10]. Studies found good sensory acceptability of cakes enriched with up to 20% green tea substituting wheat flour [9]. To date, there have been no reports on the potential physiological effects of green tea-enriched food products.

The catechins found in green tea have been shown to have potential roles in preventing cancer development, diabetes, and cardiovascular diseases [11,12]. Zhong et al. [13] found a 25% decrease in carbohydrate absorption after a consumption of green tea extract containing 300 mg of EGCG and 100 mg of ECG with a carbohydrate meal, suggesting that green tea may reduce the amount of glucose absorbed into the bloodstream, which in turn may lower the risk of developing diabetes [12,13]. Moreover, a review by Koo and Noh [14] suggested that green tea reduces the absorption of dietary fat by interfering with the processes of lipid digestion in the intestine. Studies using animal models have shown that green tea compounds can slow down lipid absorption by inhibiting the activity of pancreatic lipase [15,16]. Unno et al. [16] showed that 224 mg of green tea catechins consumed as tea infusion after meal consumption can lower the concentration of lipids in the blood by 15% and therefore may lower the risk of developing cardiovascular diseases. Studies so far have used green tea in the form of pure extracts or tea infusions to study the potential health effects, but none have used it as part of a functional food.

The aims of this study were to (1) investigate the effect of baking on the stability of catechins; (2) evaluate the sensorial acceptability of shortbread biscuits enriched with Matcha green tea powder (MGTP) and assess the effect of sugar addition on acceptability; and (3) investigate the effect of MGTP on the postprandial glucose and triglyceride response in human volunteers. We discuss the potential of MGTP-enriched biscuits as functional foods.

2. Materials and Methods

2.1. Materials

Matcha factory® Matcha green tea powder (13.2% of total phenolic content, 10% total catechin) was purchased from Chah Ltd. (Solihull, UK). Tesco® plain flour, Tate & Lyle® caster sugar, and Anchor® unsalted butter were purchased from Tesco supermarket (Leeds, UK).

HPLC (High Performance Liquid Chromatography)-grade acetonitrile and ethanol were purchased from Fisher Scientific Co. Ltd. (Leicestershire, UK). HPLC-grade methanol, (−)-epicatechin (EC), and caffeine were purchased from Sigma Aldrich Co. Ltd. (St. Louis, MI, USA). (−)-Epicatechin gallate (ECG), (−)-epigallocatechin (EGC), and (−)-epigallocatechin gallate (EGCG) were obtained from Cambridge Bioscience Ltd. (Cambridge, UK). (+)-Gallocatechin gallate (GCG) was purchased from Insight

Biotechnology Co. Ltd. (Middlesex, UK). All water refers to deionized Millipore water, Millipore Ltd. (Hertfordshire, UK).

2.2. Preparation of Shortbread Incorporated with MGTP

The dough was prepared by beating butter (83.3 g) and sugar (at three different levels, 25, 30, or 35 g 100 g^{-1} of flour) together with a mixer (KM336 Chef Classic, Kenwood Ltd., Havant, UK) for 5 min at speed 4 (180 rpm), and then flour (100 g) and MGTP were added (at the level of 2, 4, or 6 g 100 g^{-1} of flour), followed by mixing for 5 min at minimum speed (50 rpm). The dough was wrapped in clingfilm and rested for 1 h at 4 °C. The dough was rolled to 0.4 mm thickness, and then the biscuits were cut into a circle shape (4.8 cm diameter) and rested for 10 min before being placed in a conventional oven (BC190.2TCSS, Baumatic Ltd., Merthyr Tydfil, UK) at 180 °C for 15 min. After baking, the biscuits were left to cool down at room temperature.

The weight of biscuits was measured before and after baking to calculate weight loss during baking. Samples of each biscuit were prepared for sensory evaluation. For HPLC analysis, the dough and shortbread biscuit samples (made with 25 g sugar at the three levels of 2, 4, or 6 g MGTP 100 g^{-1} of flour) were ground, kept overnight in a freezer (−20 °C), and then freeze-dried (Christ Alpha 1-4 LD, SciQuip Ltd., Shropshire, UK) and packed into vacuum-sealed bags until HPLC analysis.

2.3. Defatting of Samples and Extraction of Catechins

Freeze-dried sample was weighed (1 g), mixed with 30 mL of hexane, and placed in a heat circulating water bath (Grant Instruments, Cambridge, UK) at 70 °C for 20 min. After cooling down, samples were centrifuged at 3000 rpm for 10 min. The hexane fraction was decanted. The samples were left in the fume cupboard with the light off for 2–3 h to evaporate the hexane from the samples. Defatted samples were extracted by adding 25 mL of 70% methanol with 0.3% formic acid and incubated in a water bath at 70 °C for 5 min to equilibrate to the temperature and another 45 min to extract. After cooling down, the tubes were centrifuged at 3000 rpm for 10 min and the supernatant was collected. The extraction was repeated, the supernatant was pooled together, and its volume was made to 50 mL. The samples were filtered through a 0.2 μm PTFE (Polytetrafluoroethylene) syringe filter and put in amber vials for further HPLC analysis.

2.4. HPLC Analysis of Catechins in Dough and Biscuit Samples

A method for HPLC analysis was adapted from Wang and Zhou [17]. The separation was performed on a Phenomenex C18 reverse-phase column (5 μm, 250 × 4.6 mm) (Phenomenex, Cheshire, UK) with a conventional HPLC coupled with a UV-Vis detector (SPD-20A, Shimadzu Corporation, Kyoto, Japan). A binary gradient of water with 0.1% formic acid (eluent A) and acetonitrile with 0.1% formic acid (eluent B) was used to run on the system at a flow rate of 0.5 mL·min^{-1}. The gradient started at 10% B, remained at 10% for 5 min, and increased to 15% over 9 min, then climbed to 60% over 23 min, then to 95% over 3 min, and remained at 95% for 2 min to wash the column before returning to 10% over 2 min and re-equilibrating over 6 min. The total length of the method was 45 min. The column temperature was set at 25 °C. Catechins and caffeine were detected at 275 nm. Identification of each catechin was performed by comparing the retention time and spectrum with the standard. Standard curves for quantification were prepared with standard compounds dissolved in extracting solvent (70% methanol with 0.3% formic acid) at concentrations between 2.5–100 μg·mL^{-1}. The standards were caffeine, EC, EGCG, ECG, EGC and GCG.

2.5. Sensory and Acceptability Studies

Ethical approval for the sensory evaluation study was granted by the Mathematics, Physical Sciences, and Engineering Ethical Committee at the University of Leeds (MEEC 13-026). Sensory evaluation of biscuits was conducted by human panelists, who scored the biscuits using a 9-point hedonic scale. The attributes tested were overall acceptability, appearance, aroma, colour, texture,

bitterness, and sweetness. All sensory evaluation sessions were carried out in separate booths equipped with a Compusense 5.6 sensory software (Compusense Inc., Guelph, ON, Canada), in which responses were recorded directly by the participants.

The tests evaluated 9 shortbread formulations with 3 levels of MGTP and 3 levels of sugar. Samples were assigned with 3-digit codes, and the software randomised their serving orders. Plain water was provided to rinse the mouth between samples. The evaluations were repeated in two sessions with same participants. Fifty-four participants completed the first session, and 46 participants completed the second session.

2.6. Human Intervention Study for Study of Metabolic Response

Ethical approval for this part of the study was granted by the Mathematics, Physical Sciences, and Engineering Ethical Committee at the University of Leeds (MEEC 14-040). The study was designed according to the FAO (Food and Agriculture Organization) protocol [18]. Healthy adults (n = 4 were Asian, n = 3 were South American, n = 2 were European, n = 1 was African) were recruited to the study after they met the eligibility criteria according to a health screening questionnaire (18–60 years; not allergic to any food; not pregnant or lactating; not diagnosed with chronic diseases such as diabetes, cancer, cardiovascular or digestive diseases; not taking any medication that affect the glucose and triglyceride response). The sample size was decided based on harmonized GI methodology [19] who established that 10 individuals is probably enough in most cases to obtain a significant difference between. The design of the study was a cross-over randomised control study without blinding with a one week washout period between sessions. Each participant was asked to attend following overnight fasting overnight for a least 10 h but was not asked to modify their usual diet.

2.6.1. Reference and Test Meals

Three meals (one reference and two test meals) were tested by all panelists in this study in a random order. The reference meal consisted of 100 g of plain shortbread biscuits consumed with 300 mL of warm water. The two test meals consisted of either 100 g of MGTP-enriched biscuits consumed with 300 mL of warm water or 100 g of plain shortbread biscuits consumed with 200 mL of MGTP consumed as a tea drink followed by 100 mL of warm water (total liquid volume of 300 mL). The test meals contained 54–55g of available carbohydrate, of which 16.0 g was sugar and 36 g was fat. The MGTP-enriched biscuit contained 6 g of MGTP (catechin dose of 233 mg). Plain biscuits were prepared according to exactly the same procedure but without addition of MGTP. Once the biscuits were baked and cooled down, 100 g of biscuits were weighed and packed in vacuum-seal plastic bags and used within 1 month for the human study. Matcha green tea drink was made before serving by mixing MGTP (3 g, catechin dose of 257 mg) with 200 mL of warm water. All meals contained around 54–55 g of available carbohydrate. The composition information for the biscuits tested can be found as Supplementary Material (Table S1).

2.6.2. Glucose and Triglyceride Measurement

Capillary blood glucose and triglyceride concentrations were measured from a finger-prick blood sample. A finger was sanitized with an antiseptic wipe before perforation of the skin with a Safe T pro Accu chek disposable lancet. The blood droplet was loaded onto a glucose test strip (Accu-Chek compact 17-drum test strips, Roche diagnostic Ltd., West Sussex, UK) and inserted into a glucometer (Accu-Chek® Aviva blood glucose meter, Roche diagnostic Ltd., West Sussex, UK), which returned the blood glucose concentration in $mmol{\cdot}L^{-1}$. Another blood droplet was collected by a sterile disposable pipette (15 μL Safetec Pipettes, BHR Pharmaceutical Ltd., Nuneaton, UK). The extracted blood was transferred to a triglyceride test strip (CardioChek® PTS Panel triglyceride test strips, BHR Pharmaceutical Ltd., Nuneaton, UK), which was inserted into a Cardiochek Professional analyser (CardioChek® PA Blood Analyser, BHR Pharmaceutical Ltd., Nuneaton, UK), to measure the blood triglyceride concentration in $mmol{\cdot}L^{-1}$.

Overnight fasted blood glucose and blood triglycerides were measured at baseline; then, the subject was provided the meal to be consumed within a period of 10 min. Eight blood glucose measurements were taken at 15, 30, 45, 60, 90, 120, 150 and 180 min after the start of the food consumption. Three blood triglyceride measurements were taken at 60, 120 and 180 min after the start of the food consumption.

2.6.3. iAUC Calculation

The incremental area under the curve (iAUC) of the glucose and triglyceride response was calculated according to FAO [18], using the trapezoidal rule in which all the areas of glucose response collected during the three hours period are added together, by ignoring the area beneath the baseline.

2.7. Data Analysis

Results were analysed statistically to determine mean values, standard deviations (STDs), and standard error of means (SEMs) of quantified masses of compounds obtained from HPLC in duplicate runs. The total catechins content was presented by the sum of the amounts of individual catechins (EGCG, ECG, EGC, GCG and EC). Mann-Whitney U Test was performed to determine the difference between before and after baking of catechin content.

For acceptability sensory results, one factor analysis of variance (ANOVA) with a significant level of $p < 0.05$ and Tukey's-b post-hoc test was performed to determine the difference in scores between the different biscuit formulations. Two factor ANOVA with a significant level of $p < 0.05$ and Tukey's-b post-hoc test was conducted to determine the difference of the acceptability between MGTP and sugar incorporated and their interaction effects. The response surface methodology was conducted using R program (R version 3.2.5, with R Commander package) to plot response surface and contour plot that explained the relationship between the independent variable: MGTP (X_1) and sugar (X_2); response variables; and testing acceptability attributes (Y): overall appearance, aroma, colour, texture, bitterness, and sweetness of the biscuit samples.

For the human metabolic study, one-way ANOVA and Tukey's-b post hoc test was conducted to investigate the difference between test meals that affects the glucose response and triglyceride response.
Statistical analyses were carried out using the SPSS 22.0 statistical software package (SPSS Inc., Chicago, IL, USA).

3. Results and Discussion

3.1. Stability of Catechins and Caffeine During the Baking Process

Biscuits with three different levels of MGTP were prepared (see Figure S1). Catechins and caffeine content in dough and biscuits were measured by HPLC-DAD (diode-array detector) (Figure 2, for chromatograms see Figure S2). The results indicate a significant loss of most catechins, except GCG, during the baking process, with a maximum loss of 19% in total catechins (Table 1). EGC presented the highest losses of 31% in biscuits enriched with the highest level of MGTP (6 g 100 g^{-1} of flour). However, there was an increase in GCG of up to 40% in the same biscuits, indicating that epimerization of EGC to GCG may have occurred during the baking process. Caffeine content also decreased during the baking process by up to 24%. The levels of total catechins in the highly enriched biscuits (6 g MGTP 100 g^{-1} of flour) were approximately 20–23 mg per one biscuit, which is around 9% of the amount present in a typical green tea infusion (257 mg 200 mL^{-1} cup).

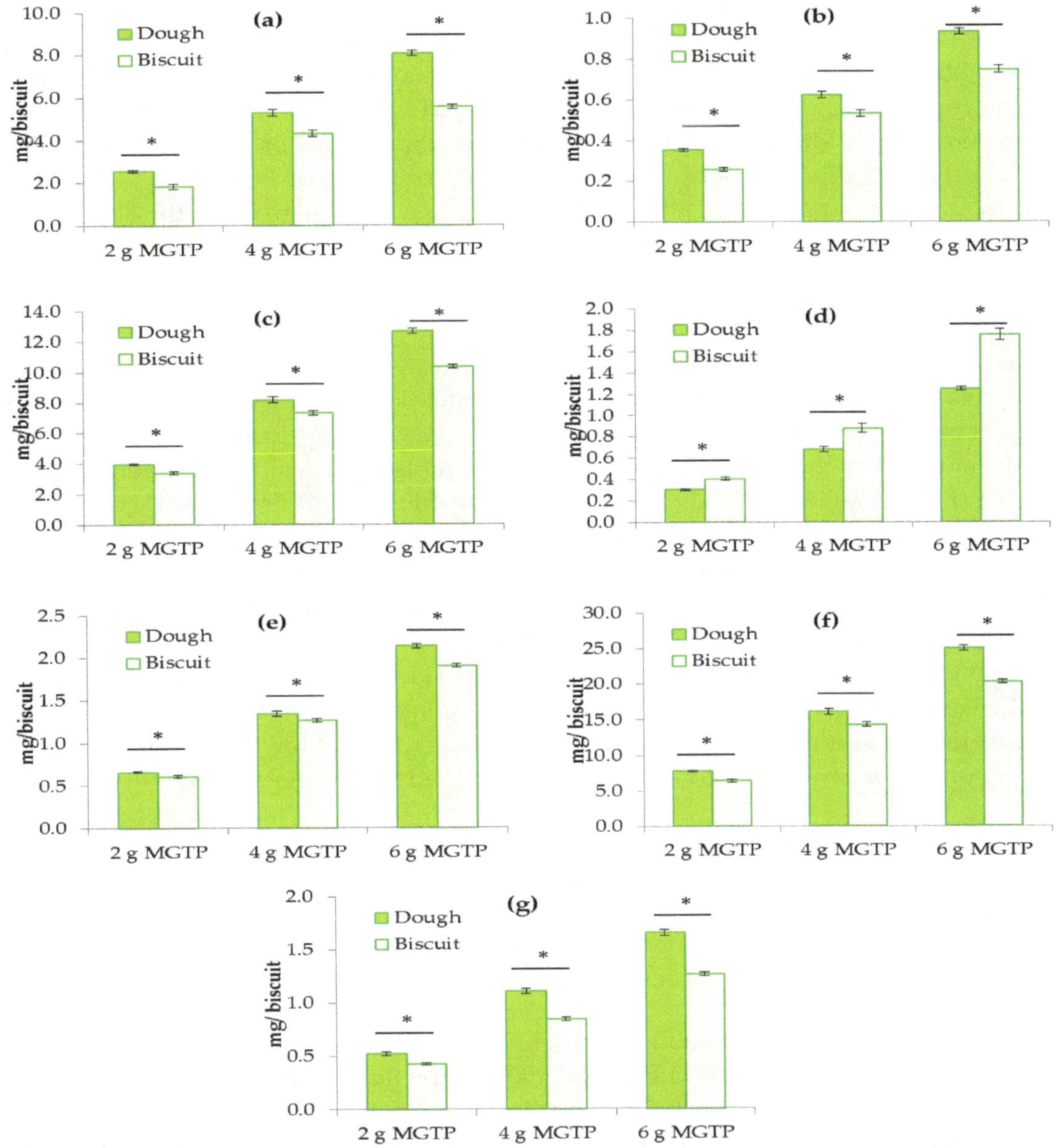

Figure 2. Amount of catechins in dough and shortbread enriched with 3 levels of MGTP (2, 4, 6 g 100 g^{-1} of flour): (**a**) EGC; (**b**) EC; (**c**) EGCG; (**d**) GCG; (**e**) ECG; (**f**) total catechins and (**g**) caffeine. Results are expressed as mg per biscuit. * indicates a significant difference ($p < 0.05$) before and after baking. The error bars represent the SEM (standard error of the mean) ($n = 12$ biscuits).

Table 1. Percentage retention of catechins and caffeine in MGTP (Matcha green tea powder)-enriched shortbread biscuits after baking as a proportion of initial content in the dough.

Compound	2 g MGTP (%)	4 g MGTP (%)	6 g MGTP (%)
(−)-epigallocatechin (EGC)	70.9 ± 9.5	81.5 ± 2.5	68.9 ± 1.6
(−)-epicatechin (EC)	72.6 ± 4.5	85.7 ± 3.5	80.2 ± 1.7
(−)-epigallocatechin gallate (EGCG)	84.9 ± 4.0	89.7 ± 2.1	81.8 ± 1.4
(+)-gallocatechin gallate (GCG)	133.0 ± 7.3	128.6 ± 11.0	140.3 ± 8.6
(−)-epicatechin gallate (ECG)	92.2 ± 3.9	94.3 ± 2.4	89.1 ± 1.2
Total catechins	82.4 ± 5.7	88.9 ± 2.5	81.1 ± 1.4
Caffeine	81.9 ± 5.0	76.3 ± 3.4	76.4 ± 1.1

The results are in agreement with the study by Wang and Zhou that showed an average retention of 83% for EGCG and 91% for ECG in green tea-enriched bread [17]. Epimerization of EGCG to GCG has been observed in bread [20]. Sharma and Zhou showed much higher losses of catechins during baking (up to 98%) [21]. The degradation followed first order kinetic parameters and could largely be prevented by acidification of the dough. Core temperatures of 120–130 °C achieved during baking would provide sufficient energy for epimerization of EGCG or EGC to GCG [21]. EGC is less stable than other catechins because of its radical scavenging hydroxyl group at the 5′ position of the B ring [22,23]. Therefore, this is could explain the increase in GCG in the MGTP-enriched biscuits.

3.2. Sensory and Overall Acceptability of Biscuits

The response surface for overall acceptability (Figure 3a) shows that biscuits with low MGTP and low sugar content received the highest acceptability. The increase in sugar in biscuit formulation did not significantly affect the acceptability of the enriched biscuits. A similar response was observed for appearance (Figure 3b), with darker green and brown colour receiving lower acceptability scores. As shown in Figure 3c, the highest response of aroma acceptability was achieved around a sugar level of 30 g 100 g^{-1} of flour. The surface response method suggested the stationary point at 1.84 g of MGTP and 27.73 g of sugar 100 g^{-1} of flour to obtain the highest response. Heat treatment can cause undesirable aromas of green tea [24]. The trained panelist detected more undesirable (described as wet wood smell) aroma of heat processed green tea at 121 °C for 1 min compared to unprocessed green tea [24]. Therefore, the aroma of shortbread biscuits containing MGTP may be affected by baking temperature at 180 °C, as it will likely cause an undesirable aroma. However, Ahmad et al. [8] found that increasing green tea powder in cookies (1–4%) increased the aroma acceptability.

As shown in Figure 3d, the highest response of colour acceptability was for the biscuits with a sugar level of 30 g 100 g^{-1} of flour and low MGTP. The colour is thought to come from chlorophyll pigments, which can degrade at high temperatures. Kim et al. [25] suggested that green tea solution became less green and deeper yellow after heating at 120 °C for 4 min. Therefore, masking the colour of biscuits by adding fresh green colouring may increase the acceptability of biscuits.

Figure 4a shows that high sugar and low content of MGTP increased the texture acceptability with an optimum score for biscuits with 30 g sugar 100 g^{-1} of flour and low MGTP. Sugar increases the crunchiness of biscuits, while MGTP increases the hardness of biscuits (data is shown in supplementary doc, Figure S3). According to Figure 4b, the bitterness acceptability was significantly affected by the level of MGTP incorporated into the biscuit ($p < 0.001$). The bitterness acceptability received a high response with biscuits that had a low level of MGTP, and sugar did not improve the acceptability. Bitterness can significantly suppress the sense of sweetness and vice versa [26]. It was found that bitterness can be perceived at a much lower concentration than sweetness at a ratio of 1:31 magnitude [27]. Finally, as shown in Figure 4c, sweetness acceptability was significantly affected by the level of MGTP in the biscuit ($p < 0.05$), with higher acceptability for sugar content of 30 g 100 g^{-1} of flour for all MGTP levels tested. This indicates that sweetness does improve the acceptability of biscuits, particularly those with high MGTP. According to the sensory trial, appearance, color, and bitterness were the most important determinants of overall acceptability.

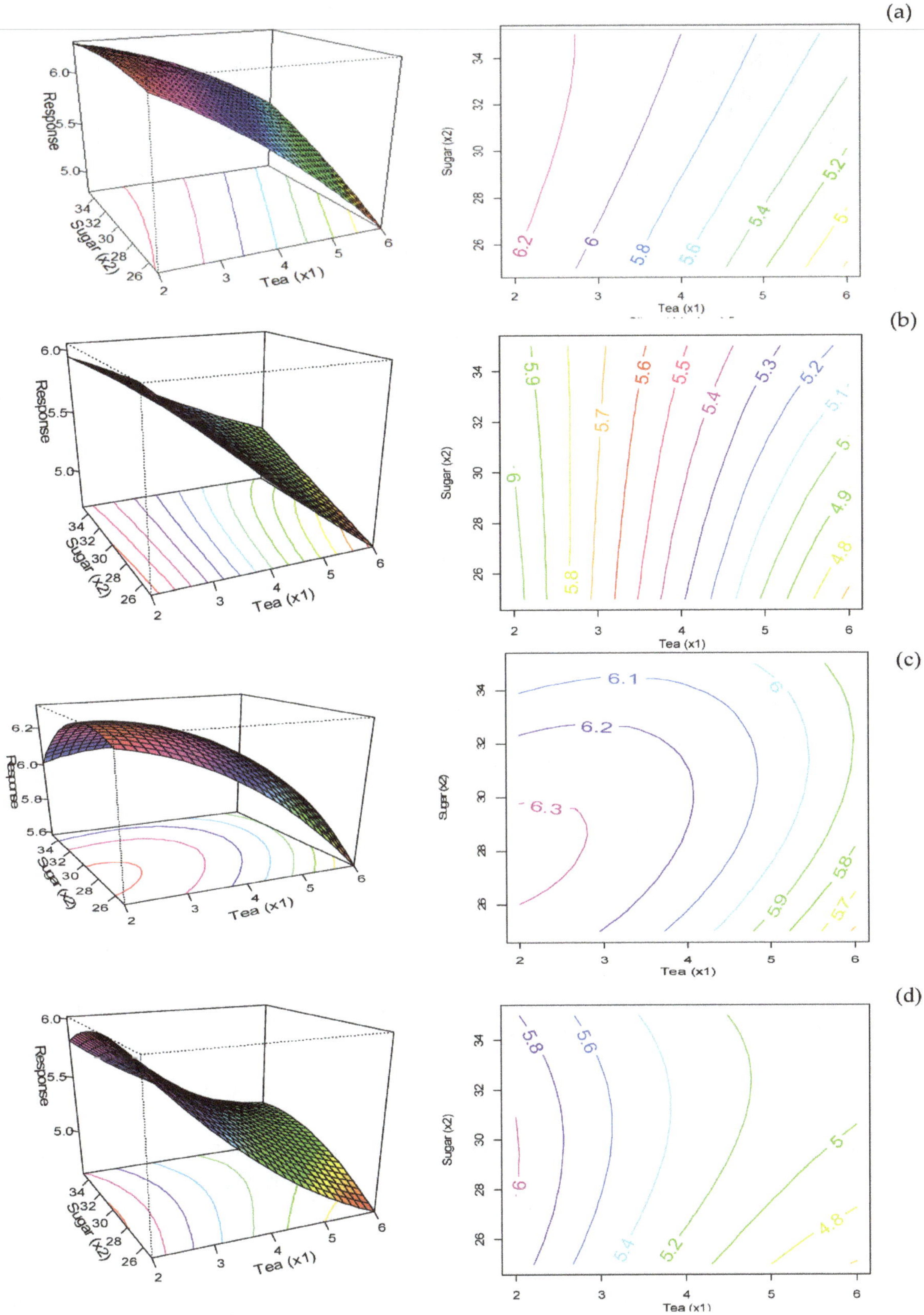

Figure 3. Response surfaces and contour plots of the effect of MGTP and sugar content incorporated (**a**) overall; (**b**) appearance; (**c**) aroma and (**d**) color acceptability of biscuits.

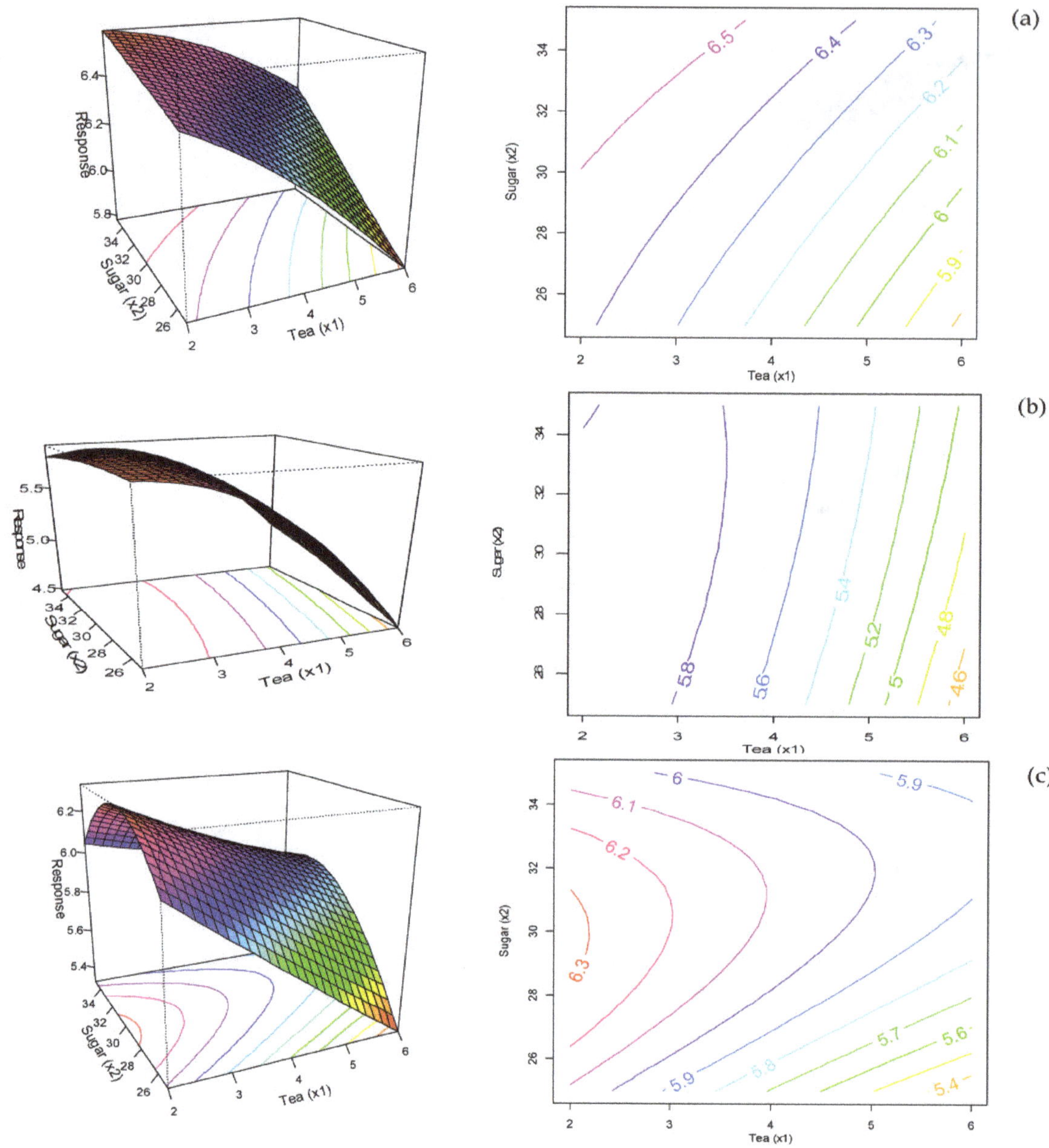

Figure 4. Response surfaces and contour plots of the effect of MGTP and sugar content incorporated (**a**) texture; (**b**) bitterness and (**c**) sweetness acceptability of biscuits.

3.3. Metabolic Response to Matcha Green Tea Biscuits

In this pilot study, 10 subjects were recruited with ages ranging from 27 to 44 years and a mean BMI of 26.67 $\pm$ 4.48 kg·m^{-2}, with a gender split of 6 females and 4 males. The portions of biscuits served to participants are shown in supplementary material (Figure S4).

3.3.1. Glucose Response

Capillary blood glucose concentration was measured at baseline and every 15 min after consumption of the control or test meals. As shown in Figure 5, the glucose response of all of the food samples peaked at 30 min after meal intake, with a slow decrease until 180 min. Consumption of the control meal consisting of plain biscuits gave the highest average iAUC (106.1 $\pm$ 63.0 mmol·min L^{-1}), followed by the test meal with MGTP-enriched biscuits (89.2 $\pm$ 44.7 mmol·min L$^{-1)}$ and the test meal with plain biscuits and a MGTP drink (81.9 $\pm$ 36.0 mmol·min L^{-1}). No significant differences in the iAUCs were observed between meals (one factor ANOVA). Although MGTP does have a tendency to lower iAUC, the variation between individuals is high. The response in the first 30 min appears to be the same amongst the foods, indicating that Matcha green tea does not affect rapidly available glucose (RAG), most probably from sucrose and rapidly digestible starch (RDS). The biggest differences appeared in later time points (>100 min), pointing to a potential inhibition of starch digestion by MGTP, whether in biscuit or tea form. There were significant differences in incremental blood glucose levels at time points 120 and 150 min post ingestion between the plain biscuits and the Matcha treatments.

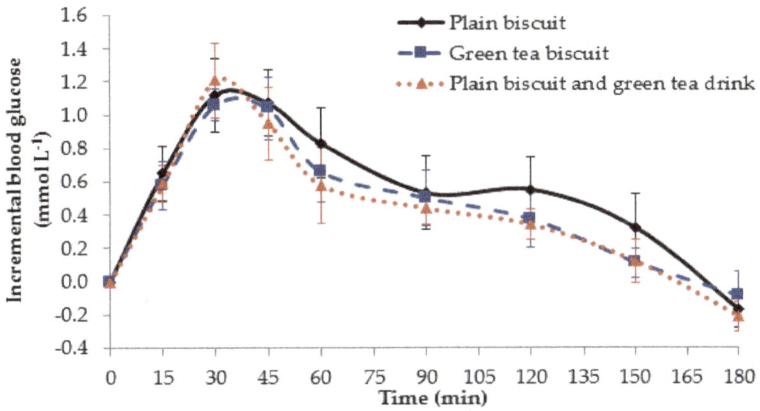

Figure 5. Mean incremental blood glucose response curves after ingestion of control and test meals over 180 min. (-◆-) represents the blood glucose curve of the control meal that consisted of plain biscuit consumed with warm water, (-■-) represents the blood glucose curve of the test meal with Matcha green tea biscuits consumed with warm water, and (..▲..) represents the blood glucose curve of the test meal with plain biscuits consumed with a Matcha green tea drink. Data expressed as the amount of blood glucose in mmol·L^{-1} and the error bars represent the SEM (n = 10).

Previous findings on the effect of green tea on glucose response have been inconclusive. Many in vivo and in vitro studies have suggested that green tea and EGCG acutely reduce postprandial blood glucose levels by inhibiting the activity of pancreatic α-amylase [28,29]. In an in vitro study, Forester et al. [28] found that EGCG non-competitively inhibited pancreatic amylase activity by 34%. Moreover, Tsuneki et al. [30] showed that glucose tolerance was significantly ($p < 0.05$) improved with tea administration compared with hot water during a glucose challenge in healthy humans. The authors speculated that the observed acute effects of green tea on blood glucose levels were mainly due to the promotion of insulin action in peripheral tissues, such as skeletal muscles and adipocytes via modification of serum protein [30]. Lochocka et al. [31] found that a single dose of green tea extract taken with a test meal significantly decreased starch digestion and absorption compared with the placebo treatment ($p = 0.003$). The study used a CO_2 starch breath test, which measures the isotope ratio of ${}_{12}CO_2/{}_{13}CO_2$ in breath samples. The starch digestion and absorption was measured based on cumulative percentage ${}_{13}C$ dose recovery [31]. They found that green tea extract (257.6 mg of catechins) decreased starch digestion and absorption in humans when consumed with a test meal. The green tea extract was used in powder form (4 g of powder containing 257.6 mg of catechins) enclosed in a starch wafer, whereas the placebo was an empty starch wafer. In our study, we observed a significant difference between responses to plain biscuits and the two green tea treatments after 120 and 150 min, suggesting that catechins may have a mild effect on starch digestion. Josic et al. [32] found that green tea infusion (150.6 mg of catechins) showed no effects on glucose or insulin levels. An animal study suggested that EGCG acutely reduces postprandial blood glucose levels in mice when co-administered with corn starch, and this may be due in part to inhibition of α-amylase [28]. Moreover, a study on the effect of green tea supplementation on insulin sensitivity in rats suggested that regular green tea infusion drink could increase insulin sensitivity [33,34]. They also suggested that the amelioration of insulin resistance by green tea is associated with increased expression of glucose transporter IV (GLUT IV) found in adipose tissue. On the other hand, Park et al. [35] proposed that gallated catechins could elevate blood glucose levels by blocking glucose uptake into tissues.

A factor that could have affected glucose response in the present study is the high fat content in shortbread biscuits. The fat content in food can lower the glucose response by slowing down gastric emptying [36]. Hence, the potential differences in starch digestion between control and test meals could have been masked by the high fat content in biscuits. In order to minimize the varied result from sugar and fat content in biscuits, the biscuits with less sugar and low fat content should be used to investigate the effect of MGTP on glucose response. We observed no effect of ethnicity on the glyceamic response to the biscuits. Previous studies have also not identified ethnicity as a significant factor to consider when testing glyceamic response [19].

3.3.2. Triglyceride Response

The incremental postprandial responses of plasma triglycerides after consumption of the control and test meals are shown in Figure 6a. When the participants consumed the control meal, plasma triglycerides rose from the baseline to reach the highest level at 120 min and almost returned back to baseline 180 min after consumption of the control meal. The concentration of triglycerides after the consumption of the test meal with Matcha green tea biscuits remained close to the baseline value until 60 min, then rose to a peak at 120 min and returned to baseline at 180 min. The reduction in iAUC after consumption of Matcha green tea biscuits (35.6 ± 44.6 mmol·min L^{-1}) was observed, compared with the consumption of plain biscuits (44.6 ± 32.1 mmol·min L^{-1}) and plain biscuits consumed with Matcha green tea drink (39.4 ± 35.7 mmol·min L^{-1}). However, statistical analysis found that there was no significant difference in iAUC between all three food samples ($p = 0.87$) due to the high variation between individuals.

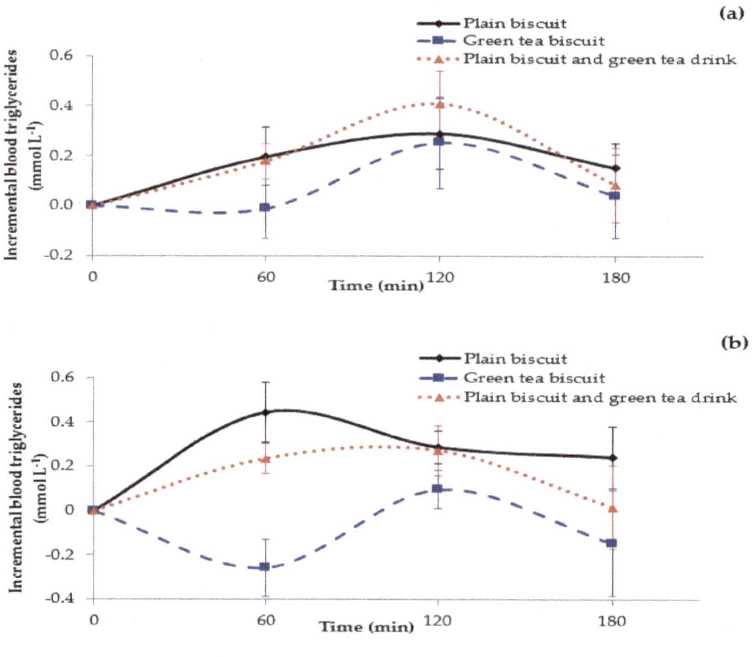

Figure 6. (**a**) The mean incremental blood triglyceride response curves after ingestion of control and test meals over 180 min (n = 10 participants); (**b**) the mean incremental blood triglyceride response curves after ingestion of control and test meals over 180 min among Asian subjects (n = 4 participants). (-◆-) represents the blood triglyceride curve of the control meal consisting of plain biscuits, (-■-) represents the blood triglyceride curve of the test meal with Matcha green tea biscuits, and (..▲..) represents the blood triglyceride curve of the test meal with plain biscuits consumed with a Matcha green tea drink. Data expressed as the amount of triglycerides in mmol L^{-1} and the error bars represent the SEM.

Figure 6b shows the incremental postprandial levels of plasma triglycerides after ingestion of the control and test meals for 4 Asian subjects compared to the other ethnicities. The curves show an average 0.26 mmol·L^{-1} decrease in plasma triglycerides following consumption of the test meal with the MGTP enriched biscuits, whereas the control meal with the plain biscuits induced an average 0.44 mmol·L^{-1} increase in plasma triglycerides. The iAUC of the test meal with Matcha green tea biscuits (8.0 ± 12.5 mmol·min L^{-1}) was significantly lower (p = 0.02) than the other meals (51.7 ± 22.3 mmol·min L^{-1} and 32.7 ± 17.6 mmol·min L^{-1}) for the control meal and test meal (plain biscuits with MGTP tea drink), respectively.

A previous study by Unno et al. [16] found that green tea drink consumed with a piece of bread covered with 20 g of butter lowered the postprandial triglyceride level compared to a meal with a control drink. In that study, there were 2 treatments of green tea; a moderate dose containing 224 mg of tea catechins and a high dose containing 674 mg of tea catechins. Both moderate and high dose treatments lowered the postprandial triglyceride levels and reduced the iAUC by 15.1% and 28.7%, respectively. Only the high dose showed a significant difference in iAUC compared to the control dose. Our findings are in agreement, as the dose of catechins (224 mg of tea catechins) reduced the iAUC by 15.1% but did not give a significant difference. The test meal used in the Unno et al. [16] study was lower in fat (18.8 g of fat) compared to our biscuits (35 g of fat).

The mechanism underlying the triglyceride lowering effect of green tea is mainly focused on the inhibition of the digestion of fat from the intestine [37]. Juhel et al. [38] found that green tea exhibits potential to inhibit gastric and pancreatic lipases. EGCG can enlarge fat droplets through interference with emulsification and micellar solubility of lipids [39–41]. Hence, the enlarged emulsion droplets can prevent the efficient emulsification of bile salt and reduce surface area for fat digestion by lipase [14,16,42,43]. Moreover, Suzuki et al. [37] proposed that catechins with gallate groups are located on the surface of the lipid emulsion and destabilize the lipid emulsion. The difference in responses according to ethnicity merits further investigation. Apolipoproteins are essential regulators of triglyeride circulation. Gene polymorphisms for the a1/c3/a4/a5 gene cluster were found to differ between Chinese and Caucasian populations [44]. Another study found that the postprandial triglyceride concentrations in South Asian men were significantly higher than European men [45]. This was indeed our observation in response to the plain biscuits with a significant effect of the green tea enrichment. These results need to be confirmed in a larger study stratified according to ethnic groups. Information about habitual diet, including catechin content, needs to be considered. Furthermore, more time points in the triglyceride time course need to be included, as triglyceride levels may take around 8 h to return to homeostatic levels.

4. Conclusions

This study showed that catechins in MGTP are relatively heat resistant, with only approximately 20% loss of total catechins during baking at 180 °C. Epimerization between EGC and GCG is thought to have occurred during biscuit baking, as the result found a decrease in EGC and an increase in GCG in the baked shortbread biscuits. The effect of MGTP on shortbread biscuit acceptability was assessed using a 9-point hedonic scale and the data was analysed with response surface methodology. With an increase in the level of green tea powder, the acceptability of biscuits decreased significantly, and sugar did not significantly improve acceptability of the enriched biscuits. The main factors affecting acceptability were colour and bitterness. The consumption of MGTP as biscuit or tea infusion did not have significant effects on acute metabolic response, but some interesting trends were observed amongst a low number of Asian participants. This indicates potential for MGTP-enriched products as functional foods. An additional study with larger sample size that takes into account the ethnicity of participants is needed to confirm the observed trends.

Supplementary Materials:
Figure S1: Plain biscuit (**a**) and green tea biscuits with 3 levels of MGTP incorporated: (**b**) 2 g, (**c**) 4 g and (**d**) 6 g of MGTP 100 g^{-1} of flour, Figure S2: Chromatograph profiles of tea catechins, (**A**) in dough; (**B**) in plain

and green tea biscuits: 1. EGC; 2. Caffeine; 3. EC; 4. EGCG; 5. GCG and 6. ECG, Figure S3: Hardness plot of biscuits with 3 levels of MGTP and sugar incorporated. The error bars represent the STDs ($n = 6$), Figure S4: Estimated nutritional data of food samples.

Acknowledgments: The authors wish to thank the Ratchabhat Phuket University for funding through Ph.D. sponsorship to BP.

Author Contributions: B.P., C.O., M.H. and L.J.M. conceived and designed the experiments; B.P. performed the experiments; B.P., C.O., M.H. and L.J.M. analysed the data, contributed reagents/materials/analysis tools, and wrote the paper.

References

1. Wang, H.; Provan, G.; Helliwell, K.; Ransom, W. The functional benefits of flavonoids: The case of tea. In *Phytochemical Functional Foods*; Johnson, I., Williamson, G., Eds.; Woodhead Publishing: Sawston, Cambridge, UK, 2003; pp. 128–159.
2. Wang, R.; Zhou, W.; Jiang, X. Reaction kinetics of degradation and epimerization of epigallocatechin gallate (EGCG) in aqueous system over a wide temperature range. *J. Agric. Food Chem.* **2008**, *56*, 694–2701. [CrossRef] [PubMed]
3. Pelillo, M.; Biguzzi, B.; Bendini, A.; Toschi, T.G.; Vanzini, M.; Lercker, G. Preliminary investigation into development of HPLC with UV and MS-electrospray detection for the analysis of tea catechins. *Food Chem.* **2002**, *78*, 369–374. [CrossRef]
4. Mennen, L.; Hirvonen, T.; Arnault, N.; Bertrais, S.; Galan, P.; Hercberg, S. Consumption of black, green and herbal tea and iron status in French adults. *Eur. J. Clin. Nutr.* **2007**, *61*, 1174–1179. [CrossRef] [PubMed]
5. Kim, Y.-K.; Jombart, L.; Valentin, D.; Kim, K.O. A cross-cultural study using Napping®: Do Korean and French consumers perceive various green tea products differently? *Food Res. Int.* **2013**, *53*, 534–542. [CrossRef]
6. Šebečić, B.; Vedrina Dragojević, I.; Vitali, D.; Hečimović, M.; Dragičević, I. Raw materials in fibre enriched biscuits production as source of total phenols. *Agric. Conspec. Sci.* **2007**, *72*, 265–270.
7. Carrillo, E.; Varela, P.; Fiszman, S. Effects of food package information and sensory characteristics on the perception of healthiness and the acceptability of enriched biscuits. *Food Res. Int.* **2012**, *48*, 209–216. [CrossRef]
8. Ahmad, M.; Baba, W.N.; Wani, T.A.; Gani, A.; Gani, A.; Shah, U.; Wani, S.M.; Masoodi, F.A. Effect of green tea powder on thermal, rheological & functional properties of wheat flour and physical, nutraceutical & sensory analysis of cookies. *J. Food Sci. Technol.* **2015**, *52*, 5799–5807. [PubMed]
9. Lu, T.M.; Lee, C.C.; Mau, J.L.; Lin, S.D. Quality and antioxidant property of green tea sponge cake. *Food Chem.* **2010**, *119*, 1090–1095. [CrossRef]
10. Li, M.; Zhang, J.H.; Zhu, K.X.; Peng, W.; Zhang, S.K.; Wang, B.; Zhu, Y.J.; Zhou, H.M. Effect of superfine green tea powder on the thermodynamic, rheological and fresh noodle making properties of wheat flour. *LWT Food Sci. Technol.* **2012**, *46*, 23–28. [CrossRef]
11. Yang, J.; Mao, Q.X.; Xu, H.X.; Ma, X.; Zeng, C.Y. Tea consumption and risk of type 2 diabetes mellitus: A systematic review and meta-analysis update. *BMJ Open* **2014**, *4*, e005632. [CrossRef] [PubMed]
12. Thielecke, F.; Boschmann, M. The potential role of green tea catechins in the prevention of the metabolic syndrome—A review. *Phytochemistry* **2009**, *70*, 11–24. [CrossRef] [PubMed]
13. Zhong, L.; Furne, J.K.; Levitt, M.D. An extract of black, green, and mulberry teas causes malabsorption of carbohydrate but not of triacylglycerol in healthy volunteers. *Am. J. Clin. Nutr.* **2006**, *84*, 551–555. [PubMed]
14. Koo, S.I.; Noh, S.K. Green tea as inhibitor of the intestinal absorption of lipids: Potential Mechanism for its Lipid-Lowering Effect. *J. Nutr. Biochem.* **2007**, *18*, 179–183. [CrossRef] [PubMed]
15. Ikeda, I.; Tsuda, K.; Suzuki, Y.; Kobayashi, M.; Unno, T.; Tomoyori, H.; Goto, H.; Kawata, Y.; Imaizumi, K.; Nozawa, A.; et al. Tea catechins with a galloyl moiety suppress postprandial hypertriacylglycerolemia by delaying lymphatic transport of dietary fat in rats. *J. Nutr.* **2005**, *135*, 155–159. [CrossRef] [PubMed]
16. Unno, T.; Tago, M.; Suzuki, Y.; Nozawa, A.; Sagesaka, Y.M.; Kakuda, T.; Egawa, K.; Kondo, K. Effect of tea catechins on postprandial plasma lipid responses in human subjects. *Br. J. Nutr.* **2005**, *93*, 543–547. [CrossRef] [PubMed]

17. Wang, R.; Zhou, W. Stability of tea catechins in the breadmaking Process. *J. Agric. Food Chem.* **2004**, *52*, 8224–8229. [CrossRef] [PubMed]
18. Food and Agriculture Organization. *Carbohydrates in Human Nutrition. Report of a Joint FAO/WHO Expert Consultation*; FAO Food Nutrition Paper; Food and Agriculture Organization of the United Nations: Rome, Itlay, 1998; Volume 66, pp. 1–140.
19. Brouns, F.; Bjorck, I.; Frayn, K.N.; Gibbs, A.L.; Lang, V.; Slama, G.; Wolever, T.M.S. Glycaemic index methodology. *Nutr. Res. Rev.* **2005**, *18*, 145–171. [CrossRef] [PubMed]
20. Wang, R.; Zhou, W.; Jiang, X. Mathematical modeling of the stability of green tea catechin epigallocatechin gallate (EGCG) during bread baking. *J. Food Eng.* **2008**, *87*, 505–513. [CrossRef]
21. Sharma, A.; Zhou, W. A stability study of green tea catechins during the biscuit making process. *Food Chem.* **2011**, *126*, 568–573. [CrossRef]
22. Guo, Q.; Zhao, B.; Shen, S.; Hou, J.; Hu, J.; Xin, W. ESR study on the structure–antioxidant activity relationship of tea catechins and their epimers. *Biochim. Biophys. Acta (BBA) Gen. Subj.* **1999**, *1427*, 13–23. [CrossRef]
23. Ananingsih, V.K.; Sharma, A.; Zhou, W. Green tea catechins during food processing and storage: A review on stability and detection. *Food Res. Int.* **2013**, *50*, 469–479. [CrossRef]
24. Wang, L.-F.; So, S.; Baik, J.H.; Kim, H.J.; Moon, K.S.; Park, S.K. Aroma changes in green tea beverage during processing and storage. In *Nutraceutical Beverages*; American Chemical Society: Washington, DC, USA, 2003; pp. 162–188.
25. Kim, E.S.; Liang, Y.R.; Jin, J.; Sun, Q.F.; Lu, J.L.; Du, Y.Y.; Lin, C. Impact of heating on chemical compositions of green tea liquor. *Food Chem.* **2007**, *103*, 1263–1267. [CrossRef]
26. Wang, R.; Zhou, W.; Isabelle, M. Comparison study of the effect of green tea extract (GTE) on the quality of bread by instrumental analysis and sensory evaluation. *Food Res. Int.* **2007**, *40*, 470–479. [CrossRef]
27. Green, B.G.; Lim, J.; Osterhoff, F.; Blacher, K.; Nachtigal, D. Taste mixture interactions: Suppression, additivity, and the predominance of sweetness. *Physiol. Behave.* **2010**, *101*, 731–737. [CrossRef] [PubMed]
28. Forester, S.C.; Gu, Y.; Lambert, J.D. Inhibition of starch digestion by the green tea polyphenol, (−)-epigallocatechin-3-gallate. *Mol. Nutr. Food Res.* **2012**, *56*, 1647–1654. [CrossRef] [PubMed]
29. Chen, N.; Bezzina, R.; Hinch, E.; Lewandowski, P.A.; Cameron-Smith, D.; Mathai, M.L.; Jois, M.; Sinclair, A.J.; Begg, D.P.; Wark, J.D.; et al. Green tea, black tea, and epigallocatechin modify body composition, improve glucose tolerance, and differentially alter metabolic gene expression in rats fed a high-fat diet. *Nutr. Res.* **2009**, *29*, 784–793. [CrossRef] [PubMed]
30. Tsuneki, H.; Ishizuka, M.; Terasawa, M.; Wu, J.B.; Sasaoka, T.; Kimura, I. Effect of green tea on blood glucose levels and serum proteomic patterns in diabetic (db/db) mice and on glucose metabolism in healthy humans. *BMC Pharmacol.* **2004**, *4*, 18. [CrossRef] [PubMed]
31. Lochocka, K.; Bajerska, J.; Glapa, A.; Fidler-Witon, E.; Nowak, J.K.; Szczapa, T.; Grebowiec, P.; Lisowska, A.; Walkowiak, J. Green tea extract decreases starch digestion and absorption from a test meal in humans: A randomized, placebo-controlled crossover study. *Sci. Rep.* **2015**, *5*, 12015. [CrossRef] [PubMed]
32. Josic, J.; Olsson, A.T.; Wickeberg, J.; Lindstedt, S.; Hlebowicz, J. Does green tea affect postprandial glucose, insulin and satiety in healthy subjects: A randomized controlled trial. *Nutr. J.* **2010**, *9*, 63. [CrossRef] [PubMed]
33. Wu, L.Y.; Juan, C.C.; Ho, L.T.; Hsu, Y.P.; Hwang, L.S. Effect of green tea supplementation on insulin sensitivity in Sprague-Dawley rats. *J. Agric. Food Chem.* **2004**, *52*, 643–648. [CrossRef] [PubMed]
34. Wu, L.Y.; Juan, C.C.; Hwang, L.S.; Hsu, Y.P.; Ho, P.H.; Ho, L.T. Green tea supplementation ameliorates insulin resistance and increase glucose transporter IV content in a fructose-fed rat model. *Eur. J. Nutr.* **2004**, *43*, 116–124. [CrossRef] [PubMed]
35. Park, J.H.; Jin, J.Y.; Baek, W.K.; Park, S.H.; Sung, H.Y.; Kim, Y.K.; Lee, J.; Song, D.K. Ambivalent role of gallated catechins in glucose tolerance in humans: A novel insight into non-absorbable gallated catechin-derived inhibitors of glucose absorption. *J. Physiol. Pharmacol.* **2009**, *60*, 101–109. [PubMed]
36. Wolever, T.M.S. *The Glycaemic Index: A Physiological Classification of Dietary Carbohydrate*; CABI Pub.: Wallingford, Oxfordshire, UK; Cambridge, MA, USA, 2006; 227p.
37. Suzuki, Y.; Unno, T.; Kobayashi, M.; Nozawa, A.; Sagesaka, Y.; Kakuda, T. Dose-dependent suppression of tea catechins with a galloyl moiety on postprandial hypertriglyceridemia in rats. *Biosci. Biotechnol. Biochem.* **2005**, *69*, 1288–1291. [CrossRef] [PubMed]

38. Juhel, C.; Armand, M.; Pafumi, Y.; Rosier, C.; Vandermander, J.; Lairon, D. Green tea extract (AR25®) inhibits lipolysis of triglycerides in gastric and duodenal medium in vitro. *J. Nutr. Biochem.* **2000**, *11*, 45–51. [CrossRef]
39. Kim, J.; Koo, S.I.; Noh, S.K. Green tea extract markedly lowers the lymphatic absorption and increases the biliary secretion of C-14-benzo a pyrene in rats. *J. Nutr. Biochem.* **2012**, *23*, 1007–1011. [CrossRef] [PubMed]
40. Chan, C.Y.; Wei, L.; Castro-Muñozledo, F.; Koo, W.L. (−)-Epigallocatechin-3-gallate blocks 3T3-L1 adipose conversion by inhibition of cell proliferation and suppression of adipose phenotype expression. *Life Sci.* **2011**, *89*, 779–785. [CrossRef] [PubMed]
41. Lee, M.-S.; Kim, C.T.; Kim, I.H.; Kim, Y. Inhibitory Effects of Green Tea Catechin on the Lipid Accumulation in 3T3-L1 Adipocytes. *Phytother. Res.* **2009**, *23*, 1088–1091. [CrossRef] [PubMed]
42. Walkowiak, J.; Bajerska, J.; Kargulewicz, A.; Lisowska, A.; Siedlerski, G.; Szczapa, T.; Kobelska-Dubiel, N.; Grzymisławski, M. Single dose of green tea extract decreases lipid digestion and absorption from a test meal in humans. *Acta Biochim. Pol.* **2013**, *60*, 481–483. [PubMed]
43. Raederstorff, D.G.; Schlachter, M.F.; Elste, V.; Weber, P. Effect of EGCG on lipid absorption and plasma lipid levels in rats. *J. Nutr. Biochem.* **2003**, *14*, 326–332. [CrossRef]
44. Liu, Z.-K.; Hu, M.; Baum, L.; Thomas, G.N.; Tomlinson, B. Associations of polymorphisms in the apolipoprotein A1/C3/A4/A5 gene cluster with familial combined hyperlipidaemia in Hong Kong Chinese. *Atherosclerosis* **2010**, *208*, 427–432. [CrossRef] [PubMed]
45. Arjunan, S.P.; Bishop, N.; Reischak-Oliveira, A.; Stensel, D.J. Exercise and coronary heart disease risk markers in South Asian and European men. *Med. Sci. Sports Exerc.* **2013**, *45*, 1261–1268. [CrossRef] [PubMed]

4

Total, Neutral and Polar Lipids of Brewing Ingredients, By-Products and Beer: Evaluation of Antithrombotic Activities

Ronan Lordan *, Eoin O'Keeffe, Alexandros Tsoupras and Ioannis Zabetakis

Department of Biological Sciences, University of Limerick, Limerick V94 T9PX, Ireland; eoin.okeeffe@ul.ie (E.O.); Alexandros.Tsoupras@ul.ie (A.T.); Ioannis.Zabetakis@ul.ie (I.Z.)

* Correspondence: Ronan.Lordan@ul.ie

Abstract: The in vitro antithrombotic properties of polar lipid constituents of malted grain (MG), pelleted hops (PH), brewer's spent grain (BSG), spent hops (SH), wort, and bottled beer from the same production line were assessed in human platelets. The total lipids (TL) were extracted according to the Bligh and Dyer method and further separated into the total neutral lipids (TNL) and total polar lipids (TPL) extracts by counter-current distribution. The TL, TNL, and TPL extracts of all samples were assessed for their ability to inhibit platelet-activating factor (PAF) and thrombin-induced human platelet aggregation. The raw materials, by-products, wort, and beer lipid extracts all exhibited antithrombotic properties against PAF and thrombin. However, the beer TPL exhibited the lowest IC_{50} values against PAF-induced (7.8 ± 3.9 μg) and thrombin-induced (4.3 ± 3.0 μg) platelet aggregation indicating that these polar lipids were the most antithrombotic. The lipid extracts tended to be more bioactive against the thrombin pathway. The fatty acid content of all the TPL extracts were assessed using GC-MS. The fatty acid composition of the most bioactive TPL extracts, the wort and the beer, shared similar fatty acid profiles. Indeed, it was noted that fermentation seems to play a role in increasing the antithrombotic properties of polar lipids against PAF and thrombin by moderately altering the polar lipid fatty acid composition. Furthermore, the use of brewing by-products as a source of functional cardioprotective lipids warrants further investigation and valorisation.

Keywords: fermentation; beer; brewer's spent grain; hops; polar lipids; platelet-activating factor; thrombin; cardiovascular disease; antithrombotic

---

1. Introduction

Cardiovascular diseases (CVD) are the leading cause of mortality globally, where diet and lifestyle are key modifiable risk factors [1]. The harmful effects of alcohol consumption have been well established, as excessive alcohol consumption has been linked to several chronic diseases, including cancer [2,3]. However, moderate alcohol consumption (up to 16 g alcohol/day) has been associated with cardiovascular health benefits, including reduced fasting glucose and blood insulin sensitivity versus non-alcoholic beer in healthy men [4]. Indeed, consumption of 1–2 alcoholic beverages/day is associated with reduced fibrinogen levels, reduced platelet aggregation, and an increase in high-density lipoprotein (HDL). These effects have mostly been attributed to the ethanol content and the presence of phenolic compounds [5–7]. Epidemiological studies demonstrate that moderate alcohol consumption reduced cardiovascular risk factors, morbidity, and mortality following a dose-effect relationship that is characterised by a J-shaped curve [6].

Atherosclerosis is the first step in the development of CVD [1]. Platelet-activating factor (PAF) is a potent platelet agonist and inflammatory mediator implicated in the onset and progression of atherosclerosis [8,9]. PAF and PAF-like molecules carry out their functions by binding to the

PAF-receptor (PAF-R), which is expressed in various cell types, including platelets, endothelial cells, neutrophils, and macrophages [1]. Activation of the PAF-R leads to the induction of multiple inflammatory pathways and platelet activation [1].

Thrombin is another important mediator of platelet activation [10]. Thrombin is a serine protease that participates in the coagulation cascade, activating factors V, VIII, XI, and XII, converting fibrinogen to fibrin, and activating other cell types [10,11]. Both PAF and thrombin are produced during coagulation and inflammation and play a crucial role in platelet activation and thrombus formation via G protein-coupled receptors [12]. Previously these two pathways were considered independent. However, recent evidence suggests that there is a crosstalk between coagulatory and inflammatory pathways during pathological processes, whereby inflammation leads to platelet activation in a reciprocal fashion [13]. Considering the important roles that PAF and thrombin hold at the nexus of coagulation and inflammation, antiplatelet and anti-inflammatory therapeutic and preventative strategies are required to prevent the development of chronic diseases such as CVD. Within this concept, several compounds of natural origin [1] can inhibit the binding of PAF to the PAF-R, which ameliorates the PAF inflammatory and prothrombotic response. Notably, polar lipid constituents of ale, lager, and stout have exhibited potent anti-PAF and antithrombotic properties [14]. However, little is known about the origin of these beer-derived antithrombotic polar lipid microconstituents and their effects against the thrombin pathway.

Beer is the most consumed alcoholic beverage globally. The raw materials used in beer production influence the different characteristics and properties of the beer [4]. Beers are produced from malted barley, water, hops (*Humulus lupulus*), and yeast (*Saccharomyces cerevisiae*). Barley (*Hordeum vulgare*) contains 2–4% (dry weight) lipid depending on various factors [15]. Commercial malts can contain up to 3.4% lipid. Approximately 70–90% of the fatty acid content of the barley and malt is triglycerides, 10–20% are sterol compounds, and approximately 10% are free fatty acids. The free lipid composition of the barley grain is approximately 68–75% neutral lipids, 7–26% glycolipids, and 9–18% phospholipids depending on the cultivar [16]. Germination of the barley and the mashing process can lead to the loss of lipid due to the release of fatty acids via the hydrolysis of triglycerides, which are then metabolised. The resulting fatty acids, mono-, and diglycerides do not tend to accumulate in the malt, and thus are not found in significant quantities in the finished product [17]. Moreover, several phospholipids can form complexes with amylose in starch before the brewing process [18]. A significant proportion of the lipid content is lost to the spent grains generated during the brewing process, and so the wort and beer contains low levels of lipid [19]. There is only a trace amount of lipid that remains in the final beer product, which are generally considered undesirable due to their impact on the formation of haze, the stability of beer foam, and the development of unfavourable flavours during conditioning [17,20].

Brewing yeasts also have the capacity to synthesise and alter several lipid species, including phospholipids and polyunsaturated fatty acids (PUFA) [21], which play a crucial role in the metabolic pathways and regulation of lipid catabolism and anabolism in yeast [17]. Furthermore, there is an increased concentration of stearic, *cis*-oleic, and linolenic acid in the wort as a result of endogenous lipase activity that releases free fatty acids from triglycerides and phospholipids in the mashing and malting process [21,22]. In addition, the composition of the malt and lauter turbidity can lead to the formation of triglycerides, diglycerides, monoglycerides, free fatty acids, phospholipids, and sphingolipids during the fermentation process [23].

The unfortunate consequence of beer production is the generation of brewing wastes and by-products, which are a significant environmental challenge, but may be valorised for the development of novel products [24]. Industrial-scale food processing by-products are increasingly being viewed as potential sources of bioactive ingredients. One such example in the brewing industry by-product previously sent to landfill is BSG [25], which is now primarily used for animal feed. The lipid content of BSG is approximately 10.0–13.5% (*w/w* of BSG samples) [26], where it is estimated that 9.1% of the total lipids are phospholipids [27].

Considering little is known about the fatty acid composition of bioactive polar lipid microconstituents of beer or brewing by-products, the aim of this study was to assess the antithrombotic properties and fatty acid composition of lipid extracts sampled at various stages of the brewing process, from the brewing raw materials (malted grain and hops), the by-products (BSG and spent hops), the wort, and the finished beer product from a commercial beer produced in Ireland.

2. Materials and Methods

2.1. Chemicals and Reagents

All glassware, chemicals, and solvents were of analytical grade and purchased from Fisher Scientific Ireland Ltd. (Dublin, Ireland). All reagents used for platelet aggregation, including bovine serum albumin (BSA), standard PAF, and standard thrombin, were high purity and purchased from Sigma-Aldrich (Wicklow, Ireland). Blood consumables, including needles (20G) and 8.2 mL sodium citrate S-monovettes, were purchased from Sarstedt Ltd. (Wexford, Ireland). For GC-MS, a pre-derivatised Supelco™ 37-component FAME standard mix, pre-derivatised heptadecanoic acid, and pre-derivatised heneicosanoic acid was purchased from Sigma-Aldrich (Wicklow, Ireland). All platelet aggregometry consumables were purchased from Labmedics LLP (Abingdon on Thames, UK). All GC-MS consumables were purchased from Apex Scientific Ltd. (Kildare, Ireland).

2.2. Beer Production and Samples Assessed

The beer, wort, raw materials, and brewing by-products used for this study were obtained from the Munster Brewery facility (Youghal, Co. Cork, Ireland). The samples assessed in this study were pelleted hops (PH), spent hops (SH), malted grains (MG), brewer's spent grains (BSG), wort, and the beer itself. All the raw materials, wort, and by-products obtained for this study correspond to the same batch and production line of the beer that was produced for and tested in this study. The beer is an organically produced Irish red ale for commercial sale under the name '12 Towers' brewed in accordance with organic standards certified by the Irish Organic Association.

The beer production is described in brief as follows. Of the malts used, approximately 90% of the overall malt was organic pale ale malt (Maris Otter malt) was kiln dried at 90–95 °C to produce the base malt of the beer with a maximum moisture content of 4.5% and a European Brewing Convention (EBC) colour scale between 7 and 10 (Castle Malting Ltd., Beloeil, Belgium). A small amount of organic roasted barley (approximately 10% of the total malt used), which was kiln dried to 230 °C that produced a roasted grain that had a maximum moisture content of 4.5% and was a colour rating between 1000–1400 EBC. Once milled by the brewery, the grains were mashed in the mash tun. To formulate the wort, 4 L of water was added per kg of crushed grain, which was steeped in the mash tun at 66 °C for 60 min. This process activated the α- and β-amylase enzymes (among others) that convert the starch to simple sugars to produce the so-called sweet wort. At the end of the mash, the lautering process begins by raising the temperature to 77–79 °C to denature the enzymes by adding heated sparge water, which also weakens the gravity of the wort runoff. This process takes approximately 3–4 h. Once Lautering was complete a sample of the BSG was stored. A brewer's hydrometer was used to measure the original gravity (OG) of the first running, which can be as high as 1.080 and also subsequently to confirm that the kettle wort is at an acceptable gravity prior to commencing boiling. The OG prior to fermentation was 1.042 and final gravity (FG) after fermentation was 1.010. These hydrometer readings are used to measure the fermentable and unfermentable substances the in wort before and during fermentation and to calculate the beers final alcoholic content (alcohol by volume or ABV) when OG is compared to the FG. Runnings from the mash tun were transferred to the kettle and once complete, the wort was heated to 100 °C and brought to the boil for 1 h, which sterilised the wort, denatured any remaining enzymes, and allowed for caramelisation of the sugars for flavour enhancement.

At the start of the boil a specific amount of organic pelleted hops (PH: Organic Goldings Hops, Charles Faram Ltd., Worcester, UK) was calculated based on flavour rating (approximately 200 g/hL) of the hops for each batch and was added to the kettle, which was boiled for a further hour. These pelleted hops are strobiles from the female hop plant that are air-dried and pelleted, and thus extremely concentrated in comparison to fresh strobiles. Thereafter, the wort underwent whirlpooling a rapid cooling process by being passed through a heat exchanger, which reduced the temperature of the wort to 20 °C. A sample of the wort was taken at this point. After whirlpooling when the wort had been moved on in the process, a sample of the SH was taken. The SH sample in reality is not purely hops, it is also known as the trub, which consists of primarily hop debris (10–20%), but is also a source of sedimented protein (50–70%), phenolic compounds (5–10%), carbohydrates (4–8%), and fatty acids (1–2%) originating from the hops and residues from the barley processing [28]. The cooled wort was transferred to the primary fermenter and was held at 20 °C. At this temperature, the yeast, a dehydrated *Saccharomyces cerevisiae* (Nottingham High Performance Ale Yeast, Lallemand Inc., Burton upon Trent, UK) was diluted in sterilised water and pitched (80–100 g per hL) into the filled fermentation tank. This is a top fermenting yeast that is commonly used to produce a wide variety of beers, including ambers, porters, stouts, and pale ales. The fermentation ran for four days. Following fermentation, a conditioning period was allowed to take place at 12 °C for approximately 7 days. After conditioning, the beer underwent cold crashing. In this process, the temperature of the conditioned beer is reduced to between 0–2 °C over 3–4 days. The process of cold crashing promotes the flocculation of yeast, which sink to the bottom of the tank due to gravity and are removed, thus increasing the clarity of the beer naturally without the need for additives. Indeed, cold crashing is also desirable due to its effects on other suspended particles, such as tannins, polyphenols, and proteins that can also flocculate and settle at the bottom of the tanks, preventing the undesirable phenomenon of chill haze. Once cold crashing was complete, the beer was bottled with a 2 g of 100% fermentable organic dextrose (Charles Faram Ltd., Worcester, UK) added to each bottle to encourage carbonation by any remaining yeast in the beer. The carbonation process takes approximately 14 days at room temperature until an optimal level of 2.2–2.5 volumes of CO_2 was achieved. Once complete the bottles were placed in cold storage (0–4 °C) for a short period of time until ready to distribute.

The finished bottled beer product, the wort, and the various by-products collected were placed in airtight containers and transported to the laboratory. The beer and wort were extracted on the day of arrival to the laboratory and the other by-products and raw materials were stored at −20 °C for a maximum of three weeks until required for extraction and analysis. All samples were taken in triplicate from different batches of the beer production process. The brewing process and sampling points are outlined in Figure 1.

2.3. Extraction and Isolation of the TL, TNL, and TPL Extracts

The total lipids (TL) of all samples were extracted in triplicate according to the Bligh and Dyer [29] method. Notably, the lipids from the brewing materials, by-products, wort, and beer were extracted from different batches of production. A tenth of each TL was stored under nitrogen at −20 °C and the remaining lipid was subjected to counter-current distribution as previously described [14] to obtain the total polar lipid (TPL) and the total neutral lipid (TNL) extracts. All extracts were stored under nitrogen at −20 °C until required for a maximum of 6 months as previously described [14].

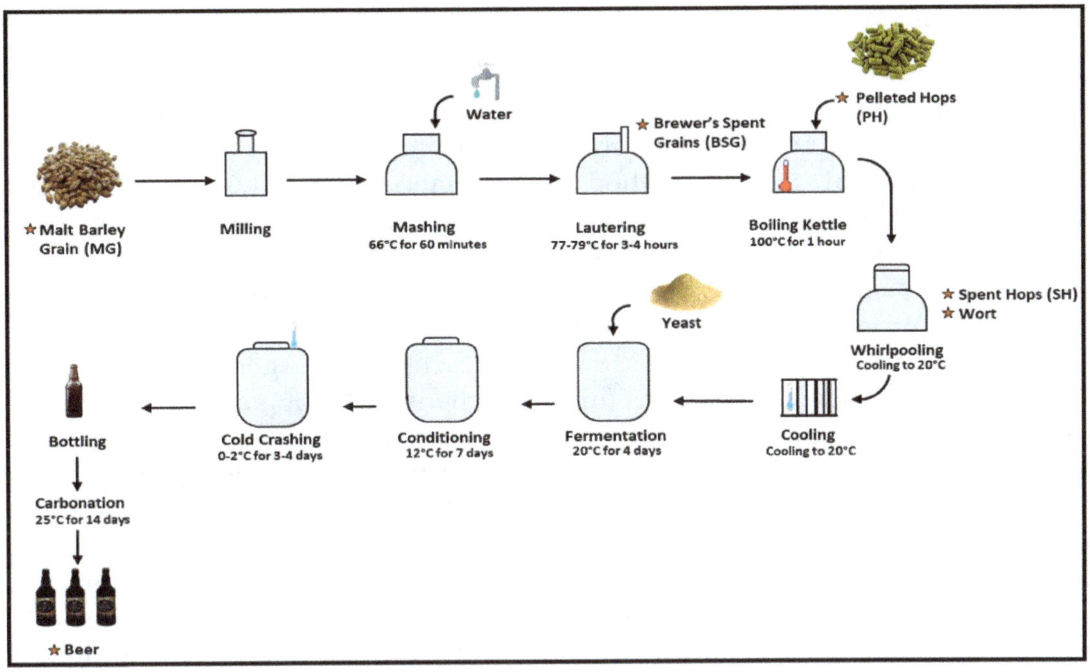

Figure 1. A schematic of the brewing process for the production of Irish red ale outlining the sampling points for the brewing materials, by-products, wort, and beer as highlighted with a star.

2.4. Platelet Aggregation Assay

The in vitro assessment of PAF and thrombin-induced platelet aggregation was carried out as previously described [14,30]. In brief, healthy human volunteers (N = 12) free from any form of antiplatelet therapy gave informed written consent and all protocols were executed in accordance with the Declaration of Helsinki following ethical approval by the University of Limerick Ethics Committee. Participants provided 50 mL or blood following an overnight fast (>8 h). The blood was drawn via venepuncture of the median cubital vein using a 20G needle into evacuated sodium citrate S-monovettes via the aspiration method (0.106 mol/L in a 1:10 ratio of citrate to blood). To obtain the platelet-rich plasma, S-monovettes were immediately centrifuged at 180× g for 18 min at 24 °C (Eppendorf 5702 R, Eppendorf Ltd, Stevenage, UK). A second centrifugation at 1500× g for 20 min at 24 °C was carried out to obtain the platelet-poor plasma (PPP). The PRP was standardised to 500,000 platelets μL^{-1} using a Shimadzu UV-1800 spectrophotometer (Kyoto, Japan), prior to analysis on a Chronolog-490 two channel platelet aggregometer (Chronolog, Havertown, PA, USA), coupled to the specialised AGGRO/LINK software package. Prior to testing, lipid samples and standard PAF were dissolved in a solution of BSA-saline (2.5 mg BSA/mL saline), while aliquots of stock solutions of active thrombin were diluted in appropriate amounts of physiological saline to obtain solutions of active thrombin with a final concentration in the aggregometer cuvette, ranging from 0.01 mU/mL NIH (National Institute of Health). The final concentration of PAF in the cuvette ranges from 1–5 × 10^{-8} M. Then, 250 µL of PRP was added to an aggregometer cuvette at 37 °C with stirring at 1000 rpm. The PRP was calibrated using the PPP as a blank. PAF and thrombin were added to the cuvettes in order to induce maximum reversible aggregation in the absence of any lipid samples. For each lipid sample, the mass of lipid required to inhibit 50% the PAF or thrombin-induced aggregation was calculated. Subsequently, the IC_{50} was calculated as previously described [14,30]. Platelet aggregation experiments for each TPL, TNL, and TL extract was carried out in triplicate against both PAF and thrombin as previously described [30,31].

2.5. Gas Chromatography-Mass Spectrometry

The preparation and analysis of the fatty acid methyl esters (FAME) were carried out in triplicate using 35 mg of the TPL samples of all samples as previously described [14]. Briefly, FAMEs were derivatised using a 0.5 M KOH CH_3OH 90% solution and extracted with n-hexane. The analysis was carried out using the internal standard method (Heneicosanoic acid—21:0) as previously described for other beverage analysis [14]. A five-point calibration curve was prepared using heneicosanoic acid (21:0 500 ppm injections) and five solutions of heptadecanoic acid (17:0—50, 100, 200, 400, and 800 ppm) methyl ester standards. Five 1 μL injections of each solution were analysed using a Varian 410-GC coupled to a Varian 210-MS equipped with a split/splitless injector (Agilent Technologies, Santa Clara, CA, USA). Separation of the FAME was conducted on an Agilent J&W DB-23 fused silica capillary column (60 m, '0.25 mm i.d.' 0.25 μm f.t.; Agilent Technologies). The ratio of the mean 17:0 to that of the internal standard (21:0) was used as the y-axis variable, while the concentration (ppm) of 17:0 was used as the x-axis variable of the calibration curve. The equation describing the curve was: $y = 0.0041x + 0.12$, with a $R^2 = 0.9969$, where the ratio of the area of the analyte peak to that of the internal standard represents the y value for the equation of the calibration curve and the x value represents the analyte concentration of a selected fatty acid in the lipid sample. The injector temperature of the Varian 410-GC and 210-MS was set at 230 °C with a split ratio of 1:20. The carrier gas was high purity helium with a liner flow rate of 1 mL/min. The oven temperature was initially programmed to 100 °C for 5 min, raised to 240 °C at 3 °C/min, and finally held isothermal at 240 °C for 10 min. Identification of FAME was achieved using a pre-derivatised standard 37-component FAME sample mix and comparison of the retention times and mass spectra of relative peaks with the aid of the Varian Star Chromatography Workstation Version 6 software (Agilent Technologies) and a NIST library of mass spectra (Gaithersburg, MD, USA). The percentage of each fatty acid was calculated using the peak area of the samples corrected by the respective response factors. Analyses were carried out in triplicate.

2.6. Statistical Analysis

All biological experimental analyses, extractions, and GC-MS analyses for each lipid sample were sample were completed in triplicate. The obtained results were expressed as a mean value ± standard deviation (SD). One-way analysis of variance (ANOVA) and the Tukey's honest significant difference (HSD) multiple comparison post-hoc test was used to determine the significant statistical differences between the analyses (SPSS Inc., Chicago, IL, USA).

3. Results

3.1. Lipid Extraction and Fractionation of Beer, and Brewing Materials

The TL, TNL, and TPL content of the beer and brewing materials are shown in Table 1 expressed in either mg/100g or g/100 g of TL, TNL, and TPL. The TNL and TPL are also expressed as a percentage of the TL. The MG and BSG were both considerably low in TL, but the TPL accounted for a substantial amount of the MG, of which just over half seems to be lost to the Brewer's spent grain in the brewing process. The largest amount of TL and TPL present in g/100 g of all samples was the PH, which was significantly higher than all the other samples. Notably the SH had a considerably lower quantity of TL and TPL than the PH, indicating that these lipids may have been extracted and diluted into the wort. However, both the wort and the beer contained extremely low amounts of lipid, the majority of which were polar lipids, results that are in accordance with previously published research [14,32,33].

Table 1. The total lipid (TL) and the total polar lipids (TPL) content of beer and brewing by-product are expressed as g/100 g and the total neutral lipid content (TNL) is expressed as mg/100 g. The TPL and TNL are also expressed as a percentage of the TL (mean ± SD, n = 3).

Sample	TL (g/100 g)	TNL (mg/100 g)	TNL (% TL)	TPL (g/100 g)	TPL (% TL)
MG	0.70 ± 0.10 [a]	100 ± 30 [a]	13.6 ± 2.9 [c]	0.52 ± 0.05 [a]	74.5 ± 3.5 [b]
BSG	1.05 ± 0.19 [a]	550 ± 110 [b]	52.6 ± 2.5 [e]	0.41 ± 0.09 [a]	38.9 ± 2.3 [a]
PH	14.17 ± 2.18 [b]	1630 ± 310 [c]	11.5 ± 3.7 [bc]	11.60 ± 1.68 [b]	79.4 ± 8.6 [bc]
SH	0.75 ± 0.06 [a]	160 ± 10 [a]	21.4 ± 3.0 [d]	0.55 ± 0.07 [a]	72.6 ± 4.1 [b]
Wort	0.03 ± 0.00 [a]	2.0 ± 1.0 [a]	5.4 ± 1.6 [ab]	0.03 ± 0.00 [a]	84.5 ± 8.9 [bc]
Beer	0.02 ± 0.00 [a]	0.3 ± 0.1 [a]	1.7 ± 0.4 [a]	0.02 ± 0.01 [a]	91.3 ± 2.7 [c]

[a,b,c,d,e] Different superscripts indicate significant differences among different lipid extracts within the same lipid class ($p < 0.05$) when means are compared using a Tukey's HSD multiple comparison test. Abbreviations: BSG = brewer's spent grain; MG = malted grain; PH = pelleted hops; SH = spent hops.

3.2. Gas Chromatography-Mass Spectrometry Analysis

While the general lipid composition of beer, wort, barley, and malts have been comprehensively characterised by Bravi and colleagues [32–34], to the best of our knowledge the fatty acid profile of the polar lipids specifically have not been previously reported. Therefore, the fatty acid profile of each TPL extract were assessed by GC-MS (Table 2). Beer consists of many volatile and non-volatile compounds that affect the beer flavour and bioactivities [14,32]. Many of the volatiles and fatty acids in beer are synthesised by yeasts during fermentation, whereas others are derived from the raw materials [32]. Research demonstrates that the dominant fatty acids in the TL of barley grains, wort, and beer are palmitic, stearic, *cis*-oleic, linoleic, and α-linolenic acids [35]. However, little is known about the fatty acid profile of the polar lipid fractions of the raw materials, wort, or the beer itself.

In this study, the MG and BSG had similar TPL fatty acid profiles. Notably, there were statistically significant differences between the MG and BSG in the percentage of palmitic and linoleic acids, where both were higher percentages in the BSG than the MG TPL. Furthermore eicosenoic acid and docosahexaenoic acids were present as a low percentage of the MG but were not detected in the BSG TPL. Additionally, there were significant differences in the TPL fatty acid composition between the MG, BSG, and the beer, namely the TPL fatty acids differed by a higher percentage of SFA and a lower percentage of monounsaturated fatty acids (MUFA) and polyunsaturated fatty acids (PUFA) in the beer TPL in contrast to the MG and BSG. While the MUFA and PUFA were present in lower amounts in the beer compared to the MG and BSG, arachidonic acid was present in the beer in notably high amounts (4.9%) but was not present in the MG or BSG. Furthermore, myristic and stearic acid were also present in a significantly high percentage of the beer TPL in contrast to the MG and BSG. The MG and the wort also differ in composition, as there was a higher percentage of palmitic, stearic, arachidonic, and eicosapentaenoic acids and a lower percentage of linoleic, arachidic, eicosenoic acid, and docosahexaenoic acid with no phytochemicals detected in the MG, BSG, or wort TPL.

Table 2. The fatty acid profile and volatile compounds detected in the total polar lipid (TPL) extracts of each sample are expressed as a percentage of the total volatile components detected by GC-MS (mean ± SD, $n = 3$).

Fatty Acids		Malt Grain	Spent Grain	Pelleted Hops	Spent Hops	Wort	Beer
8:0	Caprylic acid	ND	ND	0.04 ± 0.01^{b}	0.02 ± 0.01^{ab}	0.01 ± 0.00^{a}	ND
10:0	Capric acid	ND	ND	0.06 ± 0.00^{b}	ND	0.01 ± 0.00^{a}	0.02 ± 0.01^{a}
12:0	Lauric acid	0.17 ± 0.02^{d}	ND	0.02 ± 0.00^{a}	0.03 ± 0.01^{a}	0.09 ± 0.01^{c}	0.07 ± 0.00^{b}
12:1	*cis*-Lauroleic acid	ND	ND	0.05 ± 0.01	ND	ND	ND
14:0	Myristic acid	0.62 ± 0.06^{b}	0.69 ± 0.06^{b}	0.33 ± 0.05^{a}	1.04 ± 0.11^{c}	1.58 ± 0.04^{d}	1.55 ± 0.09^{d}
14:1	*cis*-Myristoleic acid	ND	0.41 ± 0.11	ND	ND	ND	ND
15:0	Pentadecylic acid	0.31 ± 0.04^{a}	0.22 ± 0.07^{a}	0.49 ± 0.14^{b}	0.25 ± 0.01^{a}	0.17 ± 0.02^{a}	0.16 ± 0.02^{a}
16:0	Palmitic acid	19.83 ± 0.93^{a}	27.86 ± 0.80^{b}	22.05 ± 1.23^{a}	30.38 ± 1.0^{c}	31.80 ± 0.60^{c}	32.34 ± 0.68^{c}
16:1	*cis*-Palmitoleic acid	0.39 ± 0.04^{a}	0.30 ± 0.12^{a}	2.35 ± 0.26^{c}	1.15 ± 0.15^{b}	0.60 ± 0.02^{a}	0.33 ± 0.21^{a}
17:0	Margaric acid	0.18 ± 0.02^{a}	ND	1.24 ± 0.03^{d}	0.46 ± 0.03^{c}	0.24 ± 0.02^{b}	0.23 ± 0.01^{ab}
17:1	*cis*-Heptadecenoic acid	0.09 ± 0.01^{a}	ND	0.75 ± 0.04^{d}	0.36 ± 0.03^{c}	0.20 ± 0.01^{b}	0.20 ± 0.03^{b}
18:0	Stearic acid	2.63 ± 0.62^{ab}	2.23 ± 0.25^{a}	2.85 ± 0.08^{abc}	3.85 ± 0.18^{d}	3.61 ± 0.09^{cd}	3.32 ± 0.10^{bcd}
18:1 c9	*cis*-Oleic acid	9.04 ± 0.19^{d}	8.81 ± 0.44^{d}	4.39 ± 0.11^{a}	6.67 ± 0.26^{d}	6.12 ± 0.24^{bc}	5.62 ± 0.18^{b}
18:1 t13	*trans*-Oleic acid	0.66 ± 0.02^{a}	1.01 ± 0.09^{ab}	1.27 ± 0.16^{bc}	1.82 ± 0.24^{d}	1.42 ± 0.09^{c}	1.26 ± 0.14^{bc}
18:2 c9, c12	Linoleic acid	56.67 ± 0.77^{e}	51.83 ± 1.59^{d}	25.46 ± 1.5^{a}	40.68 ± 0.34^{b}	44.78 ± 0.06^{c}	43.48 ± 1.55^{bc}
18:3 c6, c9, c12	γ-Linolenic acid	ND	ND	0.58 ± 0.02^{b}	0.12 ± 0.01^{a}	ND	ND
18:3 c9, c12, c15	α-Linolenic acid	6.80 ± 0.95^{abc}	5.87 ± 0.54^{ab}	23.42 ± 1.4^{d}	8.83 ± 0.92^{c}	7.72 ± 0.71^{bc}	5.13 ± 0.26^{a}
20:0	Arachidic acid	0.58 ± 0.10^{ab}	0.78 ± 0.17^{bc}	1.02 ± 0.04^{c}	0.48 ± 0.07^{a}	ND	ND
20:1 c13	Eicosenoic acid	ND	ND	0.25 ± 0.05^{a}	0.54 ± 0.04^{c}	0.39 ± 0.02^{b}	ND
20:2 c11, c14	Eicosadienoic acid	ND	ND	1.00 ± 0.05^{c}	0.49 ± 0.07^{b}	0.27 ± 0.01^{a}	0.31 ± 0.04^{a}
20:4 c5, c8, c11, c14	Arachidonic acid	ND	ND	ND	ND	0.52 ± 0.06	4.93 ± 0.02
20:5 c5, c8, c11, c14, c17	Eicosapentaenoic acid	ND	ND	0.53 ± 0.01^{b}	0.16 ± 0.03^{a}	0.41 ± 0.10^{b}	ND
22:0	Behenic acid	0.30 ± 0.04^{a}	ND	1.32 ± 0.32^{c}	0.72 ± 0.13^{b}	0.41 ± 0.02^{ab}	0.29 ± 0.07^{a}
22:1	Erucic acid	0.32 ± 0.09^{a}	ND	0.41 ± 0.06^{a}	0.34 ± 0.09^{a}	ND	ND
22:6 c4, c7, c10, c13, c16, c19	Docosahexaenoic acid	0.47 ± 0.09^{a}	ND	1.46 ± 0.17^{b}	0.43 ± 0.13^{a}	ND	ND
Σ_{SFA}		24.43 ± 0.70^{a}	31.79 ± 0.94^{b}	29.40 ± 1.32^{b}	37.23 ± 0.91^{c}	37.94 ± 0.60^{c}	37.97 ± 0.54^{c}
Σ_{MUFA}		10.67 ± 0.14^{c}	10.53 ± 0.41^{c}	9.47 ± 0.48^{b}	10.86 ± 0.37^{c}	9.13 ± 0.21^{b}	7.42 ± 0.45^{a}
Σ_{PUFA}		63.95 ± 1.53^{c}	57.69 ± 1.09^{b}	52.87 ± 2.66^{a}	50.71 ± 0.67^{a}	53.69 ± 0.60^{a}	53.75 ± 1.76^{a}

Table 2. *Cont.*

Fatty Acids	Malt Grain	Spent Grain	Pelleted Hops	Spent Hops	Wort	Beer
Volatiles						
Hexanedioic acid	ND	ND	ND	ND	0.28 ± 0.04	1.12 ± 0.21
Aromadendrene oxide	ND	ND	1.77 ± 0.39	0.11 ± 0.02	ND	ND
2,4-Di-*tert*-butylphenol	ND	ND	ND	ND	ND	0.12 ± 0.01
β-Caryophyllene	ND	ND	2.02 ± 0.37 ^{b}	0.37 ± 0.05 ^{a}	ND	0.07 ± 0.01 ^{a}
2-Dodecanone	ND	ND	0.07 ± 0.05	0.04 ± 0.01	ND	ND
Cubenol	ND	ND	0.24 ± 0.18	ND	ND	ND
Tau-Cadinol	ND	ND	0.14 ± 0.08	ND	ND	ND
Tau-Muurolol	ND	ND	0.29 ± 0.02	ND	ND	0.08 ± 0.00
$\Sigma_{Volatiles}$	ND	ND	8.90 ± 0.32 ^{b}	0.95 ± 0.32 ^{a}	0.28 ± 0.04	1.37 ± 0.22 ^{a}

^{a,b,c,d,e} Mean values ± SD (n = 3), different letters in the same row indicate statistically significant differences between the lipid compositions when means are compared using Tukey's HSD multiple comparison test ($p \leq 0.05$). Abbreviations: c = *cis*; MUFA = monounsaturated fatty acids; ND: non-detectable; PUFA = polyunsaturated fatty acids; SFA = saturated fatty acids; t = *trans*.

Another contributing factor to the fatty acid composition of beer is the hops. Hops are known for their high concentrations of volatile components that can impart bitter flavours and aroma to the wort and final product in the brewing process [36]. However, there is relatively little literature addressing the fatty acid compositions of the TL or TPL of hops. In this study, there were significant differences between the fatty acid compositions of the TPL of the PH and the SH. While the total percentage of PUFA in the TPL of the PH and SH were similar, there was a significant increase in the percentage of SFA and MUFA in the SH. However, this is most likely not due to an actual rise in the levels of these fatty acids in the TPL, but may be due to the fact that the PH TPL extract contained a high amount of volatile components that seemed to significantly reduce in the SH. Considering these levels of volatile phytochemicals were not present in the wort or beer in any significant percentages, it is likely that these volatiles were lost during the boiling of the wort, which has been documented previously in studies [37]. Generally, there was a lower percentage of palmitoleic, margaric, and α-linolenic, arachidic, eicosadienoic, docosahexaenoic acids in the SH in contrast to the PH, whereas there was a significantly higher percentage of myristic, palmitic, stearic, *cis*-oleic, *trans*-oleic, and linoleic acids in the SH in contrast to the PH. Furthermore, there was a high percentage of caryophyllene and aromadendrene oxide in the PH TPL.

While the intention of this analysis was to assess the fatty acid profile of the TPL extract, volatile phytochemicals and other constituents were also detected in the TPL extracts of beer, PH, and SH in low percentages. The beer TPL extract contained the highest percentage of phytochemicals at 1.37%, which can mainly be attributed to the detection of adipic acid (or hexanedioic acid). Other compounds identified in the final beer TPL extract were β-caryophyllene, 2,4-Di-*tert*-butylphenol, and tau-muurolol in low percentages. β-caryophyllene and other essential oils were also present in the PH TPL extracts, including tau-muurolol, a cadinene sesquiterpenoid that is a plant metabolite, fungicide, and volatile oil [38], which is commonly found in hops [39]. The PH also contains β-caryophyllene, a bicyclic sesquiterpene that was also present in the beer and SH. β-caryophyllene is a characteristic essential oil of hops that is usually in high abundance in comparison to other phytochemicals [36,40] and is the most abundant phytochemical in the PH and SH TPL extract.

3.3. Platelet Aggregation Assay Analysis

The TL, TNL, and TPL of each extract were assessed for their ability to inhibit PAF and thrombin-induced platelet aggregation in human PRP. The results of the platelet aggregometry assay for all lipid samples are expressed as an IC_{50} value, which is the mass of the lipid sample in micrograms (μg) required to inhibit half (50%) the maximum-reversible PAF/thrombin-induced platelet aggregation. The IC_{50} results for each extract tested against PAF-induced platelet aggregation are presented in Table 3. It is clear from the data presented that overall the TL and TPL are the most bioactive fractions in the various brewing-related extracts. Overall, the TNL extracts generally exhibited poor bioactivity. Notably in the MG, the TNL was slightly more bioactive than the TL, but was less bioactive than the TPL. Furthermore, the BSG TL had an exceedingly low IC_{50}, and thus a higher anti-PAF effect, in comparison to the relative effect of the TNL and TPL. It is not known why this may be the case and further research is required to ascertain whether there may be synergistic effects between the compounds extracted in the TL of the BSG. In terms of the hop extracts, TL, TNL, and TPL IC_{50} values were similar and did not show any statistically significant differences between the PH and the SH. The wort and final beer product were generally the most bioactive TL, TNL, and TPL extracts, although not statistically significantly different from each other.

The IC_{50} results for each lipid extract assessed against thrombin-induced platelet aggregation are presented in Table 4. Similarly to the results of the PAF-induced platelet aggregation assay, it is clear that overall the TL and TPL are the most bioactive fractions in the various brewing-related extracts. The IC_{50} values of the TNL of the MG, BSG, PH, and SH were high, indicating poor inhibition against thrombin. However, the TNL IC_{50} values for the wort and beer were comparable to each other and were considerably lower, and thus more effective against thrombin than the TNL extracts from all other sources. Like the TNL extracts, the TPL of the MG, BSG, PH, and SH were high, indicating poor thrombin inhibition. However, the wort and the beer exhibited extremely low IC_{50} values that were not statistically significantly different from each other. Notably, the TL extracts of the MG, BSG, PH, and SH also possess considerable inhibitory properties against thrombin, although not as potent as the beer or the wort.

Table 3. The in vitro biological activities of the total lipids (TL), total neutral lipids (TNL), and total polar lipids (TPL) of the beer and brewing by-products against platelet-activating factor (PAF)-induced human platelet aggregation, expressed as an IC_{50} in micrograms (μg) of the sample extract. The hPRP concentration was approximately 500,000 platelets μL^{-1}. The final concentration of PAF in the cuvette was 2.6×10^{-8} M. All experimental analyses were carried out in triplicate (mean ± SD, $n = 3$).

Sample	TL	TNL	TPL
MG	495 ± 105 [b]	298 ± 89 [a]	191 ± 58 [ab]
BSG	69 ± 33 [a]	610 ± 136 [b]	617 ± 184 [c]
PH	453 ± 109 [b]	1088 ± 172 [c]	473 ± 280 [c]
SH	519 ± 81 [b]	924 ± 166 [c]	436 ± 142 [bc]
Wort	70 ± 29 [a]	175 ± 61 [a]	58 ± 11 [a]
Beer	6.4 ± 4.5 [a]	248 ± 66 [a]	7.8 ± 3.9 [a]

[a,b,c] Different superscripts indicate significant differences among different lipid extracts within the same lipid class ($p < 0.05$), when means are compared using ANOVA and Tukey's HSD multiple comparison test. Abbreviations: BSG = brewer's spent grain; hPRP = human platelet-rich plasma; MG = malt grain PAF = platelet-activating factor; PH = pelleted hops; SH = spent hops; TL = total lipids; TNL = total neutral lipids; TPL = total polar lipids.

Table 4. The in vitro biological activities of the total lipids (TL), total neutral lipids (TNL), and total polar lipids (TPL) of the beer and brewing by-products against thrombin-induced human platelet aggregation. Results are expressed as an IC_{50} in micrograms (μg) of each lipid extract. The hPRP concentration was approximately 500,000 platelets μL^{-1}. The final concentration of thrombin in the cuvette was 0.1–1.0 mU/mL. All experimental analyses were carried out in triplicate (mean ± SD, $n = 3$).

Sample	TL	TNL	TPL
MG	112 ± 21 [b]	433 ± 77 [b]	247 ± 39 [b]
BSG	87 ± 10 [b]	409 ± 30 [b]	203 ± 49 [b]
PH	221 ± 42 [c]	478 ± 97 [b]	207 ± 51 [b]
SH	155 ± 56 [bc]	572 ± 76 [b]	396 ± 62 [c]
Wort	10 ± 3.7 [a]	165 ± 61 [a]	24 ± 17 [a]
Beer	2.4 ± 0.9 [a]	206 ± 73 [a]	4.3 ± 3.0 [a]

[a,b,c] Different superscripts indicate significant differences among different lipid extracts within the same lipid class ($p < 0.05$), when means are compared using ANOVA with Tukey's HSD multiple comparison test. Abbreviations: BSG = brewer's spent grain; hPRP = human platelet-rich plasma; PAF = platelet-activating factor; MG = malt grain; PH = pelleted hops; SH = spent hops; TL = total lipids; TNL = total neutral lipids; TPL = total polar lipids.

4. Discussion

Previous research has demonstrated that commercial ale, lager, and stout possess potent anti-PAF activities as demonstrated through PAF-induced platelet aggregation assays [14]. Therefore, the aim of this study was to assess the antithrombotic activities and fatty acid composition of brewing raw materials, by-products, wort, and beer from a single production line in an active brewery.

In this study the TL, TNL, and TPL were extracted from the raw materials (MG and PH), by-products (BSG and SH), wort, and Irish red ale, all originating from the same production line. The raw materials used in beer production contain a significant amount of lipids, particularly from the malted barley and hops. However, only trace amounts remain in the final beer product [19]. The lipid content of the MG mix used as a raw material in this study was considerably low (0.7 g/100 g), where other ale malts can possess higher lipid levels between 2.8–3.4 g/100 g as reported by Anness [41]. There are several reasons why the lipid content of the MG was low in this study, including that the lipids of barley tend to form complex interactions making them tightly bound to starch [18], thus making them difficult to extract. It is possible that much of the lipid was not efficiently extracted using the Bligh and Dyer [29] method. This extraction method does not use harsh acid or heat treatments and therefore does not efficiently extract all of the lipids but was chosen for this study as an efficient method for extracting bioactive lipids against platelet aggregation. Indeed, studies have demonstrated a large variation of lipid yield between different extraction procedures, including some being more efficient than others for co-extracting non-lipid substances as part of the crude lipid content [42]. Other studies have also acknowledged that barley lipids are poorly extractable without the use of hot alcoholic extraction [43]. Therefore, further studies should consider the use of other extraction methods.

Notably, the BSG had a non-statistically significant higher lipid content than the malt, but a statistically lower TPL content (~39% of the total lipids). This is in accordance with previous research that estimates that 30% of the barley lipid content is lost during the germination of barley due to the hydrolysis of triglycerides, which are subsequently metabolised [41].

The greatest amount of lipid extracted from any sample was the PH (14.7 g/100 g) with 79% being polar compounds. In hops generally, there is a limited amount of fatty acids (1–2%) present [28]. However, the essential oil content of air-dried female hop flowers (strobiles) is generally around 0.5–3%, whereas waxes and steroids are generally present in trace to high amounts (25%) [44]. Considering that the hops used in this study were dried and pelleted, the oil and fatty acid content was highly concentrated, thus explaining the high lipid content as per Table 1. The hops were added during the boiling process to allow the essential oils present in the hops to contribute to beer flavour and aroma [40]. However, much of the essential oils present in these bittering hops are highly volatile and some are lost during the boiling process to evaporation [37], while any that remain are dispersed in the wort, but may be filtered out during clarification of the wort. At the end of the boiling process, the SH are collected within the trub. As demonstrated in Table 1, the SH contains low levels of lipids. This is most likely due to the pelleted hops being dispersed and rehydrated within the wort and the loss of some volatile compounds from the essential oils during the boiling process. Notably, there was a high percentage of caryophyllene and aromadendrene oxide in the PH TPL. Aromadendrene oxide is an oxygenated sesquiterpene that is considered an essential oil, which exhibits anticancer properties [45].

During the brewing process, a significant proportion of the lipid content is lost to the spent grains [17]. Indeed, in this study the lipid content of the beer and wort were considerably low, but the low beer TL is in accordance with previously published research [14,41]. The presence of lipids in beer is generally considered as a negative proponent due to their effect on foam stabilisation and flavour. Therefore, the reduction of lipid levels is actively reduced where possible through various parts of the clarification processes used by breweries. The low lipid content of beer generally may also be due to the fact that barley contains polar lipids and fatty acids that are closely associated with polysaccharides that create amylose-lipid complexes that are difficult to fully extract [23]. Considering the high TL and TPL content of the BSG, it is likely that this is the case and that these lipids are lost to the BSG.

The fatty acid composition of the TPL extracts of all the brewing ingredients, by-products, wort and beer was determined. While the intention of the GC-MS analysis was to assess the fatty acid profile of the TPL extract, volatile phytochemicals and other constituents were also detected in the TPL extracts of the beer, PH, and SH in low but considerable percentages. The beer TPL extract contained the highest percentage of phytochemicals at 1.37%, which can mainly be attributed to the detection of adipic acid, an unusual non-volatile, alcohol soluble, dicarboxylic acid found sparsely in nature but is used as a food additive (E355) as a firming or raising agent, which has tart flavour and is safe for human consumption in low doses [46]. As it was not an intentional additive in the production of the beer, it is not known where in the brewing process the adipic acid originates from or if it was a contaminant as it was only found in the TPL of the wort and the final beer product.

Phenolic compounds play a significant role in aroma and flavour development in beer production [47]. Present in beer, 2,4-Di-*tert*-butylphenol is a phenolic compound that is produced by a variety of plants, but can also synthesised enzymatically by *S. cerevisiae* from organic acids [48]. Interestingly it is a bioactive compound with potential anticancer effects [49], antioxidant activities, and may be preventative against the neuroinflammatory effects of amyloid beta (Aβ) in animal models of Alzheimer's disease [50]. Considering some phenolic compounds have antiplatelet properties [51], it is yet to be determined whether 2,4-Di-*tert*-butylphenol contributed to the antithrombotic activities observed in this study. Tau-muurolol was also detected, which is a cadinene sesquiterpenoid that is a plant metabolite, fungicide, and volatile oil [52] that was detected in the beer and PH TPL extracts. β-caryophyllene, a bicyclic sesquiterpene was also present in the beer, PH, and SH. β-caryophyllene is a characteristic essential oil of hops that is usually in high abundance in comparison to other phytochemicals [36,40] and is the most abundant phytochemical in the PH and SH TPL extract. Notably, caryophyllene compounds may possess anticancer, analgesic, antioxidant, antimicrobial, and anti-inflammatory activities [53]. Indeed, caryophyllene molecules were present in abundance in essential oil extracts from 25 species of plants that demonstrated anti-platelet activity against adenosine diphosphate (ADP), arachidonic acid, and the thromboxane A_2 agonist U46619-induced platelet aggregation in guinea pig and rat plasma [54].

PAF and thrombin-induced platelet aggregation assays were used to assess the antithrombotic activity of the TL, TNL, and TPL extracts of the brewing raw materials, by-products, wort, and beer. Generally, the TPL extracts were the most potent against PAF-induced platelet aggregation. The TL extracts exhibited considerable anti-PAF and anti-thrombin effects, but generally the TPL extracts were more potent against PAF, whereas in the case of thrombin, the TL in cases were considerably more antithrombotic than the TNL and moderately more potent that the TPL extracts. Considering, the overall poorer inhibitory effects of both the TNL and TPL extracts of the MG, BSG, PH, and SH against thrombin, the compounds present in the combined TL extract may induce synergistic effects that improve the antithrombotic properties of these extracts, as has previously been demonstrated in beer [14] and other extracts of natural origin marine extracts [55]. It can be suggested that coextracted microconstituents such as phenolic compounds and phytochemicals with potential antithrombotic activities may in part be responsible for these observations as previously demonstrated [51]. Indeed, considering the BSG possessed potent anti-PAF and anti-thrombin activities, these by-products of the brewing industry could potentially be used in the development of nutraceuticals or functional foods and animal feeds, as has previously been demonstrated using by-products of the olive oil industry [56]. Indeed, BSG contains other significant bioactive microconstituents such as peptides and phenolic compounds that exhibit antioxidant activity [26] that supports the need for further research into the valorisation of BSG as a functional product for human health.

The beer and wort extracts were the most bioactive fractions against PAF and thrombin. While not deemed statistically significantly different, the bioactivity of the TL and TPL of the wort seemed to increase considerably following fermentation. Previous studies in dairy products have shown that the fermentation process may play a role in the biosynthesis of functional antithrombotic lipids [57]. However, it has yet to be confirmed whether *S. cerevisiae* can indeed biosynthesise antithrombotic polar lipids, but this study does demonstrate that yeasts may affect the fatty acid composition of the polar lipids. Further structure activity relationship studies are required to confirm this notion.

As depicted in Table 2, there is a statistically significant increase in the percentage of polar lipids bearing fatty acids arachidonic acid and eicosapentaenoic acid (EPA) in their structures as a result or the wort fermentation. Various studies have demonstrated that polar lipids of natural origin that bear these fatty acids in their structures along with stearic, cis-oleic, and linoleic acids, all of which are present in abundance in the beer and wort TPL, exhibit potent antithrombotic properties against PAF-induced platelet aggregation [9]. Similarly, the beer (red ale) TL and TPL IC_{50} values obtained in this study were similar to those published for Smithwick's red ale TL and TPL against PAF-induced platelet aggregation using the same methods [27]. The fatty acid compositions of the wort and beer TPL share structural resemblance to the classical PAF structure, which is generally composed of palmitic (68%), stearic (27%), or oleic (4%) acids at the *sn*-1 position, with acetic acid esterified to the *sn*-2 position, and a phosphocholine group at the *sn*-3 position [58]. Juxtaposed, the most abundant fatty acids of the TPL of the wort were palmitic (31.8%), stearic (3.6%), oleic (6.1%), and linoleic (44.8%)

acids and the most abundant fatty acids present in the TPL of the beer were palmitic (32.3%), stearic (3.3%), oleic (5.6%), and linoleic (43.4%) acids. Further research is required to confirm whether there is structural homology between some polar lipids and PAF, which facilitates their binding to the PAF-R, which may account for their potent biological actions against PAF.

In contrast to the wealth of evidence demonstrating that polar lipids can inhibit the biological actions of PAF, there is little published research demonstrating the mechanisms for the antiplatelet effects of food-derived polar lipids against thrombin-induced platelet aggregation. It seems that the amphiphilic properties of these bioactive polar lipid moieties expedite their transfer from blood lipoproteins to the membranes of circulating platelets. Thus such bioactive polar lipids can either directly affect several platelet membrane receptors related to platelet activation (i.e. binding of polar lipids to the PAF-R) [31] or indirectly affect these platelet receptors. Polar lipids may indirectly affect platelet receptors through altering the microenvironment and polarisation of the phospholipid membrane, which potentially alters the affinity of a ligand to a receptor relating to platelet activation, such as thrombin [9,31,59,60]. However, further research is required to verify these potential mechanisms and to discern the structures of these compounds, in order to fully elucidate the structure activity relationships between bioactive polar lipid extracts and their overall antiplatelet effects.

5. Conclusions

The antithrombotic activities of lipid extracts from brewing raw materials, by-products, wort, and beer were assessed. The most bioactive anti-PAF and anti-thrombin polar lipid extracts originated from the wort and the final beer product. While not statistically significantly different, it is apparent that fermentation of the wort may play a key role in increasing the anti-PAF bioactivity of polar lipids extracted from beer. These findings are in accordance with previous studies demonstrating that fermentation plays a key role in altering the bioactivity of anti-PAF polar lipids during milk fermentation. Indeed, this research supports and furthers previously published research demonstrating the presence of potent anti-PAF polar lipids in red ale. It was also observed that some phytochemicals and phenolic compounds may contribute to antithrombotic properties of these lipid extracts. Furthermore, this is the first study to demonstrate the anti-thrombin activities of beer polar lipids, but further research is required to discern the exact structures and mechanisms responsible for these observations. Moreover, it was determined that the BSG may be a suitable brewing industry by-product for valorisation as potential nutraceuticals or functional foods for improved human cardiovascular health.

Author Contributions: The study was conceptualized by I.Z., R.L., and A.T. The methods were developed by R.L. and A.T.; All experiments and interpretation of results were performed by E.O., R.L., and A.T. The manuscript was prepared by R.L. and A.T. and all authors reviewed and approved the final submission.

Acknowledgments: The authors would like to express their sincere gratitude to Padraig Hyde and Adrian Hyde of Munster Brewery for their kind donation of their time, expertise, beer, and brewing materials for this study. The authors would also like to thank all the volunteers for their donations, Elaine Ahern for her phlebotomy support, and the Department of Biological Science, University of Limerick, Ireland for their continued support.

References

1. Tsoupras, A.; Lordan, R.; Zabetakis, I. Inflammation, not cholesterol, is a cause of chronic disease. *Nutrients* **2018**, *10*, 604. [CrossRef] [PubMed]
2. Schwarzinger, M.; Thiébaut, S.P.; Baillot, S.; Mallet, V.; Rehm, J. Alcohol use disorders and associated chronic disease—A national retrospective cohort study from france. *BMC Public Health* **2017**, *18*, 43. [CrossRef]
3. Lordan, R.; Tsoupras, A.; Zabetakis, I. The potential role of dietary platelet-activating factor inhibitors in cancer prevention and treatment. *Adv. Nutr.* **2019**, *10*, 148–164. [CrossRef] [PubMed]
4. Nogueira, L.C.; do Rio, R.F.; Lollo, P.C.B.; Ferreira, I.M.P.L.V.O. Moderate alcoholic beer consumption: The effects on the lipid profile and insulin sensitivity of adult men. *J. Food Sci.* **2017**, *82*, 1720–1725. [CrossRef] [PubMed]

5. Arranz, S.; Chiva-Blanch, G.; Valderas-Martínez, P.; Medina-Remón, A.; Lamuela-Raventós, R.M.; Estruch, R. Wine, beer, alcohol and polyphenols on cardiovascular disease and cancer. *Nutrients* **2012**, *4*, 759. [CrossRef]
6. De Gaetano, G.; Costanzo, S.; Di Castelnuovo, A.; Badimon, L.; Bejko, D.; Alkerwi, A.; Chiva-Blanch, G.; Estruch, R.; La Vecchia, C.; Panico, S.; et al. Effects of moderate beer consumption on health and disease: A consensus document. *Nutr. Metab. Cardiovasc. Dis.* **2016**, *26*, 443–467. [CrossRef]
7. Lombardi, G.; Vannini, S.; Blasi, F.; Marcotullio, M.C.; Dominici, L.; Villarini, M.; Cossignani, L.; Moretti, M. In vitro safety/protection assessment of resveratrol and pterostilbene in a human hepatoma cell line (HepG2). *Nat. Prod. Commun.* **2015**, *10*, 1403–1408. [CrossRef]
8. Lordan, R.; Nasopoulou, C.; Tsoupras, A.; Zabetakis, I. The anti-inflammatory properties of food polar lipids. In *Bioactive Molecules in Food*; Mérillon, J.M., Ramawat, K.G., Eds.; Springer International Publishing: Cham, Switzerland, 2018; pp. 1–34.
9. Lordan, R.; Tsoupras, A.; Zabetakis, I. Phospholipids of animal and marine origin: Structure, function, and anti-inflammatory properties. *Molecules* **2017**, *22*, 1964. [CrossRef]
10. Jaberi, N.; Soleimani, A.; Pashirzad, M.; Abdeahad, H.; Mohammadi, F.; Khoshakhlagh, M.; Khazaei, M.; Ferns, G.A.; Avan, A.; Hassanian, S.M. Role of thrombin in the pathogenesis of atherosclerosis. *J. Cell. Biochem.* **2019**, *120*, 4757–4765. [CrossRef]
11. Li, Z.; Delaney, M.K.; O'Brien, K.A.; Du, X. Signaling during platelet adhesion and activation. *Arterioscler. Thromb. Vasc. Biol.* **2010**, *30*, 2341–2349. [CrossRef]
12. Tsopanoglou, N.E.; Maragoudakis, M.E. Thrombin's central role in angiogenesis and pathophysiological processes. *Eur. Cytokine Netw.* **2009**, *20*, 171–179.
13. Jennings, L.K. Mechanisms of platelet activation: Need for new strategies to protect against platelet-mediated atherothrombosis. *Thromb. Haemost.* **2009**, *101*, 248–257. [CrossRef]
14. Lordan, R.; O'Keeffe, E.; Dowling, D.; Mullally, M.; Heffernan, H.; Tsoupras, A.; Zabetakis, I. The in vitro antithrombotic properties of ale, lager, and stout beers. *Food Biosci.* **2019**, *28*, 83–88. [CrossRef]
15. Seefeldt, H.F.; Larsen, F.H.; Viereck, N.; Petersen, M.A.; Engelsen, S.B. Lipid composition and deposition during grain filling in intact barley (hordeum vulgare) mutant grains as studied by ^{1}H HR MAS NMR. *J. Cereal Sci.* **2011**, *54*, 442–449. [CrossRef]
16. Shewry, P.R. Chapter 7-minor components of the barley grain: Minerals, lipids, terpenoids, phenolics, and vitamins. In *Barley*, 2nd ed.; Shewry, P.R., Ullrich, S.E., Eds.; AACC International Press: St. Paul, MI, USA, 2014; pp. 169–192.
17. Cozzolino, D.; Degner, S. An overview on the role of lipids and fatty acids in barley grain and their products during beer brewing. *Food Res. Int.* **2016**, *81*, 114–121. [CrossRef]
18. Marion, D.; Dubreil, L.; Douliez, J.-P. Functionality of lipids and lipid-protein interactions in cereal-derived food products. *OCL* **2003**, *10*, 47–56. [CrossRef]
19. Olšovská, J.; Vrzal, T.; Štěrba, K.; Slabý, M.; Kubizniaková, P.; Čejka, P. The chemical profiling of fatty acids during the brewing process. *J. Sci. Food Agric.* **2019**, *99*, 1772–1779. [CrossRef]
20. Bamforth, C.W. Progress in brewing science and beer production. *Annu. Rev. Chem. Biomol. Eng.* **2017**, *8*, 161–176. [CrossRef]
21. Moonjai, N.; Verstrepen, K.J.; Shen, H.Y.; Derdelinckx, G.; Verachtert, H.; Delvaux, F.R. Linoleic acid supplementation of a cropped brewing lager strain: Effects on subsequent fermentation performance with serial repitching. *J. I. Brew.* **2003**, *109*, 262–272. [CrossRef]
22. Moonjai, N.; Verstrepen, K.J.; Delvaux, F.R.; Derdelinckx, G.; Verachtert, H. The effects of linoleic acid supplementation of cropped yeast on its subsequent fermentation performance and acetate ester synthesis. *J. Inst. Brew.* **2002**, *108*, 227–235. [CrossRef]
23. Gordon, R.; Power, A.; Chapman, J.; Chandra, S.; Cozzolino, D. A review on the source of lipids and their interactions during beer fermentation that affect beer quality. *Fermentation* **2018**, *4*, 89. [CrossRef]
24. Olajire, A.A. The brewing industry and environmental challenges. *J. Clean. Prod.* **2012**. [CrossRef]
25. Mussatto, S.; Dragone, G.; Roberto, I. Brewers' spent grain: Generation, characteristics and potential applications. *J. Cereal Sci.* **2006**, *43*, 1–14. [CrossRef]
26. Connolly, A.; Piggott, C.O.; FitzGerald, R.J. Characterisation of protein-rich isolates and antioxidative phenolic extracts from pale and black brewers' spent grain. *Int. J. Food Sci. Technol.* **2013**, *48*, 1670–1681. [CrossRef]
27. Niemi, P.; Tamminen, T.; Smeds, A.; Viljanen, K.; Ohra-aho, T.; Holopainen-Mantila, U.; Faulds, C.B.;

Poutanen, K.; Buchert, J. Characterization of lipids and lignans in brewer's spent grain and its enzymatically extracted fraction. *J. Agric. Food Chem.* **2012**, *60*, 9910–9917. [CrossRef] [PubMed]

28. Dos Santos Mathias, T.R.; de Mello, P.P.M.; ervulo, E.F.C. Solid wastes in brewing process: A review. *J. Brew. Distill.* **2014**, *5*, 1–9.
29. Bligh, E.G.; Dyer, W.J. A rapid method of total lipid extraction and purification. *Can. J. Biochem. Physiol.* **1959**, *37*, 911–917. [CrossRef] [PubMed]
30. Tsoupras, A.; Zabetakis, I.; Lordan, R. Platelet aggregometry assay for evaluating the effects of platelet agonists and antiplatelet compounds on platelet function in vitro. *MethodsX* **2019**, *6*, 63–70. [CrossRef]
31. Tsoupras, A.; Lordan, R.; Shiels, K.; Saha, S.K.; Nasopoulou, C.; Zabetakis, I. In vitro antithrombotic properties of salmon (*salmo salar*) phospholipids in a novel food-grade extract. *Mar. Drugs* **2019**, *17*, 62. [CrossRef]
32. Bravi, E.; Marconi, O.; Sileoni, V.; Perretti, G. Determination of free fatty acids in beer. *Food Chem.* **2017**, *215*, 341–346. [CrossRef]
33. Bravi, E.; Benedetti, P.; Marconi, O.; Perretti, G. Determination of free fatty acids in beer wort. *Food Chem.* **2014**, *151*, 374–378. [CrossRef]
34. Bravi, E.; Marconi, O.; Perretti, G.; Fantozzi, P. Influence of barley variety and malting process on lipid content of malt. *Food Chem.* **2012**, *135*, 1112–1117. [CrossRef]
35. Evans, D.E.; Goldsmith, M.; Redd, K.S.; Nischwitz, R.; Lentini, A. Impact of mashing conditions on extract, its fermentability, and the levels of wort free amino nitrogen (fan), β-glucan, and lipids. *J. Am. Soc. Brew. Chem.* **2012**, *70*, 39–49. [CrossRef]
36. Michiu, D.; Socaci, S.A.; Jimborean, M.A.; Mudura, E.; Fărcaş, A.C.; Biriş-Dorhoi, S.E.; Tofană, M. Determination of volatile markers from magnum hops in beer by in-tube extraction—gas chromatography-mass spectrometry. *Anal. Lett.* **2018**, *51*, 2967–2980. [CrossRef]
37. Praet, T.; Van Opstaele, F.; De Causmaecker, B.; Aerts, G.; De Cooman, L. Heat-induced changes in the composition of varietal hop essential oils via wort boiling on a laboratory scale. *J. Am. Soc. Brew. Chem.* **2016**, *74*, 212–223. [CrossRef]
38. Yoon, M.-Y.; Cha, B.; Kim, J.-C. Recent trends in studies on botanical fungicides in agriculture. *Plant Pathol. J.* **2013**, *29*, 1–9. [CrossRef]
39. Bocquet, L.; Sahpaz, S.; Hilbert, J.L.; Rambaud, C.; Rivière, C. Humulus lupulus l., a very popular beer ingredient and medicinal plant: Overview of its phytochemistry, its bioactivity, and its biotechnology. *Phytochem. Rev.* **2018**, *17*, 1047–1090. [CrossRef]
40. Eyres, G.; Dufour, J.-P. 22-hop essential oil: Analysis, chemical composition and odor characteristics. In *Beer in Health and Disease Prevention*; Preedy, V.R., Ed.; Academic Press: San Diego, CA, USA, 2009; pp. 239–254.
41. Anness, B.J. Lipids of barley, malt and adjuncts. *J. I. Brew.* **1984**, *90*, 315–318. [CrossRef]
42. Blasi, F.; Montesano, D.; Simonetti, M.S.; Cossignani, L. A simple and rapid extraction method to evaluate the fatty acid composition and nutritional value of goji berry lipid. *Food Anal. Method.* **2017**, *10*, 970–979. [CrossRef]
43. Morrison, W.R.; Coventry, A.M. Extraction of lipids from cereal starches with hot aqueous alcohols. *Starch Stärke* **1985**, *37*, 83–87. [CrossRef]
44. Almaguer, C.; Schönberger, C.; Gastl, M.; Arendt, E.K.; Becker, T. Humulus lupulus—A story that begs to be told. A review. *J. I. Brew.* **2014**, *120*, 289–314. [CrossRef]
45. Pavithra, P.S.; Mehta, A.; Verma, R.S. Aromadendrene oxide 2, induces apoptosis in skin epidermoid cancer cells through ROS mediated mitochondrial pathway. *Life Sci.* **2018**, *197*, 19–29. [CrossRef]
46. Kennedy, G.L. Toxicity of adipic acid. *Drug Chem. Toxicol.* **2002**, *25*, 191–202. [CrossRef]
47. Lentz, M. The impact of simple phenolic compounds on beer aroma and flavor. *Fermentation* **2018**, *4*, 20. [CrossRef]
48. Shinohara, T.; Kubodera, S.; Yanagida, F. Distribution of phenolic yeasts and production of phenolic off-flavors in wine fermentation. *J. Biosci. Bioeng.* **2000**, *90*, 90–97. [CrossRef]
49. Varsha, K.K.; Devendra, L.; Shilpa, G.; Priya, S.; Pandey, A.; Nampoothiri, K.M. 2,4-di-tert-butyl phenol as the antifungal, antioxidant bioactive purified from a newly isolated lactococcus sp. *Int. J. Food Microbiol.* **2015**, *211*, 44–50. [CrossRef] [PubMed]
50. Choi, S.J.; Kim, J.K.; Kim, H.K.; Harris, K.; Kim, C.-J.; Park, G.G.; Park, C.-S.; Shin, D.-H. 2,4-di-tert-butylphenol

from sweet potato protects against oxidative stress in pc12 cells and in mice. *J. Med. Food* **2013**, *16*, 977–983. [CrossRef]

51. Bijak, M.; Ziewiecki, R.; Saluk, J.; Ponczek, M.; Pawlaczyk, I.; Krotkiewski, H.; Wachowicz, B.; Nowak, P. Thrombin inhibitory activity of some polyphenolic compounds. *Med. Chem. Res.* **2014**, *23*, 2324–2337. [CrossRef] [PubMed]
52. Policegoudra, R.S.; Goswami, S.; Aradhya, S.M.; Chatterjee, S.; Datta, S.; Sivaswamy, R.; Chattopadhyay, P.; Singh, L. Bioactive constituents of homalomena aromatica essential oil and its antifungal activity against dermatophytes and yeasts. *J. Mycol. Med.* **2012**, *22*, 83–87. [CrossRef]
53. Fidyt, K.; Fiedorowicz, A.; Strządała, L.; Szumny, A. Β-caryophyllene and β-caryophyllene oxide-natural compounds of anticancer and analgesic properties. *Cancer Med.* **2016**, *5*, 3007–3017. [CrossRef]
54. Tognolini, M.; Barocelli, E.; Ballabeni, V.; Bruni, R.; Bianchi, A.; Chiavarini, M.; Impicciatore, M. Comparative screening of plant essential oils: Phenylpropanoid moiety as basic core for antiplatelet activity. *Life Sci.* **2006**, *78*, 1419–1432. [CrossRef]
55. Nasopoulou, C.; Karantonis, H.C.; Andriotis, M.; Demopoulos, C.A.; Zabetakis, I. Antibacterial and anti-PAF activity of lipid extracts from sea bass (Dicentrarchus labrax) and gilthead sea bream (Sparus aurata). *Food Chem.* **2008**, *111*, 433–438. [CrossRef]
56. Sioriki, E.; Smith, T.K.; Demopoulos, C.A.; Zabetakis, I. Structure and cardioprotective activities of polar lipids of olive pomace, olive pomace-enriched fish feed and olive pomace fed gilthead sea bream (*Sparus aurata*). *Food Res. Int.* **2016**, *83*, 143–151. [CrossRef]
57. Lordan, R.; Walsh, A.M.; Crispie, F.; Finnegan, L.; Cotter, P.D.; Zabetakis, I. The effect of ovine milk fermentation on the antithrombotic properties of polar lipids. *J. Funct. Foods* **2019**, *54*, 289–300. [CrossRef]
58. Demopoulos, C.A.; Karantonis, H.C.; Antonopoulou, S. Platelet-activating factor—A molecular link between atherosclerosis theories. *Eur. J. Lipid Sci. Technol.* **2003**, *105*, 705–716. [CrossRef]
59. Mori, T.A.; Beilin, L.J.; Burke, V.; Morris, J.; Ritchie, J. Interactions between dietary fat, fish, and fish oils and their effects on platelet function in men at risk of cardiovascular disease. *Arterioscler. Thromb. Vasc. Biol.* **1997**, *17*, 279–286. [CrossRef]
60. Yoshida, K.; Nagatoishi, S.; Kuroda, D.; Suzuki, N.; Murata, T.; Tsumoto, K. Phospholipid membrane fluidity alters ligand binding activity of a g protein-coupled receptor by shifting the conformational equilibrium. *Biochemistry* **2019**, *58*, 504–508. [CrossRef]

5

Isolation of *Penicillium citrinum* from Roots of *Clerodendron cyrtophyllum* and Application in Biosynthesis of Aglycone Isoflavones from Soybean Waste Fermentation

Duy Tien Doan [1], Duc Phuong Luu [1], Thanh Duong Nguyen [1], Bich Hoang Thi [2], Hong Minh Pham Thi [2,3], Huu Nghi Do [2,3], Van Huyen Luu [4], The Dan Pham [2,5], Van Thai Than [6], Hai Ha Pham Thi [7,*], Minh Quan Pham [2,3] and Quoc Toan Tran [2,3,*]

1. Institute of Chemistry, Vietnam Academy of Science and Technology, 18 Hoang Quoc Viet St., Cau Giay Dist., Hanoi 10072, Vietnam; doanduytien@yahoo.com (D.T.D.); luuphuongtheday@gmail.com (D.P.L.); ntduong182@gmail.com (T.D.N.)
2. Institute of Natural Products Chemistry, Vietnam Academy of Science and Technology, 18 Hoang Quoc Viet St., Cau Giay Dist., Hanoi 10072, Vietnam; bichhoang.inpc@gmail.com (B.H.T.); minhhcsh@gmail.com (H.M.P.T.); dohnghi@gmail.com (H.N.D.); danpt.bi9064@st.usth.edu.vn (T.D.P.); minhquanaries@gmail.com (M.Q.P.)
3. Graduate University of Science and Technology, Vietnam Academy of Science and Technology, Hanoi 10072, Vietnam
4. Hanoi University of Natural Resources and Environment, Hanoi 10072, Vietnam; lvhuyen@hunre.edu.vn
5. Vietnam Academy of Science and Technology, University of Science and Technology of Hanoi, Hanoi 10072, Vietnam
6. NTT Institute of High Technology, Nguyen Tat Thanh University, Ho Chi Minh City 700000, Vietnam; tvthai@ntt.edu.vn
7. Faculty of Biotechnology, Nguyen Tat Thanh University, Ho Chi Minh City 700000, Vietnam

* Correspondence: pthha@ntt.edu.vn (H.H.P.T.); tranquoctoan2010@gmail.com (Q.T.T.)

Abstract: Soybeans offer an abundant source of isoflavones, which confer useful bioactivities when existing in aglycone forms. The conversion of isoflavones into aglycones via fermentation of soybean products is often realized by β-glucosidase, an enzyme produced by fungi. In this study, a filamentous fungus, *Clerodendron cyrtophyllum*, was isolated from root of *Clerodendron cyrtophyllum* Turcz, which was able to produce the highest activity of β-glucosidase up to 33.72 U/mL at 144 h during fermentation on Potato Dextrose Broth (PDB). The obtained fungus was grown on isoflavones-rich soybean extract to produce genistein and daidzein, achieving the conversion rate of 98.7%. Genistein and daidzein were isolated and purified by column chromatography using hexane/acetone (29:1/1:1), reaching purities of over 90% of total isoflavones, as identified and determined by TLC, LC-MS/MS, and ^1H and ^{13}C NMR spectroscopy. These results imply that the isolated *P. citrinum* is a potential fungal strain for industrial-scale production of genistein and daidzein from isoflavones-containing soybean extracts. These products may serve as potential raw materials for manufacture of functional foods that are based on aglycones.

Keywords: *Penicillium citrinum*; β-glucosidase; soybean extract; fermentation; isoflavones; aglycones

1. Introduction

Isoflavones are polyphenolics that exert estrogen-like effects and have been widely utilized in manufacture of foods and cosmetics [1]. Isoflavones exhibit a myriad of bioactivities including protecting against colon cancer and aging skin, easing postmenopausal symtoms in women, reducing the risk of osteoporosis, preventing cardiovascular disease, having antimutagenic, antioxidant, and anti-inflammatory effects, and acting as tyrosine kinase enzyme inhibitors [1,2]. Since the intestinal absorption of isoflavone in aglycone form, particularly geistein, is more expedited than in the glycosylated form, most beneficial biological properties have been suggested to originate from aglycone isoflavone [2]. However, the content of aglycones is significantly lower than that of the glycoside counterpart, accounting for only 5% of total isoflavones. Structurally, the phenolic group of isoflavones is bonded to glycosides and primary hydroxyl group of glucose moiety is bonded to 6-O-acetyl or 6-O-malonyl derivatives. It has been shown that isoflavones existed in 12 isomers: three free isoflavones (aglycones) and nine linked isoflavones (glucosides) [3–6].

In traditional Asian diets, the main supply of isoflavones is from soybean (*Glycine max*) [7]. Soybean contains a large amount of bioactive subtances such as isoflavones, saponin, phytosterol, protease inhibitor, inositol hexaphosphate, and trypsin inhibitors [8]. As the bioavailability of soy isoflavone aglycones is superior to that of the glycoside forms, the isolation of isoflavone aglycones from soy products as well as production of aglycones for pharmaceutical and functional food applications have attracted research interest recently [9,10].

Industrial production of soybean oil generates byproducts such as soapstocks and soy cakes. While the former, which is rich in fatty acids [11], could be utilized in production of animal feeds, soap, nonpetroleum waxes, and biofuels, the latter was recently suggested to play an important part in the biotechnological production of several high-added value chemicals, such as fumaric acid by fungi, carotenoids by yeasts, and polyol esters and wax esters by the enzymatic synthesis [12–14]. The production of such soybean-derived products are realized via various techniques including saponification [15], esterification, and enzymatic hydrolysis [16].

The common production technique of aglycones involves hydrolysis of isoflavone glucosides using chemical catalysts (e.g., bases or acids) [8]. Alternatively, the transformation of isoflavones glycosides to aglycones can be also achieved during soybean germination as a natural occurence or by selective enzymatic hydrolysis and fermentation with β-glucosidase-producing microorganisms [17–21]. The latter has attracted considerable attention by researchers as a green approach.

β-Glucosidase (β β -D-glucoside glucohydrolase; EC 3.2.1.21), an exocellulase responsible for the hydrolysis of the O-glycosyl linkage of terminal nonreducing β-D-glucosyl residues releasing β-D-glucose, e.g., the bond in cellobiose, has been the enzyme of interest in large scale production via fermentation with microbes [22,23]. To be specific, feasible microbes that have been utilized in β-glucosidase production include *Aspergillus* niger [24,25], *A. oryzae* [26], *Penicillium* brasilianum [27], *Phanerochaete chrysosporium* [28], *Aspergillus* oryzae [29], *Thermofilum pendens* [30], yeasts (mostly *Candida* sp.) and several bacterial species. Even though fermentation to produce β-glucosidase for hydrolysis using *A. niger*, a filamentous fungus, is popular and has been the standard in commercial β-glucosidase production [31], emerging approaches utilize various strains from the *Penicillium* genus [27]. These new techniques also produce lipase and esterase, which act as catalysts for hydrolysis of ester groups of 6-O-acetyl and 6-O-malonyl isoflavones derivatives for activation of hydrolysis of glycosides by β-glucosidase.

In this work, multiple β-glucosidases-producing fungi were isolated and screened from roots of the *Clerodendron cyrtophyllum* Turcz plant. The fungal strain that exhibited the highest β-glucosidase activity was selected and then used for fermentation of isoflavones-rich soybean extract to produce aglycones, genistein, and daidzein. The products were identified and determined by thin layer chromatography (TLC), liquid chromatography-tandem mass spectrometry (LC-MS/MS), and nuclear magnetic resonance (NMR).

2. Materials and Methods

2.1. Materials

Sabouraud-2% dextrose Broth (SDB), Sabouraud-4% glucose-Agar (SA), potato dextrose broth (PDB), potato dextrose agar (PDA), p-nitrophenyl-β-D-glucopyranoside (pNPG), p-nitrophenol (pNP), and methylene blue were purchased from Merck KGaA (Darmstadt, Germany). Roots of *Clerodendron cyrtophyllum* Turcz, locally collected at Hoai Duc ward, Hanoi, Vietnam, were coarsely ground to the size of 5 mm and then were divided equally to two parts. One part was subjected to sun drying and sterilization using UV light for 10 min while the other part was stored in gunny bags. The sized *C. cyrtophyllum* Turcz's roots were used for isolation of the β-glucosidase-producing fungi. Oil-extracted soybean residue (dry form) (*Glycine max* L.) was purchased from T&H Agriculture and Technology, JSC (Hanoi, Vietnam).

2.2. Isolation of Microorganisms

Fungal strains were isolated by serial dilution [32]. Briefly, 1 g of the sized *C. cyrtophyllum* Turcz's roots was mixed with 10 mL of sterile deionized water. The following serial dilution was performed to 10^{-5} and 0.1 mL of the suspension was dispersed onto the sterilized PDA agar plates, which were allowed to stand for 72 h at 30 °C to promote fungal growth. Different types of fungi were isolated. They were then subcultured on sterilized PDA plates several times to obtain pure cultures, which were maintained at 4 °C for further study.

2.3. Fungal Identification

The fungal cultures were obtained by repeatedly transferring onto sterilized PDA plates and inoculated at 30 °C for 72 h. After inoculation, characteristics such as color and size of colonies during the growth was monitored and recorded. A little amount of mycelial mat was placed on clean glass slide and then stained with methylene blue. These slides were microscopically analyzed for morphological characteristics. Fungal isolates were identified by comparing these characteristics with those listed in standard reference book [33].

To prepare DNA, each fungal strain was cultured and incubated on PDA plates for three days at 30 °C. Purelink Genomic DNA Kits (Life Technology, ThermoFisher Scientific, Massachusetts, USA) was used to obtain DNA from the hyphae of the isolate. Two primer pairs, ITS1 (5′-TCCGTAGGTGAACCTGCGG-3′) and ITS4 (5′-TCCTCCGCTTATTTGATATGC-3′) were used to perform the amplification of the the internal transcribed spacer region (ITS) of the nuclear ribosomal DNA operon [34]. PCR experiments were performed as follows. First, a 20 μL mixture containing 5–50 ng of DNA, AccuPrep PCR premix (Bioneer, Daejeon, South Korea), and 5 pmol of each primer was created. The mixture was first denatured at 95 °C for 5 min. Afterwards, a total of 30 cycles of denaturation, annealing, and extension took place with the elapsed time of 30 s in each cycle. Temperature for the three processes was 95, 48, and 72 °C, respectively. The protocol concluded with extension at 72 °C for 7 min. Electrophoretic characterization of the obtained PCR products was performed in 1% agarose gel. Obtained genomic sequences were referenced to GenBank via BLAST search tool (http://blast.ncbi.nlm.nih.gov/Blast.cgi) and were found to be in line with reported sequences.

2.4. Enzymatic Activity

Fungal strains were maintained on PDA at 30 °C with periodic transfer of five days. Inoculum was prepared by growing the fungal mycelium in 100 mL sterilized basal medium, which consisted of 2 g/L $(NH_4)_2SO_4$, 1 g/L KH_2PO_4, 0.4 g/L $MgSO_4{\cdot}7H_2O$, and 0.5 g/L $CaCl_2$ (pH = 5.6) and 10% (*w/v*) PDB as carbon source in 250 mL Erlenmeyer conical flasks. Incubation was carried out at 120 rpm using a rotary shaker, at 30 °C for 72 h. After incubation, β-glucosidases produced by different fungi strains in flasks were extracted by supplementing with potassium phosphate buffer 20 mM (pH = 6), followed by shaking at 200 rpm for 1 h and then filted by using membrane Supro 450 size 0.45 um (Pall, Ann Arbor, MI, USA). The obtained filtrates were used as crude enzymes. The hydrolysis of p-nitrophenyl-β-D-glucopyranoside (pNPβG) substrate was taken as the measure for β-glucosidase activity of fungi [35]. The reaction mixture contained 30 μL of appropriately aliquot (the filtrate) from incubated flask, 60 μL of pNPβG and 210 μL of acetate buffer. The reaction commenced at 50 °C for 60 min, followed by addition of 300 μL of 1 M Na_2CO_3. The resultant release of p-nitrophenol (pNP) caused color change, which was measured spectrophotometrically at 410 nm. The enzyme quantity required to maintain the pNP release rate of 1 μmol per minute is equivalent to one unit of β-glucosidase activity.

2.5. *Optimization of the β-Glucosidase Production*

The incubation of *Penicillium citrinum* was carried out in a 250 mL Erlenmeyer flask containing 100 mL of described basal medium under rotary shaking at 120 rpm at 30 °C for seven days. β-glucosidase activity was determined at different intervals starting from the beginning of incubation, including 24, 48, 72, 96, 120, 144, and 168 h, using the aforementioned procedure.

Effect of carbon sources on growth and enzyme production were evaluated by the following procedure. First, 1 mL aliquot of SDP-grown *Penicillium* sp. was placed into a 250 mL Erlenmeyer flasks containing 100 mL the basal medium with adding 0.75% $(NH_4)_2SO_4$, 50 mM KH_2PO_4. Afterwards, different carbon sources including either PDB, corn, potato, barley, and Czapek's Dox (Cz) were supplemented at the concentration of 3% (*w/v*). Incubation of flasks was carried out using a rotary shaker (120 rpm) at 30 °C for the optimum time obtained in the previous section.

2.6. *Fermentation of Soybean Residual Using P. citrinium*

First, 50 g of soybean residue collected after the extraction process of soybean oil, accruing from the extraction process of soybean oil, was used as a feedstock for isoflavones extraction by using 100 mL of ethanol/water (70/30, *v/v*) and 70 °C for 2 h. The extracted mixture was filtered to obtain filtrate. The extraction experiment was repeated three times and the filtrates were pooled together before ethanol removal by vacuum distillation to obtain the final extract (designated as CDN) containing concentrated isoflavones for fermentation experiments. The fermentation mixture was made up by mixing 20% (*w/v*) glucose and 5–20% (*v/v*) of CDN extract, 0.75% (*w/v*) $(NH_4)_2SO_4$, 50 mM KH_2PO_4, pH 4.5 followed by sterilization at 121 °C for 20 min. A fungal amount of 2% (*v/v*) of *P. citrinium* was used to inoculate the medium prepared in 250 mL Erlenmeyer flasks and incubation at 30 °C for 120 h with shaking rate of 180 rpm. Samples were regularly taken at 24, 48, 72, 96, and 120 h of fermentation, followed by addition of ethanol, vortexing, and centrifugation to obtain supernatants for the determination of the conversion of glucosides, genistin, and daidzin into aglycones and corresponding glycosides.

Hydrolysis rate was calculated by the following equation:

$$H = \frac{\text{isoflavone glycosides in control samples} - \text{isoflavone glycosides in hydrolyzed samples}}{\text{isoflavone glycosides in control samples}} \times 100$$

Isoflavone aglycones in the hydrolyzed mixture were isolated and purified by means of column chromatography (Mini-C, diameter of 70 mm) on silica gel (Merck 60, 15–40 μm, height loaded of 10 cm) using hexane/acetone (29:1/1:1).

2.7. *Determination of Glucosides and Aglycones Using TLC, LC-MS/MS, NMR*

To perform TLC (thin layer chromatography) analysis, silica gel 60 F_{254} plates were used. The employed developing solvent was a mixture of chloroform/methanol/water (80:20:2, *v/v/v*, lower phase). The revelation of spots were performed by spraying with $FeCl_3$ 5% or 1% $Ce(SO_4)_2/H_2SO_4$, followed by exposure to UV lamp with wavelength of 254 nm till spots were clearly observed. Identification of glucosides and aglycones was made by comparison with reference standards. An LC instrument (Agilent 1100 system, Santa Clara, CA, USA) was employed to perform LC analysis at a detection wavelength of 260 nm, the injection volume of 20 μL with the reverse phase C25 ODS-2 (250 mm × 4.6 mm, 5 μm) column. Two solvents, A (acetonitrile 100%) and B (formic acid 0.15%), were used as the mobile phase. The gradient conditions were as follows. [100–50% B, 0–50 min]; [50–20% B, 50–52 min]; [20–0% B, 52–60 min] with a flow rate of 1.0 mL/min. Mass spectra of Electron Spray Ionisation (ESI) were recorded on the Agilent 1100 Series mass spectrometer connected with Varian 320-MS (LabWrench, Midland,

Canada). ^{1}H-NMR spectra were recorded by 500 MHz (Bruker XL-500, Billerica, MA, USA) with DMSO-d_6 or acetone-d_6 as solvents and tetramethylsilane as an internal standard. ^{13}C-NMR spectra were recorded at 125 MHz (Bruker XL-500) with DMSO-d_6 or acetone-d_6 as solvents and as internal standard.

2.8. Statistical Anaylsis

Experiments were carried out in triplicate for the accuracy of data. Statistical significant differences were realized at $p < 0.05$ via Student's t-test. Statistical analysis was performed in the JMP Pro 13.2 software.

3. Results

3.1. Isolation and Screening of β-Glucosidase-Producing Microorganisms

Roots from *Clerodendron cyrtophyllum* Turcz sp. were used as microbial sources to isolate fungi with β-glucosidase activity on PDA medium. At 10^{-5} dilution, colonies were isolated separately. They were then subcultured on sterilized PDA plates several times to obtain pure culture for identification and β-glucosidase enzyme assay. After several subcultures at 30 °C for 72 h, 10 fungi were isolated with different morphological characteristics of colony. Five fungi were isolated from fresh samples (designated as BC) of *C. cyrtophyllum* Turcz's while five other fungi were isolated from dried plant samples (designated as BSD).

For enzymatic screening and fungal selection, the ten fungal isolates were tested for their capability of enzyme production. The β-glucosidase activity of these fungi is shown in the Figure 1. The strains BC2 and BSD5 were determined as the most potential fungi for enzyme production (5.41 ± 0.27 and 8.53 ± 0.20 U/mL, respectively) in comparison with other strains (<0.63 U/mL) and were therefore selected for further studies.

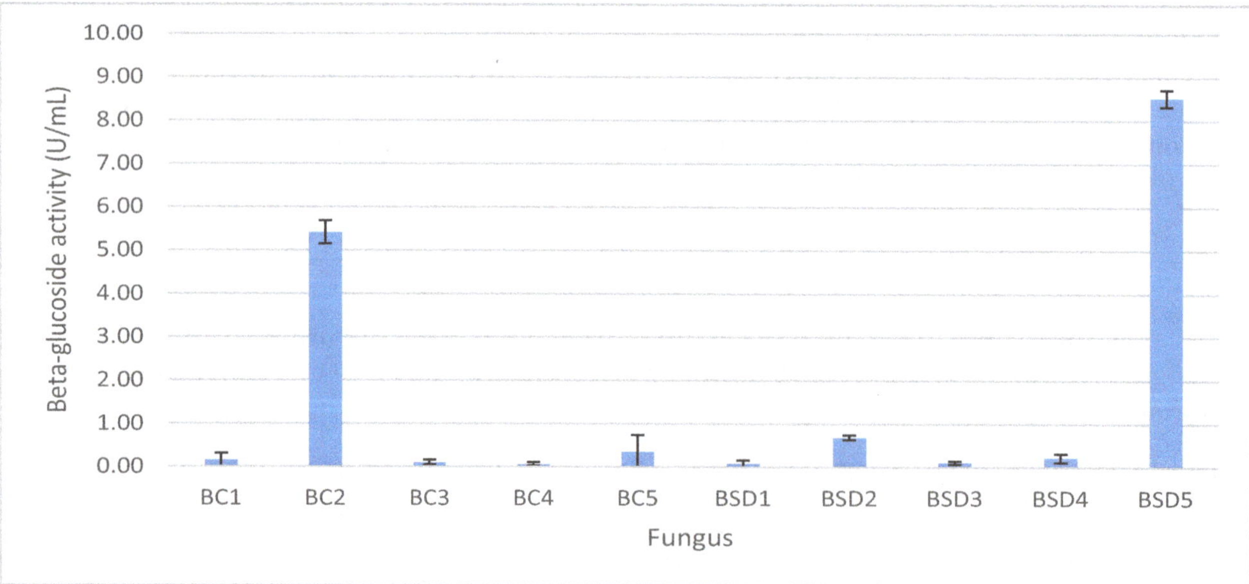

Figure 1. β-glucosidase activity of the isolated fungi.

3.2. Isolation and Screening of β-Glucosidase-Producing Microorganisms

On SA medium, colonies of BC2 grew fast and displayed a compact green or yellow basal felt enclosed by a layer of white of erect conidiophores. The diameter of colonies was approximately measured as 2.4 cm. Microscopically, conidiophore stipes are long and smooth-walled and the color of hyaline turned dark towards the vesicle. Conidial heads were biseriate, large, globose, and showed tendency to radiate, splitting into several loose columns with age. Additionally, phialides, usually in the form of septate metulae, were also observed. These morphological characteristics affirm that this fungus belongs to the *Aspergillus* species.

The shade of colonies of BSD5 growing on SA medium was green in color and a dense felt of conidiophores was observed. The average diameter of colonies after three days of incubation was 1.2 cm. Observing under a microscope, conidiophores were hyaline and smooth-walled. In addition, terminal verticils, carrying 3–5 metulae each, were observed on conidiophores. In each metula, around 3–7 phialides were recognized. Regarding conidia, they are smooth-walled and their shape appeared to be globose or subglobose. In addition, the production of conidia was basipetal from the phialides. Therefore, the described fungus belonged to the *Penicillium* species.

After identification by morphological characteristics, genomic DNA of the *Penicillium* sp. was identified to ensure that this fungus belonged to *Penicillium* sp. Figure 2 shows the PCR products on agarose gel 1% in which lane 1 is marker proteins and lane 2 is DNA of the fungus. It can be demonstrated that the molecular mass of this fungus is 540 bp. By using ITS method, the genome DNA of the *Penicillium* sp. was sequenced as:

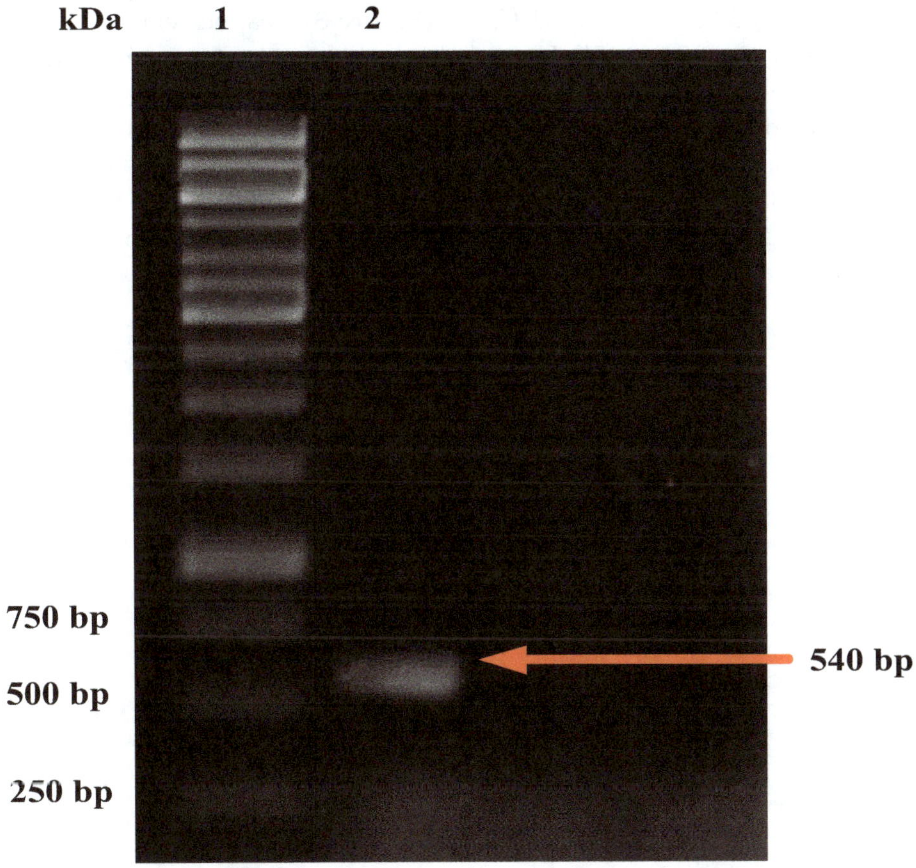

Figure 2. PCR amplification of genomic DNA of *P. citrinum* (lane 2) on agarose gel 1%. Lane 1—DNA size marker.

"CATGCTCCGGCCGCCATGGCGGCCGCGGGAATTCGATTTCCGTAGGTGAACCTGCGGAA GGATCATTACCGAGTGCGGGCCCCTCGGGGCCCAACCTCCCACCCGTGTTGCCCGAACCTATGT TGCCTCGGCGGGCCCCGCGCCCGCCGACGGCCCCCCTGAACGCTGTCTGAAGTTGCAGTCTGA GACCTATAACGAAATTAGTTAAAACTTTCAACAACGGATCTCTTGGTTCCGGCATCGATGAAG AACGCAGCGAAATGCGATAACTAATGTGAATTGCAGAATTCAGTGAATCATCGAGTCTTTGAA CGCACATTGCGCCCTCTGGTATTCCGGAGGGCATGCCTGTCCGAGCGTCATTGCTGCCCTCAAG CCCGGCTTGTGTGTTGGGCCCCGTCCCCCCCGCCGGGGGACGGGCCCGAAAGGCAGCGGCG

GCACCGCGTCCGGTCCTCGAGCGTATGGGGCTTCGTCACCCGCTCTAGTAGGCCCGGCCGGCG CCAGCCGACCCCCAACCTTTAATTATCTCAGGTTGACCT".

To gain insights into the evolutionary relationship, two methods for creation of the phylogenetic trees, namely Neighbor Joining (NJ) and Maximum Parsimony (MP), were employed, resulting in almost identical topologies. The aligned dataset consisted of 42 taxa and 100 characters. Our sequence (marked as unknown) achieved 100% matching with those of *Penicillium citrinum* existing in the database, as evidenced by the excellent bootstrap results. Therefore, the examined fungus presumably belonged to the *Penicillium* genus and firmly aligned with the *P. citrinum* species, as demonstrated by the the strong sequence similarities with the said species.

3.3. *Optimization of β-Glucosidase Production by P. citrinum*

The optimum incubation time is the time interval at which the highest β-glusosidase activity was attained. After incubation for 24, 48, 72, 96, 120, 144, and 168 h, β-glusosidase activity was 0.23, 2.56, 8.16, 21.25, 23.55, 33.37, and 23.23 U/mL (Figure 3), respectively. This indicates that the highest β-glucosidase activity of 33.63 U/mL was achieved at 144 h of the fermentation time and that prolonged incubation time seemed to reduce enzyme yield. This could be explained by the reduced quantities of nutrients, in both micro and macro forms, existing in the medium after an extended period of fermentation. The phenomenon highlights the role of fungal physiology in inactivating secretary machinery of the enzymes. In addition, the rapid enzyme production in the initial period might be attributable to the high resistance to microbial hydrolysis of the materials, which was later diminished as the fermentation time elapsed.

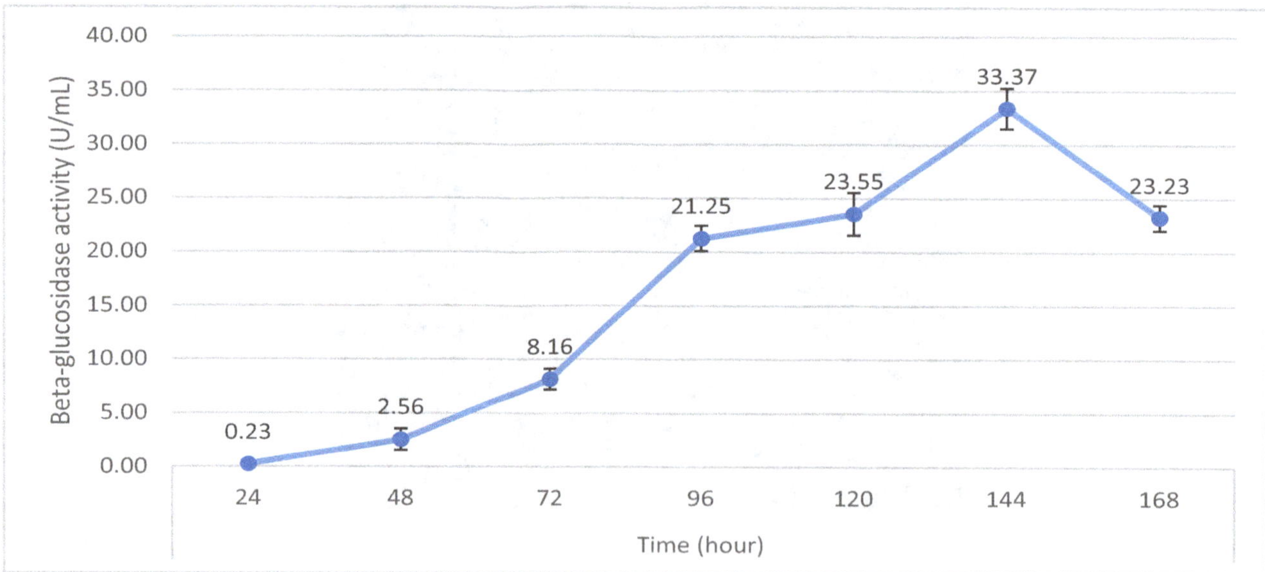

Figure 3. Effect of fermentation time on β-glucosidase activity of *P. citrinum*.

Carbon source is a critical factor affecting the production of enzymes. Therefore, *P. citrinum* was tested to grow in fermentation medium containing various carbon sources under the temperature of 30 °C, agitation speed of 200 rpm, and for six days. Figure 4 shows that the highest β-glucosidase activity of 32.97 U/mL was achieved on potato, and the lower β-glucosidase activities of 4.39, 1.80, and 12.17 U/mL were recorded on barley, corn, and Cz sources, respectively.

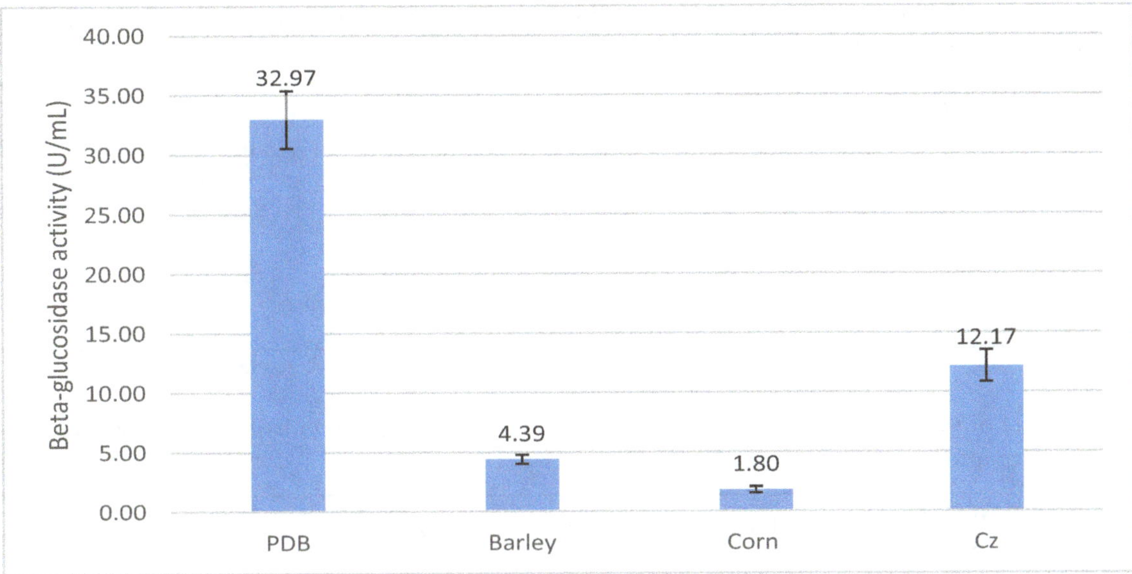

Figure 4. Effect of different carbon sources on β-glucosidase activity of *P. citrinum.*

3.4. Fermentation of Soybean Residual Extract by P. citrinum for Aglycones (Genistein, Daidzein) Production

Figure 5 and Table 1 show that soybean residual extract originally contained glucosides, which were still dominant in the first 24 h fermentation, but partly hydrolyzed after 48 h and completely converted to aglycones after 72 h fermentation. Moreover, the data revealed that at 10–20% (*v/v*) volumetric ratio of *P. citrinum* inoculum to CDN substrate, the transformation into aglycones from glucoside forms complete took place during 72 h of fermentation (Table 2). This indicates that the optimal conditions for fermentation of soybean residual extract to aglycones was 10% (*v/v*) of *P. citrinum* enzyme to CDN with fermentation time of 72 h at 30 °C.

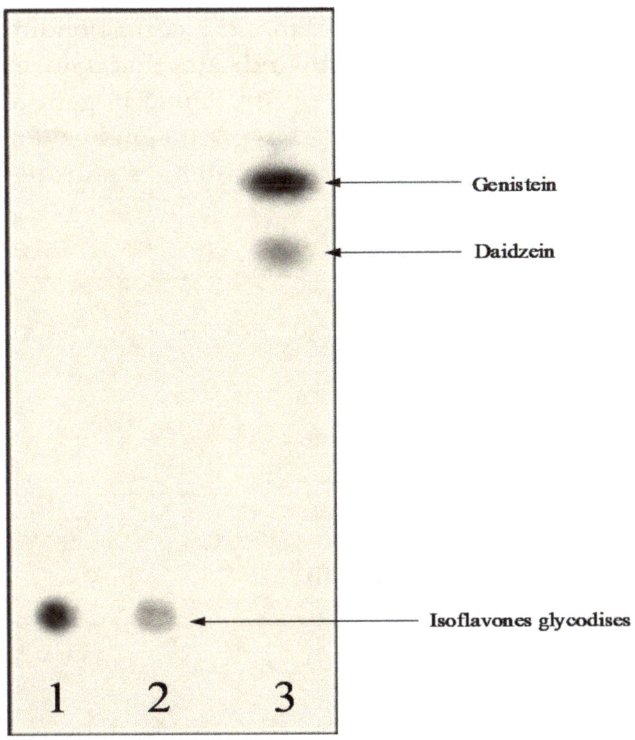

Figure 5. TLC results of fermentation of soybean residual extract using *P. citrinium* at 30 °C during (1) 2 h, (2) 48 h, and (3) 72 h.

Table 1. Effect of hydrolysis time of soybean residual extract on isoflavon glucosides and aglycones formation by *P. citrinium* at 30 °C.

Fermentation Time (h)	Isoflavone Glucosides	Aglycones	Remark
0	++++	-	Original soybean extract without addition of enzyme
24	++++	-	
48	+++	+	
72	-	++++	
96	-	++++	
120	-	++++	

Note: ++++, dark stain; +++, medium stain; +, weak stain; -, no stain.

Table 2. Effect of volumetric ratio of soybean residual extract/enzyme on isoflavone glucosides and aglycones formation by *P. citrinium* at 30 °C.

Soybean Residual Extract/Enzyme Ratio (*v*/*v*, %)	Isoflavone Glucosides	Aglycones	Remark
0	++++	-	Original soybean extract without addition of enzyme
5	-	+	
10	-	+++	
15	+	+++	
20	++	+++	

Note: ++++, dark strain; +++, medium stain; ++, medium-weak stain; +, weak stain; -, no stain.

3.5. Identification and Characterization of Aglycones Using LC-MS/MS, TLC, and NMR

LC-MS/MS results reveal that in the first stage of fragmentation in the negative ion mode, one ion of high intensity at m/z 253 (Figure 6A) was observed, which corresponded to the elemental composition of ($C_{15}H_{10}O_4$, daidzein) with molecular weight of 254.23 (Figure 6B). On the other hand, in the positive ion mode, the highest intensity fragment appeared at m/z 255, corresponding to the same ion having an elemental chemical composition of ($C_{15}H_{10}O_4$). Data indicates that daidzein obtained after extraction and purification from fermentation broth is of high purity. Similarly, genistein ion fragments appeared at m/z 269.0 (Figure 6C) and m/z 271.1 (Figure 6D), having the highest intensity in the negative and positive mode, respectively. These findings are in line with the results of the standard reagents and of previously reported works [3,7].

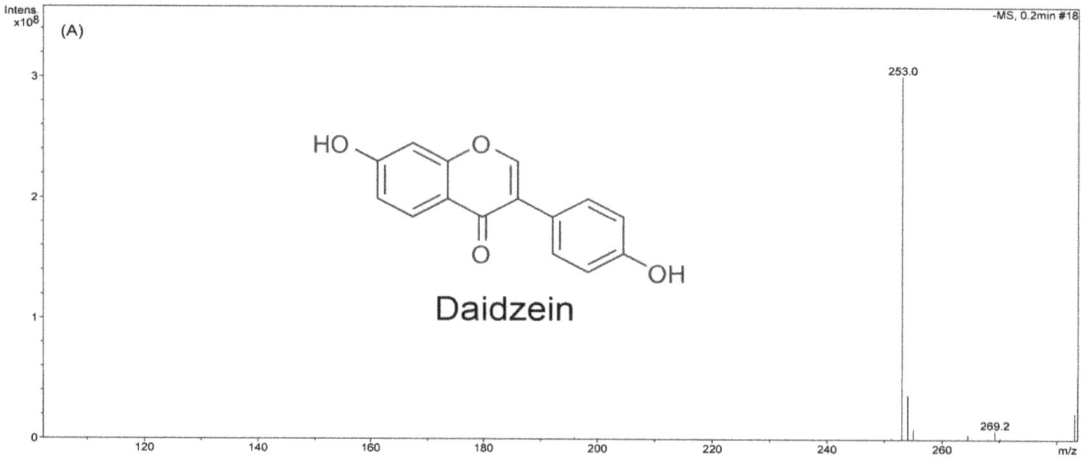

Figure 6. *Cont.*

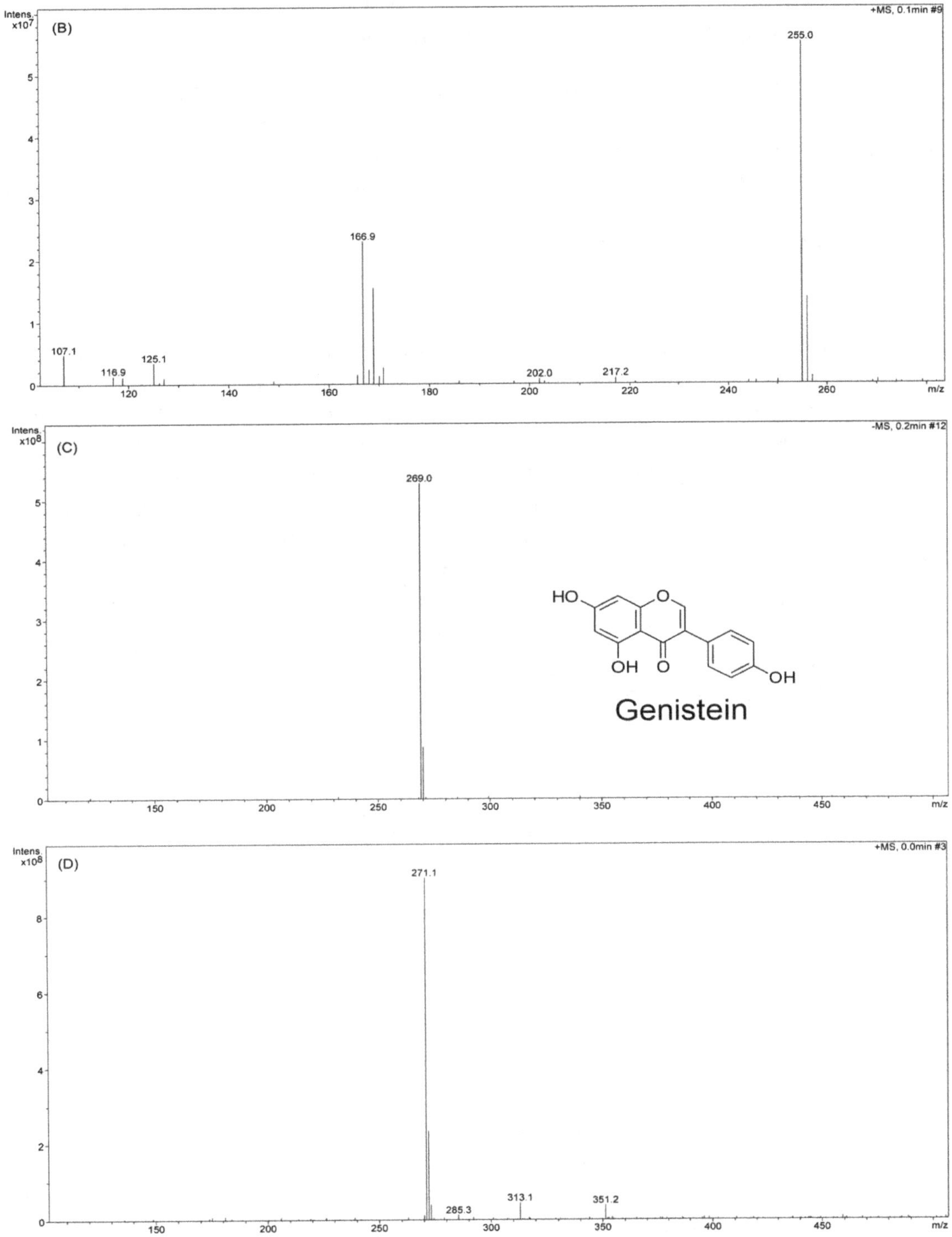

Figure 6. LC-MS/MS spectra of daidzein and genistein. Negative mode of daidzein at m/z 253 (**A**), positive mode of daidzein at m/z 255 (**B**), negative mode of genistein at m/z 269.0 (**C**), and positive mode of genistein at m/z 271.1 (**D**).

For genistein (DTE1, 99.80 mg, purity 90%), light yellow needle crystals, $R_f = 0.37$ (TLC, silica gel, solvent n-hexan/acetone (7/3, *v/v*)) appeared as yellow-brown with 5% $FeCl_3$ and dark green with $Ce(SO_4)_2$ (data not shown). ^{1}H-NMR (Acetone, 500 Hz): δ (ppm) 6.28 (1H, d, J = 2 Hz, H6), 6.41 (1H, d, J = 2.5 Hz, H8), 6.90 (2H, dd, J = 2 Hz, H3′, H5′), 7.46 (2H, dd, J = 2 Hz, H2′, H6′), 8.163 (1H, d, J = 1.5 Hz, H2), 13.03 (1H, s, OH). ^{13}C-NMR (Acetone, 125 Hz): δ (ppm) 94.15 (s, C8),

99.52 (s, C6), 105.87 (s, C10), 115.65 (d, C3′, C5′), 122.75 (s, C1′), 123.76 (d, C3), 130.86 (d, C2′, C6′), 153.98 (s, C2), 163.64 (d, C5), 158.76 (d, C9), 158.13 (t, C4), 164.70 (t, C7), 181.35 (t, C7).

For daidzein (DTE2, 300.58 mg, purity 90%); white needle crystals, R_f = 0.30 (TLC, silica gel, solvent n-hexan/acetone (7/3, *v*/*v*)) appeared as dark-green with $Ce(SO_4)_2$ and colorless with 5% $FeCl_3$ (data not shown). ^{1}H-NMR (Acetone, 500 Hz): δ (ppm) 6.89 (3H, dd, J = 2 Hz, 9 Hz, H3′, H5′, OH4′), 6.98 (1H, m, H8), 7.47 (2H, dd, J = 5.5 Hz, 2 Hz, H2′, H6′), 8.06 (1H, d, J = 8.5 Hz, H6), 8.14 (1H, s, H2). ^{13}C-NMR (DMSO, 125 Hz): δ (ppm) 102.04 (s, C8), 115.07 (d, C6), 116.58 (d, C5′, C3′), 123.43 (d, C3), 127.23 (t, C1′), 129.99 (d, C5), 125.74 (s, C2), 157.11 (d, C4′), 157.37 (d, C9), 162.45 (t, C7), 174.63 (s, C4).

4. Discussion

It was reported that β-glucosidase can be produced on different carbon sources by fungi with different activities [36]. Lachke et al. [37] found that the maximum β-glucosidase activity of *Penicillium funiculosum* was 30–36 U/mL, achieved on 3% rice bran or defatted oil cakes after 288 h fermentation. By stark contrast, the peak activity was found at a much lower level of 2.8 U/mL with *Penicillium miczynskii* cultured on 3% pineapple peel within 216 h of fermentation (Table 3) [38]. Furthermore, the investigation of Jeya et al. [39] resulted in the highest β-glucosidase activity of 26.4 U/mL in *P. purpurogenum* produced on rice straw, while Ng et al. [40] achieved the highest β-glucosidase activity of 57.5 U/g solid when rice bran was used via solid fermentation. Although other variables (e.g., temperature, pH, etc.) have not been optimized in this study, β-glucosidase produced by the isolated *P. citrinum* was reached 33.63–33.72 U/mL, listing *P. citrinum* as the top fungal strain among the reported fungi producing highest activity of β-glucosidase. In terms of scalability, β-glucosidase holds the potential to be cloned into other hosts such as *Escherichia coli* for large-scale industrial production [41].

Table 3. β-glucosidase production of several fungal strains.

Fungal Strain	Fermentation Conditions	β-Glucosidase Activity (U/mL)	Ref.
P. funiculosum	Substrate: Rice bran, defatted oil cakes Temperature: 20 °C pH: 4.5 Fermentation time: 288 h	30–36	[34]
P. miczynskii	Substrate: Pineapple peel Temperature: 30 °C pH: 5.5 Fermentation time: 216 h	2.82	[35]
P. purpurogenum KJS506	Substrate: Rice straw Temperature: 32 °C pH: 4 Fermentation time: 144 h	26.4	[36]
P. citrinium YS40-5	Substrate: Rice bran Temperature: 70 °C pH: 6.0 Fermentation time: 96 h	57.5 U/g	[37]
P. citrinium	Substrate: PDB Temperature: 30 °C pH: 4.5 Fermentation time: 144 h	33.72	Current study

The hydrolysis yield of soybean waste extract (rich in isoflavone glycosides) to their aglycones by *P. citrinum* was estimated to be 98.7%, which is comparable to aglycone rates of 94.22 and 97.14% achieved by *D. hansenii* UFV-1 immobilized cells containing β-glycosidase and free enzyme, respectively [42], on soy molasses. However, our reported hydrolysis rate is higher than the rate of 93% achieved in deglycosylation of extracts of soybean flour and embryo in β-glucosidase derived from *Paecilomyces thermophila* J18 [43]. Moreover, the biotransformation rate is also higher than that by a marine *Streptomyces* sp. 060524, which achieved only 90% on the same substrate during 108 h fermentation [5].

Isoflavone aglycones can be derived from soybean waste by extraction with ethanol/water solvent followed by acid hydrolysis and purification [44], reaching purity of 92%. Alternatively, the soybean extract can be hydrolyzed by cellulase to produce crude aglycone isoflavones, followed by purification, to obtain purity of 80.38–87.21%. Experimental data obtained in this study showed that the purity of genistein and daidzein reached over 90%, which is comparable to the purity obtained by the reported methods, demonstrating raw materials with potential for utilization in industrial applications, e.g., pharmaceutics and functional foods, with minimum refining [3].

5. Conclusions

The *P. citrinum* fungus strain that produces the highest β-glucosidase activity of 33.72 U/mL, thus placing it amongst the most active fungi in this regard, has been successfully isolated from roots of *Clerodendron cyrtophyllum* Turcz. The fungus demonstrated a catalytic capacity to hydrolyze isoflavones-rich soybean extract into aglycones (e.g., genistein and daidzein) with a hydrolysis yield of 98.7% after 72 h of fermentation at 30 °C. Purification of the hydrolyzed mixture (rich in genistein and daidzein) by column chromatography using hexane/acetone (29:1/1:1) resulted in aglycone products with purity of over 90%. These results imply that soybean extract is a promising raw material for manufacture of functional foods derived from aglycones. Our study demonstrated a potential pathway for the production of aglycones from residual soybean extract via fermentation with an isolated fungi as a biocatalyst, with applciations in the pharmaceutical and functional food industries.

Author Contributions: Investigation, D.T.D., D.P.L., T.D.N., B.H.T., H.M.P.T., H.N.D., V.H.L., T.D.P., V.T.T., M.Q.P. and H.H.P.T.; Supervision, Q.T.T.; Writing–Original draft, D.T.D.

References

1. Anderson, J.J.B.; Garner, S.C. Phytoestrogens and human function. *Nutr. Today* **1997**, *32*, 232. [CrossRef]
2. Markovic, R.; Baltic, M.Z.; Pavlovic, M.; Glisic, M.; Radulovic, S.; Djordjevic, V.; Sefer, D. Isoflavones-from biotechnology to functional foods. *Procedia Food Sci.* **2015**, *5*, 176–179. [CrossRef]
3. Yatsu, F.K.J.; Koester, L.S.; Bassani, V.L. Isoflavone-aglycone fraction from Glycine max: A promising raw material for isoflavone-based pharmaceutical or nutraceutical products. *Rev. Bras. Farmacogn.* **2016**, *26*, 259–267. [CrossRef]
4. Hong, J.L.; Qin, X.Y.; Shu, P.; Wang, Q.; Zhou, Z.F.; Wang, G.K.; Lin, B.B.; Wang, Q.; Qin, M.J. Comparative study of isoflavones in wild and cultivated soybeans as well as bean products by high-performance liquid chromatography coupled with mass spectrometry and chemometric techniques. *Eur. Food Res. Technol.* **2011**, *233*, 869. [CrossRef]
5. Hu, S.C.; Hong, K.; Song, Y.C.; Liu, J.Y.; Tan, R.X. Biotransformation of soybean isoflavones by a marine Streptomyces sp. 060524 and cytotoxicity of the products. *World J. Microbiol. Biotechnol.* **2008**, *25*, 115. [CrossRef]
6. Baú, T.R.; Ida, E.I. Soymilk processing with higher isoflavone aglycone content. *Food Chem.* **2015**, *183*, 161–168. [CrossRef] [PubMed]
7. Delmonte, P.; Perry, J.; Rader, J.I. Determination of isoflavones in dietary supplements containing soy, red clover and kudzu: Extraction followed by basic or acid hydrolysis. *J. Chromatogr. A* **2006**, *1107*, 59–69. [CrossRef] [PubMed]
8. Rostagno, M.A.; Villares, A.; Guillamón, E.; García-Lafuente, A.; Martínez, J.A. Sample preparation for the analysis of isoflavones from soybeans and soy foods. *J. Chromatogr. A* **2009**, *1216*, 2–29. [CrossRef] [PubMed]
9. Handa, C.L.; Couto, U.R.; Vicensoti, A.H.; Georgetti, S.R.; Ida, E.I. Optimisation of soy flour fermentation parameters to produce β-glucosidase for bioconversion into aglycones. *Food Chem.* **2014**, *152*, 56–65. [CrossRef]
10. Chun, J.; Kim, G.M.; Lee, K.W.; Choi, I.D.; Kwon, G.H.; Park, J.Y.; Jeong, S.J.; Kim, J.S.; Kim, J.H. Conversion

of isoflavone glucosides to aglycones in soymilk by fermentation with lactic acid bacteria. *J. Food Sci.* **2007**, *72*, M39–M44. [CrossRef]

11. Aguieiras, E.C.G.; Cavalcanti-Oliveira, E.D.; de Castro, A.M.; Langone, M.A.P.; Freire, D.M.G. Simultaneous enzymatic transesterification and esterification of an acid oil using fermented solid as biocatalyst. *J. Am. Oil Chem. Soc.* **2017**, *94*, 551–558. [CrossRef]
12. Papadaki, A.; Kopsahelis, N.; Mallouchos, A.; Mandala, I.; Koutinas, A.A. Bioprocess development for the production of novel oleogels from soybean and microbial oils. *Food Res. Int.* **2019**, *126*, 108684. [CrossRef]
13. Papadaki, A.; Androutsopoulos, N.; Patsalou, M.; Koutinas, M.; Kopsahelis, N.; Castro, A.; Papanikolaou, S.; Koutinas, A. Biotechnological production of fumaric acid: The effect of morphology of rhizopus arrhizus NRRL 2582. *Fermentation* **2017**, *3*, 33. [CrossRef]
14. Papadaki, A.; Papapostolou, H.; Alexandri, M.; Kopsahelis, N.; Papanikolaou, S.; de Castro, A.M.; Freire, D.M.G.; Koutinas, A.A. Fumaric acid production using renewable resources from biodiesel and cane sugar production processes. *Environ. Sci. Pollut. Res.* **2018**, *25*, 35960–35970. [CrossRef]
15. Haas, M.J. Improving the economics of biodiesel production through the use of low value lipids as feedstocks: Vegetable oil soapstock. *Fuel Process. Technol.* **2005**, *86*, 1087–1096. [CrossRef]
16. Aguieiras, E.C.G.; Papadaki, A.; Mallouchos, A.; Mandala, I.; Sousa, H.; Freire, D.M.G.; Koutinas, A.A. Enzymatic synthesis of bio-based wax esters from palm and soybean fatty acids using crude lipases produced on agricultural residues. *Ind. Crops Prod.* **2019**, *139*, 111499. [CrossRef]
17. Fujita, A.; Alencar, S.M.; Park, Y.K. Conversion of isoflavone glucosides to aglycones by partially purified β-glucosidases from microbial and vegetable sources. *Appl. Biochem. Biotechnol.* **2015**, *176*, 1659–1672. [CrossRef]
18. Ahn-Jarvis, J.H.; Teegarden, M.D.; Schwartz, S.J.; Lee, K.; Vodovotz, Y. Modulating conversion of isoflavone glycosides to aglycones using crude beta-glycosidase extracts from almonds and processed soy. *Food Chem.* **2017**, *237*, 685–692. [CrossRef]
19. da Silva, L.H.; Celeghini, R.M.S.; Chang, Y.K. Effect of the fermentation of whole soybean flour on the conversion of isoflavones from glycosides to aglycones. *Food Chem.* **2011**, *128*, 640–644. [CrossRef]
20. Xie, L.; Hettiarachchy, N.S.; Cai, R.; Tsuruhami, K.; Koikeda, S. Conversion of Isoflavone Glycosides to Aglycones in SoyLife and Soymeal Using β-glycosidase. *J. Food Sci.* **2003**, *68*, 427–430. [CrossRef]
21. Chang, F.; Xue, S.; Xie, X.; Fang, W.; Fang, Z.; Xiao, Y. Carbohydrate-binding module assisted purification and immobilization of β-glucosidase onto cellulose and application in hydrolysis of soybean isoflavone glycosides. *J. Biosci. Bioeng.* **2018**, *125*, 185–191. [CrossRef] [PubMed]
22. Molina, G.; de Lima, E.A.; Borin, G.P.; de Barcelos, M.C.S.; Pastore, G.M. Chapter 7—Beta-Glucosidase From Penicillium. In *New and Future Developments in Microbial Biotechnology and Bioengineering*; Gupta, V.K., Rodriguez-Couto, S., Eds.; Elsevier: Amsterdam, The Netherlands, 2018; pp. 137–151.
23. Yan, F.; Xia, W.; Zhang, X.; Chen, S.; Nie, X.; Qian, L. Characterization of β-glucosidase from Aspergillus terreus and its application in the hydrolysis of soybean isoflavones. *J. Zhejiang Univ. Sci. B* **2016**, *17*, 455–464. [CrossRef] [PubMed]
24. Chang, K.H.; Jo, M.N.; Kim, K.T.; Paik, H.D. Evaluation of glucosidases of Aspergillus niger strain comparing with other glucosidases in transformation of ginsenoside Rb1 to ginsenosides Rg3. *J. Ginseng Res.* **2014**, *38*, 47–51. [CrossRef] [PubMed]
25. Baraldo Junior, A.; Borges, D.G.; Tardioli, P.W.; Farinas, C.S. Characterization of β-Glucosidase Produced by Aspergillus niger under Solid-State Fermentation and Partially Purified Using MANAE-Agarose. *Biotechnol. Res. Int.* **2014**, *2014*, 317092. [CrossRef] [PubMed]
26. Langston, J.; Sheehy, N.; Xu, F. Substrate specificity of Aspergillus oryzae family 3 β-glucosidase. *Biochim. Biophys. Act. BBA Proteins Proteom.* **2006**, *1764*, 972–978. [CrossRef]
27. Krogh, K.B.R.M.; Harris, P.V.; Olsen, C.L.; Johansen, K.S.; Hojer-Pedersen, J.; Borjesson, J.; Olsson, L. Characterization and kinetic analysis of a thermostable GH3 β-glucosidase from Penicillium brasilianum. *Appl. Microbiol. Biotechnol.* **2010**, *86*, 143–154. [CrossRef] [PubMed]
28. Tsukada, T.; Igarashi, K.; Yoshida, M.; Samejima, M. Molecular cloning and characterization of two intracellular β-glucosidases belonging to glycoside hydrolase family 1 from the basidiomycete Phanerochaete chrysosporium. *Appl. Microbiol. Biotechnol.* **2006**, *73*, 807. [CrossRef]
29. Kudo, K.; Watanabe, A.; Ujiie, S.; Shintani, T.; Gomi, K. Purification and enzymatic characterization of secretory glycoside hydrolase family 3 (GH3) aryl β-glucosidases screened from Aspergillus oryzae

genome. *J. Biosci. Bioeng.* **2015**, *120*, 614–623. [CrossRef]

30. Li, D.; Li, X.; Dang, W.; Tran, P.L.; Park, S.H.; Oh, B.C.; Hong, W.S.; Lee, J.S.; Park, K.H. Characterization and application of an acidophilic and thermostable β-glucosidase from Thermofilum pendens. *J. Biosci. Bioeng.* **2013**, *115*, 490–496. [CrossRef]
31. Dekker, R.F.H. Kinetic, inhibition, and stability properties of a commercial β-D-glucosidase (cellobiase) preparation from *aspergillus niger* and its suitability in the hydrolysis of lignocellulose. *Biotechnol. Bioeng.* **1986**, *28*, 1438–1442. [CrossRef]
32. Tendulkar, S.R.; Saikumari, Y.K.; Patel, V.; Raghotama, S.; Munshi, T.K.; Balaram, P.; Chattoo, B.B. Isolation, purification and characterization of an antifungal molecule produced by Bacillus licheniformis BC98, and its effect on phytopathogen Magnaporthe grisea. *J. Appl. Microbiol.* **2007**, *103*, 2331–2339. [CrossRef] [PubMed]
33. Kidd, S.; Halliday, C.L.; Alexiou, H.; Ellis, D.H. *Descriptions of Medical Fungi*; CutCut Digital: Richmond, VA, USA, 2016.
34. White, T.J.; Bruns, T.; Lee, S.J.W.T.; Taylor, J. Amplification and direct sequencing of fungal ribosomal RNA genes for phylogenetics. In *PCR Protocols: A Guide to Methods and Applications*; Innis, M.A., Gelfand, D.H., Sninsky, J.J., White, T.J., Eds.; Academic Press: Cambridge, MA, USA, 1990; pp. 315–322.
35. Cai, Y.J.; Buswell, J.A.; Chang, S.T. β-Glucosidase components of the cellulolytic system of the edible straw mushroom, Volvariella volvacea. *Enzyme Microb. Technol.* **1998**, *22*, 122–129. [CrossRef]
36. So, J.H.; Kim, W.C.; Shin, J.H.; Yu, C.B.; Rhee, I.K. Purification and characterization of a β-glucosidase capable of hydrolyzing soybean isoflavone glycosides from Pichia guilliermondii K123-1. *Food Sci. Biotechnol.* **2010**, *19*, 1373–1379. [CrossRef]
37. Lachke, A.H.; Bastawde, K.B.; Powar, V.K.; Srinivasan, M.C. Enhanced production of extracellular β-glucosidase by penicillium funiculosum in submerged culture. *Biotechnol. Lett.* **1983**, *5*, 649–652. [CrossRef]
38. Beitel, S.M.; Knob, A. Penicillium miczynskii β -glucosidase: A Glucose-Tolerant Enzyme Produced Using Pineapple Peel as Substrate. *Ind. Biotechnol.* **2013**, *9*, 293–300. [CrossRef]
39. Jeya, M.; Joo, A.R.; Lee, K.M.; Tiwari, M.K.; Lee, K.M.; Kim, S.H.; Lee, J.K. Characterization of β-glucosidase from a strain of Penicillium purpurogenum KJS506. *Appl. Microbiol. Biotechnol.* **2010**, *86*, 1473–1484. [CrossRef] [PubMed]
40. Ng, I.S.; Li, C.W.; Chan, S.P.; Chir, J.L.; Chen, P.T.; Tong, C.G.; Yu, S.M.; Ho, T.H.D. High-level production of a thermoacidophilic β-glucosidase from Penicillium citrinum YS40-5 by solid-state fermentation with rice bran. *Bioresour. Technol.* **2010**, *101*, 1310–1317. [CrossRef]
41. Xue, Y.; Song, X.; Yu, J. Overexpression of β-glucosidase from Thermotoga maritima for the production of highly purified aglycone isoflavones from soy flour. *World J. Microbiol. Biotechnol.* **2009**, *25*, 2165–2172. [CrossRef]
42. Maitan-Alfenas, G.P.; de A Lage, L.G.; de Almeida, M.N.; Visser, E.M.; de Rezende, S.T.; Guimarães, V.M. Hydrolysis of soybean isoflavones by Debaryomyces hansenii UFV-1 immobilised cells and free β-glucosidase. *Food Chem.* **2014**, *146*, 429–436. [CrossRef]
43. Yang, S.; Wang, L.; Yan, Q.; Jiang, Z.; Li, L. Hydrolysis of soybean isoflavone glycosides by a thermostable β-glucosidase from Paecilomyces thermophila. *Food Chem.* **2009**, *115*, 1247–1252. [CrossRef]
44. Nemitz, M.C.; Teixeira, H.F.; von Poser, G.L. A new approach for the purification of soybean acid extract: Simultaneous production of an isoflavone aglycone-rich fraction and a furfural derivative-rich by-product. *Ind. Crops Prod.* **2015**, *67*, 414–421. [CrossRef]

6

Systematic Review and Meta-Analysis of a Proprietary Alpha-Amylase Inhibitor from White Bean (*Phaseolus vulgaris* L.) on Weight and Fat Loss in Humans

Jay Udani *, Ollie Tan and Jhanna Molina

Medical Private Practice, Agoura Hills, CA 91301, USA; ollietan124@yahoo.com (O.T.); jhannamolina@gmail.com (J.M.)

* Correspondence: drjayu2016@gmail.com

Abstract: The aim of this meta-analysis was to examine the evidence for the effectiveness of a proprietary alpha-amylase inhibitor from white bean (*Phaseolus vulgaris* L.) supplementation interventions in humans on modification of body weight and fat mass. A systematic literature search was performed using three databases: PubMed, the Cochrane collaboration, and Google Scholar. In addition, the manufacturer was contacted for internal unpublished data, and finally, the reference section of relevant original research and review papers were mined for additional studies. Eleven studies were selected for the meta-analysis of weight loss (a total of 573 subjects), and three studies for the meta-analysis of body fat reduction (a total of 110 subjects), as they fulfilled the inclusion criteria. *Phaseolus vulgaris* supplementation showed an average effect on weight loss difference of −1.08 kg (95% CI (confidence interval), −0.42 kg to −1.16 kg, $p < 0.00001$), and the average effect on body fat reduction was 3.26 kg (95% CI, −2.35 kg to −4.163 kg, $p = 0.02$). This meta-analysis found statistically significant effects of *Phaseolus vulgaris* supplementation on body weight and body fat.

Keywords: weight loss; fat loss; obesity; alpha-amylase inhibitor; meta-analysis; *Phaseolus vulgaris* L.

---

1. Introduction

There are many dietary interventions available to counteract the epidemic of overweight and obesity which play a major role in the development of insulin resistance and type 2 diabetes mellitus [1]. One strategy is based on lowering the excessive intake of carbohydrates, especially, the refined ones [2]. This could be achieved by lowering the portions or replacing the carbohydrates with more fats or by adding soluble fiber to the diet which is thought to slow down the absorption of carbohydrates [3]. Lowering the glycemic index through the usage of fiber in the diet is not favored by most people due to potential taste preferences and adverse reactions resulting in gastrointestinal problems such as gas and diarrhea. Therefore, another strategy becomes more and more promising to impact the carbohydrate absorption by using bioactive ingredients which block or slow the carbohydrate absorption in the gastrointestinal tract via inhibiting the necessary enzymes, amylase and glucosidase [4]. Amylase breaks down complex carbohydrates, such as starch, into oligosaccharides and glucosidase enzymes further convert these to monosaccharides.

There are the different forms of amylase inhibitors, namely, Alpha-amylase inhibitor isoform 1 (Alpha-AI1), Alpha-AI2, and Alpha-AIL which can be found in in the embryonic axes and cotyledons in the seed of common beans (*Phaseolus* spp.) [5]. These so-called glycoproteins bind to alpha-amylase non-covalently, mainly through hydrophobic interaction, by completely blocking access to the active site of the alpha-amylase [6,7]. The Alpha-AI1 isoform is the one with anti-amylase bioactivity in humans, and therefore, inhibits the starch digestion [8]. This blocking affect is also dependent on pH, temperature, incubation time and the presence of particular ions which have been optimized for the specific and proprietary product named Phase2® brand *Phaseolus vulgaris* White Bean product (Pharmachem Laboratories, Kearny, NJ, USA) [9,10]. This particular dietary supplement has demonstrated its potential and ability to cause weight loss in numerous clinical trials in humans [11].

Phase2® brand *Phaseolus vulgaris* White Bean extract is made by a standardized water extract of non-GMO (Genetically Modified Organism) whole dried beans (*Phaseolus vulgaris*) which is made through a proprietary process. The white-to-beige powder consists of *Phaseolus vulgaris* (~90%) and Gum Arabic (~10%). It has at least 3000 alpha-amylase inhibiting units (AAIU) per gram when tested at a pH 6.8 using potato starch as the substrate and pancreatin as the enzyme source. The Phase2® brand products are used in dietary supplements in various forms, including powders, tablets, capsules and chewables for the application of weight control and weight loss. In addition, it is also incorporated in food products like chewing gum, mashed potatoes, yeast-raised dough (bread, pizza, etc.) without losing bioactivity or changing the appearance, texture or taste of the food [12–14].

The aim of this meta-analysis was to examine the evidence for the effectiveness of a proprietary alpha-amylase inhibitor from white bean (*Phaseolus vulgaris*) supplementation interventions on modification of body weight and fat mass.

2. Methods

This review was performed according to the PRISMA (preferred reporting items for systematic reviews and meta-analyses) statement for quality of reporting a meta-analysis [15].

2.1. Literature Search

Literature searches in PubMed, the Cochrane collaboration, and Google Scholar were undertaken using the following keywords: *Phaseolus vulgaris*, Alpha-amylase inhibitor/inhibition, Phase2®, White bean extract, kidney bean, starch blocker, weight loss, body weight, body fat, BMI (body mass index), anthropometric measures, obesity, overweight and safety.

In addition, the manufacturer was contacted for internal unpublished data, and finally, the reference section of relevant original research and review papers were mined for additional studies. No age, sex, geographic, time or publication status restrictions were imposed on the initial search.

2.2. Study Selection Criteria

Studies were eligible for inclusion if they met the following PICOS' (Participants, Intervention, Control, Outcome measurements, and Study design) criteria: (a) Participants: overweight or obese individuals; (b) Intervention: Phase2® brand *Phaseolus vulgaris* white bean extract, at least 1200 mg per day, for at least 4 weeks; (c) Control: studies comparing the experimental group (*Phaseolus vulgaris* supplementation) with a control/placebo group (no *Phaseolus vulgaris* supplementation), or against baseline; (d) Outcome measurements: studies needed to include measurements of body mass or fat mass; (e) Study design: Studies needed to be either randomized, double-blind, placebo-controlled parallel or crossover trial, or open-label studies.

2.3. Assessment of Risk of Bias

For the quality assessment of randomized controlled trials (RCTs), we used the Delphi list, which includes eight questions with three response options "yes", "no", or "do not know" depending on compliance with key methodological components, and produces a quality score of maximum 9 points that provides an overall estimate of RCT quality [16].

2.4. Data Extraction and Quality Assessment

Two reviewers independently extracted the following data from the selected articles: publication year, number of participants (*Phaseolus vulgaris* and control group), baseline characteristics of the participants, methodological characteristics of the study, pre- and post-values and standard deviation for body mass and fat mass, and statistical information.

2.5. Statistical Analysis

A meta-analysis to estimate the overall treatment effect of *Phaseolus vulgaris* supplementation relative to control groups was performed. Standardized Mean Difference (d) was used in the determination of effect size. In getting the Standardized Mean Difference (d), Cramer's v (which shows the magnitude size) and 95% CI (confidence interval) for each d was computed. The following guideline was used in reading magnitude effect size for Cramer's v: $v < 0.1$ small effect, $0.1 < v < 0.3$ medium effect, $v > 0.3$ large effect. Weighted effect size on all studies was done using the Hunter–Schmidt approach. Weights are objectively assigned based from sample sizes of the studies. Hence, studies with bigger sample size ($n = 60$ [17]) had higher weight, compared to studies with smaller sample size ($n = 10$ [18]). p-values of individual studies are transformed (logarithmic) and aggregated using Chi-square.

3. Results

3.1. Article Selection

One hundred and sixty-five articles were identified. From this list, 54 human studies were identified, and 5 of these were determined to be duplicates, leaving 49 unique studies. Of these 49 studies, only 13 involved the Phase2® *Phaseolus vulgaris* ingredient and one of the following outcomes: weight loss, body fat loss, or anthropometric measures (reductions in waist, hip or thigh measurements). A meta-analysis which included studies which did and did not use the Phase2® *Phaseolus vulgaris* ingredient was excluded. In addition, one of the studies was excluded as it did not provide means, standard deviations, nor p-values [19]. The meta-analysis for weight loss includes 11 studies (see prisma flow diagram, Figure 1), with a total of 573 subjects (see Table 1). The meta-analysis for fat loss includes 3 studies [18,20,21] with a total of 110 subjects (see Table 2). Three studies were excluded, as they did not measure fat mass [22–24]. One study was excluded as it only reported fat loss in percent and not in kilogram [25].

Table 1. Effects of *Phaseolus vulgaris* on body weight. The overall p-value was determined using Chi-square (Chi-square value (W) = 80.02).

Study	Treatment Group			Control Group			p	Weight	Effect (d)	Weighted Mean Difference (Fixed) 95% CI	
	n	Mean	SD	n	Mean	SD				Lower	Upper
Udani et al. 2007 [11]	13	−6.0		12	−4.7		0.424	4%	−0.33	−0.46	1.12
Asano [26]	9	−2.9						3%	−0.19	−1.06	0.67
Koike et al. 2005 [18]	10	−1.8					0.002	3%	−1.61	−0.61	−2.62
Grube et al. 2014 [17]	60	−2.9	2.6	60	−0.9	2.0	0.001	19%	−0.85	−0.48	−1.12
Osorio et al. 2009 [23]	49	−2.3		49	2.21		0.001	15%	−1.00	−0.41	−1.60
Rothacker (week 12) 2003 [27]	30	−6.9		60	0.8		0.029	9%	−0.58	−0.62	−1.09
Wu et al. 2010 [24]	50	−1.9	−0.2	51	−0.4	−0.1	0.049	15%	−0.40	-0.00	−0.79
Celleno et al. 2007 [20]	20	−2.9	−1.2	30	−0.4	0.4		9%	−2.99	−2.25	−3.73
Thom et al. 2000 [21]	20	−3.5		20	2.0		0.001	6%	−1.13	−0.46	−0.12
Udani et al. 2004 [28]	20	−3.8		19	−1.65		0.35	6%	−0.30	−0.33	−0.93
Yamada et al. [25]	33	−0.8	0.2	33			0.01	10%	−0.97	−0.24	−1.68
Total	314			259			0.001	100%	−1.08	−0.43	−1.16

SD: standard deviation, CI: confidence interval.

Table 2. Effects of *Phaseolus vulgaris* on body fat. The overall *p*-value was determined using Chi-square (Chi-square value (*W*) = 36.84).

Study	Treatment Group			Control Group			*p*	Weight	Effect (d)	Weighted Mean Difference (Fixed) 95% CI	
	n	Mean	SD	*n*	Mean	SD				Lower	Upper
Koike et al. 2005 [18]	10	−1.2	−0.4				0.001	17%	−1.58	−2.58	−0.57
Celleno et al. 2007 [20]	30	−2.4	−0.67	30	−0.16	−0.33	0.001	50%	−4.24	−5.15	−3.33
Thom et al. 2000 [21]	20	−2.3	−1.5	20	0.7	−0.6	0.01	33%	−2.63	−3.47	−1.78
Total	60			50			0.02	100%	−3.26	−4.16	−2.35

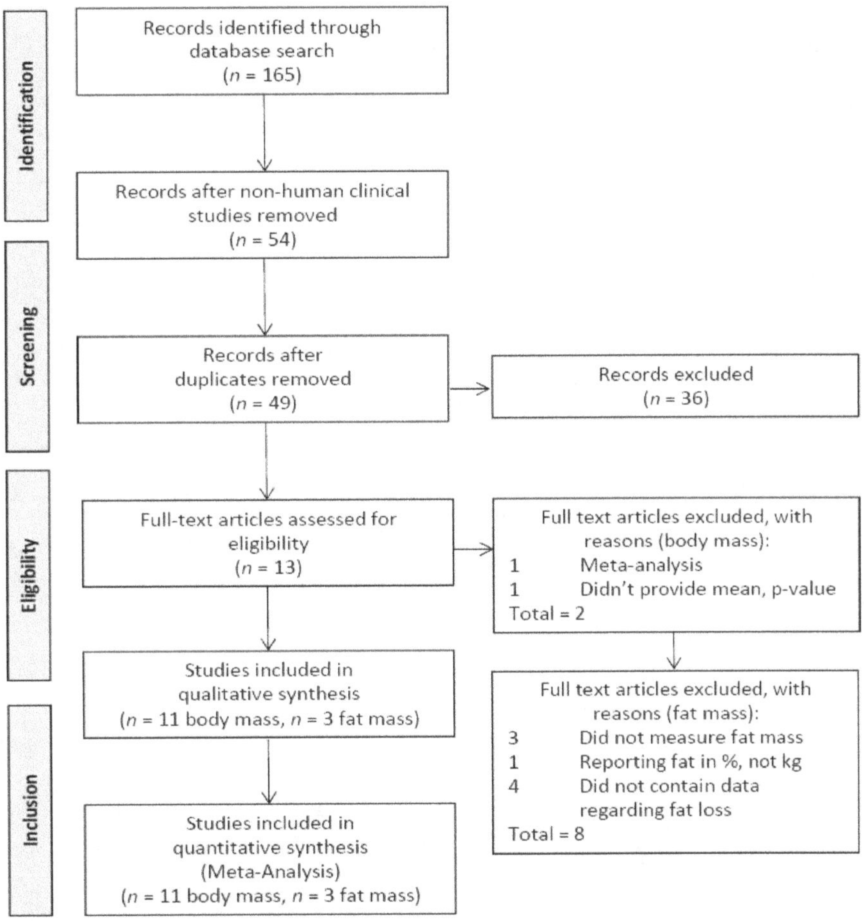

Figure 1. Prisma flow diagram for *Phaseolus vulgaris* and body mass, fat mass.

3.2. *Phaseolus vulgaris* Doses and Duration of Supplementation

The most common dose of *Phaseolus vulgaris* was 3000 mg per day, divided into three doses of 1000 mg (6/11). One study used 3000 mg per day, divided into two doses of 1500 mg [18], and one study used 2000 mg per day, divided into two doses of 1000 mg [11]. Two studies used 400 mg [21], and 445 mg [20] *Phaseolus vulgaris*, respectively, as part of a multi-ingredient blend. One study did not specify the amount of *Phaseolus vulgaris* used [25]. *Phaseolus vulgaris* was supplemented for 1 month (3/11) [11,20,23], 2 months (5/11) [18,24–26,28], or 3 months (3/11) (see Table 3) [17,21,27].

Table 3. Characteristics of the 11 clinical studies included in the meta-analysis.

Study	Participants		Intervention				Comparison	Methods		Study Design	
	Country	Subjects Information	Dose	Diet Intervention	Duration of Intervention	*n* Phase 2	*n* Control	Weight	Fat Mass	Design	Delphi-Score
Asano et al. [26]	Japan	5:1 female to male ratio; average age 36.3 + 12.7; BMI > 25; average BMI = 31.6	3000 mg per day (1000 mg per meal)	no caloric restriction	2 months	9	0	Scale	n/a	Open-Label	2
Udani et al. 2007 [22]	USA	0.3:1 female to male ratio; age 18-40; average BMI = 26	2000 mg per day (1000 mg at breakfast & lunch)	maintain a caloric intake of 1800 per day	4 weeks	13	12	Scale	-	RDBPC	8
Koike et al. 2005 [18]	Japan	1:1 female to male ratio; mean age 41.1 and BMI range 23–30	2× per day 1500 mg Phase 2, 400 mg Clove, 40 mg Lysine 40 mg, 40 mg Arginine, 40 mg Alanine	no caloric restriction	8 weeks	10	0	Scale	n/a	Open-Label	1
Grube et al. 2014 [17]	Germany	3:1 female to male ratio; mean age 46; BMI range 25–35	3000 mg per day (1000 mg per meal)	hypocaloric (500 kcal), providing 40% of energy as carbohydrates	12 weeks	60	57	Scale	BIA	RDBPC	9
Osorio et al. 2009 [23]	Mexico	obese and overweight (age range 18–75 years)	3000 mg per day (1000 mg per meal)	no caloric restriction besides carbohydrate-rich meals	30 days	37	0	Scale	-	Open-Label	1
Rothacker 2003 [27]	USA	24 male; 36 female; mean age 33.2; BMI range 24–32	3000 mg per day (1000 mg per meal)	no caloric restriction	12 weeks	34	26	Scale	BIA	RDBPC	8
Wu et al. 2010 [24]	China	1:1 female to male ratio; age 20-50; BMI range 25–40	3000 mg per day (1000 mg per meal)	no caloric restriction	8 weeks	51	50	Scale	-	RDBPC	8
Celleno et al. 2007 [20]	Italy	2.5:1 female to male ratio; mean age 34; average BMI = 26	3× per day 445 mg of Phase 2, 56 mg vitamin B3, and 0.5 mg chromium	carbohydrate-rich meals (100–200g)	30 days	30	29	Scale	BIA	RDBPC	8
Thom et al. 2000 [21]	Norway	9:1 female to male ratio; mean age 45.6; average BMI = 31	3× per day 400 mg Phase 2, 400 mg inulin, and 100 mg Garcinia cambogia	no caloric restriction	12 weeks	20	20	Scale	BIA	RDBPC	8
Udani et al. 2004 [28]	USA	9:1 female to male ratio; mean age 36.5; average weight of 193.1 pounds	3000 mg per day (1000 mg per meal)	no caloric restriction	8 weeks	20	19	Scale	BIA	RDBPC	8
Yamada et al. [25]	Japan	1:1 female to male ratio; age 25–60; no BMI information	Twice a day proprietary functional food containing Phase 2	no caloric restriction	8 weeks	23	24	Scale	n/a	Open-Label	4

BMI: body mass index; RDBPC: Randomized, Double-Blind, Placebo-Controlled; n/a: method not described; BIA: bioelectrical impedance analysis; -: not measured.

3.3. Control Groups

Participants of the control group had similar characteristics to the intervention groups, but they did not receive *Phaseolus vulgaris* supplementation. In most studies, placebo capsules were administered.

3.4. Effects on Body Weight

Table 1 summarizes the effects of *Phaseolus vulgaris* on body mass. *Phaseolus vulgaris* supplementation showed an average effect on weight loss difference of −1.08 kg (95% CI, −0.42 kg to −1.16 kg, $p < 0.00001$).

3.5. Effects on Fat Loss

Table 2 summarizes the effects of *Phaseolus vulgaris* on fat mass. The average effect of *Phaseolus vulgaris* supplementation on body fat reduction was 3.26 kg (95% CI, −2.35 kg to −4.163 kg, $p = 0.02$).

3.6. Risk of Bias and Publication Bias

Table 4 shows Delphi scores of each reviewed study. The Delphi scores varied between 1 and 9, the mean being 5.9 and the standard deviation ±3.2. Four studies obtained a score below the mean: Asano [26], Koike et al. 2005 [18], Osorio et al. 2009 [23], and Yamada et al. [25], with Asano [26], Koike et al. [18] and Osorio et al. [23] being open-label studies.

Table 4. Delphi-Scores.

Delphi-Scores/Studies	Asano et al. [26]	Udani et al. 2007 [11]	Grube et al. 2014 [17]	Rothacker et al. 2003 [27]	Wu et al. 2010 [24]	Celleno et al. 2007 [20]	Thom et al. 2000 [21]	Udani et al. 2004 [28]	Koike et al. 2005 [18]	Osorio et al. 2009 [23]	Yamada et al. [25]
1. Treatment allocation (a) Was a method of randomization performed?	0	1	1	1	1	1	1	1	0	0	1
(b) Was the treatment allocation concealed?	0	1	1	1	1	1	1	1	0	0	0
2. Were the groups similar at baseline regarding the most important prognostic indicators?	0	1	1	1	1	1	1	1	0	0	1
3. Where the eligibility criteria specified?	1	1	1	1	1	1	1	1	0	0	1
4. Was the outcome assessor blinded?	0	1	1	1	1	1	1	1	0	0	0
5. Was the care provider blinded?	0	1	1	1	1	1	1	1	0	0	0
6. Was the patient blinded?	0	1	1	1	1	1	1	1	0	0	0
7. Were point estimates and measures of variability presented for the primary outcome measures?	1	1	1	1	1	1	1	1	1	1	1
8. Did the analysis include an intention-to-treat analysis?	0	0	1	0	0	0	0	0	0	0	0
Total Delphi Score	2	8	9	8	8	8	8	8	1	1	4

4. Discussion

The aim of this meta-analysis was to determine the effectiveness of Phase2® (*Phaseolus vulgaris*) to support weight loss and to reduce body fat. The overall meta-analysis revealed a significant difference in change in body weight, and body fat between Phase2® (*Phaseolus vulgaris*) and placebo.

Barret et al. conducted a review of clinical studies with Phase 2 brand *Phaseolus vulgaris* White Bean product on weight loss and glycemic control [29]. The analysis identified ten clinical studies which have demonstrated weight loss over time following administration of Phase 2 when taken concurrently with meals containing carbohydrates. Three of these clinical studies revealed significant loss of body weight with Phase 2 compared to a placebo control in people who are overweight or obese. In addition, three clinical trials showed a reduction in serum triglycerides over time. Nine of these clinical studies reported by Barret et al. have been used in this systematic review and meta-analysis. The study by Vinson et al. was not taken into consideration due to its focus on glycemic index and blood glucose investigations without looking into weight loss parameters [30].

While our meta-analysis revealed a significant difference in weight loss over placebo, a previous meta-analysis of *Phaseolus vulgaris* [31] showed a non-significant difference in weight loss between *Phaseolus vulgaris* and placebo groups. This can be explained by the fact that the Onakpoya et al. meta-analysis included not only studies performed with Phase 2, but all studies on *Phaseolus vulgaris*. Both meta-analyses showed significant effects on fat loss. The importance of this work was to isolate the effects of the Phase 2 brand *Phaseolus vulgaris* White Bean from the body of literature. By using unpublished data and all arms of all studies available to us, we were able to demonstrate statistically significant effects on weight and body fat. Part of this importance is in the supplement industry, there is an assumed "generic equivalence" which we know to be false. The prior meta-analysis assumed such a generic equivalence and therefore came up with negative results. In this case, by limiting to only Phase 2, it does appear that there is significant weight and body fat loss with an excellent safety profile.

Low carbohydrate diets have been linked to weight loss, even when not consciously restricting calories, improved triglyceride levels, a reduction in blood glucose levels and improved insulin sensitivity, a decrease in blood pressure. Very low carbohydrate diets (ketogenic diets), with fewer than 50 g of carbohydrate per day, have been linked to weight loss and specific health benefits including neurological disorders. Adaptations to a ketogenic diet is often difficult and nutritional aids have been shown to be useful for entering into nutritional ketosis [32]. A recently concluded study indicated that both low-fat and low-carb diets can work for weight loss, and that there is no "best diet" when it comes to low-carb vs. low-fat diets. In total, 263 males and 346 premenopausal females were assigned to either a low-fat diet or a low-carb diet for 12 months. At 12 months, the low-fat group had lost 5.3 kg and the low-carb group 6.0 kg and this difference is neither statistically significant nor clinically relevant. The healthy diet that will work for you is the one you can stick to, and that varies by individual [33].

5. Conclusions

This meta-analysis found significant effect of Phase2® *Phaseolus vulgaris* supplementation on body weight and body fat.

Acknowledgments: This review was financially supported by Pharmachem Laboratories, Kearny, NJ, USA.

Author Contributions: J.U. was the primary author and was responsible for the design of the review and meta-analysis. J.M. was responsible for organizing references and extracting data from references into evidence tables. O.T. was responsible for the design and execution of meta-analyses. All authors reviewed and approved the final manuscript.

References

1. De Toro-Martín, J.; Arsenault, B.J.; Després, J.P.; Vohl, M.C. Precision Nutrition: A Review of Personalized Nutritional Approaches for the Prevention and Management of Metabolic Syndrome. *Nutrients* **2017**, *9*, 913. [CrossRef] [PubMed]
2. Preuss, H.G.; Bagchi, D. Nutritional therapy of impaired glucose tolerance and diabetes mellitus. In *Nutritional Aspects and Clinical Management of Chronic Disorders and Diseases*; Bronner, F., Ed.; CRC Press: Boca Raton, FL, USA, 2002; pp. 69–91. ISBN 9781420041286.
3. Bell, S.J.; Sears, B. Low-Glycemic-Load Diets: Impact on Obesity and Chronic Diseases. *Crit. Rev. Food Sci. Nutr.* **2003**, *43*, 357–377. [CrossRef] [PubMed]
4. Fukagawa, N.K.; Anderson, J.W.; Hageman, G.; Young, V.R.; Ninaker, K.L. High-carbohydrate, high-fiber diets increase peripheral insulin sensitivity in healthy young and old adults. *Am. J. Clin. Nutr.* **1990**, *52*, 524–528. [CrossRef] [PubMed]
5. Bowman, D.E. Amylase inhibitor of navy bean. *Science* **1945**, *102*, 358–359. [CrossRef] [PubMed]
6. Santimone, M.; Koukiekolo, R.; Moreau, Y.; Le Berre, V.; Rouge, P.; Marchis-Mouren, G.; Desseaux, V. Porcine pancreatic a-amylase inhibition by the kidney bean (*Phaseolus vulgaris*) inhibitor (α-AI1) and structural changes in the α-amylase inhibitor complex. *Biochim. Biophys. Acta* **2004**, *1696*, 181–190. [CrossRef] [PubMed]
7. Bompard-Gilles, C.; Rousseau, P.; Rouge, P.; Payan, F. Substrate mimicry in the active center of a mammalian α-amylase: Structural analysis of an enzyme-inhibitor complex. *Structure* **1996**, *4*, 1441–1452. [CrossRef]
8. Payan, F. Structural basis for the inhibition of mammalian and insect α-amylases by plant protein inhibitors. *Biochim. Biophys. Acta* **2004**, *1696*, 171–180. [CrossRef] [PubMed]
9. Le Berre-Anton, V.; Bompard-Gilles, C.; Payan, F.; Rouge, P. Characterization and functional properties of the α-amylase inhibitor (α-AI) from kidney bean (*Phaseolus vulgaris*) seeds. *Biochim. Biophys. Acta* **1997**, *1343*, 31–40. [CrossRef]
10. Lajolo, F.M.; Finardi-Filho, F. Partial characterization of the amylase inhibitor of black beans (*Phaseolus vulgaris*), variety Rico 23. *J. Agric. Food Chem.* **1985**, *33*, 132–138. [CrossRef]
11. Udani, J.; Hardy, M.; Kavoussi, B. Dietary supplement carbohydrate digestion inhibitors: A review of the literature. In *Obesity. Epidmiology, Pathophysiology, and Prevention*; Bagchi, D., Preuss, H.G., Eds.; CRC Press: Boca Raton, FL, USA, 2007; pp. 279–298.
12. Udani, K. *The Mighty Bean*; European Baker: Bucharest, Romania, 2005.
13. Phase 2®/StarchLite. Available online: www.phase2info.com/pdf/Phase2_Study13.pdf (accessed on 5 January 2018).
14. Phase 2®/StarchLite in Chewing Gum. Available online: http://www.phase2info.com/pdf/Phase2_Study14.pdf (accessed on 5 January 2018).
15. Moher, D.; Liberati, A.; Tetzlaff, J.; Altman, D.G.; the PRISMA Group. Preferred Reporting Items for Systematic Reviews and Meta-Analyses: The PRISMA Statement. *Ann. Intern. Med.* **2009**, *151*, 264–269. [CrossRef] [PubMed]
16. Verhagen, A.P.; de Vet, H.C.W.; de Bie, R.A.; Kessels, A.G.; Boers, M.; Bouter, L.M.; Knipschild, P.G. The Delphi list: A criteria list for quality assessment of randomized clinical trials for conducting systematic reviews developed by Delphi consensus. *J. Clin. Epidemiol.* **1998**, *51*, 1235–1241. [CrossRef]
17. Grube, B.; Chong, W.; Chong, P.; Riede, L. Weight Reduction and Maintenance with IQP-PV-101: A 12-Week Randomized Controlled Study with a 24-Week Open Label Period. *Obesity* **2014**, *22*, 645–651. [CrossRef] [PubMed]
18. Koike, T.; Koizumi, Y.; Tang, L.; Takahara, K.; Saitou, Y. The antiobesity effect and the safety of taking "Phaseolamin(TM) 1600 diet". *J. New Rem. Clin.* **2005**, *54*, 1–16.
19. Erner, S.; Meiss, D. The Effect of Thera-Slim on Weight, Body Composition and Select Laboratory Parameters in Adults with Overweight and Mild-Moderate Obesity. Unpublished work. 2003.
20. Celleno, L.; Tolaini, M.V.; D'Amore, A.; Perricone, N.V.; Preuss, H.G. A dietary supplement containing standardized Phaseolus vulgaris extract influences body composition of overweight men and women. *Int. J. Med. Sci.* **2007**, *49*, 45–52. [CrossRef]
21. Thom, E. A randomized, double-blind, placebo-controlled trial of a new weight-reducing agent of natural origin. *J. Int. Med. Res.* **2000**, *28*, 229–233. [CrossRef] [PubMed]

22. Udani, J.; Singh, B. Blocking Carbohydrate Absorption and Weight Loss: A Clinical Trial Using a Proprietary Fractionated White Bean Extract. *Altern. Ther. Health Med.* **2007**, *13*, 32–37. [PubMed]
23. Osorio, L.; Gamboa, J. Random Multi-Center Evaluation to Test the Efficacy of *Phaseolus vulgaris* (Precarb) in Obese and Overweight Individuals. Unpublished work. 2005.
24. Wu, X.; Xiaofeng, X.; Shen, J.; Perricone, N.; Preuss, H. Enhanced Weight Loss From a Dietary Supplement Containing Standardized *Phaseolus vulgaris* Extract in Overweight Men and Women. *J. Appl. Res.* **2010**, *10*, 73–79.
25. Yamada, J.; Yamamoto, T.; Hideyo, Y. Effects of Combination of Functional Food Materials on Body Weight, Body Fat Percentage, Serum Triglyceride and Blood Glucose. Unpublished work. 2007.
26. Asano, N. The Report of the Test Regarding the Efficacy of Phaseolamine on Weight Loss. Unpublished work, 2009.
27. Rothacker, D. Reduction in body weight with a starch blocking diet aid: StarchAway comparison with placebo. *Leiner Health Prod.* **2003**. Unpublished work.
28. Udani, J.; Hardy, M.; Madsen, D.C. Blocking carbohydrate absorption and weight loss: A clinical trial using Phase 2 brand proprietary fractionated white bean extract. *Altern. Med. Rev.* **2004**, *99*, 63–69.
29. Barrett, M.L.; Udani, J.K. A proprietary alpha-amylase inhibitor from white bean (*Phaseolus vulgaris*): A review of clinical studies on weight loss and glycemic control. *Nutr. J.* **2011**, *10*, 24. [CrossRef] [PubMed]
30. Vinson, J.; Al Kharrat, H.; Shuta, D. Investigation of an amylase inhibitor on human glucose absorption after starch consumption. *Open Nutraceuticals J.* **2009**, *2*, 88–91. [CrossRef]
31. Onakpoya, I.; Aldaas, S.; Terry, R.; Ernst, E. The efficacy of Phaseolus vulgaris as a weight-loss supplement: A systematic review and meta-analysis of randomised clinical trials. *Br. J. Nutr.* **2011**, *106*, 196–202. [CrossRef] [PubMed]
32. Harvey, C.J.D.C.; Schofield, G.M.; Williden, M. The use of nutritional supplements to induce ketosis and reduce symptoms associated with keto-induction: A narrative review. *PeerJ* **2018**, *16*, e4488. [CrossRef] [PubMed]
33. Gardner, C.D.; Trepanowski, J.F.; Del Gobbo, L.C.; Hauser, M.E.; Rigdon, J.; Ioannidis, J.P.A.; Desai, M.; King, A.C. Effect of Low-Fat vs Low-Carbohydrate Diet on 12-Month Weight Loss in Overweight Adults and the Association With Genotype Pattern or Insulin Secretion. *JAMA* **2018**, *319*, 667–679. [CrossRef] [PubMed]

7

Lactic Acid Bacteria from Kefir Increase Cytotoxicity of Natural Killer Cells to Tumor Cells

Takuya Yamane [1,2,3,*], Tatsuji Sakamoto [1,2], Takenori Nakagaki [3] and Yoshihisa Nakano [1,2]

1. Center for Research and Development Bioresources, Organization for Research Promotion, Osaka Prefecture University, Sakai, Osaka 599-8570, Japan; sakamoto@biochem.osakafu-u.ac.jp (T.S.); nakano@biochem.osakafu-u.ac.jp (Y.N.)
2. Department of Applied Life Sciences, Graduate School of Life and Environmental Sciences, Osaka Prefecture University, Sakai, Osaka 599-8531, Japan
3. Institute of Food Sciences, Nakagaki Consulting Engineer and Co., Ltd., Nishi-ku, Sakai 593-8328, Japan; tnakagaki@nakagaki.co.jp

* Correspondence: tyt29194@osakafu-u.ac.jp

Abstract: The Japanese fermented beverage, homemade kefir, contains six lactic acid bacteria: *Lactococcus. lactis* subsp. *Lactis*, *Lactococcus. lactis* subsp. *Cremoris*, *Lactococcus. Lactis* subsp. *Lactis biovar diacetylactis*, *Lactobacillus plantarum*, *Leuconostoc meseuteroides* subsp. *Cremoris* and *Lactobacillus casei*. In this study, we found that a mixture of the six lactic acid bacteria from kefir increased the cytotoxicity of human natural killer KHYG-1 cells to human chronic myelogenous leukemia K562 cells and colorectal tumor HCT116 cells. Furthermore, levels of mRNA expression and secretion of IFN-γ (interferon gamma) increased in KHYG-1 cells that had been treated with the six lactic acid bacteria mixture from kefir. The results suggest that the six lactic acid bacteria mixture from kefir has strong effects on natural immunity and tumor cell cytotoxicity.

Keywords: kefir; lactic acid bacteria; natural killer cell; cytotoxicity

---

1. Introduction

The fermented beverage kefir has many health benefits, including its antibacterial, anticarcinogenic, wound healing, antiallergenic, immunomodulation, and gastrointestinal immunity effects [1]. The fermented beverage, homemade kefir, has been available for more than 20 years in Japan. Homemade kefir contains six lactic acid bacteria: *Lactococcus. lactis* subsp. *Lactis* [2–12], *Lactococcus. lactis* subsp. *Cremoris* [8,9,13], *Lactococcus. Lactis* subsp. *Lactis biovar diacetylactis* [4], *Lacto bacillus planterun* [4,14–16], *Leuconostoc meseuteroides* subsp. *Cremoris* [7,9], and *Lacto bacillus casei* [2,5,12,16]. Kefir is able to offer health benefits through modulation of the gastrointestinal immune system, and previous studies showed that kefir increases the levels of some proinflammatory cytokines including TNF-α (tumor necrosis factor alpha), IFN-γ (interferon gamma) and IL-12 (interleukin 12) [1]. Lactic acid bacteria have beneficial effects with respect to diarrhea [17,18], food allergies [19], and inflammatory bowel disease [20–22]. Lactic acid bacteria also play an important role in the prevention of colorectal cancer [23,24], and *Lacto bacillus casei* Shirota increases the activity of natural killer (NK) cells [25,26]. However, the effect of homemade kefir on NK cell activity is not clear. In this study, we found that a six lactic acid bacteria mixture from homemade kefir increases NK cell activity, including cytotoxic activity against human colorectal tumor HCT116 cells. These results suggest that the mixture of six lactic acid bacteria from homemade kefir has important effects on innate immunity and tumor cell cytotoxicity.

2. Materials and Methods

2.1. Materials

Homemade kefir was provided by Nakagaki Consulting Engineer and Co., Ltd. (Osaka, Japan). Roswell Park Memorial Institute (RPMI) 1640 medium, Dulbecco's modified Eagle's medium (DMEM), and human interleukin-2 were purchased from Wako Pure Chemical Industries, Ltd. (Osaka, Japan). All other reagents were of analytical grade.

2.2. Cell Culture

KHYG-1 and K562 cells were provided by JCRB Cell Bank (Osaka, Japan), and HCT116 cells were purchased from American Tissue Culture Collection (ATCC) (Manassas, VA, USA). KHYG-1 cells were cultured in RPMI 1640 medium with 10% fetal bovine serum (Sigma, St. Louis, MO, USA) and 1 μg/mL IL-2. K562 and HCT116 cells were cultured in RPMI 1640 medium and in Dulbecco's modified Eagle's medium (DMEM), respectively, with 10% fetal bovine serum.

2.3. Preparation of Lactic Acid Bacteria Mixture

One gram of homemade kefir powder was added to 1 L of de Man, Rogosa and Sharpe (MRS) broth and cultured for 24 h at 22.5 °C. The cultured solution was centrifuged at 3000 rpm for 30 min at 4 °C using a TOMY centrifugation apparatus (TOMY SEIKO, Tokyo, Japan), and the six lactic acid bacteria mixture was obtained from the precipitates. A lactic acid bacteria mixture from killed bacteria was prepared by autoclaving at 120 °C for 15 min. Identification of the lactic acid bacteria cultured in the MRS broth was performed by polymerase chain reaction (PCR) using DNA from the six lactic acid bacteria as templates. After PCR, amplified DNA was separated on 2.0% agarose gels and stained with ethidium bromide. The PCR conditions and primers used are shown in Table 1.

2.4. Measurement of NK Cell Activity and Tumor Cytotoxicity

KHYG-1 cells were treated with the six lactic acid bacteria mixture for 24 h at 37 °C in a 5% CO_2 incubator. The cells that had been treated with the six lactic acid bacteria mixture were reacted with K562 cells or with HCT116 cells for 4 h at 37 °C in a 5% CO_2 incubator. NK cell activity and tumor cytotoxicity were measured using an LDH Cytotoxicity Detection Kit (Takara, Shiga, Japan).

2.5. RT-PCR (Reverse Transcription Polymerase Chain Reaction)

Nucleotide sequences of primers used for RT-PCR were as follows: hIFNγ-F: 5′-GAATGTCCAACGCAAAGCAA-3′, hIFNγ-R: 5′-GCTGCTGGCGACAGTTCAG-3′, hACTB-F: 5′-CTTCCTGGGCATGGAGTC-3′, and hACTB-R: 5′-GGATGTCCACGTCACACTTC-3′. The full RNAs were prepared from cells and subjected to semi-quantitative RT-PCR analyses. PCR conditions were 1 min at 94 °C, 30 s at 94 °C, 30 s at 60 °C, and 35 cycles of 1 min at 72 °C for IFNγ and ACTB. After the reactions, PCR products were separated on 2.0% agarose gels and stained with SAFELOOK™ Pregreen (Wako, Osaka, Japan). Intensities of the bands were quantified using Image J software (https://imagej.nih.gov/ij/). β-actin mRNA was also amplified as a control.

2.6. IFN-γ Measurement

IFN-γ was measured using a Human IFN-γ ELISA (enzyme-linked immunosorbent assay) Development Kit (PeproTech, Rocky Hill, NJ, USA) according to the manufacturer's instructions.

2.7. Statistical Analysis

Data are expressed as means ± S.E (standard error). Statistical analyses were performed with an analysis of variance (one-way ANOVA) followed by an unpaired Student's *t*-test.

Table 1. Polymerase chain reaction (PCR) primers and reacting conditions.

Strain	Primer Sequence		PCR Condition	Ref.
L. lactis subsp. *Lactis*	sense antisense	5′-CGTTATGGATTTGATGGATATAAAGC-3′ 5′-ACTCTTCTTAAGAACAAGTTTAACAGC-3′	94 °C 9 min, 94 °C 30 s, 50 °C 30 s, 72 °C 60 s × 45 cycles, 72 °C 7 min	[27]
L. lactis subsp. *Cremoris*	sense antisense	5′-CGTTATGGATTTGATGGATATAAAGC-3′ 5′-ACTCTTCTTAAGAACAAGTTTAACAGC-3′	94 °C 9 min, 94 °C 30 s, 50 °C 30 s, 72 °C 60 s × 45 cycles, 72 °C 7 min	
L. lactis subsp. *lactis biovar diacetylactis*	sense antisense	5′-CTTCGTTATGATTTTACA-3′ 5′-AATATCAACAATTCCATG-3′	94 °C 30 s, 94 °C 30 s, 46 °C 60 s, 72 °C 60 s × 30 cycles, 72 °C 2 min	[28,29]
Leuconostoc mesenteroides subsp. *Cremoris* (Genus-specific primers for *Leuconostoc*)	sense antisense	5′-AACTTAGTGTCGCATGAC-3′ 5′-AGTCGAGTTACAGACTACAA-3′	94 °C 5 min, 94 °C 60 s, 60 °C 60 s, 72 °C 60 s × 30 cycles, 72 °C 10 min	[30]
Lactobacillus plantarum	sense antisense	5′-CCGTTTATGCGGAACACCTA-3′ 5′-TCGGGATTACCAAACATCAC-3′	94 °C 3 min, 94 °C 30 s, 54 °C 10 s, 72 °C 30 s × 30 cycles, 72 °C 5 min	[31]
Lactobacillus casei	sense	5-TGCACTGAGATTCGACTTAA-3	94 °C 3 min, 94 °C 45 s, 45 °C 45 s, 72 °C 60 s × 30 cycles, 72 °C 5 min	[32]

3. Results and Discussion

3.1. Induction of NK Activity by the Six Lactic Acid Bacteria from Homemade-Kefir

As shown in Figure 1, the six lactic acid bacteria from homemade kefir were detected in MRS broth cultures and identified using PCR with the bacteria's DNA as templates. The cytotoxicity of KHYG-1 cells that had been treated with the six lactic acid bacteria mixture, against K562 cells, increased in a cell number-dependent manner (Figure 2). As shown in Figure 3A, KHYG-1 cells were activated by the six lactic acid bacteria mixture and increased their cytotoxicity against K562 cells in a dose-dependent manner. Lactic acid bacteria have many effects on biological activities such as apoptosis induction, antioxidant activities, and immune response improvement [33]. Nagao et al. reported that *Lactobacillus casei Shirota* enhanced NK cell activity [25]. *Lacto bacillus plantarum C4* isolated from kefir has also been shown to prevent infection with *Yersinia enterocolitice* O9 in the intestine in mice. Additionally, a concentrated supernatant from the cultured medium of *Lacto bacillus plantarum C4* has antibacterial and anti-tumor activities [34]. Since the six lactic acid bacteria mixture from homemade kefir includes *Lacto bacillus plantarum* and *Lacto bacillus casei*, it is thought that these lactic acid bacteria contribute to the induction of NK cell activity.

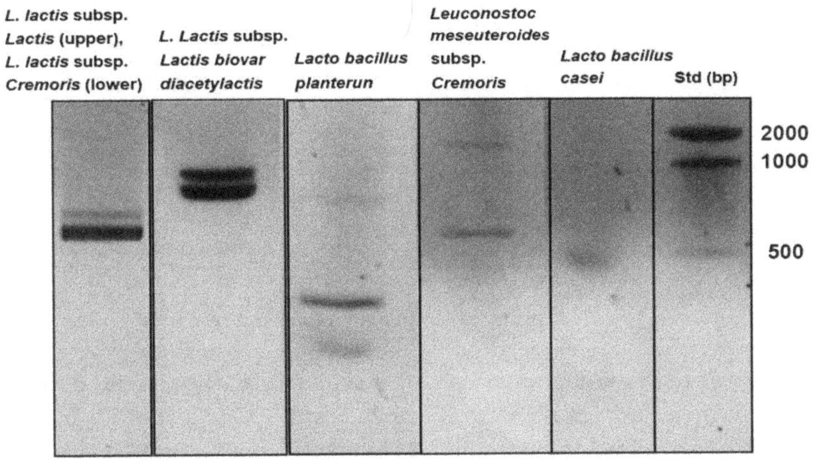

Figure 1. Identification of the six lactic acid bacteria cultured in de Man, Rogosa and Sharpe (MRS) broth using polymerase chain reaction (PCR) as described in the Materials and Methods. The amplified DNA after PCR were separated on agarose gels.

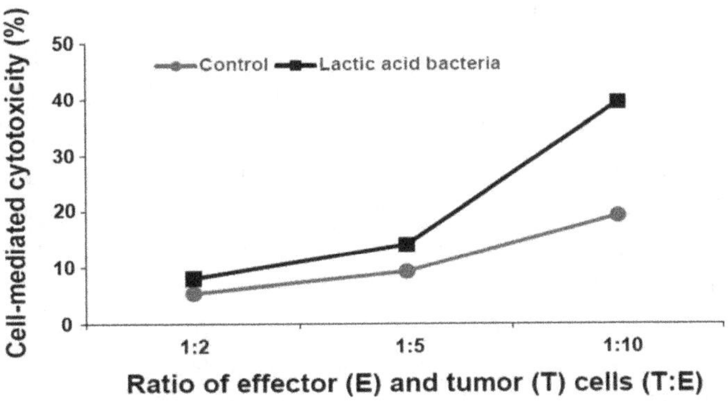

Figure 2. Cell-mediated cytotoxicity of natural killer (NK) cells by a six lactic acid bacteria mixture. KHYG-1 cells were treated with a six lactic acid bacteria mixture for 24 h at 37 °C in a 5% CO_2 incubator. The treated cells were reacted with K562 cells for 4 h at 37 °C in a 5% CO_2 incubator. Cell-mediated cytotoxicity increased for KHYG-1 cells that had been treated with the six lactic acid bacteria mixture.

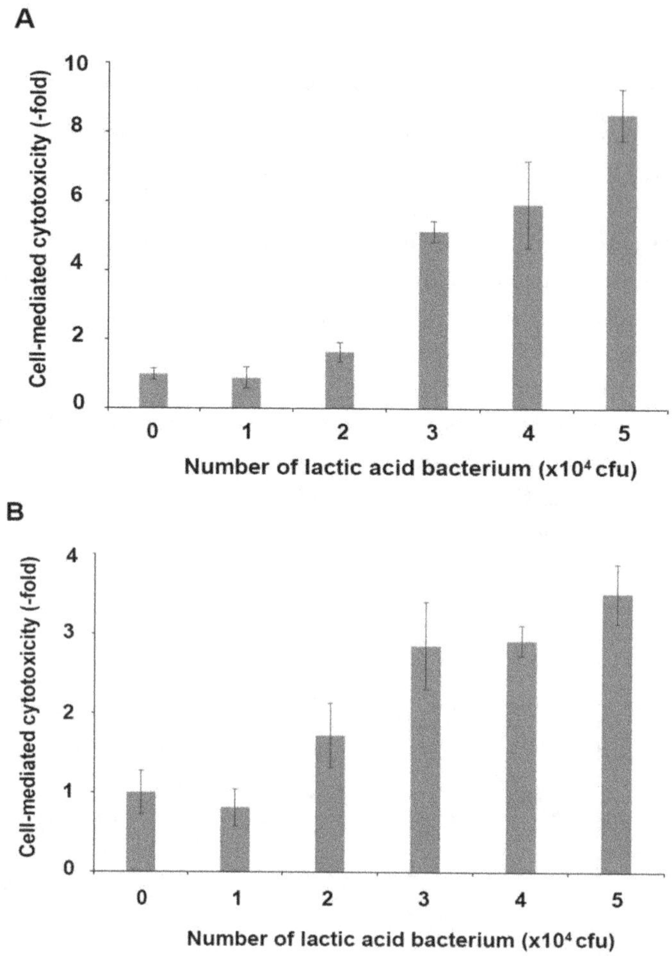

Figure 3. Induction of cell-mediated cytotoxicity by a six lactic acid bacteria mixture. KHYG-1 cells were treated with a six lactic acid bacteria mixture for 24 h at 37 °C in a 5% CO_2 incubator. The treated cells were reacted with K562 cells (**A**) or with HCT116 cells (**B**) for 4 h at 37 °C in a 5% CO_2 incubator. In both cases, cell-mediated cytotoxicity was increased by KHYG-1 cells that had been treated with the six lactic acid bacteria mixture in a dose-dependent manner.

3.2. Induction of Cytotoxicity by the Six Lactic Acid Bacteria Against Human Colorectal Tumor Cells

Cytotoxic activity of KHYG-1 cells against HCT116 cells was increased by the six lactic acid bacteria mixture in a dose-dependent manner (Figure 3B). NK cells have the intrinsic ability to detect and kill cancer cells [35]. The lytic functions of NK cells mediated by granzyme B and perforin have dominated investigations of the role of NK cells in anti-cancer defense [36]. The effector function of NK cells is tightly regulated by activating and inhibiting receptors. Tumor cells can evade the anti-tumor activity of NK cells by modifying the expression of NK cell receptors. In colorectal carcinoma, for instance, the expression of activating receptors—such as CD16 (FCGR3A, Fc fragment of IgG receptor IIIa), NKp46 (NCR1, natural cytotoxicity triggering receptor 1), NKp30 (NCR3, natural cytotoxicity triggering receptor 3), and NKG2D (KLRK1, killer cell lectin like receptor K1)—is decreased. Additionally, the expression of inhibiting receptors, such as KIR3DL1 (killer cell immunoglobulin-like receptor 3DL1) and NKG2A (killer cell lectin like receptor C1), is increased [37]. The six lactic acid bacteria mixture or its secretory compounds may regulate the expression of these receptor genes and inhibit tumor formation by escaping from NK cell-mediated cytotoxicity. Lactic acid bacteria have indeed been demonstrated to have a host of properties for preventing the development of a colorectal tumor, specifically by inhibiting its initiation or progression. In the pathway of the anticancer immune response, lactic acid bacteria also stimulate NK cell activity [33]. Furthermore, a seminal 11-year prospective cohort study conducted in Japan showed an inverse correlation between increase of cancer incidence and the level of NK cell cytotoxicity [38]. These results indicate that the six lactic acid bacteria mixture from homemade kefir reacts with human colorectal tumor HCT116 cells through activation of the immunity of NK cells.

3.3. *Induction of Cytotoxicity of KHYG-1 Cells by the Killed Lactic Acid Bacteria Mixture*

To examine the distinct effects of live and dead lactic acid bacteria on NK cell activation, KHYG-1 cells were treated with the live and the killed six lactic acid bacteria mixtures and cytotoxicity assays were carried out. As shown in Figure 4A, activation of KHYG-1 cells was increased by treatment with both the live and killed mixtures. Cytotoxicity of KHYG-1 cells against HCT116 cells was also increased by both mixtures (Figure 4B). Previous studies, on the other hand, have shown that 40% to 62% of several strains of *L. plantarum* survive under the low pH conditions in a simulated intestine [39], and that 81% to 93% of several strains of *L. casei* can also survive at pH 2.0 for 2 h [40]. The present and previous results, therefore, suggest that both lactic acid bacteria that have been killed by gastric acid and live lactic acid bacteria have effects on NK cell activation in the intestine after the administration of homemade kefir.

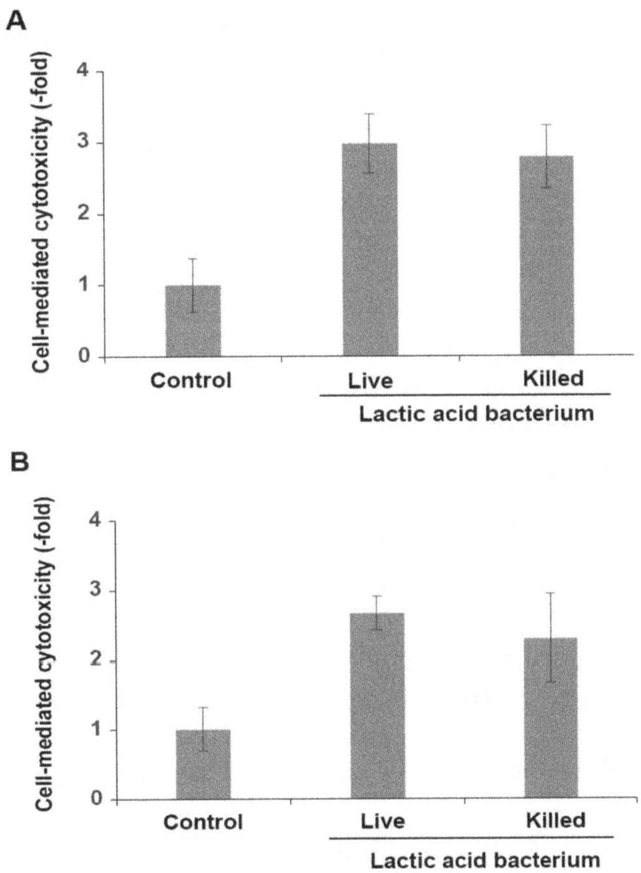

Figure 4. Induction of cell-mediated cytotoxicity of KHYG-1 cells by the live and the killed lactic acid bacteria mixtures. KHYG-1 cells were treated with both mixtures (3×10^4 cfu) for 24 h at 37 °C in a 5% CO_2 incubator. The treated cells were reacted with K562 cells (**A**) or with HCT116 cells (**B**) for 4 h at 37 °C in a 5% CO_2 incubator. In both cases, cell-mediated cytotoxicity was increased in KHYG-1 cells that had been treated with both the live and the killed lactic acid bacteria mixtures.

3.4. Increased Expression and Secretion Levels of IFN-γ in KHYG-1 Cells

IFN-γ mRNA and IFN-γ secretion were both increased in KHYG-1 cells that had been treated by the six lactic acid bacteria mixture (Figure 5A,B). NK cells regulate various immune cells through the secretion of IFN-γ and they perform tumor surveillance [41]. Increased IFN-γ expression and secretion induced by the mixture of six lactic acid bacteria from homemade kefir may provide a synergistic effect on anti-tumor activity.

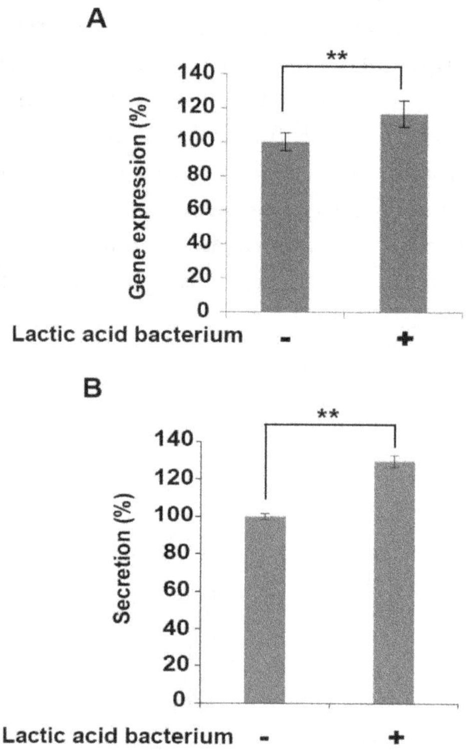

Figure 5. Increased expression and secretion levels of IFN-γ. (**A**) The expression level of IFN-γ mRNA was increased in KHYG-1 cells that had been treated with the six lactic acid bacteria mixture (3×10^4 cfu) for 4 h at 37 °C in a 5% CO_2 incubator ($n = 3$, ** $p < 0.01$). (**B**) The secretion level of IFN-γ mRNA was increased in the same, treated, KHYG-1 cells ($n = 6$, ** $p < 0.01$).

4. Conclusions

This study showed that the cytotoxicity of NK cells and the expression and secretion of IFN-γ in NK cells were increased after treatment of the cells with a six lactic acid bacteria mixture. Further in vitro and in vivo studies using animal models of colorectal cancer are needed to investigate the mechanisms underlying the effects of the six lactic acid bacteria mixture.

Author Contributions: Takuya Yamane, Tatsuji Sakamoto, Takenori Nakagaki and Yoshihisa Nakano conceptualized the study; Takuya Yamane carried out experiments; Takuya Yamane conducted the analyses; and Takuya Yamane wrote the manuscript.

References

1. Bourrie, B.C.; Willing, B.P.; Cotter, P.D. The Microbiota and Health Promoting Characteristics of the Fermented Beverage Kefir. *Front. Microbiol.* **2016**, *7*, 647. [CrossRef] [PubMed]
2. Angulo, L.; Lopez, E.; Lema, C. Microflora present in kefir grains of the Galician region (North-West of Spain). *J. Dairy Res.* **1993**, *60*, 263–267. [CrossRef] [PubMed]

3. Pintado, M.E.; Da Silva, J.A.L.; Fernandes, P.B.; Malcata, F.X.; Hogg, T.A. Microbiological and rheological studies on Portuguese kefir grains. *Int. J. Food Sci. Technol.* **1996**, *31*, 15–26. [CrossRef]
4. Garrote, G.L.; Abraham, A.G.; De Antoni, G.L. Chemical and microbiological characterisation of kefir grains. *J. Dairy Res.* **2001**, *68*, 639–652. [CrossRef] [PubMed]
5. Simova, E.; Beshkova, D.; Angelov, A.; Hristozova, T.; Frengova, G.; Spasov, Z. Lactic acid bacteria and yeasts in kefir grains and kefir made from them. *J. Ind. Microbiol. Biotechnol.* **2002**, *28*, 1–6. [CrossRef] [PubMed]
6. Witthuhn, R.C.; Schoeman, T.; Britz, T.J. Isolation and characterization of the microbial population of different South African kefir grains. *Int. J. Dairy Technol.* **2004**, *57*, 33–37. [CrossRef]
7. Witthuhn, R.; Schoeman, T.; Britz, T. Characterisation of the microbial population at different stages of Kefir production and Kefir grain mass cultivation. *Int. Dairy J.* **2005**, *15*, 383–389. [CrossRef]
8. Yüksekdağ, Z.; Beyatli, Y.; Aslim, B. Determination of some characteristics coccoid forms of lactic acid bacteria isolated from Turkish kefirs with natural probiotic. *LWT Food Sci. Technol.* **2004**, *37*, 663–667. [CrossRef]
9. Mainville, I.; Robert, N.; Lee, B.; Farnworth, E.R. Polyphasic characterization of the lactic acid bacteria in kefir. *Syst. Appl. Microbiol.* **2006**, *29*, 59–68. [CrossRef] [PubMed]
10. Chen, H.-C.; Wang, S.-Y.; Chen, M.-J. Microbiological study of lactic acid bacteria in kefir grains by culture-dependent and culture-independent methods. *Food Microbiol.* **2008**, *25*, 492–501. [CrossRef] [PubMed]
11. Garofalo, C.; Osimani, A.; Milanović, V.; Aquilanti, L.; De Filippis, F.; Stellato, G.; Di Mauro, S.; Turchetti, B.; Buzzini, P.; Ercolini, D.; et al. Bacteria and yeast microbiota in milk kefir grains from different Italian regions. *Food Microbiol.* **2015**, *49*, 123–133. [CrossRef] [PubMed]
12. Zanirati, D.F.; Abatemarco, M.; de Cicco Sandes, S.H.; Nicoli, J.R.; Nunes, Á.C.; Neumann, E. Selection of lactic acid bacteria from Brazilian kefir grains for potential use as starter or probiotic cultures. *Anaerobe* **2015**, *32*, 70–76. [CrossRef] [PubMed]
13. Korsak, N.; Taminiau, B.; Leclercq, M.; Nezer, C.; Crevecoeur, S.; Ferauche, C.; Detry, E.; Delcenserie, V.; Daube, G. Short communication: Evaluation of the microbiota of kefir samples using metagenetic analysis targeting the 16S and 26S ribosomal DNA fragments. *J. Dairy Sci.* **2015**, *98*, 3684–3689. [CrossRef] [PubMed]
14. Santos, A.; San Mauro, M.; Sanchez, A.; Torres, J.M.; Marquina, D. The antimicrobial properties of different strains of *Lactobacillus* spp. isolated from kefir. *Syst. Appl. Microbiol.* **2003**, *26*, 434–437. [CrossRef] [PubMed]
15. Da Cruz Pedrozo Miguel, M.G.; Cardoso, P.G.; de Assis Lago, L.; Schwan, R.F. Diversity of bacteria present in milk kefir grains using culture-dependent and culture-independent methods. *Food Res. Int.* **2010**, *43*, 1523–1528. [CrossRef]
16. Nalbantoglu, U.; Cakar, A.; Dogan, H.; Abaci, N.; Ustek, D.; Sayood, K.; Can, H. Metagenomic analysis of the microbial community in kefir grains. *Food Microbiol.* **2014**, *41*, 42–51. [CrossRef] [PubMed]
17. Chouraqui, J.P.; Van Egroo, L.D.; Fichot, M.C. Acidified milk formula supplemented with *Bifidobacterium lactis*: Impact on infant diarrhea in residential care settings. *J. Pediatr. Gastroenterol. Nutr.* **2004**, *38*, 288–292. [CrossRef] [PubMed]
18. Gaón, D.; García, H.; Winter, L.; Rodríguez, N.; Quintás, R.; González, S.N.; Oliver, G. Effect of *Lactobacillus strains* and *Saccharomyces boulardii* on persistent diarrhea in children. *Medicina (Buenos Aires)* **2003**, *63*, 293–298.
19. Pohjavuori, E.; Viljanen, M.; Korpela, R.; Kuitunen, M.; Tiittanen, M.; Vaarala, O.; Savilahti, E. *Lactobacillus* GG effect in increasing IFN-gamma production in infants with cow's milk allergy. *J. Allergy Clin. Immunol.* **2004**, *114*, 131–136. [CrossRef] [PubMed]
20. Bourlioux, P.; Koletzko, B.; Guarner, F.; Braesco, V. The intestine and its microflora are partners for the protection of the host: Report on the Danone Symposium "The Intelligent Intestine," held in Paris, June 14, 2002. *Am. J. Clin. Nutr.* **2003**, *78*, 675–683. [CrossRef] [PubMed]
21. Azcárate-Peril, M.A.; Sikes, M.; Bruno-Bárcena, J.M. The intestinal microbiota, gastrointestinal environment and colorectal cancer: A putative role for probiotics in prevention of colorectal cancer? *Am. J. Physiol. Gastrointest. Liver Physiol.* **2011**, *301*, G401–G424. [CrossRef] [PubMed]
22. Del Carmen, S.; de LeBlanc, A.M.; Miyoshi, A.; Rocha, C.S.; Azevedo, V.; LeBlanc, J.G. Potential application of probiotics in the prevention and treatment of inflammatory bowel diseases. *Ulcers* **2011**, *2011*, 841651. [CrossRef]
23. Rafter, J.J. The role of lactic acid bacteria in colon cancer prevention. *Scand. J. Gastroenterol.* **1995**, *30*, 497–502. [CrossRef] [PubMed]

24. Hirayama, K.; Rafter, J. The role of lactic acid bacteria in colon cancer prevention: Mechanistic considerations. *Antonie Van Leeuwenhoek* **1999**, *76*, 391–394. [PubMed]
25. Nagao, F.; Nakayama, M.; Muto, T.; Okumura, K. Effects of a fermented milk drink containing *Lactobacillus casei* strain Shirota on the immune system in healthy human subjects. *Biosci. Biotechnol. Biochem.* **2000**, *64*, 2706–2708. [CrossRef] [PubMed]
26. Dong, H.; Rowland, I.; Tuohy, K.M.; Thomas, L.V.; Yaqoob, P. Selective effects of *Lactobacillus casei* Shirota on T cell activation, natural killer cell activity and cytokine production. *Clin. Exp. Immunol.* **2010**, *161*, 378–388. [CrossRef] [PubMed]
27. Nomura, M.; Kobayashi, M.; Okamoto, T. Rapid PCR-Based Method Which Can Determine Both Phenotype and Genotype of *Lactococcus lactis* Subspecies. *Appl. Environ. Microbiol.* **2002**, *68*, 2209–2213. [CrossRef] [PubMed]
28. Beimfohr, C.; Ludwig, W.; Schleifer, K.H. Rapid Genotypic Differentiation of *Lactococcus lactis* Subspecies and Biovar. *Syst. Appl. Microbiol.* **1997**, *20*, 216–221. [CrossRef]
29. Feutry, F.; Torre, P.; Arana, I.; Garcia, S.; Desmasures, N.; Casalta, E. *Lactococcus lactis* strains from raw ewe's milk samples from the PDO Ossau-Iraty cheese area: Levels, genotypic and technological diversity. *Dairy Sci. Technol.* **2012**, *92*, 655–670. [CrossRef]
30. Kahala, M.; Maki, M.; Lehtovaara, A.; Tapanainen, J.M.; Katiska, R.; Juuruskorpi, M.; Juhola, J.; Joutsjoki, V. Characterization of starter lactic acid bacteria from the Finnish fermented milk product viili. *J. Appl. Microbiol.* **2008**, *105*, 1929–1938. [CrossRef] [PubMed]
31. Torriani, S.; Felis, G.E.; Dellaglio, F. Differentiation of *Lactobacillus plantarum*, *L. pentosus*, and *L. paraplantarum* by *recA* gene sequence analysis and multiplex PCR assay with *recA* gene-derived primers. *Appl. Environ. Microbiol.* **2001**, *67*, 3450–3454. [CrossRef] [PubMed]
32. Ward, L.J.H.; Timmins, M.J. Differentiation of *Lactobacillus casei*, *Lactobacillus paracasei* and *Lactobacillus rhamnosus* by polymerase chain reaction. *Lett. Appl. Microbiol.* **1999**, *29*, 90–92. [CrossRef] [PubMed]
33. Zhong, L.; Zhang, X.; Covasa, M. Emerging roles of lactic acid bacteria in protection against colorectal cancer. *World J. Gastroenterol.* **2014**, *20*, 7878–7886. [CrossRef] [PubMed]
34. De Montijo-Prieto, S.; Moreno, E.; Bergillos-Meca, T.; Lasserrot, A.; Ruiz-López, M.D.; Ruiz-Bravo, A.; Jiménez-Valera, M.A. *Lactobacillus plantarum* strain isolated from kefir protects against intestinal infection with *Yersinia enterocolitica* O9 and modulates immunity in mice. *Res. Microbiol.* **2015**, *166*, 626–632. [CrossRef] [PubMed]
35. Nicholson, S.E.; Keating, N.; Belz, G.T. Natural killer cells and anti-tumor immunity. *Mol. Immunol.* **2017**, in press. [CrossRef] [PubMed]
36. Voskoboinik, I.; Whisstock, J.C.; Trapani, J.A. Perforin and granzymes: Function, dysfunction and human pathology. *Nat. Rev. Immunol.* **2015**, *15*, 388–400. [CrossRef] [PubMed]
37. Lee, H.H.; Kang, H.; Cho, H. Natural killer cells and tumor metastasis. *Arch. Pharm. Res.* **2017**, *40*, 1037–1049. [CrossRef] [PubMed]
38. Imai, K.; Matsuyama, S.; Miyake, S.; Suga, K.; Nakachi, K. Natural cytotoxic activity of peripheral-blood lymphocytes and cancer incidence: An 11-year follow-up study of a general population. *Lancet* **2000**, *356*, 1795–1799. [CrossRef]
39. Tokatlı, M.; Gülgör, G.; Bağder Elmacı, S.; Arslankoz İşleyen, N.; Özçelik, F. In Vitro Properties of Potential Probiotic Indigenous Lactic Acid Bacteria Originating from Traditional Pickles. *BioMed Res. Int.* **2015**, *2015*, 315819. [CrossRef] [PubMed]
40. Zhang, B.; Wang, Y.; Tan, Z.; Li, Z.; Jiao, Z.; Huang, Q. Screening of Probiotic Activities of Lactobacilli Strains Isolated from Traditional Tibetan Qula, A Raw Yak Milk Cheese. *Asian-Australas. J. Anim. Sci.* **2016**, *29*, 1490–1499. [CrossRef] [PubMed]
41. Ikeda, H.; Old, L.J.; Schreiber, R.D. The roles of IFN gamma in protection against tumor development and cancer immunoediting. *Cytokine Growth Factor Rev.* **2002**, *13*, 95–109.

8

Effects of Two Doses of Curry Prepared with Mixed Spices on Postprandial Ghrelin and Subjective Appetite Responses

Sumanto Haldar [1], Joseph Lim [1], Siok Ching Chia [1], Shalini Ponnalagu [1] and Christiani Jeyakumar Henry [1,2,*]

1 Clinical Nutrition Research Centre (CNRC), Singapore Institute for Clinical Sciences (SICS), Agency for Science Technology and Research (A*STAR), 30 Medical Drive, Singapore 117609, Singapore; sumanto_haldar@sics.a-star.edu.sg (S.H.); joseph_lim@sics.a-star.edu.sg (J.L.); smileychiasc@gmail.com (S.C.C.); Shalini_Ponnalagu@sics.a-star.edu.sg (S.P.)

2 Department of Biochemistry, National University of Singapore, Singapore 119077, Singapore

* Correspondence: jeya_henry@sics.a-star.edu.sg

Abstract: Spices are known to provide orosensory stimulation that can potentially influence palatability, appetite, and energy balance. Previous studies with individual spices have shown divergent effects on appetite and energy intake measures. In a real-life context, however, several spices are consumed in combinations, as in various forms of curries. Therefore, we investigated changes in postprandial appetite and plasma ghrelin in response to the intake of two doses of curry prepared with mixed spices. The study was undertaken in healthy Chinese men, between 21 and 40 years of age and body mass index $\leq$27.5 kg/m^2. Appetite was measured using visual analogue scales (VAS) and plasma ghrelin was measured using multiplex assay. Compared with the control meal (Dose 0 Control (D0C), 0 g mixed spices), we found significantly greater suppression in 'hunger' (both $p < 0.05$, after Bonferroni adjustments) as well in 'desire to eat' (both $p < 0.01$) during the Dose 1 Curry (D1C, 6 g mixed spices) and Dose 2 Curry (D2C, 12 g mixed spices) intake. There were no differences, however, in plasma ghrelin or in other appetite measures such as in 'fullness' or in 'prospective eating' scores. Overall, the results of our study indicate greater inter-meal satiety due to mixed spices consumption, independent of any changes in plasma ghrelin response.

Keywords: spices; curry; ghrelin; appetite response

---

1. Introduction

Spices and related flavor compounds consumed worldwide are known to provide orosensory stimulation which can potentially influence palatability and appetite. This in turn can modulate ingestive behavior within meals and between meals and thereby have the potential to alter energy balance [1]. It is an established fact that taste and smell can influence satiety and hunger responses [2,3], although the associations can be divergent, depending on the individual food types [4], as well as on the optimal dosing of sensory intensity [5]. The literature on the intake of individual spices *per se* indicate that the associations between sensory, appetite, and energy intake to be rather equivocal, with some studies showing an increased palatability/liking of foods when spices are added to them [6], whereas other studies finding no such differences [7]. Similarly, regarding appetite response, the findings have been rather variable, with some studies showing no differences in appetite ratings when pepper, ginger, horseradish, etc. were individually added to a mixed dish [8],whereas a recent animal study found appetite enhancing effects of essential oils from both cinnamon and ginger [9]. Similarly, increased use of spices have also been reported in individuals with compromised chemosensory function in order to compensate for the loss of appetite [10], supporting the appetite modulating ability of spices.

In the recently completed 'Polyspice study' we found significant improvements in postprandial glucose homeostasis as well as increases in glucagon like peptide- (GLP-1) response [11,12]. Given the equivocal nature of findings in the current literature regarding spice intake and appetite response, we further explored whether the subjective appetite response will differ between two doses of curry, made with polyphenol rich mixed spices, in comparison with non-curry control within the same Polyspice study cohort. Furthermore, while it is reasonably well established that postprandial ghrelin response can differ depending on the macronutrient composition of the meals [13,14], less is known regarding the effects of dietary bioactive phytochemicals on ghrelin response. Evidence is beginning to emerge that polyphenol content of foods may influence postprandial ghrelin response [15–17], with different polyphenols suggested to have divergent effects [18]. Therefore, we additionally investigated the postprandial ghrelin response to two different doses of curry made with polyphenol rich mixed spices and vegetables. To the best of our knowledge, this is the first dose-response study of its kind exploring the effects of dietary relevant doses of curry intake, made with mixed spices, on postprandial appetite and ghrelin response.

2. Materials and Methods

The details of the study design have been described previously [11]. In brief, the study was undertaken in healthy Chinese men between 21 and 40 years of age and body mass index $\leq$27.5 kg/m^2. The study was approved by the Domain Specific Research Board (DSRB) ethics committee, Singapore (Reference: C/2015/00729) and was registered on clinicaltrials.gov (Identifier No. NCT02599272). This was a 3-way randomized crossover trial, with each volunteer completing three separate study sessions: Dose 0 Control (D0C), or Dose 1 Curry (D1C), or Dose 2 Curry (D2C) treatments. Twenty volunteers completed D0C and D2C sessions, whereas 17 volunteers completed the D1C (optional) session. During the individual study sessions, each volunteer consumed the test meals for breakfast, after an overnight fast following a standardized dinner the evening before. D0C meal contained no (0 g) spices, D1C meal consisted 6 g of mixed spices, and D2C meal consisted of 12 g mixed spices. The mixed spices preparations for D1C and D2C were identical and were prepared by thoroughly mixing dried powders of different spices consisting of turmeric, coriander seeds, cumin seeds (all Everest Spices, Mumbai, India), dried Indian gooseberry (*'amla'*, *emblica officinalis*, Ramdev Spices, Ahmedabad, India), cayenne pepper (Robertson's, Durban, South Africa), cinnamon (McCormick's, Baltimore, MD, USA), and clove (Robertson's, Durban, South Africa) and were mixed in the ratio of 8:4:4:4:2:1:1, respectively. Test meals were consumed with a portion of white rice, providing a total of approximately 100 g available carbohydrates each and were balanced for total energy, protein, fat, dietary fiber, and total vegetables content. The mean total energy contents for each test meal was approximately 605 kilocalories consisting around 67%, 7%, and 27% energy from carbohydrate, protein, and fat, respectively. Volunteers were asked to consume their meals within 15 min of serving.

Visual analogue scales (VAS) were used to rate subjective appetite sensations as validated previously [19,20]. The VAS consisted of 100 mm long horizontal lines with two ends describing "extremely ... " (coded as 100 mm) and "not at all ... " (coded as 0 mm) with each scale measuring 'hunger', 'fullness', 'desire to eat', and 'prospective eating'. Volunteers were asked to capture their appetite sensations during various times, at regular intervals, by putting vertical mark along the four horizontal lines. These measurements were undertaken immediately prior to the consumption of test meals (baseline, 0 h) followed by 7 postprandial time points at various regular intervals (0.25 h, 0.5 h, 1.0 h, 1.5 h, 2.0 h, 2.5 h, 3 h). Blood samples were also obtained for plasma ghrelin measurements via an intravenous cannula collected during the same times as the appetite response measurements (except for 0.25 h time point). Blood samples were collected in 2 mL K_2 Ethylenediaminetetraacetic acid (EDTA) vacutainer tube (BD, Franklin Lakes, NJ, USA) pre-treated with cOmplete™, Mini, EDTA-free protease inhibitor cocktail tablet (Roche, Basel, Switzerland), stored cool on ice, and were centrifuged within 45 min of collection at 1500× g for 10 min at 4 °C. Plasma samples were then immediately stored at −80 °C until analyses. Luminex® bead-based multiplex assays, based on Luminex® xMAP® technology, were used to measure total ghrelin concentration in plasma according to manufacturer's protocol (ProcartaPlex, Thermo Fisher Scientific, Waltham, MA, USA).

Statistical analysis was performed using SPSS, version 24 (IBM Inc., Armonk, North Castle, NY, USA). Data were analyzed using the mixed effects model with the doses as the fixed effect using a compound symmetry covariance structure to test for the overall effect of the doses. Change from baseline response for plasma ghrelin and appetite measures were calculated as the change from baseline areas under the curve (ΔAUC). Post-hoc pairwise comparisons, using Bonferroni corrections, were used to compare differences in change from baseline AUCs between various doses. Furthermore, to test the overall effect of the doses on total AUC data for plasma ghrelin, the corresponding baseline values (fasting values) of the subjects at each of the doses were added as a covariate, with the doses as the fixed effects using a compound symmetry covariance structure. However, for the overall tests of the change from baseline AUCs, no covariates were used. Square root transformations of the data were undertaken to achieve normal distribution, where necessary.

3. Results

There were no reported adverse reactions to the test meals, and the volunteers consumed their served meal portions in full within the suggested time allocated, indicating a satisfactory tolerance. Postprandial ghrelin response to the three test meals is shown in Figure 1. There were no significant differences in either the change from baseline AUC (ΔAUC) or in the total areas under the curve (total AUC) between the D0C, D1C, and D2C meals. The mean change from baseline (0 h) of subjective appetite ratings including 'hunger', 'fullness', 'desire to eat', and 'prospective eating' are shown in Figure 2. Compared with the control (D0C) test meal, D1C and D2C led to significantly greater suppressions in 'hunger' (by approximately 54% and 51% during D1C and D2C, respectively, as compared with D0C control meal, both $p < 0.05$, after Bonferroni corrections) as well as in the 'desire to eat' (by approximately 62% and 60% in D1C and D2C, respectively, as compared with D0C control meal, both $p < 0.01$, after Bonferroni corrections), as calculated using the areas under the curve of the change from baseline measurements. The summary data are shown in Table 1. Moreover, even though the mean change from baseline AUC (ΔAUC) of postprandial 'fullness' was also greater by about 20% during D1C and D2C meals as compared with the D0C meal, indicating increased 'fullness', none of the differences reached statistical significance. Similarly, there were no statistical differences in the 'prospective eating' rating between test meals.

Table 1. Postprandial changes from baseline (ΔAUC) over 3 h periods in plasma ghrelin concentration and appetite response measures during three test meals (D0C, D1C, and D2C).

Measurement	D0C (Mean ± SD) (n = 20)	D1C (Mean ± SD) (n = 17)	D2C (Mean ± SD) (n = 20)	Pairwise Comparison *
Total Ghrelin (ΔAUC)	−78,098.98 ± 41,101.98	−76,549.46 ± 41,482.70	−78,883.94 ± 40,022.88	ND
'Hunger' (ΔAUC)	−4659.45 ± 3272.36	−7179.61 ± 3782.34	−7020.96 ± 3871.20	D0C vs. D1C (p = 0.017) D0C vs. D2C (p = 0.028)
'Fullness' (ΔAUC)	6393.71 ± 3681.80	7764.54 ± 3908.07	7850.15 ± 3581.19	ND
'Desire to Eat'(ΔAUC)	−4495.00 ± 3194.31	−7268.09 ± 4053.52	−7194.88 ± 3849.50	D0C vs. D1C (p = 0.002) D0C vs. D2C (p = 0.005)
'Prospective eating' (ΔAUC)	−4913.78 ± 3401.05	−6095.76 ± 3612.99	−5883.42 ± 3506.46	ND

* Pairwise comparisons after Bonferroni correction. Δ AUC—changes from baseline area under the curve, ND—no significant difference, D0C—Dose 0 Control, D1C—Dose 1 Curry, D2C—Dose 2 Curry (D2C—), SD—standard deviation.

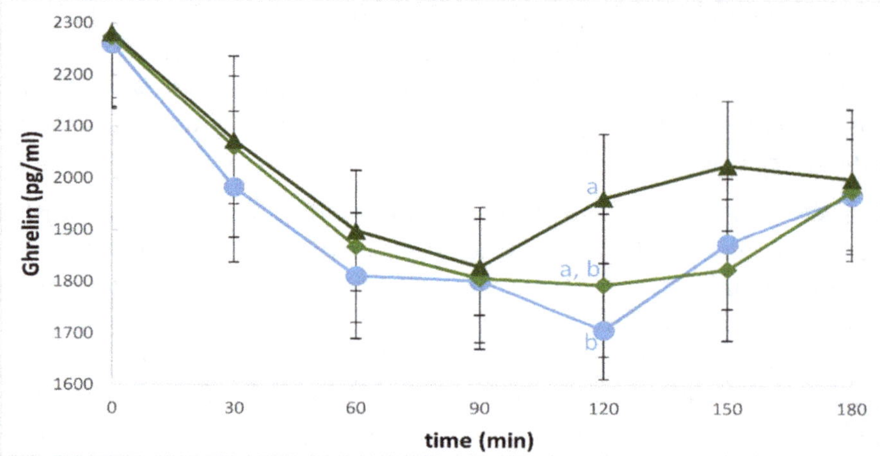

Figure 1. Mean (±Standard Error of Mean) postprandial plasma ghrelin concentration in response to the intake of three test meals: ●Dose 0 Control (D0C), ♦ Dose 1 Curry (D1C), ▲ Dose 2 Curry (D2C). The differences between the treatments at each time point were measured after controlling for the baseline values. Treatments that were significantly different from each other (p-value < 0.05) are represented by different letters. At time 120 min, there was a significant main effect of the treatment, although there was only marginal significance observed between Dose 0 and Dose 2 (p-value = 0.056), as shown in the figure above.

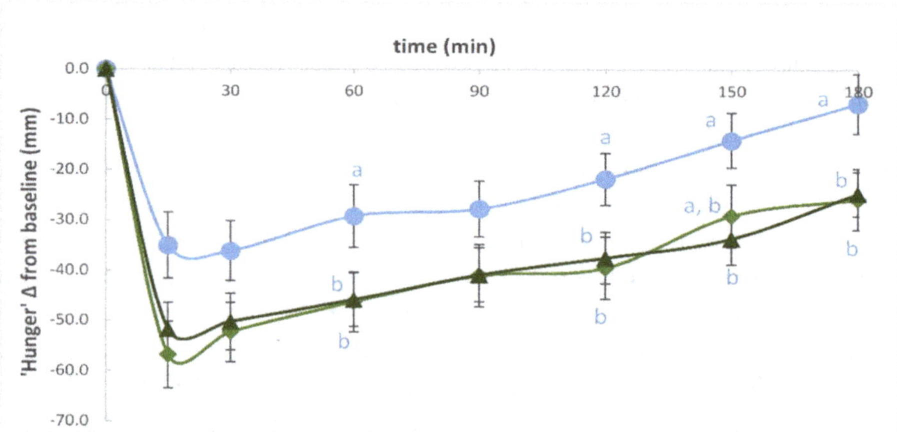

(**a**)

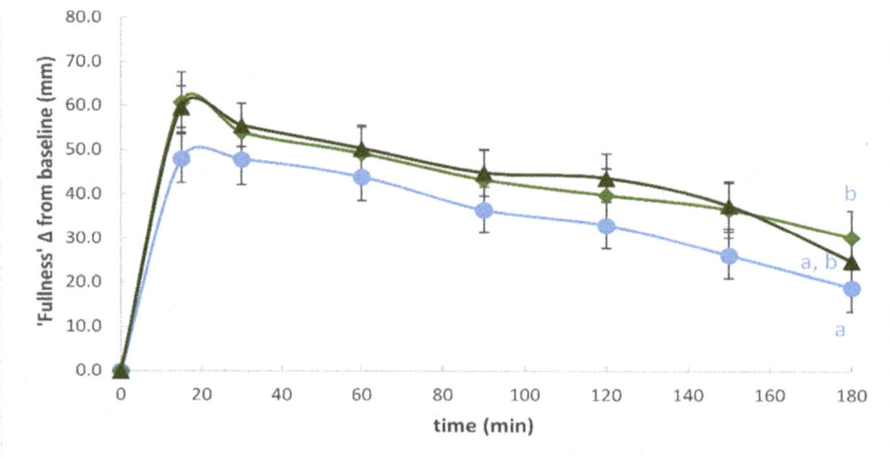

(**b**)

Figure 2. *Cont.*

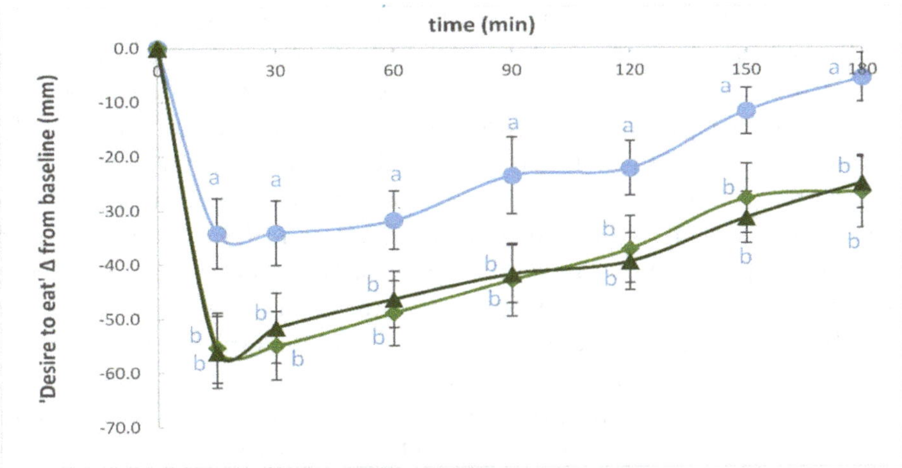

(c)

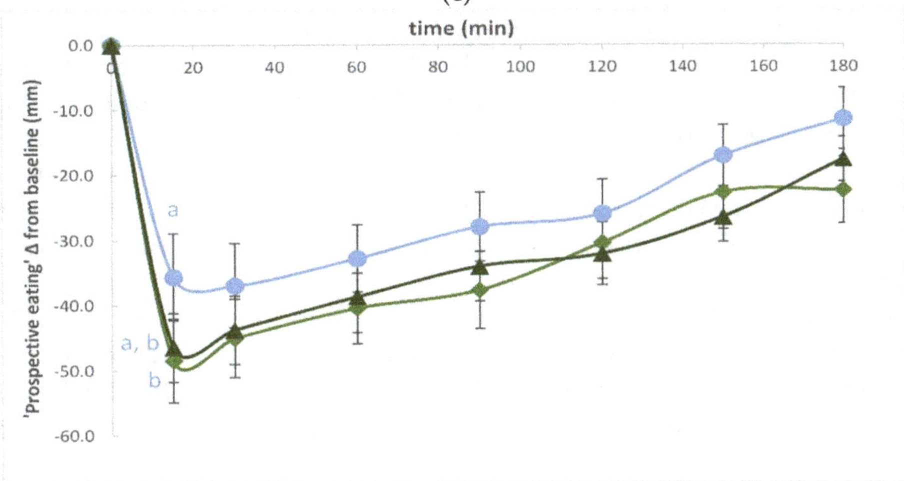

(d)

Figure 2. Mean (±SEM) in subjective appetite ratings over a 3 h period following consumption of three test meals. (**a**) 'Hunger'; (**b**) 'Fullness'; (**c**) 'Desire to eat'; (**d**) 'Prospective eating'. ● Dose 0 Control (D0C), ♦ Dose 1 Curry (D1C), ▲ Dose 2 Curry (D2C). In all the appetite ratings, the main effect of time and treatment were significantly different (p-value < 0.05). Treatments that were significantly different from each other (p-value < 0.05) are represented by different letters at each given time point.

4. Discussion

It is generally believed that glucose homeostasis is associated with appetite and/or incretin hormone response and vice-versa [21–23]. While several studies have investigated these effects simultaneously by modulating macronutrient compositions of meals, a limited number of studies have explored the effects of mixed spices in humans using a controlled dose-response trial [1]. Given that we have previously shown beneficial effects of curry made with mixed spices on glucose homeostasis [11], in this additional investigation, we wanted to explore the influence of dose-dependent increases in the intake of curry made with mixed spices on appetite and ghrelin responses. The strengths of our study design were the use of dietary relevant doses of mixed spices that are typically consumed in Indian curries and that the study was deliberately undertaken in a Chinese population, who would not usually consume large amounts of Indian curries, thereby avoiding any potential residual effects due to habituation. Moreover, we also balanced the total energy, macronutrients, and total vegetable contents across the three test meals.

Despite all the test meals being well tolerated, we found significant increases in 'hunger' suppression and in the suppression of 'desire to eat' with the mixed spice containing curry doses as compared with the control meal. This indicates that the consumption of spices may increase inter-meal satiety, which ties-in with our previously reported finding within the same study of an increase in plasma GLP-1 concentration with increasing curry doses [12], which can partly lead to appetite suppression. Other studies have also shown that consumption of individual spices can lead to increases in plasma GLP-1 [24] as well as in peptide YY (PYY) [25] concentrations. Furthermore, the lack of any difference in postprandial ghrelin response between the various test meals in our study is similar to the observation made with two doses of cinnamon added to 300 g of rice pudding [24]. The consistencies in these findings may suggest that the appetite suppression effects of spices may be via the increases in the in vivo concentrations of anorexigenic gut hormones such as GLP-1 and PYY, rather than via an increased suppression of the orexigenic hormone ghrelin. In further support of our findings, a recent study also found appetite suppressing effects of individual spices (e.g., turmeric, cinnamon, ginger) [25]. All these spices (and more) were used together in the mixed spice containing test meals in our study. In contrast to our findings, however, another study investigating the effects of individual spices such as mustard, horseradish, black pepper, and ginger found negligible effects on appetite response [8]. Therefore, different spices are likely to give rise to divergent effects. As such, spices such as chili have been shown to demonstrate appetite stimulating effects [26]. The 'appetizer effects' of spices have also been previously shown by adding them in low salt-foods [27] as well as to reduced fat foods [6]. The contrasting effects of different spices on appetite could be resulting from the diverse ways by which individual spices can affect the sensory and molecular pathways, as have been reviewed in detail elsewhere [1].

Within our study population we found a modest inter-individual variability in the subjective appetite ratings as a result of mixed spice consumption at the various doses, as observed through the large standard deviations in appetite rating measures (Table 1). This could partly be due to differences in prior familiarities and likings, since it has been shown in a recent study that familiarity of spices can determine pleasantness response which in turn can affect appetite [28]. Indeed, prior preference for an individual to sweet or savory foods has been shown to determine the quantity of either sweet or savory foods that is eaten in an experimental setting [29]. There are also indications that behavioral variables including risk taking and different personality traits could also influence the motivation to consume spicy foods [30], and although this previous study was undertaken within the Western dietary context, we used Chinese males who may also have different affiliations towards eating Indian curries. In our study, however, we did not gather any information on prior familiarity, liking, or on personally traits which could directly or indirectly explain part of the inter-individual variabilities in appetite responses.

We did not find any obvious dose-response associations with appetite measures in our study, since both the curry doses seemed to have exerted similar effects as compared with the non-curry control meal. This was despite previous studies suggesting an inverted U-shaped (Wundt) curve between sensory intensity and appetite response as discussed in more detail by McCrickerd et al. [5]. More specifically, both palatability [31] as well as appetite in response to dose-dependent increases in flavor/taste intensities observed this inverted U-shaped phenomenon by several investigators [32,33], although we did not find such effects. These differences in findings could be explained by the fact that the "preferred" taste intensity for spices could have varied between individuals, which may have contributed to the moderate inter-individual variability in appetite response seen in our study. This in turn could lead to lack of any obvious dose-response effects. Moreover, we measured neither the volunteers' innate taste preference nor the palatability of the test meals, which were some of the limitations of this study. Additionally, the volunteers were required to consume the entire amount of test meals served, irrespective of their within meal satiation. Furthermore, the study could have been more objective if we provided them an *ad libitum* meal for lunch and measured the volunteers' actual food intake rather than solely measuring subjective appetite response between meals. Since the primary objective of our study was to investigate metabolic response to standardized, fixed amounts of foods, the study of *ad libitum* food intake measurement was not an option. Finally, in addition to taste, the aroma from the release of volatile compounds from spices could have also contributed to greater appetite suppression. It is well recognized that aroma from foods and non-food materials reaching the olfactory epithelium via the orthonasal and the retronasal routes can lead to appetite suppression [34,35].

5. Conclusions

The results from our study indicate that mixed spices consumption can lead to greater increases in inter-meal satiety through suppression in both 'hunger' as well as in 'desire to eat' in the period immediately subsequent to the meal. Both differences in taste intensities as well as aroma from the addition of mixed spices may have contributed to a greater satiety value of the mixed spice containing meals. These changes in postprandial appetite responses seem to be independent of changes in plasma ghrelin concentration, although could potentially have been related to the increase in postprandial plasma GLP-1 concentration, as found within the same cohort previously. The postprandial effects of individual spices or mixed spices on other appetite hormones remain to be established. It should be noted that this was a single-meal, acute feeding study and any long-term effects remain to be further investigated.

Acknowledgments: This project was funded by the Singapore Institute for Clinical Sciences, Agency for Science Technology and Research (A*STAR), Singapore. The authors would like to thank Keri McCrickerd for the fruitful discussions and the volunteers for taking part in this study.

Author Contributions: S.H. and C.J.H. conceived and designed the experiments; S.C.C. and S.H. performed the experiments; S.H., J.L., and S.P. analyzed the data; S.H., J.L., and S.P. wrote the paper. All authors have read and approved the manuscript.

References

1. Mattes, R.D. Spices and energy balance. *Physiol. Behav.* **2012**, *107*, 584–590. [CrossRef] [PubMed]
2. Warwick, Z.S.; Hall, W.G.; Pappas, T.N.; Schiffman, S.S. Taste and smell sensations enhance the satiating effect of both a high-carbohydrate and a high-fat meal in humans. *Physiol. Behav.* **1993**, *53*, 553–563. [CrossRef]
3. Masic, U.; Yeomans, M.R. Does monosodium glutamate interact with macronutrient composition to influence subsequent appetite? *Physiol. Behav.* **2013**, *116–117*, 23–29. [CrossRef] [PubMed]
4. Sørensen, L.B.; Møller, P.; Flint, A.; Martens, M.; Raben, A. Effect of sensory perception of foods on appetite and food intake: A review of studies on humans. *Int. J. Obes.* **2003**, *27*. [CrossRef] [PubMed]
5. McCrickerd, K.; Forde, C.G. Sensory influences on food intake control: Moving beyond palatability. *Obes. Rev.* **2016**, *17*, 18–29. [CrossRef] [PubMed]
6. Peters, J.C.; Polsky, S.; Stark, R.; Zhaoxing, P.; Hill, J.O. The influence of herbs and spices on overall liking of reduced fat food. *Appetite* **2014**, *79*, 183–188. [CrossRef] [PubMed]
7. Manero, J.; Phillips, C.; Ellison, B.; Lee, S.-Y.; Nickols-Richardson, S.M.; Chapman-Novakofski, K.M. Influence of seasoning on vegetable selection, liking and intent to purchase. *Appetite* **2017**, *116*, 239–245. [CrossRef] [PubMed]
8. Gregersen, N.T.; Belza, A.; Jensen, M.G.; Ritz, C.; Bitz, C.; Hels, O.; Frandsen, E.; Mela, D.J.; Astrup, A. Acute effects of mustard, horseradish, black pepper and ginger on energy expenditure, appetite, ad libitum energy intake and energy balance in human subjects. *Br. J. Nutr.* **2012**, *109*, 556–563. [CrossRef] [PubMed]
9. Ogawa, K.; Ito, M. Appetite-enhancing effects of curry oil. *Biol. Pharm. Bull.* **2016**, *39*, 1559–1563. [CrossRef] [PubMed]
10. Mattes, R.D.; Cowart, B.J. Dietary assessment of patients with chemosensotyr disorders. *J. Acad. Nutr. Diet.* **1994**, *94*, 50–56. [CrossRef]
11. Haldar, S.; Chia, S.C.; Lee, S.H.; Lim, J.; Leow, M.K.-S.; Chan, E.C.Y.; Henry, C.J. Polyphenol-rich curry made with mixed spices and vegetables benefits glucose homeostasis in Chinese males (polyspice study): A dose–response randomized controlled crossover trial. *Eur. J. Nutr.* **2017**. [CrossRef] [PubMed]

12. Haldar, S.; Chia, S.C.; Henry, C.J. Polyphenol-rich curry made with mixed spices and vegetables increases postprandial plasma GLP-1 concentration in a dose-dependent manner. *Eur. J. Clin. Nutr.* **2018**, *72*, 297–300. [CrossRef] [PubMed]
13. Gibbons, C.; Caudwell, P.; Finlayson, G.; Webb, D.-L.; Hellström, P.M.; Näslund, E.; Blundell, J.E. Comparison of postprandial profiles of ghrelin, active GLP-1, and total PYY to meals varying in fat and carbohydrate and their association with hunger and the phases of satiety. *J. Clin. Endocrinol. Metab.* **2013**, *98*, E847–E855. [CrossRef] [PubMed]
14. Jakubowicz, D.; Froy, O.; Wainstein, J.; Boaz, M. Meal timing and composition influence ghrelin levels, appetite scores and weight loss maintenance in overweight and obese adults. *Steroids* **2012**, *77*, 323–331. [CrossRef] [PubMed]
15. Gruendel, S.; Garcia, A.L.; Otto, B.; Mueller, C.; Steiniger, J.; Weickert, M.O.; Speth, M.; Katz, N.; Koebnick, C. Carob pulp preparation rich in insoluble dietary fiber and polyphenols enhances lipid oxidation and lowers postprandial acylated ghrelin in humans. *J. Nutr.* **2006**, *136*, 1533–1538. [CrossRef] [PubMed]
16. Panickar, K.S. Effects of dietary polyphenols on neuroregulatory factors and pathways that mediate food intake and energy regulation in obesity. *Mol. Nutr. Food Res.* **2013**, *57*, 34–47. [CrossRef] [PubMed]
17. Kaliora, A.C.; Kanellos, P.T.; Gioxari, A.; Karathanos, V.T. Regulation of gip and ghrelin in healthy subjects fed on sun-dried raisins: A pilot study with a crossover trial design. *J. Med. Food* **2017**, *20*, 301–308. [CrossRef] [PubMed]
18. Serrano, J.; Casanova-Martí, À.; Depoortere, I.; Blay, M.T.; Terra, X.; Pinent, M.; Ardévol, A. Subchronic treatment with grape-seed phenolics inhibits ghrelin production despite a short-term stimulation of ghrelin secretion produced by bitter-sensing flavanols. *Mol. Nutr. Food Res.* **2016**, *60*, 2554–2564. [CrossRef] [PubMed]
19. Hill, A.J.; Magson, L.D.; Blundell, J.E. Hunger and palatability: Tracking ratings of subjective experience before, during and after the consumption of preferred and less preferred food. *Appetite* **1984**, *5*, 361–371. [CrossRef]
20. Flint, A.; Raben, A.; Blundell, J.E.; Astrup, A. Reproducibility, power and validity of visual analogue scales in assessment of appetite sensations in single test meal studies. *Int. J. Obes.* **2000**, *24*. [CrossRef]
21. Chapman, I.M.; Goble, E.A.; Wittert, G.A.; Morley, J.E.; Horowitz, M. Effect of intravenous glucose and euglycemic insulin infusions on short-term appetite and food intake. *Am. J. Physiol.* **1998**, *274*, R596–R603. [CrossRef] [PubMed]
22. Falkén, Y.; Hellström, P.M.; Sanger, G.J.; Dewit, O.; Dukes, G.; Grybäck, P.; Holst, J.J.; Näslund, E. Actions of prolonged ghrelin infusion on gastrointestinal transit and glucose homeostasis in humans. *Neurogastroenterol. Motil.* **2010**, *22*, e192–e200. [CrossRef] [PubMed]
23. Edholm, T.; Degerblad, M.; Grybäck, P.; Hilsted, L.; Holst, J.J.; Jacobsson, H.; Efendic, S.; Schmidt, P.T.; Hellström, P.M. Differential incretin effects of GIP and GLP-1 on gastric emptying, appetite, and insulin-glucose homeostasis. *Neurogastroenterol. Motil.* **2010**, *22*. [CrossRef] [PubMed]
24. Hlebowicz, J.; Hlebowicz, A.; Lindstedt, S.; Björgell, O.; Höglund, P.; Holst, J.J.; Darwiche, G.; Almér, L.-O. Effects of 1 and 3 g cinnamon on gastric emptying, satiety, and postprandial blood glucose, insulin, glucose-dependent insulinotropic polypeptide, glucagon-like peptide 1, and ghrelin concentrations in healthy subjects. *Am. J. Clin. Nutr.* **2009**, *89*, 815–821. [CrossRef] [PubMed]
25. Zanzer, Y.C.; Plaza, M.; Dougkas, A.; Turner, C.; Björck, I.; Östman, E. Polyphenol-rich spice-based beverages modulated postprandial early glycaemia, appetite and pyy after breakfast challenge in healthy subjects: A randomized, single blind, crossover study. *J. Funct. Foods* **2017**, *35*, 574–583. [CrossRef]
26. Maji Amal, K.; Banerji, P. Phytochemistry and gastrointestinal benefits of the medicinal spice, capsicum annuum l (chilli): A review. *J. Complement. Integr. Med.* **2016**, *13*, 97–122. [CrossRef] [PubMed]
27. Ghawi, S.K.; Rowland, I.; Methven, L. Enhancing consumer liking of low salt tomato soup over repeated exposure by herb and spice seasonings. *Appetite* **2014**, *81*, 20–29. [CrossRef] [PubMed]
28. Knaapila, A.; Laaksonen, O.; Virtanen, M.; Yang, B.; Lagström, H.; Sandell, M. Pleasantness, familiarity, and identification of spice odors are interrelated and enhanced by consumption of herbs and food neophilia. *Appetite* **2017**, *109*, 190–200. [CrossRef] [PubMed]
29. Griffioen-Roose, S.; Mars, M.; Finlayson, G.; Blundell, J.E.; de Graaf, C. Satiation due to equally palatable sweet and savory meals does not differ in normal weight young adults. *J. Nutr.* **2009**, *139*, 2093–2098. [CrossRef] [PubMed]

30. Byrnes, N.K.; Hayes, J.E. Behavioral measures of risk tasking, sensation seeking and sensitivity to reward may reflect different motivations for spicy food liking and consumption. *Appetite* **2016**, *103*, 411–422. [CrossRef] [PubMed]
31. Yeomans, M.R. Palatability and the micro-structure of feeding in humans: The appetizer effect. *Appetite* **1996**, *27*, 119–133. [CrossRef] [PubMed]
32. Yeomans, M.R. Taste, palatability and the control of appetite. *Proc. Nutr. Soc.* **1998**, *57*, 609–615. [CrossRef] [PubMed]
33. Bolhuis, D.P.; Lakemond, C.M.M.; de Wijk, R.A.; Luning, P.A.; de Graaf, C. Both longer oral sensory exposure to and higher intensity of saltiness decrease ad libitum food intake in healthy normal-weight men. *J. Nutr.* **2011**, *141*, 2242–2248. [CrossRef] [PubMed]
34. Ramaekers, M.G.; Luning, P.A.; Ruijschop, R.M.A.J.; Lakemond, C.M.M.; Bult, J.H.F.; Gort, G.; van Boekel, M.A.J.S. Aroma exposure time and aroma concentration in relation to satiation. *Br. J. Nutr.* **2013**, *111*, 554–562. [CrossRef] [PubMed]
35. Ruijschop, R.M.A.J.; Boelrijk, A.E.M.; de Graaf, C.; Westerterp-Plantenga, M.S. Retronasal aroma release and satiation: A review. *J. Agric. Food Chem.* **2009**, *57*, 9888–9894. [CrossRef] [PubMed]

9

How Fermentation affects the Antioxidant Properties of Cereals and Legumes

Michela Verni [1,*], Vito Verardo [2,3] and Carlo Giuseppe Rizzello [1]

1 Department of Soil, Plant and Food Science, University of Bari Aldo Moro, 70126 Bari, Italy
2 Department of Nutrition and Food Science, University of Granada, Campus Universitario de Cartuja, E-18071 Granada, Spain
3 Institute of Nutrition and Food Technology 'José Mataix', Biomedical Research Centre, University of Granada, Avenida del Conocimiento s/n, E-18071 Granada, Spain
* Correspondence: michela.verni@uniba.it

Abstract: The major role of antioxidant compounds in preserving food shelf life, as well as providing health promoting benefits, combined with the increasing concern towards synthetic antioxidants, has led the scientific community to focus on natural antioxidants present in food matrices or resulting from microbial metabolism during fermentation. This review aims at providing a comprehensive overview of the effect of fermentation on the antioxidant compounds of vegetables, with emphasis on cereals- and legumes- derived foods. Polyphenols are the main natural antioxidants in food. However, they are often bound to cell wall, glycosylated, or in polymeric forms, which affect their bioaccessibility, yet several metabolic activities are involved in their release or conversion in more active forms. In some cases, the antioxidant properties in vitro, were also confirmed during in vivo studies. Similarly, bioactive peptides resulted from bacterial and fungal proteolysis, were also found to have ex vivo protective effect against oxidation. Fermentation also influenced the bioaccessibility of other compounds, such as vitamins and exopolysaccharides, enabling a further improvement of antioxidant activity in vitro and in vivo. The ability of fermentation to improve food antioxidant properties strictly relies on the metabolic activities of the starter used, and to further demonstrate its potential, more in vivo studies should be carried out.

Keywords: Lactic acid bacteria; fungi; phenolic compounds; bioactive peptides; grains

---

1. Antioxidant Compounds in Food Matrices

The increasing interest towards healthier food and lifestyles has steered the scientific community to pay great attention to the field of free radicals and antioxidant compounds. Free radicals are atoms, molecules, or ions containing an unpaired electron, which makes them unstable and highly reactive [1]. The generation of free radicals in our body occurs as consequence of exposure to different physiochemical conditions or pathological states. Free radicals are responsible for damaging biologically relevant molecules and lipids, nucleic acids, and proteins are the major targets [2]. They are generated continuously; however, they are also involved in inter-cellular and intra-cellular signaling systems and enzymatic reactions essential to intermediary metabolic processes of life [3], therefore, their daily production must be balanced. If free radicals overcome the body's ability to regulate them, and the ratio between free radical generation and antioxidant defenses is unbalanced, a condition known as oxidative stress ensues. Being the oxidative stress responsible for an enormous number of conditions, including cancer, cardiovascular and neurodegenerative diseases, atherosclerosis, inflammatory state, and many others [2,4], preventing it by enhancing the intake of dietary antioxidants represents the most feasible way of protection against free radicals. Antioxidants need to be capable of delaying or inhibiting the oxidation of a substrate, yet an important property they should also have, is the ability to form a new radical that is stable through intramolecular hydrogen bonding on further oxidation [1]. Several mechanisms of action can be responsible for their activity. Antioxidants can (i) scavenge species that initiate peroxidation, (ii) donate a hydrogen or an electron, (iii) chelate metal ions preventing the generation of reactive species or lipid peroxides de-composition, (iv) quench the radical O_2^- preventing peroxides formation, (v) breaking autoxidative chain reaction, (vi) inhibit pro-oxidative enzymes, and/or (vii) reduce localized O_2 concentrations [1,5]. From a technological point of view, antioxidants are designed to prevent food from spoiling through oxidation, thus reducing loss of nutrients, and maintaining texture, color pigments, taste, freshness, functionality, and aroma [3]. Therefore, antioxidants are an important category of food preservatives and can be divided into natural or synthetic. Natural antioxidants include flavonoids, phenolic acids, carotenoids, and tocopherols [1]; however, other protein derived compounds, such as amino acids and bioactive peptides, have received great attention for their displayed antioxidant properties [6–8]. Both natural and synthetic antioxidants, act by similar mechanisms and their chemical structure and polarity influence the antioxidant activity [5]. Antioxidants efficiency generally increases with the increase of their concentration; however, the dependence is not linear, and when the maximum activity is reached, it may also decrease [9]. Except for carotenes, tocopherols, and their esters, natural antioxidants are mostly much more polar than synthetic ones. They are also less active and substrate specific, and their antioxidant activity depends highly on synergists factors [9].

This review aims at providing a comprehensive overview of the effect of fermentation on the antioxidant activity of vegetable matrices. The literature is full of articles claiming the potential of food fermentation in improving antioxidant properties; however, the method used to quantify phenolic compounds, unless performed by chromatographic analysis is the classic Folin-Ciocalteu, which suffers from several drawbacks. The test is sensitive to pH, temperature, and reaction time; inorganic and non-phenolic organic substances, including reducing agents, react with Folin reagent, causing overestimations of the phenolic content [10,11]. For this reason, all the examples reported in this review were chosen among those in which a characterization of the phenolic profile was performed. Moreover, among vegetable matrices, only grains were considered since (i) diets in developing countries are primarily based on cereals and legumes, whereas in Western society there is an increasing interest in strictly vegetarian diets [12]; (ii) cereals are often consumed as refined products, yet most of the bioactive compounds are in the outer layers of the grains, and get lost during milling [13,14]; (iii) legumes consumption is often limited by the presence of antinutritional compounds which fermentation has proven to diminish [13,14]. After an extensive research on multiple databases, 76 research articles, half of which published in the last five years, highlighting the effect of fermentation on grains antioxidant properties were selected for this review. Respectively, 39 and 17 papers reported phenolic and proteic compounds as responsible for the antioxidant activity. Moreover, such activity was demonstrated in vivo in about 15% of the studies considered.

1.1. Phenolic Compounds

The antioxidant activity of phenolic compounds lies in their ideal chemical structure, facilitating the hydrogen or electron donation from hydroxyl groups positioned along the aromatic ring and conferring radical scavenging activities and metal-chelating potential. Phenolics have the ability of stabilizing and delocalizing the un-paired electron within their aromatic rings [15]. Phenolics are composed of at least one aromatic ring with at least one hydroxyl group and may be classified based on the number of phenol rings and the structural elements that are bound to the rings [16]. Phenolic acids, flavonoids, tannins, stilbenes, and lignans are the main groups of phenolics.

Phenolic acids are divided into hydroxybenzoic acids and hydroxycinnamic acids and usually act as antioxidants by trapping free radicals. Flavonoids, instead, can scavenge free radicals and chelate metals [5,15]. The common characteristic of flavonoids is the basic 15-carbon flavan structure. They are arranged in three rings (A, B, and C) and the different classes vary for the level of saturation of the C ring, whereas compounds within the same class differ for the level of substitution of A and B rings [5]. Polyphenols stability and free radical scavenging potential depend on both the number and location of the free OH group. The antioxidant activity increases with the increase of the hydroxyl groups, especially if positioned in ortho-3,4 [17].

Based on their chemical structure, tannins are defined as hydrolysable or condensed (proanthocyanidins). Condensed tannins are oligomers and polymers of flavan-3-ols, whereas hydrolysable tannins are glycosylated gallic and ellagic acid derivatives [18]. It was proven that free radicals scavenging activity of both hydrolysable and condensed tannins involves a fast and a slow step [19]. The fast scavenging reaction is inhibited by complexation of the tannin with protein, a very tight bond between the phenolic group of tannins and the NH group of proteins, which prevents their hydrolysis and digestion in the stomach [19]. Nevertheless, the overall capacity of the tannin-protein complex for scavenging seems to be similar to that of the free tannin [18,19].

1.2. *Antioxidant Peptides and Protein Derivatives*

Besides their nutritional, physicochemical, and sensory properties, proteins can be responsible for health promoting benefits, mainly attributed to biologically active peptides [20]. Bioactive peptides are produced by digestive enzymes during gastrointestinal digestion, or by proteolytic enzymes during food processing (ripening, fermentation, cooking), storage, or in vitro hydrolysis [7]. These peptides may play various roles (antimicrobial, antihypertensive, hypocholesterolemic, immunomodulatory, antioxidative, antithrombotic, antitumoral) and can be released from native proteins that derive from vegetable or animal matrices [7,8].

Peptides displaying antioxidant activity usually contain 5–16 amino acid residues [21]. The exact mechanism behind it has not fully been understood, yet several studies reported that they are inhibitors of lipid peroxidation, scavengers of free radicals and chelators of transition metal ions. [8,21]. Tyrosine, tryptophan, methionine, lysine, cysteine, and histidine are examples of amino acids displaying antioxidant activity. Synthesized peptides containing the active fragments have been proven to inhibit lipid peroxidation, while the tripeptides, Tyr-HisTyr, and Pro-His-His were found to be effective in stabilizing radical and non-radical oxygen species, including peroxynitrite and lipid peroxide [22]. Amino acids with aromatic residues can donate protons to electron deficient radicals, whereas histidine-containing peptides, thanks to the imidazole group, have been found to have hydrogen-donating, lipid peroxyl radical trapping, and metal ion-chelating abilities [8]. On the other hand, sulphur containing amino acids, have antioxidant action due to the direct interaction of thiol group with radicals. Cysteine and homocysteine inhibit LDL (low-density lipoprotein) oxidation by hemin and copper, methionine residues, instead, scavenge oxidizing agents [6]. Besides the presence of the proper amino acids, their specific positioning in the sequence plays an important role in antioxidant activity of peptides as well as other factors, such as the structure, amino acids configuration, hydrophobicity, and concentration [8].

1.3. *Synthetic Antioxidants*

Synthetic antioxidants were developed to prolong food shelf life but also because of the need to have a standard measurement system to compare with natural antioxidants. There are numerous compounds used in food, animal, and cosmetic applications to prevent oxidation; some also have antifungal properties and possess at least one phenolic ring in the structure. Butylated hydroxyanisole (BHA), butylated hydroxytoluene (BHT), tert-butylhydroquinone, propyl gallate, octyl gallate, 2,4,5-Trihydroxy butyrophenone, nordihydroguaiaretic acid, and 4-Hexylresorcinol are some examples [1]. Among these, BHT and BHA, alone or in combination with others, are the most commonly employed [2] and synergistic effects were also reported [23]. Today, almost all processed foods contain synthetic antioxidants and, despite being reported safe in the past, several studies have addressed their danger for human health, among which liver, kidney, and lungs damages, mutagenesis, carcinogenesis, and many others [19]. For this reason, between 2011 and 2012, the European food safety authority re-evaluated their maximum levels of intake in adults and children [24,25]. Considering the increasing risk factors related to synthetic antioxidants, there has been a global trend toward the use and the search for effective natural substance as therapeutic antioxidants.

2. Bioaccessibility and Bioavailability of Antioxidant Compounds

The research around antioxidants has grown exponentially, but there are still limitations that need to be considered before the real potential of these molecules is properly appreciated. All the bioactive compounds, to exert their biological properties, must be available in the target tissue, which is why, when addressing a specific property, it is important to consider their absorption in the gastro-intestinal tract. The absorption depends on the compound bioaccessibility and bioavailability. Only polyphenols that reach the gut, released from the food matrix by the action of digestive enzymes and gut microbiota, are bioaccessible, and therefore, potentially bioavailable [26].

Among polyphenol classes, their physicochemical characteristics play a significant role in the overall availability. It was observed that the absorption of phenolic acids, having small-molecular weight, as well as flavones, catechins, and quercetin glucosides results easier compared to larger polyphenols such as proanthocyanidins, which need to be degraded into monomer or dimer units before being absorbed [27,28]. Anthocyanins can be absorbed as glycosides and appear as such in blood [29], whereas galloylated monomeric flavonols do not seem to undergo extensive metabolism [30]. Another important factor to consider when assessing polyphenols bioavailability is their metabolism and the biotransformation reactions they can undergo once absorbed. As a result of the changes in their structure they may or may not still exert the biological action [28].

As for peptides, their ability to resist enzymatic digestion in the gastrointestinal tract is necessary to ensure their bioactivity within the human body. Since peptides' potential properties strictly depend on the amino acid composition, the loss of amino acid residues as a result of proteolysis in the gastrointestinal tract can lead to changes in the activity. Although it is more likely that small molecules get absorbed without undergoing further digestion, studies have showed that peptides with higher molecular weight can pass to the plasma without modifications and it seems that the amino acids composition is a factor of key importance in the resistance during the digestion tract [31].

Even though the use of in vitro tests has generated a controversy over the last years, these methods are still of great importance in the selection of potential antioxidant compounds. Therefore, in vitro assays are still necessary to screen among the thesis, yet major effort should be put into validate in vivo the bioaccessibility of such compounds. Despite the high reliability recognized to the in vivo studies, the problems related to the approval for the ethical committee, the long times and the high costs and the dependence on the individual response, pushed the development of in vitro methods simulating human digestion. The most widely used procedure for screening bioaccessibility is the in vitro static gastro-intestinal method. However, this method does not include a colonic phase where compounds may be metabolized by the colonic microbiota. A more reliable assessment can be obtained with dynamic gastro-intestinal models, which include the biological environment of the intestine [26].

3. Estimation of the Antioxidant Activity in Foods

3.1. *In Vitro Assays*

Although dozens of methods exist to investigate antioxidant activity, only a few are commonly employed to assess food antioxidant potential (for a review see Alam et al. [4]). Among scavenging activity assays, ABTS (2,20-azino-bis (3-ethylbenzothiazoline-6-sulfonic acid)) and DPPH (2,2-diphenyl-1-picrylhydrazyl) are colorimetric assays where the radicals decolorize in the presence of antioxidants [1]. In the hydroxyl radical scavenging, activity fluorescein is used as a probe and the fluorescence decay curve is monitored in the presence and absence of the antioxidants. ORAC (oxygen radical absorbance capacity) is a test performed using Trolox (a water-soluble analog of Vitamin E) as a standard and is based on the generation of free radical and measurement of decrease in fluorescence in the presence of free radical scavengers [4]. Another assay commonly used is the ferric reducing-antioxidant power

(FRAP), characterized by the reduction of Fe^{3+} to Fe^{2+} followed by the alteration of color from yellow to blue and analyzed through a spectrophotometer [4]. Several other assays, among which thiobarbituric reactive substances (TBARS) and glutathione peroxidase (GSHPx) methods, evaluate the inhibition of lipid peroxidation [1]. Considering the limitations of in vitro methods: (i) presence in the extracts of pigments and fluorophores interfering with absorbance and fluorescence readings, (ii) failure to evaluate radical scavenging rate, and (iii) lack of biological relevance due to the use of artificial radicals not found in food or biological systems; antioxidant activity should not be concluded based on a single antioxidant test model [11].

3.2. Ex Vivo Assays

Since in vitro assays fail to predict the antioxidant activity in vivo and testing a substance directly on animals or human is not an easy approach, methods comprising cellular models for a rapid initial screening have been developed. The hemolysis inhibition assay includes the use of plasma as substrate of oxidation. When exposed to ROS (reactive oxygen species), the oxidation of protein (hemoglobin) and lipid (mainly cholesteryl ester) begins, leading to destruction of the cell shape and membrane structure and ultimately hemolysis. The degree of hemolysis is determined spectrophotometrically measuring the concentration of released hemoglobin in the solution and the inhibition of hemolysis by antioxidants calculated by comparing with a control containing no antioxidants [11]. In cell culture models, human or animal cell lines such as keratinocyte or fibroblasts are subjected to oxidative-induced stress and then incubated for a certain amount of time with the substance to test. At the end of incubation, MTT (3-(4,5-dimethylthiazol-2-yl)-2,5- diphenyltetrazolium bromide) assay, which evaluates the ability of succinate dehydrogenase to convert MTT into formazan crystals in viable cells is performed [32,33]. Otherwise, in cellular antioxidant assays, a fluorescent probe is introduced into the cell cultures and in the presence of ROS or RNS (reactive nitrogen species), the substance is excited emitting fluorescence. The fluorescence intensity measured is proportional to the level of oxidation. Antioxidants absorbed into the cells scavenge the radicals, resulting in lower degree of oxidation observed as attenuated fluorescence increase [11]. Besides cellular assays, for the ex vivo evaluation of antioxidant activity, other biological systems exist, such as the inhibition of LDL and DNA oxidation assays. In the LDL-cholesterol assay, oxidation is induced by transition metals or peroxyl radical, and LDL is incubated with the samples. Then, the extent of the oxidation is determined by measuring the generated amount of lipid peroxides and by the TBARS assay [4]. DNA oxidation assay is based on a similar principle, but in this case, the DNA strand breaking is induced by hydroxyl or peroxyl radicals because they are the major sources responsible for DNA oxidative damage, especially mitochondrial [11].

3.3. In Vivo Assays

In vivo protocols commonly include the administration of antioxidants to testing animals for a specified period of time, after which the animals are sacrificed, and blood or tissues analyzed [4]. The lipid peroxidation (LPO) assay, which measures spectrophotometrically the end products of LPO process in the tested tissue, is one of the most used. GSHPx, instead, catalyzes the reduction of hydroperoxides. GSHPx measurement is performed especially in patients who are under oxidative stress; low activity of this enzyme is one of the early consequences of a disturbance of the prooxidant/antioxidant balance. While the FRAP assay, which was originally applied to plasma, is one of the most rapid tests and very useful for routine analysis [4].

4. Effect of Microbial Fermentation on the Antioxidant Activity

4.1. Metabolic Activities Affecting Phenolics

Plant phenolics are known to possess antimicrobial properties against bacteria, fungi, and yeasts; therefore, the ability to metabolize them comes from the need of detoxifying such compounds that, if present at high concentrations negatively affect the integrity of the cell wall and membrane, dissipate the pH gradient, delay the metabolism of carbohydrates and denature proteins [34–37]. Whether it is carried out by fungi, yeasts, or bacteria, microbial fermentation has an impact on the phenolic compounds characterizing food matrices and metabolic activities are species- or strains-specific and depend on their portfolio of enzymes. A schematization of the major effects of fermentation on phenolic compounds is reported in Table 1.

Table 1. Main effect of polyphenols metabolism on the antioxidant activity of fermented cereals and legumes.

Matrix	Microorganisms Employed	Process Parameters	Effect	Reference
Wheat bran	Baker's yeast	20 °C for 20 h	Release of phenolic acids and improved bioaccessibility and colonic metabolism of phenolic acids	[38]
	Spontaneous fermentation conducted mainly by *Lactobacillus*, *Leuconostoc* and *Pediococcus* spp.	Backslopping for 13 days at 18 °C	Release of ferulic acid	[39]
	Baker's yeast and LAB	20 °C for 24 h in anaerobic condition	Conversion of ferulic and caffeic acids into their derivatives and increase in sinapic acid.	[40]
	Hericium erinaceus and enzymes	25 °C for 7 days	Release of ferulic acid	[41]
Kamut bread	Baker's yeast and spontaneously fermented sourdough	30 °C for 1.5 h	Response to oxidative stress in in vivo studies with rats.	[42]
Rice bran	*Rhizopus oryzae* CTT 1217	30 °C for 120 h	Increase ferulic acid and DPPH scavenging activity. Inhibition of peroxidase and polyphenol oxidase.	[43]
	Rhizopus oligosporus F0020 *Monascus purpureus* F0061	32 °C for 12 days	Release of phenolic acids and increase of FRAP	[44]
Rye bran	*Bacillus subtilis* subsp. *subtilis* NRRL NRS-744	37 °C for 8 days	Release of phenolic acids	[45]
	Baker's yeast	25 °C for 14 h	Increase of phenolic acids	[46]
	Baker's yeast	20 °C for 24 h	Release of phenolic acids but no improved bioaccessibility in in vitro digestive systems	[47,48]
Sorghum flour	*Lactobacillus plantarum* FUA3171, *Lactobacillus casei* FUA3166, *Lactobacillus fermentum* FUA3165 *Lactobacillus reuteri* FUA3168	34 °C for 24 h	Release of phenolic acids and flavonoids	[49]
Tef pancake	Spontaneously fermented sourdough	25 °C for 24-120 h	Solubilization of bound phenolics and improved antioxidant potentials on FRAP and ABTS	[50]
Malt based beverage	*Lb. plantarum* Lp758, Lp765, Lp725, *Lactobacillus brevis* Lb986, *Lactobacillus amylolyticus* LaTL3, LaT15	30 °C for 72 h	Decarboxylation of phenolic acids.	[51]

Table 1. *Cont.*

Matrix	Microorganisms Employed	Process Parameters	Effect	Reference
Soy	*Bacillus subtilis* SHZ	30 °C for 36 h	Superoxide radical scavenging activity and reducing power potential	[52]
	B. subtilis MTCC5480, MTCC1747	42 °C for 24 h	Increase in the antioxidant activity due to both phenolic compounds and peptides	[53]
	Aspergillus oryzae ATCC 1011 *Rhizopus oryzae* ATCC 24563 *Bacillus subtilis* ATCC 6051	30 °C for 48 h	Increase in phenolic acids and flavonoids	[54]
	Bacillus pumilus HY1	37 °C for 60 h	Increase in phenolic acids, flavonoids and tannins monomeric forms	[55]
	Aspergillus awamori *Aspergillus niger* *Aspergillus niveus*	30 °C for 5 days	Increase in phenolic acids and flavonoids as consequence of β-glucosidase activity	[56]
	R. oligosporus	Room temperature for 20 days	Increase in phenolic acids and flavonoids	[57]
	Lentinus edodes CY-35	Room temperature for 50 days	Increase in phenolic acids and flavonoids as consequence of laccase and β-glucosidase activities	[58]
	Bacillus natto	37 °C for 48 h	Increase in phenolic acids and flavonoids	[59]
	Lactobacillus plantarum CECT 748 T	30 °C for 48 h	Increase in phenolic acids and flavonoids	[60]
	Pool of selected LAB	37 °C for 48 h	Increase in phenolic acids, flavonoids, saponins, phytosterols, and tocopherols	[61]
	Lactobacillus casei *Lactobacillus acidophilus*	32 °C for 15 h	Increased of the aglycones/glycosylated isoflavones ratio and bound phenolics	[62]
	Lactobacillus casei 0979 after germination	30 °C for 24 h	Increase in isoflavones glycosides and aglycones	[63]
	Kefir grains containing LAB and yeasts	30 °C for 24 h	Increase of isoflavones and improved antioxidant activities on DPPH and ABTS	[64]
	Lb. plantarum DPPMA24W, DPPMASL33 *Lb. fermentum* DPPMA114 *Lactobacillus rhamnosus* DPPMAAZ1	30 °C for 96 h	Increase of isoflavone aglycones especially equol	[65]
Cowpeas	Spontaneously fermented *Lb. plantarum* ATCC 14917	37 °C for 48 h	Increase of phenolic acids derivatives and flavonoids. Improved antioxidant activity on DPPH	[66]
Lentils	*Lb. plantarum* CECT 748 and commercial protease	37 °C for 15 h	Reduction of ROS on RAW 264.7 cells	[67]
	Spontaneously fermented	35 °C for 4 days	Decrease of condensed tannin and increase of monomers.	[68]

4.1.1. Metabolic Activities Affecting Phenolic Acids

Phenolic acids are by far the most important food phenolics in terms of quantity, they represent one-third of dietary phenolics and can be present in soluble form within the cytoplasm or bounded to the cell wall [69]. Hydroxybenzoic and hydroxycinnamic acids may be decarboxylated by lactic acid bacteria (LAB) to the corresponding phenol or vinyl derivatives or hydrogenated by phenolic acid reductases [70]. Metabolites of phenolic acids conversion, compared to their precursors, have reduced antimicrobial activity [36] and it was also hypothesized that LAB use hydroxycinnamic acids as external acceptors of electrons, which allow them to gain one extra mole of ATP [71,72]. Strains of *Lactobacillus rossiae*, *Lactobacillus brevis*, and *Lactobacillus curvatus* have followed one of the two paths (decarboxylation or reduction), whereas strains of *Leuconostoc mesenteroides* and *Lactobacillus fermentum* were found not capable of metabolizing hydroxycinnamic acids [71]. Phenolic acids metabolism is influenced by the composition and intrinsic factors of the matrices, therefore, depending on the substrate, the metabolism can shift from decarboxylase to reductase [72]; nevertheless, the derivatives exert higher biological activities than their precursors [73].

Phenolic acid reductase and phenolic acid decarboxylase activities contributed to polyphenol metabolism in red sorghum fermented with *Lactobacillus plantarum* and *Lb. fermentum*. Ferulic acid was reduced to dihydroferulic acid, and caffeic acid was metabolized to vinylcatechol and ethylcatechol but also dihydrocaffeic acid [49]. Similar results were obtained during the fermentation of a malt-based beverage with a pool of LAB including *Lb. plantarum*, *Lb. brevis*, and *Lactobacillus amylolyticus* [51]. Savolainen et al. [40] studied the role of oxygen during the fermentation of a liquid wheat bran sourdough. It was observed that anaerobic conditions, in which lactic acid bacteria and endogenous heterotrophic bacteria grew better, induced the conversion of ferulic and caffeic acids into their corresponding derivatives, and increased the amount of sinapic acid. Aerobic conditions, which favored yeasts growth, was characterized by the presence of dihydroxyphenyl ethanol and hydroxyphenylacetaldehyde.

Phenolic acid metabolism was also reported in yeasts and fungi. Cinnamate caboxy-lyase activity, which transforms coumaric and ferulic acids into their vinyl derivatives, was reported in *S. cerevisiae* strains [74]. Species belonging to *Aspergillus*, *Fusarium*, and *Pycnoporus* genera as well as *Pseudomonas* were responsible for the decarboxylation of ferulic acid and eugenol and their further metabolization, through a lyase, to vanillin, vanillic, and protocatechuic acids [75,76].

As mentioned above, phenolic acids are often bound, as dimers, trimers and/or oligomers, to the plant cell wall polysaccharides such as xylan and pectin. Another class of enzymes involved in their metabolism is represented by feruloyl esterases which are capable of releasing ferulic acid and other cinnamic acid. Feruloyl esterases have been described in lactic acid bacteria, mostly *Lactobacillus plantarum* strains [69,77], in fungi of the genus *Aspergillus* and *Penicillium* [78,79], as well as in some *Bacillus*, *Pseudomonas*, and *Pseudoalteromonas* strains [77,79,80], and it was also hypothesized in *S. cerevisiae* [81]. Several authors studied the impact of bioprocessing with baker's yeast, LAB, and fungi, with or without the addition of commercial enzymes, on phenolic acids release in wheat bran [39–41,81], rye bran [46–48], rice bran [43,44], sorghum [49], and tef [51]. In all cases, substantial increases, especially of ferulic acid, were observed. Ferulic acid antioxidant properties are ascribed to its ability to inhibit lipid peroxidation and LDL oxidation greater than other hydroxycinnamic acids [82]. Anson et al. [38] fermented wheat bran with baker's yeast and used it to produce a fortified bread having ferulic, *p*-coumaric, and sinapic acids content up to three-fold higher than unprocessed bran. Breads were subjected to gastro-intestinal digestion in vitro, although phenolic compounds bioavailability substantial increased, most of them were recovered from the jejunal compartment; only a small part of them was further metabolized in the colon section. Slightly different results were obtained by Koistinen et al. [83], who fermented rye bran with baker's yeast. Despite the extensive phenolic acid release caused by the bioprocessing (up to 30-fold higher than unfermented sample), when subjected to in vitro colon model, no differences were observed among the thesis.

Among fermented legumes, phenolic acid decarboxylase and esterase activities were reported in fermented cowpeas [66], lentils [67,68], and chickpea [84]. Soy phenolic composition, on the other hand, has been extensively characterized [85], as well as its changes during fermentation with bacterial [55,59–61] and fungal strains [54,56,58,86]. Dueñas et al. [54] observed that despite hydroxycinnamic acids content was higher than hydroxybenzoic in unfermented soy flour, hydroxybenzoic acids significantly increased during fermentation, up to seven-fold when *Aspergillus oryzae* was used. On the other hand, *p*-hydroxyphenylacetic acid, which was not detected in raw flours, reached up to 30 μg/g after fermentation [54]. Riciputi et al. [62] also characterized the bound phenolic profile of soymilk fermented with *Lactobacillus casei* and *Lb. acidophilus* to prepare a fermented version of tofu. Bound phenolics were mostly phenolic acids, of which syringic represented more than 30%, followed by *p*-coumaric, ferulic, and *p*-cumaroyl-hexose derivatives, which all increased compared to soybean flour and traditional tofu [62].

4.1.2. Metabolic Activities Affecting Flavonoids

Flavonoids, the other big group of food phenolics, are often glycosylated and several enzymes, belonging to the class of hydrolases, are produced by a great number of microorganisms, both bacteria and fungi [57]. Glycosyl hydrolases convert flavonoid glycosides to the corresponding aglycones, which show higher bioactivity in humans than their precursor glycosides [60]. Glucosidase activity from *Lactobacillus* spp. was responsible for the reduction of flavonoids glycosides in red sorghum, which corresponded to the increase of the aglycones, taxifolin, eriodictyol, and naringenin [49]. Bhanja et al. [87] suggested that besides β-glucosidases, different carbohydrate cleaving enzymes among which amylase and xylanase are responsible for the release of phenolics during solid state fermentation of wheat by *A. oryzae* and *Aspergillus awamori*. Among flavonoids, soy isoflavones are the most extensively studied for their health benefits. As for most flavonoids, they normally occur as glucoside-bound moieties, yet it is the aglycone form that is metabolically active, showing higher antioxidant activity and being absorbed in the intestines faster than their glucoside bound forms [85]. Fermentation with *Lb. casei* and *Lb. acidophilus* enabled the increased of the aglycones/glycosylated ratio in fermented tofu more than 10- and five-fold higher compared to soybean flour and traditional tofu, respectively. Fermentation also increased the content of genistein and daidzein, the major isoflavones found in soybean [62]. Di Cagno et al. [65] fermented soymilk with a pool of LAB strains selected for the high β-glucosidase activity, registering the increase of daidzein, genistein, glycitein, and especially equol. β-glucosidase is the major enzyme involved in isoflavones release and its activity was responsible for the improvement of the scavenging activity on DPPH radical in many soy-products fermented by *Bacillus* spp. [55,85], *Aspergillus* spp. [54,56], *Rhizopus* spp. [54,86], *Lactobacillus* spp. [60,61,63], and *Lentinus edodes* [58]. Dueñas et al. [54] reported that fungal fermentation acted more intensively in releasing isoflavones aglycones compared to flavanones and flavonols. In addition to the β-glucosidase activity, McCue et al. [58] also ascribed the increase of phenolic compounds to a laccase, an enzyme involved in lignin biodegradation by white-rot fungi, suggesting the possibility of a direct activity on polymeric phenolic substrate. In a recent study, instead, the effect of fermentation on soy and chickpea isoflavones was evaluated after legumes seeds were germinated [63]. The authors evaluated the effect of different process parameters adopted during germination. An increase in isoflavones glycosides and aglycones was already observed on sprouts, however, after incubation with *Lb. casei*, especially when seeds were germinated with blue light, a substantial boost in their content was observed.

4.1.3. Metabolic Activities Affecting Tannins

Tannase, which specifically breaks the galloyl ester bonds of hydrolyzable tannins, was first reported for several fungal species of the genus *Aspergillus*. Over the last two decades, many bacterial species of the genera, including *Streptococcus*, *Lonepinella*, *Bacillus*, and *Lactobacillus*, have also been reported to possess tannase activity [88]. However, tannase acting on condensed tannins was also described [89]. An example of this enzymatic activity was reported during a spontaneous fermentation of lentils [68]. Eight catechin and epicatechin dimers, trimers and tetramers were identified in raw lentils. Their content was halved after a spontaneous fermentation with a consequent increase, of the monomeric forms. A similar outcome, was observed during the fermentation of a soy product with *Bacillus pumilus* [55], nevertheless, lactobacilli, and bifidobacteria from gut microbiota as well as a strain of *Lb. plantarum* isolated from cheese, were found to cleave the heterocyclic ring of monomeric flavan-3-ols, giving rise to 1-(3′,4′-dihydroxyphenyl)-3-(2″,4″,6″-trihydroxyphenyl)propan-2-ol (3,4-diHPP-2-ol) [90]. This compound, which can be further degraded by the gut microbiota in several other substances, was recently studied for its antioxidant properties [91]. The authors found that 3,4-diHPP-2-ol had scavenging activity on ABTS and DPPH radicals higher than its precursor, as well as than other phenolic compounds. In addition, 3,4-diHPP-2-ol also showed the ability to reduce Fe^{3+} to Fe^{2+}, higher than Trolox.

4.2. Release of Antioxidant Peptides

With the bioactive peptides crypted in the native protein, the active amino acid sequences need to be released through proteolytic microorganisms. Most of the studies involving the formation of bioactive peptides by fermentation are carried out by lactic acid bacteria which own a complex system of proteases and peptidases. Their proteolytic system consists of an extracellular proteinase, a transport system specific for small peptides, and a multitude of intracellular specific, generic, endo-, and eso-peptidases [92]. A pool of selected lactic acid bacteria (comprising *Lactobacillus alimentarius*, *Lb. brevis*, *Lb. sanfranciscensis*, and *Lactobacillus hilgardii*) was selected to ferment several cereal flours [32]. The highest antioxidant activity on DPPH and inhibition of linoleic acid autoxidation were found for fermented whole wheat, spelt, rye, and kamut. Twenty-five peptides (8-57 amino acid residues), identified by nano-liquid chromatography-electrospray ionization-tandem mass spectrometry (nano-LC-ESI-MS/MS), showed ex vivo antioxidant activity on mouse fibroblasts artificially subjected to oxidative stress [32]. Galli et al. [93] adopted the same experimental design selecting 23 out of 131 LAB strains to singly inoculate wheat flour doughs. The sourdough extracts reduced ROS formation in several cell lines (RAW 264.7 murine macrophage, murine H-end endothelium cells and Human intestinal Caco-2 cells). Another recent study exploited the effect of fermentation with *Lb. plantarum* and a commercial protease on lentils [67]. Due to the flavonoids liberated during the bioprocessing, a reduction of ROS on RAW 264.7 macrophage cell line was observed. Bioprocessed lentils were later subjected to simulated gastro-intestinal digestion and, since it was observed an increase in the inhibition of ROS formation, the authors suggested that the pH changes caused structure modifications of both phenolics and peptides, releasing even more bioactive sequences [67].

Twenty-seven selected LAB were also used to ferment quinoa flours and screened for the ability to improve antioxidant activity [33]. The highest scavenging activity on DPPH radical (more than 80%) was found when fermentation was carried out with *Lb. plantarum* T6B4, T6C16, and T0A10, whereas only *Lb. plantarum* T1B6, T6B4, and T0A10 showed antioxidant activity on ABTS radical. Since the last strain also enabled the highest inhibition of linoleic acid autoxidation, it was the only extract further subjected to the purification and characterization of antioxidant peptide fractions. Five peptides, with sizes from 5 to 9 amino acid residues, identified by nano-LC-ESI-MS/MS, showed antioxidant activity on human keratinocytes NCTC 2544 artificially subjected to oxidative stress and resulted resistant to further hydrolysis by digestive enzymes [33]. Ex vivo antioxidant properties of extracts of quinoa seed fermented with *Rhizopus oligosporus* were also evaluated by Matsuo [94]. The extracts increased both activities of superoxide dismutase and glutathione peroxidase ex vivo, therefore, they were used to feed rats for 13 days, confirming the results in vivo.

Several studies reported the ability of *Bacillus* sp., during soybean and wheat germ fermentation, to improve the in vitro antioxidant activity on DPPH and ABTS radicals. However, the activity was only ascribed to peptides; it was not demonstrated on purified fractions, nor were the sequences identified [95–98]. Conversely, rice proteins, residues from starch extraction, were hydrolyzed with a mixture of commercial proteolytic enzymes and *Bacillus pumilus* AG1, showing antioxidant activity towards ABTS radical. Almost all the peptides contained in the hydrolysate showed one or more features typical of well-known antioxidant peptides, most probably conferring a synergic antioxidant effect to the mixture with the potential to be used as functional ingredient [99].

Nevertheless, fungal eso- and endo-proteases play an important role in physiology and development of fungi, they are widely used in food industry [100], and examples of antioxidant peptides obtained by fungal fermentation were also reported (Table 2). Fermentation of soy flour with *Aspergillus oryzae* enabled the hydrolysis of native proteins into small molecular weight peptides, 90% of which were less than 3 kDa. The fermented soy was found to have antioxidant activity on DPPH radical higher than that of the positive controls (α-tocopherol and γ-oryzanol). It also inhibited 51.2% of linoleic acid oxidation, which was equivalent to 77% of the antioxidant activity of α-tocopherol [101].

As for phenolic compounds, several research papers focused on the antioxidant properties of soybean peptides as a result of fermentation with *Bacillus subtilis* [52,53], *Lb. plantarum* [102], *R. microspores* [103], *A. oryzae* [104], *Bifidobacterium* sp. [105]. Among the properties evaluated, the peptides possessed strong Cu^{2+} chelation ability, superoxide radical scavenging activity, reducing power potential and some of the peptides considered also resisted simulated gastro-intestinal digestion [53]. In one case, after assessing the radical scavenging activities on DPPH and ABTS, and the chelating ability of ferrous ions in vitro, the antioxidant properties of fermented soy were proven in vivo on rats, confirming the increase of superoxide dismutase activity in liver and kidney, and glutathione peroxidase activity in kidney [104]. A very recent study exploited the nutritional properties of a traditional soy-based Indonesian fermented food bought at local business with different level of sanitation [106]. The sanitation conditions clearly influence the microflora involved in the fermentation therefore affecting the formation of functional peptides. The identified peptides from the three different stores, differing in both number and molecular weight, showed similar and dissimilar features regarding amino acid sequences and functionalities. Yet, it was the cleanest production facility that had the highest number of peptides associated with functional properties including antioxidant activity [106]. Hence, this study enlightened the considerable impact of the starter in the success of the fermentation process.

Table 2. Main effect of bioactive peptides and amino acids derivatives on the antioxidant activity of fermented cereals, pseudocereals, and legumes.

Matrix	Microorganisms Employed	Process Parameters	Effect	Reference
Wheat flour	*Lactobacillus farciminis* A11, A19, H3, *Lactobacillus rossiae* A20, Gd40, *Lactobacillus sanfranciscensis* B3, I4, *Lactobacillus plantarum* O4, *Lactobacillus brevis* A7	30 °C for 24 h	Reduction of ROS on RAW 264.7, H-end and Caco-2 cells	[93]
Defatted wheat germ	*Bacillus subtilis* B1	37 °C for 24 h	Unidentified peptides	[96]
Rice protein	*Bacillus pumilus* AG1	37 °C for 72 h	Identified peptide sequences with high antioxidant activity	[99]
Wheat, spelt, rye, and kamut flours	Pool of selected LAB	37 °C for 24 h	Identified peptide sequences with high antioxidant activity	[32]
Quinoa	*Rhizopus oligosporus* NRRL2710	36 °C for 24 h	Increased ex vivo and in vivo activities of superoxide dismutase, GSHPx, and TBARS	[94]
	L. plantarum T0A10	37 °C for 24 h	Identified peptides with antioxidant activity on human keratinocytes NCTC 2544	[33]

Table 2. *Cont.*

Matrix	Microorganisms Employed	Process Parameters	Effect	Reference
Soy	*R. oligosporus* ATCC 64063 *Aspergillus oryzae* DSM 1861 *Neurospora intermedia* DSM 1965	31 °C for 6 days 25 °C for 6 days 30 °C for 5 days	Increase of OH and ABTS radical scavenging activity due to potentially bioactive peptides	[107]
	Spontaneously sourdough containing *Rhizopus* spp., LAB and yeasts	Room temperature for 2 days	Identified peptide sequences with potential antioxidant activity	[106]
	B. subtilis SHZ	30 °C for 36 h	Superoxide radical scavenging activity and reducing power potential	[52]
	B. subtilis MTCC5480, MTCC1747	42 °C for 24 h	Increase in the antioxidant activity due to both phenolic compounds and peptides	[53]
	Lb, plantarum Lp6	30 °C for 24 h	Identified peptide sequences with high antioxidant activity	[102]
	Aspergillus orizae	30 °C for 3 days 45 °C for 4 days	Unidentified low molecular weight peptides	[100]
	Rhizopus microsporus	36 °C for 25 h	Improvement in the antioxidant activity attributed to amino acids and peptides	[97]
	Bifidobacterium sp.	37 °C for 48 h	Inhibition of ascorbate autoxidation, superoxide radical scavenging activity and reducing power potential peroxide	[105]
	Aspergillus oryzae	30 °C for 60 h	Superoxide dismutase and glutathione peroxidase activities *in vivo*	[104]
Kidney beans	*B. subtilis* CECT 39T *Lb. plantarum* CECT 748T	30 °C for 96 h 37 °C for 96 h	Improved antioxidant activity on ORAC-FL	[108]
Lentils	*Lb. plantarum* CECT 748 and commercial protease	37 °C for 15 h	Reduction of ROS on RAW 264.7 cells	[67]

4.3. Secondary Effects of Fermentation

4.3.1. Vitamins

The ability of fermentation to modify phenolic and protein composition strictly relies on the metabolic activities of the specific starter used; however, the effect of acidification on endogenous proteinases or other enzymes involved in phenolics and protein metabolism cannot be excluded [69,92], as well as improving phenol solubility [49]. Few authors have also reported changes in vitamin content during fermentation [42,61,109] (Table 3). Vitamin E, also known as tocopherol, is an important antioxidant, which, due to a chroman group, halts lipid peroxidation by donating its phenolic hydrogen to peroxyl radicals forming tocopheroxyl radicals that are unreactive and unable to continue the oxidative chain reaction [1]. However, only photosynthetic microorganisms are known to accumulate detectable amounts of tocopherols; therefore, other factors participate to its increase during some food fermentations [110]. Fermented soy germ extracts exhibited a higher inhibition effect against the superoxide anion radical and lesser but significant ferric-reducing and DPPH radical scavenging effects compared to raw soy germ, which was ascribed to an increase in phenolic acids and isoflavones but also to tocopherols [61]. On the contrary, a decrease in tocopherol was observed in lupins fermentation, both spontaneous and inoculated with a strain of *Lb. plantarum* [111], Małgorzata et al. [112] instead, observed a decrease in the scavenging activity on ABTS of buckwheat fermented with *R. oligosporus*, despite the increase of tocopherol content. When *Cordyceps sinensis*, a fungus used in Chinese traditional medicine, was used to ferment stale rice, vitamin E concentration was doubled compared to unfermented rice and superoxide dismutase activity increased. Fermented rice was administrated to mice for 40 days inhibiting oxidative enzymes in brain and liver therefore delaying senescence [109]; and similar effects were also obtained by feeding rabbits with extracts of red bean fermented with *B. subtilis* [113]. To a combined action of polyphenols and vitamins was ascribed the protective effect against oxidative stress in mice after the consumption of bread made with Kamut sourdough [42,114]. However, Kamut breads, especially those with sourdough had a high content of selenium, which is known to participate in cells oxidative stress protection [114].

Table 3. Secondary effect of fermentation on the antioxidant activity of cereals and legumes.

Matrix	Microorganisms Employed	Process Parameters	Effect	Reference
Stale rice	*Cordyceps sinensis*	25 °C for 7 days	Increase of tocopherol and superoxide dismutase activity in mice	[109]
Rice medium	*Lactobacillus kefiranofaciens*		EPS responsible of atherosclerosis prevention	[115]
Wheat distillers' grains	*Preussia aemulans*	Room temperature for 7 days	EPS formation with high radical scavenging activity and metal ions chelating ability	[116]
Wheat germ and bran	Yeasts and lactobacilli		High vitamin content responsible for in vivo antioxidant activity in liver and kidney	[117]
Kidney beans	*Bacillus subtilis* IMR-NK1	30 °C for 48 h	Improved antioxidant activity on DPPH, reducing power potential and Fe^{2+} chelating ability	[118]
	Bacillus subtilis BCRC 14716	30 °C for 48 h	Increased vitamin E levels in liver and brain of rabbit, and superoxide dismutase activity in the brain	[113]

Great attention has gained a preparation known as Lisosan G®, a mineral- and vitamin-rich powder registered as nutritional supplement, which consists in wheat germ and bran fermented with a mix of lactobacilli and yeast strains [119]. Its antioxidant activity in vitro was confirmed after supplementation in the diet of 40 rabbits for 60 days. Lisosan G was found to reduce reactive oxygen metabolites and increase vitamin A and E concentrations in the blood. In addition, it caused the induction of antioxidant enzymes in the liver and kidney of the treated rabbits [117].

4.3.2. Production of Exopolysaccharides

Exopolysaccharides (EPS) are long-chain polysaccharides produced by microorganisms, as a response to environmental stress, using various sugars as substrates. EPS are either associated with cell surfaces or secreted into the environment and can be classified as homo- or hetero-exopolysaccharides, depending on the composing sugar units [120]. The EPS biosynthetic pathway is very complex and includes several enzymes and glucose-6-phosphate appears to be a key intermediate linking between the anabolic pathways of EPS production and the catabolic pathways of sugar degradation [121]. EPS can be produced by bacteria, yeasts, or filamentous fungi and their physiological role depends on the microorganism producing them [120]. EPS are mostly employed in food industry as texture modifiers; however, fungal and bacterial EPS have been proved to have anticancer, antimicrobial, hypocholesterolemic, hypoglycemic, and also antioxidant activity [122]. It was suggested that their radical scavenging ability is associated to the molecular weight and the number of hydroxyl and amino groups, yet the relationship between antioxidant activity and physico-chemical properties or structural features is still uncertain due to opposite results [122]. Many purified EPS produced during fermentation with species of the genera *Lactobacillus* [123–126], *Lactococcus* [127,128], *Cordyceps* [129,130], *Aspergillus* [131] were found to have antioxidant activity in vitro and in vivo. Scavenging activity towards DPPH, ABTS and OH radicals, metal ion chelating ability, and inhibition of linoleic acid peroxidation, as well as protective effect against Caco-2 cells oxidative stress and increased superoxide dismutase in mice are among the properties demonstrated; however, there are few studies that have confirmed it during food fermentation. A study conducted few years ago, explored the potential of wheat distillers' grains water extract fermentation to produce EPS by *Preussia aemulans* [116]. Compared to the unfermented extract, the fermented one had 36% of EPS higher and the scavenging activity against DPPH, ABTS, and OH radicals were assessed. One of the EPS fractions showed antioxidant activity comparable to that of ascorbic acid, as well as high ability to chelate metal ions and these properties were found to be dose-dependent [116]. Uchida et al. [115] studied the effect of rice kefiran, an EPS produced in a rice medium by *Lactobacillus kefiranofaciens*, on the diet of rabbits. The authors concluded that kefiran prevents the onset of atherosclerosis in hypercholesterolemic rabbits through antinflamatory and antioxidant actions [118].

5. Conclusions

The increasing interest in nutraceuticals reflects consumers' attention towards studies indicating that specific diets or components in the diet are associated with lower risk of certain disease. Consequentially, consumer trends have shifted towards super foods that not only fulfill basic nutritious requirement, but also exert any number of functional features while being natural without additives. The major role of antioxidant compounds in preserving food shelf life, as well as providing health promoting benefits, combined with the increasing concern towards synthetic antioxidants, has led many authors to look for natural ways of increasing their content through fermentation. Phenolic compounds are the most studied substances displaying such properties, nevertheless, also peptides and protein derivatives, vitamins, and EPS, released or produced by the complex microbial enzymatic system, have been proven to exert antioxidant activities in vitro, ex vivo and in vivo (Figure 1).

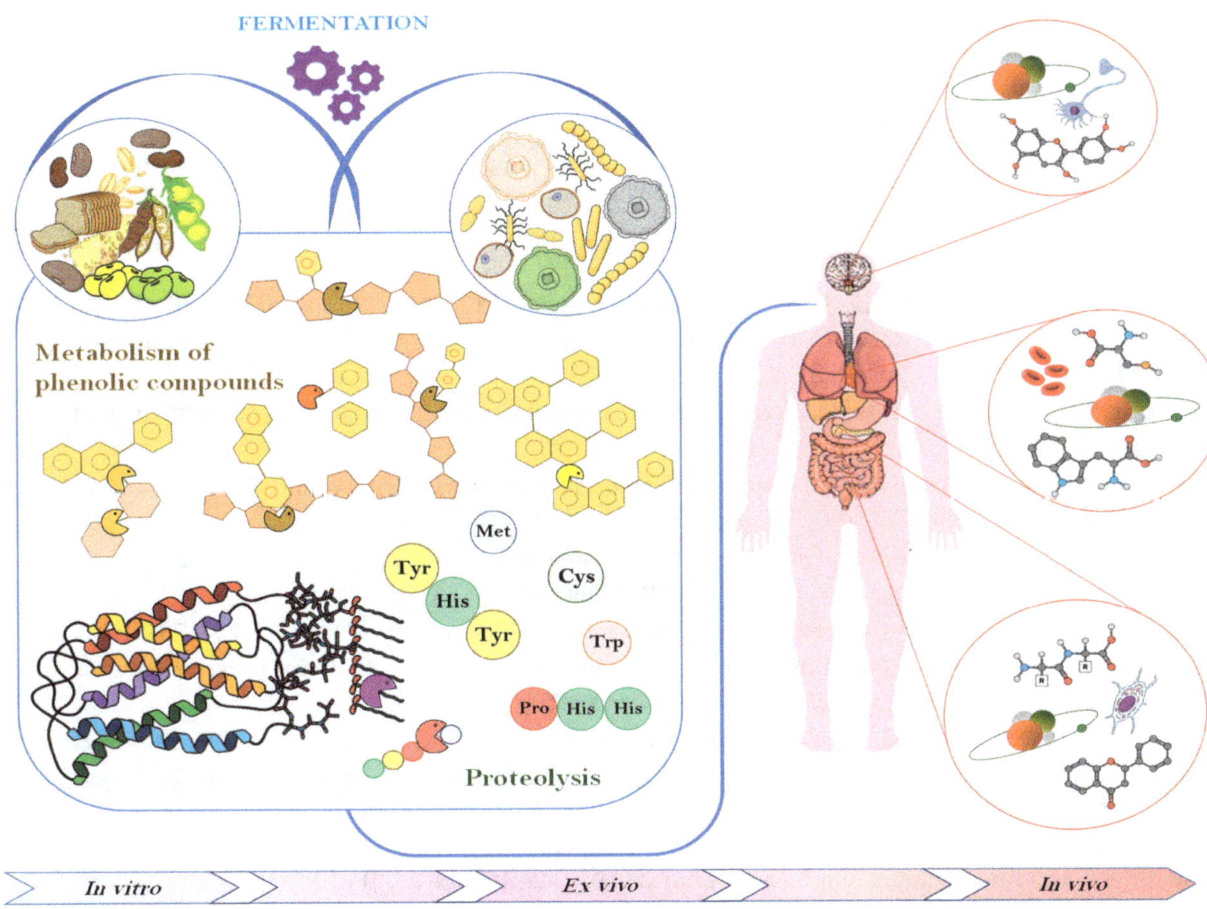

Figure 1. Schematic representation of the main effects of fermentation on food antioxidant compounds and consequent impact on human body.

Since most of the metabolic activities responsible for the antioxidant properties highlighted above are species- or strain- specific, starters selection is a pivotal step, and, even though the strains employed in these fermentations are recognized as safe, process parameters as well as many other factors, both affecting microbial and nutritional quality of fermented foods, need to be considered. Furthermore, as previously elucidated, an activity in vitro does not always correspond to an actual physiological function in vivo due to modifications occurring during the gastrointestinal digestion, therefore affecting the potential bioavailability of such compounds. Fermentation has the potential to meet consumers' requirements, yet more in vivo studies are needed.

Author Contributions: M.V. collected literature and wrote the manuscript, V.V., and C.G.R. reviewed and edited the manuscript. All the authors read and approved the manuscript.

Acknowledgments: V.V. thanks the Spanish Ministry of Economy and Competitiveness (MINECO) for "Ramon y Cajal" contract (RYC-2015-18795).

References

1. Carocho, M.; Ferreira, I.C. A review on antioxidants, prooxidants and related controversy: Natural and synthetic compounds, screening and analysis methodologies and future perspectives. *Food Chem. Toxicol.* **2013**, *51*, 15–25. [CrossRef] [PubMed]
2. Lobo, V.; Patil, A.; Phatak, A.; Chandra, N. Free radicals, antioxidants and functional foods: Impact on human health. *Pharmacogn. Rev.* **2010**, *4*, 118. [CrossRef] [PubMed]
3. Griffiths, K.; Aggarwal, B.; Singh, R.; Buttar, H.; Wilson, D.; De Meester, F. Food antioxidants and their anti-inflammatory properties: A potential role in cardiovascular diseases and cancer prevention. *Diseases* **2016**, *4*, 28. [CrossRef] [PubMed]
4. Alam, M.N.; Bristi, N.J.; Rafiquzzaman, M. Review on in vivo and in vitro methods evaluation of antioxidant activity. *Saudi Pharm. J.* **2013**, *21*, 143–152. [CrossRef] [PubMed]
5. Brewer, M.S. Natural antioxidants: Sources, compounds, mechanisms of action, and potential applications. *Compr. Rev. Food Sci. Food Saf.* **2011**, *10*, 221–247. [CrossRef]
6. Atmaca, G. Antioxidant effects of sulfur-containing amino acids. *Yonsei Med. J.* **2004**, *45*, 776–788. [CrossRef] [PubMed]
7. Rizzello, C.G.; Tagliazucchi, D.; Babini, E.; Rutella, G.S.; Saa, D.L.T.; Gianotti, A. Bioactive peptides from vegetable food matrices: Research trends and novel biotechnologies for synthesis and recovery. *J. Funct. Foods* **2016**, *27*, 549–569. [CrossRef]
8. Sarmadi, B.H.; Ismail, A. Antioxidative peptides from food proteins: A review. *Peptides* **2010**, *31*, 1949–1956. [CrossRef]
9. Pokorný, J. Are natural antioxidants better–and safer–than synthetic antioxidants? *Eur. J. Lipid Sci. Technol.* **2007**, *109*, 629–642. [CrossRef]
10. Box, J.D. Investigation of the Folin-Ciocalteau phenol reagent for the determination of polyphenolic substances in natural waters. *Water Res.* **1983**, *17*, 511–525. [CrossRef]
11. Shahidi, F.; Zhong, Y. Measurement of antioxidant activity. *J. Funct. Foods* **2015**, *18*, 757–781. [CrossRef]
12. Singh, B.; Singh, J.P.; Kaur, A.; Singh, N. Phenolic composition and antioxidant potential of grain legume seeds: A review. *Food Res. Int.* **2017**, *101*, 1–16. [CrossRef] [PubMed]
13. Gobbetti, M.; De Angelis, M.; Di Cagno, R.; Calasso, M.; Archetti, G.; Rizzello, C.G. Novel insights on the functional/nutritional features of the sourdough fermentation. *Int. J. Food Microbiol.* **2019**, *302*, 103–113. [CrossRef] [PubMed]
14. Verni, M.; Rizzello, C.G.; Coda, R. Fermentation biotechnology applied to cereal industry by-products: Nutritional and functional insights. *Front. Nutr.* **2019**, *6*, 42. [CrossRef] [PubMed]
15. Dey, T.B.; Chakraborty, S.; Jain, K.K.; Sharma, A.; Kuhad, R.C. Antioxidant phenolics and their microbial production by submerged and solid state fermentation process: A review. *Trends Food Sci. Technol.* **2016**, *53*, 60–74.

16. Manach, C.; Scalbert, A.; Morand, C.; Rémésy, C.; Jiménez, L. Polyphenols: Food sources and bioavailability. *Am. J. Clin. Nutr.* **2004**, *79*, 727–747. [CrossRef] [PubMed]
17. Lupea, A.X.; Pop, M.; Cacig, S. Structure-radical scavenging activity relationships of flavonoids from *Ziziphus* and *Hydrangea* extracts. *Rev. Chim.* **2008**, *59*, 309–313.
18. Shahidi, F.; Naczk, M. *Phenolics in Food and Nutraceuticals*; CRC press: Boca Raton, FL, USA, 2003; pp. 1–558.
19. Shahidi, F.; Ambigaipalan, P. Phenolics and polyphenolics in foods, beverages and spices: Antioxidant activity and health effects–A review. *J. Funct. Foods* **2015**, *18*, 820–897. [CrossRef]
20. Shahidi, F.; Zhong, Y. Bioactive peptides. *J. AOAC Int.* **2008**, *91*, 914–931.
21. Chen, H.M.; Muramoto, K.; Yamauchi, F.; Fujimoto, K.; Nokihara, K. Antioxidative properties of histidine-containing peptides designed from peptide fragments found in the digests of a soybean protein. *J. Agric. Food Chem.* **1998**, *46*, 49–53. [CrossRef]
22. Sánchez, A.; Vázquez, A. Bioactive peptides: A review. *Food Qual. Saf.* **2017**, *1*, 29–46. [CrossRef]
23. Nanditha, B.; Prabhasankar, P. Antioxidants in bakery products: A review. *Crit. Rev. Food Sci. Nutr.* **2008**, *49*, 1–27. [CrossRef]
24. EFSA. Panel on food additives and nutrient sources added to food (ANS); Scientific opinion on the reevaluation of butylated hydroxyanisole—BHA (E 320) as a food additive. *EFSA J.* **2011**, *9*, 2392. [CrossRef]
25. EFSA. Panel on food additives and nutrient sources added to food (ANS); Scientific opinion on the reevaluation of butylated hydroxytoluene BHT (E 321) as a food additive. *EFSA J.* **2012**, *10*, 2588. [CrossRef]
26. Carbonell-Capella, J.M.; Buniowska, M.; Barba, F.J.; Esteve, M.J.; Frígola, A. Analytical methods for determining bioavailability and bioaccessibility of bioactive compounds from fruits and vegetables: A review. *Compr. Rev. Food Sci. Food Saf.* **2014**, *13*, 155–171. [CrossRef]
27. Martin, K.R.; Appel, C.L. Polyphenols as dietary supplements: A double-edged sword. *Nutr. Diet. Suppl.* **2010**, *2*, 1–12. [CrossRef]
28. Hackman, R.M.; Polagruto, J.A.; Yan Zhu, Q.; Sun, B.; Fujii, H.; Keen, C.L. Flavanols: Digestion, absorption and bioactivity. *Phytochem. Rev.* **2008**, *7*, 195–208. [CrossRef]
29. D'Archivio, M.; Filesi, C.; Di Benedetto, R.; Gargiulo, R.; Giovannini, C.; Masella, R. Polyphenols, dietary sources and bioavailability. *Ann. Ist. Super. Sanita* **2007**, *43*, 348.
30. Cermak, R.; Durazzo, A.; Maiani, G.; Böhm, V.; Kammerer, D.R.; Carle, R.; Wiczkowski, W.; Piskula, M.K.; Galensa, R. The influence of postharvest processing and storage of foodstuffs on the bioavailability of flavonoids and phenolic acids. *Mol. Nutr. Food Res.* **2009**, *53*, S184–S193. [CrossRef]
31. García-Mora, P.; Martín-Martínez, M.; Bonache, M.A.; González-Múniz, R.; Peñas, E.; Frias, J.; Martinez-Villaluenga, C. Identification, functional gastrointestinal stability and molecular docking studies of lentil peptides with dual antioxidant and angiotensin I converting enzyme inhibitory activities. *Food Chem.* **2017**, *221*, 464–472. [CrossRef]
32. Coda, R.; Rizzello, C.G.; Pinto, D.; Gobbetti, M. Selected lactic acid bacteria synthesize antioxidant peptides during sourdough fermentation of cereal flours. *Appl. Environ. Microbiol.* **2012**, *78*, 1087–1096. [CrossRef]
33. Rizzello, C.G.; Lorusso, A.; Russo, V.; Pinto, D.; Marzani, B.; Gobbetti, M. Improving the antioxidant properties of quinoa flour through fermentation with selected autochthonous lactic acid bacteria. *Int. J. Food Microbiol.* **2017**, *241*, 252–261. [CrossRef]
34. Filannino, P.; Di Cagno, R.; Gobbetti, M. Metabolic and functional paths of lactic acid bacteria in plant foods: Get out of the labyrinth. *Curr. Opin. Biotechnol.* **2018**, *49*, 64–72. [CrossRef]
35. Jiménez, N.; Esteban-Torres, M.; Mancheño, J.M.; de las Rivas, B.; Muñoz, R. Tannin degradation by a novel tannase enzyme present in some *Lactobacillus plantarum* strains. *Appl. Environ. Microbiol.* **2014**, *80*, 2991–2997. [CrossRef]
36. Raccach, M. The antimicrobial activity of phenolic antioxidant in food: A review. *J. Food Saf.* **1984**, *6*, 141–170. [CrossRef]
37. Sánchez-Maldonado, A.F.; Schieber, A.; Gänzle, M.G. Structure—function relationships of the antibacterial activity of phenolic acids and their metabolism by lactic acid bacteria. *J. Appl. Microbiol.* **2011**, *111*, 1176–1184. [CrossRef]
38. Anson, N.M.; Selinheimo, E.; Havenaar, R.; Aura, A.M.; Mattila, I.; Lehtinen, P.; Bast, A.; Poutanen, K.; Haenen, G.R. Bioprocessing of wheat bran improves in vitro bioaccessibility and colonic metabolism of phenolic compounds. *J. Agric. Food Chem.* **2009**, *57*, 6148–6155. [CrossRef]

39. Manini, F.; Brasca, M.; Plumed-Ferrer, C.; Morandi, S.; Erba, D.; Casiraghi, M.C. Study of the chemical changes and evolution of microbiota during sourdoughlike fermentation of wheat bran. *Cereal Chem.* **2014**, *91*, 342–349. [CrossRef]
40. Savolainen, O.I.; Coda, R.; Suomi, K.; Katina, K.; Juvonen, R.; Hanhineva, K.; Poutanen, K. The role of oxygen in the liquid fermentation of wheat bran. *Food Chem.* **2014**, *153*, 424–431. [CrossRef]
41. Xie, C.Y.; Gu, Z.X.; You, X.; Liu, G.; Tan, Y.; Zhang, H. Screening of edible mushrooms for release of ferulic acid from wheat bran by fermentation. *Enz. Microb. Technol.* **2010**, *46*, 125–128. [CrossRef]
42. Benedetti, S.; Primiterra, M.; Tagliamonte, M.C.; Carnevali, A.; Gianotti, A.; Bordoni, A.; Canestrari, F. Counteraction of oxidative damage in the rat liver by an ancient grain (Kamut brand khorasan wheat). *Nutrition* **2012**, *28*, 436–441. [CrossRef]
43. Schmidt, C.G.; Gonçalves, L.M.; Prietto, L.; Hackbart, H.S.; Furlong, E.B. Antioxidant activity and enzyme inhibition of phenolic acids from fermented rice bran with fungus *Rizhopus oryzae*. *Food Chem.* **2014**, *146*, 371–377. [CrossRef]
44. Razak, D.L.A.; Rashid, N.Y.A.; Jamaluddin, A.; Sharifudin, S.A.; Long, K. Enhancement of phenolic acid content and antioxidant activity of rice bran fermented with *Rhizopus oligosporus* and *Monascus purpureus*. *Biocatal. Agric. Biotechnol.* **2015**, *4*, 33–38. [CrossRef]
45. Webber, D.M.; Hettiarachchy, N.S.; Li, R.; Horax, R.; Theivendran, S. Phenolic profile and antioxidant activity of extracts prepared from fermented heat-stabilized defatted rice bran. *J. Food Sci.* **2014**, *79*, H2383–H2391. [CrossRef]
46. Katina, K.; Laitila, A.; Juvonen, R.; Liukkonen, K.H.; Kariluoto, S.; Piironen, V.; Landberg, R.; Aman, P.; Poutanen, K. Bran fermentation as a means to enhance technological properties and bioactivity of rye. *Food Microbiol.* **2007**, *24*, 175–186. [CrossRef]
47. Koistinen, V.M.; Katina, K.; Nordlund, E.; Poutanen, K.; Hanhineva, K. Changes in the phytochemical profile of rye bran induced by enzymatic bioprocessing and sourdough fermentation. *Food Res. Intern.* **2016**, *89*, 1106–1115. [CrossRef]
48. Nordlund, E.; Katina, K.; Aura, A.M.; Poutanen, K. Changes in bran structure by bioprocessing with enzymes and yeast modifies the in vitro digestibility and fermentability of bran protein and dietary fibre complex. *J. Cereal Sci.* **2013**, *58*, 200–208. [CrossRef]
49. Svensson, L.; Sekwati-Monang, B.; Lutz, D.L.; Schieber, A.; Ganzle, M.G. Phenolic acids and flavonoids in nonfermented and fermented red sorghum (*Sorghum bicolor* (L.) *Moench*). *J. Agric. Food Chem.* **2010**, *58*, 9214–9220. [CrossRef]
50. Shumoy, H.; Gabaza, M.; Vandevelde, J.; Raes, K. Soluble and bound phenolic contents and antioxidant capacity of tef injera as affected by traditional fermentation. *J. Food Compos. Anal.* **2017**, *58*, 52–59. [CrossRef]
51. Dongmo, S.N.; Sacher, B.; Kollmannsberger, H.; Becker, T. Key volatile aroma compounds of lactic acid fermented malt based beverages–impact of lactic acid bacteria strains. *Food Chem.* **2017**, *229*, 565–573. [CrossRef]
52. Yu, B.; Lu, Z.X.; Bie, X.M.; Lu, F.X.; Huang, X.Q. Scavenging and anti-fatigue activity of fermented defatted soybean peptides. *Eur. Food Res. Technol.* **2008**, *226*, 415–421. [CrossRef]
53. Sanjukta, S.; Rai, A.K.; Muhammed, A.; Jeyaram, K.; Talukdar, N.C. Enhancement of antioxidant properties of two soybean varieties of Sikkim Himalayan region by proteolytic *Bacillus subtilis* fermentation. *J. Funct. Foods* **2015**, *14*, 650–658. [CrossRef]
54. Dueñas, M.; Hernández, T.; Lamparski, G.; Estrella, I.; Muñoz, R. Bioactive phenolic compounds of soybean (*Glycine max* cv. *Merit*): Modifications by different microbiological fermentations. *Pol. J. Food Nutr. Sci.* **2012**, *62*, 241–250.
55. Cho, K.M.; Hong, S.Y.; Math, R.K.; Lee, J.H.; Kambiranda, D.M.; Kim, J.M.; Islam, S.A.; Yun, M.G.; Cho, J.J.; Lim, W.J.; et al. Biotransformation of phenolics (isoflavones, flavanols and phenolic acids) during the fermentation of cheonggukjang by *Bacillus pumilus* HY1. *Food Chem.* **2009**, *114*, 413–419. [CrossRef]
56. Georgetti, S.R.; Vicentini, F.T.M.C.; Yokoyama, C.Y.; Borin, M.D.F.; Spadaro, A.C.C.; Fonseca, M.J.V. Enhanced in vitro and in vivo antioxidant activity and mobilization of free phenolic compounds of soybean flour fermented with different β-glucosidase-producing fungi. *J. Appl. Microbiol.* **2009**, *106*, 459–466. [CrossRef]
57. Avila, M.; Jaquet, M.; Moine, D.; Requena, T.; Pelaez, C.; Arigoni, F.; Jankovic, I. Physiological and biochemical characterization of the two α-L-rhamnosidases of *Lactobacillus plantarum* NCC245. *Microbiology* **2009**, *155*, 2739–2749. [CrossRef]

58. McCue, P.; Horii, A.; Shetty, K. Mobilization of phenolic antioxidants from defatted soybean powders by *Lentinus edodes* during solid-state bioprocessing is associated with enhanced production of laccase. *Innov. Food Sci. Emerg. Technol.* **2004**, *5*, 385–392. [CrossRef]
59. Hu, Y.; Ge, C.; Yuan, W.; Zhu, R.; Zhang, W.; Du, L.; Xue, J. Characterization of fermented black soybean natto inoculated with *Bacillus natto* during fermentation. *J. Sci. Food Agric.* **2010**, *90*, 1194–1202. [CrossRef]
60. Landete, J.M.; Hernández, T.; Robredo, S.; Duenas, M.; de las Rivas, B.; Estrella, I.; Munoz, R. Effect of soaking and fermentation on content of phenolic compounds of soybean (*Glycine max* cv. *Merit*) and mung beans (*Vigna radiata* L. *Wilczek*). *Int. J. Food Sci. Nutr.* **2015**, *66*, 203–209. [CrossRef]
61. Hubert, J.; Berger, M.; Nepveu, F.; Paul, F.; Daydé, J. Effects of fermentation on the phytochemical composition and antioxidant properties of soy germ. *Food Chem.* **2008**, *109*, 709–721. [CrossRef]
62. Riciputi, Y.; Serrazanetti, D.I.; Verardo, V.; Vannini, L.; Caboni, M.F.; Lanciotti, R. Effect of fermentation on the content of bioactive compounds in tofu-type products. *J. Funct. Foods* **2016**, *27*, 131–139. [CrossRef]
63. Budryn, G.; Klewicka, E.; Grzelczyk, J.; Gałązka-Czarnecka, I.; Mostowski, R. Lactic acid fermentation of legume seed sprouts as a method of increasing the content of isoflavones and reducing microbial contamination. *Food Chem.* **2019**, *285*, 478–484. [CrossRef]
64. Fiorda, F.A.; de Melo Pereira, G.V.; Thomaz-Soccol, V.; Medeiros, A.P.; Rakshit, S.K.; Soccol, C.R. Development of kefir-based probiotic beverages with DNA protection and antioxidant activities using soybean hydrolyzed extract, colostrum and honey. *LWT-Food Sci. Technol.* **2016**, *68*, 690–697. [CrossRef]
65. Di Cagno, R.; Mazzacane, F.; Rizzello, C.G.; Vincentini, O.; Silano, M.; Giuliani, G.; De Angelis, M.; Gobbetti, M. Synthesis of isoflavone aglycones and equol in soy milks fermented by food-related lactic acid bacteria and their effect on human intestinal Caco-2 cells. *J. Agric. Food Chem.* **2010**, *58*, 10338–10346. [CrossRef]
66. Dueñas, M.; Fernández, D.; Hernández, T.; Estrella, I.; Muñoz, R. Bioactive phenolic compounds of cowpeas (*Vigna sinensis* L). Modifications by fermentation with natural microflora and with *Lactobacillus plantarum* ATCC 14917. *J. Sci. Food Agric.* **2005**, *85*, 297–304. [CrossRef]
67. Bautista-Expósito, S.; Peñas, E.; Dueñas, M.; Silván, J.M.; Frias, J.; Martínez-Villaluenga, C. Individual contributions of Savinase and *Lactobacillus plantarum* to lentil functionalization during alkaline pH-controlled fermentation. *Food Chem.* **2018**, *257*, 341–349. [CrossRef]
68. Bartolomé, B.; Estrella, I.; Hernandez, T. Changes in phenolic compounds in lentils (*Lens culinaris*) during germination and fermentation. *Z. Lebensm Unters Forsch. A* **1997**, *205*, 290–294. [CrossRef]
69. Gänzle, M.G. Enzymatic and bacterial conversions during sourdough fermentation. *Food Microbiol.* **2014**, *37*, 2–10. [CrossRef]
70. Rodríguez, H.; Curiel, J.A.; Landete, J.M.; de las Rivas, B.; de Felipe, F.L.; Gómez-Cordovés, C.; Mancheño, J.M.; Muñoz, R. Food phenolics and lactic acid bacteria. *Int. J. Food Microbiol.* **2009**, *132*, 79–90. [CrossRef]
71. Filannino, P.; Gobbetti, M.; De Angelis, M.; Di Cagno, R. Hydroxycinnamic acids used as external acceptors of electrons: An energetic advantage for strictly heterofermentative lactic acid bacteria. *Appl. Environ. Microbiol.* **2014**, *80*, 7574–7582. [CrossRef]
72. Filannino, P.; Bai, Y.; Di Cagno, R.; Gobbetti, M.; Gänzle, M.G. Metabolism of phenolic compounds by *Lactobacillus* spp. during fermentation of cherry juice and broccoli puree. *Food Microbiol.* **2015**, *46*, 272–279. [CrossRef]
73. Senger, D.R.; Li, D.; Jaminet, S.C.; Cao, S. Activation of the Nrf2 cell defense pathway by ancient foods: Disease prevention by important molecules and microbes lost from the modern western diet. *PLoS ONE* **2016**, *11*, e0148042. [CrossRef]
74. Chatonnet, P.; Dubourdieu, D.; Boidron, J.N.; Lavigne, V. Synthesis of volatile phenols by *Saccharomyces cerevisiae* in wines. *J. Sci. Food Agric.* **1993**, *62*, 191–202. [CrossRef]
75. Gasson, M.J.; Kitamura, Y.; McLauchlan, W.R.; Narbad, A.; Parr, A.J.; Parsons, E.L.H.; Payne, J.; Rhodes, M.J.C.; Walton, N.J. Metabolism of ferulic acid to vanillin. A bacterial gene of the enoyl-SCoA hydratase/isomerase superfamily encodes an enzyme for the hydration and cleavage of a hydroxycinnamic acid SCoA thioester. *J. Biol. Chem.* **1998**, *273*, 4163–4170. [CrossRef]
76. Longo, M.A.; Sanromán, M.A. Production of food aroma compounds: Microbial and enzymatic methodologies. *Food Technol. Biotechnol.* **2006**, *44*, 335–353.
77. Donaghy, J.; Kelly, P.F.; McKay, A.M. Detection of ferulic acid esterase production by *Bacillus* spp. and lactobacilli. *Appl. Microbiol. Biotechnol.* **1998**, *50*, 257–260. [CrossRef]

78. Benoit, I.; Danchin, E.G.; Bleichrodt, R.J.; de Vries, R.P. Biotechnological applications and potential of fungal feruloyl esterases based on prevalence, classification and biochemical diversity. *Biotechnol. Lett.* **2008**, *30*, 387–396. [CrossRef]
79. Mathew, S.; Abraham, T.E. Ferulic acid: An antioxidant found naturally in plant cell walls and feruloyl esterases involved in its release and their applications. *Crit. Rev. Biotechnol.* **2004**, *24*, 59–83. [CrossRef]
80. Aurilia, V.; Parracino, A.; Saviano, M.; D'Auria, S. The psychrophilic bacterium *Pseudoalteromonas halosplanktis* TAC125 possesses a gene coding for a cold-adapted feruloyl esterase activity that shares homology with esterase enzymes from γ-proteobacteria and yeast. *Gene* **2007**, *397*, 51–57. [CrossRef]
81. Coghe, S.; Benoot, K.; Delvaux, F.; Vanderhaegen, B.; Delvaux, F.R. Ferulic acid release and 4-vinylguaiacol formation during brewing and fermentation: Indications for feruloyl esterase activity in *Saccharomyces cerevisiae*. *J. Agric. Food Chem.* **2004**, *52*, 602–608. [CrossRef]
82. Anson, N.M.; Hemery, Y.M.; Bast, A.; Haenen, G.R. Optimizing the bioactive potential of wheat bran by processing. *Food. Funct.* **2012**, *3*, 362–375. [CrossRef]
83. Koistinen, V.M.; Nordlund, E.; Katina, K.; Mattila, I.; Poutanen, K.; Hanhineva, K.; Aura, A.M. Effect of bioprocessing on the in vitro colonic microbial metabolism of phenolic acids from rye bran fortified breads. *J. Agric. Food Chem.* **2017**, *65*, 1854–1864. [CrossRef]
84. Xiao, Y.; Xing, G.; Rui, X.; Li, W.; Chen, X.; Jiang, M.; Dong, M. Enhancement of the antioxidant capacity of chickpeas by solid state fermentation with *Cordyceps militaris* SN-18. *J. Funct. Foods* **2014**, *10*, 210–222. [CrossRef]
85. McCue, P.; Shetty, K. Health benefits of soy isoflavonoids and strategies for enhancement: A review. *Crit. Rev. Food Sci. Nutr.* **2004**, *44*, 361–367. [CrossRef]
86. Randhir, R.; Vattem, D.; Shetty, K. Solid-state bioconversion of fava bean by *Rhizopus oligosporus* for enrichment of phenolic antioxidants and L-DOPA. *Inn. Food Sci. Emerg. Technol.* **2004**, *5*, 235–244. [CrossRef]
87. Bhanja, T.; Kumari, A.; Banerjee, R. Enrichment of phenolics and free radical scavenging property of wheat koji prepared with two filamentous fungi. *Bioresour. Technol.* **2009**, *100*, 2861–2866. [CrossRef]
88. Iwamoto, K.; Tsuruta, H.; Nishitaini, Y.; Osawa, R. Identification and cloning of a gene encoding tannase (tannin acylhydrolase) from *Lactobacillus plantarum* ATCC 14917T. *Syst. Appl. Microbiol.* **2008**, *31*, 269–277. [CrossRef]
89. Ramírez-Coronel, M.A.; Viniegra-Gonzalez, G.; Darvill, A.; Augur, C. A novel tannase from *Aspergillus niger* with β-glucosidase activity. *Microbiology* **2003**, *149*, 2941–2946. [CrossRef]
90. Sánchez-Patán, F.; Tabasco, R.; Monagas, M.; Requena, T.; Peláez, C.; Moreno-Arribas, M.V.; Bartolomé, B. Capability of *Lactobacillus plantarum* IFPL935 to catabolize flavan-3-ol compounds and complex phenolic extracts. *J. Agric. Food Chem.* **2012**, *60*, 7142–7151. [CrossRef]
91. Gleńsk, M.; Hurst, W.J.; Glinski, V.B.; Bednarski, M.; Gliński, G.A. Isolation of 1-(30,40-Dihydroxyphenyl)-3-(2″,4″,6″-trihydroxyphenyl)-propan-2-ol from grape seed extract and evaluation of its antioxidant and antispasmodic potential. *Molecules* **2019**, *24*, 2466. [CrossRef]
92. Gobbetti, M.; De Angelis, M.; Corsetti, A.; Di Cagno, R. Biochemistry and physiology of sourdough lactic acid bacteria. *Trends Food Sci. Technol.* **2005**, *16*, 57–69. [CrossRef]
93. Galli, V.; Mazzoli, L.; Luti, S.; Venturi, M.; Guerrini, S.; Paoli, P.; Vincenzini, M.; Granchi, L.; Pazzagli, L. Effect of selected strains of lactobacilli on the antioxidant and anti-inflammatory properties of sourdough. *Int. J. Food Microbiol.* **2018**, *286*, 55–65. [CrossRef]
94. Matsuo, M. In vivo antioxidant activity of methanol extract from quinoa fermented with *Rhizopus oligosporus*. *J. Nutr. Sci. Vitaminol.* **2005**, *51*, 449–452. [CrossRef]
95. Apostolidis, E.; Kwon, Y.I.; Ghaedian, R.; Shetty, K. Fermentation of milk and soymilk by *Lactobacillus bulgaricus* and *Lactobacillus acidophilus* enhances functionality for potential dietary management of hyperglycemia and hypertension. *Food Biotechnol.* **2007**, *21*, 217–236. [CrossRef]
96. Niu, L.Y.; Jiang, S.T.; Pan, L.J. Preparation and evaluation of antioxidant activities of peptides obtained from defatted wheat germ by fermentation. *J. Food Sci. Technol.* **2013**, *50*, 53–61. [CrossRef]
97. Watanabe, N.; Fujimoto, K.; Aoki, H. Antioxidant activities of the water-soluble fraction in tempeh-like fermented soybean (GABA-tempeh). *Int. J. Food Sci. Nutr.* **2007**, *58*, 577–587. [CrossRef]
98. Zhu, Y.P.; Fan, J.F.; Cheng, Y.Q.; Li, L.T. Improvement of the antioxidant activity of Chinese traditional fermented okara (Meitauza) using *Bacillus subtilis* B2. *Food Control* **2008**, *19*, 654–661. [CrossRef]

99. Dei Più, L.; Tassoni, A.; Serrazanetti, D.I.; Ferri, M.; Babini, E.; Tagliazucchi, D.; Gianotti, A. Exploitation of starch industry liquid by-product to produce bioactive peptides from rice hydrolyzed proteins. *Food Chem.* **2014**, *155*, 199–206. [CrossRef]
100. Yike, I. Fungal proteases and their pathophysiological effects. *Mycopathologia* **2011**, *171*, 299–323. [CrossRef]
101. Lee, J.S.; Rho, S.J.; Kim, Y.W.; Lee, K.W.; Lee, H.G. Evaluation of biological activities of the short-term fermented soybean extract. *Food Sci. Biotechnol.* **2013**, *22*, 973–978. [CrossRef]
102. Amadou, I.; Gbadamosi, O.S.; Shi, Y.; Kamara, M.T.; Jin, S. Identification of antioxidative peptides from *Lactobacillus plantarum* Lp6 fermented soybean protein meal. *Res. J. Microbiol.* **2010**, *5*, 372–380. [CrossRef]
103. Gibbs, B.F.; Zougman, A.; Masse, R.; Mulligan, C. Production and characterization of bioactive peptides from soy hydrolysate and soy-fermented food. *Food Res. Int.* **2004**, *37*, 123–131. [CrossRef]
104. Wang, D.; Wang, L.J.; Zhu, F.X.; Zhu, J.Y.; Chen, X.D.; Zou, L.; Saito, M. In vitro and in vivo studies on the antioxidant activities of the aqueous extracts of Douchi (a traditional Chinese salt-fermented soybean food). *Food Chem.* **2008**, *107*, 1421–1428. [CrossRef]
105. Tamam, B.; Syah, D.; Suhartono, M.T.; Kusuma, W.A.; Tachibana, S.; Lioe, H.N. Proteomic study of bioactive peptides from tempeh. *J. Biosci. Bioeng.* **2019**, in press. [CrossRef]
106. Starzyńska-Janiszewska, A.; Stodolak, B.; Gómez-Caravaca, A.M.; Mickowska, B.; Martin-Garcia, B.; Byczyński, Ł. Mould starter selection for extended solid-state fermentation of quinoa. *LWT-Food Sci. Technol.* **2019**, *99*, 231–237. [CrossRef]
107. Limón, R.I.; Peñas, E.; Torino, M.I.; Martínez-Villaluenga, C.; Dueñas, M.; Frias, J. Fermentation enhances the content of bioactive compounds in kidney bean extracts. *Food Chem.* **2015**, *172*, 343–352. [CrossRef]
108. Zhang, Z.; Lei, Z.; Yun, L.; Zhongzhi, L.; Chen, Y. Chemical composition and bioactivity changes in stale rice after fermentation with *Cordyceps sinensis*. *J. Biosci. Bioeng.* **2008**, *106*, 188–193. [CrossRef]
109. Ogbonna, J.C. Microbiological production of tocopherols: Current state and prospects. *Appl. Microbiol. Biotechnol.* **2009**, *84*, 217–225. [CrossRef]
110. Wang, Y.C.; Yu, R.C.; Chou, C.C. Antioxidative activities of soymilk fermented with lactic acid bacteria and bifidobacteria. *Food Microbiol.* **2006**, *23*, 128–135. [CrossRef]
111. Frias, J.; Miranda, M.L.; Doblado, R.; Vidal-Valverde, C. Effect of germination and fermentation on the antioxidant vitamin content and antioxidant capacity of *Lupinus albus* L. var. *Multolupa*. *Food Chem.* **2005**, *92*, 211–220. [CrossRef]
112. Małgorzata, W.; Joanna, H.; Konrad, P.M. Effect of solid-state fermentation with *Rhizopus oligosporus* on bioactive compounds and antioxidant capacity of raw and roasted buckwheat groats. *It. J. Food Sci.* **2015**, *27*, 424–431.
113. Chou, S.T.; Chung, Y.C.; Peng, H.Y.; Hsu, C.K. Improving antioxidant status in aged mice by 50% ethanol extract from red bean fermented by *Bacillus subtilis*. *J. Sci. Food Agric.* **2013**, *93*, 2562–2567. [CrossRef]
114. Gianotti, A.; Danesi, F.; Verardo, V.; Serrazanetti, D.I.; Valli, V.; Russo, A.; Riciputi, Y.; Tossani, N.; Caboni, M.F.; Guerzoni, M.E.; et al. Role of cereal type and processing in whole grain in vivo protection from oxidative stress. *Front. Biosci.* **2011**, *16*, 1609–1618. [CrossRef]
115. Uchida, M.; Ishii, I.; Inoue, C.; Akisato, Y.; Watanabe, K.; Hosoyama, S.; Toida, T.; Ariyoshi, N.; Kitada, M. Kefiran reduces atherosclerosis in rabbits fed a high cholesterol diet. *J. Atheroscler. Throm.* **2010**, 1006100247. [CrossRef]
116. Li, Y.T.; Meng, S.L.; Wang, L.B.; Wang, Y.P.; Zu, X.Y.; Yang, Y.N.; Zhang, Z.Y. Antioxidative activity of exopolysaccharide extract from fermented wheat distillers. *Adv. J. Food Sci. Technol.* **2014**, *6*, 1067–1075. [CrossRef]
117. Pozzo, L.; Vizzarri, F.; Ciardi, M.; Nardoia, M.; Palazzo, M.; Casamassima, D.; Longo, V. The effects of fermented wheat powder (Lisosan G) on the blood lipids and oxidative status of healthy rabbits. *Food Chem. Toxicol.* **2015**, *84*, 1–7. [CrossRef]
118. Chung, Y.C.; Chang, C.T.; Chao, W.W.; Lin, C.F.; Chou, S.T. Antioxidative activity and safety of the 50 ethanolic extract from red bean fermented by *Bacillus subtilis* IMR-NK1. *J. Agric. Food Chem.* **2002**, *50*, 2454–2458. [CrossRef]
119. La Marca, M.; Beffy, P.; Pugliese, A.; Longo, V. Fermented wheat powder induces the antioxidant and detoxifying system in primary rat hepatocytes. *PLoS ONE* **2013**, *8*, e83538. [CrossRef]
120. Donot, F.; Fontana, A.; Baccou, J.C.; Schorr-Galindo, S. Microbial exopolysaccharides: Main examples of synthesis, excretion, genetics and extraction. *Carbohydr. Polym.* **2012**, *87*, 951–962. [CrossRef]

121. Welman, A.D.; Maddox, I.S. Exopolysaccharides from lactic acid bacteria: Perspectives and challenges. *Trends Biotechnol.* **2003**, *21*, 269–274. [CrossRef]
122. Wang, J.; Hu, S.; Nie, S.; Yu, Q.; Xie, M. Reviews on mechanisms of in vitro antioxidant activity of polysaccharides. *Oxid. Med. Cell. Longev.* **2016**. [CrossRef]
123. Adesulu-Dahunsi, A.T.; Jeyaram, K.; Sanni, A.I.; Banwo, K. Production of exopolysaccharide by strains of *Lactobacillus plantarum* YO175 and OF101 isolated from traditional fermented cereal beverage. *PeerJ* **2018**, *6*, e5326. [CrossRef]
124. Liu, C.F.; Tseng, K.C.; Chiang, S.S.; Lee, B.H.; Hsu, W.H.; Pan, T.M. Immunomodulatory and antioxidant potential of *Lactobacillus* exopolysaccharides. *J. Sci. Food Agric.* **2011**, *91*, 2284–2291. [CrossRef]
125. Patten, D.A.; Laws, A.P. *Lactobacillus*-produced exopolysaccharides and their potential health benefits: A review. *Benef. Microbes* **2015**, *6*, 457–471. [CrossRef]
126. Zhang, L.; Liu, C.; Li, D.; Zhao, Y.; Zhang, X.; Zeng, X.; Yang, Z.; Li, S. Antioxidant activity of an exopolysaccharide isolated from *Lactobacillus plantarum* C88. *Int. J. Biol. Macromol.* **2013**, *54*, 270–275. [CrossRef]
127. Guo, Y.; Pan, D.; Li, H.; Sun, Y.; Zeng, X.; Yan, B. Antioxidant and immunomodulatory activity of selenium exopolysaccharide produced by *Lactococcus lactis* subsp. *lactis*. *Food Chem.* **2013**, *138*, 84–89. [CrossRef]
128. Pan, D.; Mei, X. Antioxidant activity of an exopolysaccharide purified from *Lactococcus lactis* subsp. *lactis* 12. *Carbohydr. Polym.* **2010**, *80*, 908–914. [CrossRef]
129. Leung, P.H.; Zhao, S.; Ho, K.P.; Wu, J.Y. Chemical properties and antioxidant activity of exopolysaccharides from mycelial culture of *Cordyceps sinensis* fungus Cs-HK1. *Food Chem.* **2009**, *114*, 1251–1256. [CrossRef]
130. Yan, J.K.; Li, L.; Wang, Z.M.; Leung, P.H.; Wang, W.Q.; Wu, J.Y. Acidic degradation and enhanced antioxidant activities of exopolysaccharides from *Cordyceps sinensis* mycelial culture. *Food Chem.* **2009**, *117*, 641–646. [CrossRef]
131. Chen, Y.; Mao, W.; Tao, H.; Zhu, W.; Qi, X.; Chen, Y.; Li, H.; Zhao, C.; Yang, Y.; Hou, Y.; et al. Structural characterization and antioxidant properties of an exopolysaccharide produced by the mangrove endophytic fungus *Aspergillus* sp. Y16. *Biores. Technol.* **2011**, *102*, 8179–8184. [CrossRef]

10

Improved Lycopene Production from Different Substrates by Mated Fermentation of *Blakeslea Trispora*

Ayse Sevgili and Osman Erkmen *

Department of Food Engineering, Faculty of Engineering, University of Gaziantep, 27310 Gaziantep, Turkey; aysesevgili8@gmail.com
* Correspondence: erkmen@gantep.edu.tr

Abstract: The production of lycopene from different substrates by *Blakeslea trispora* in fermentation was investigated. Lycopene productions from 4 and 6% glucose (pH 6.5) in shake flask fermentation were 77.7 and 28.1 mg L^{-1}. Increasing the glucose concentration to 6% resulted in a decrease in lycopene production by 36.2%. A maximum lycopene concentration of 944.8 mg L^{-1} was detected with 4% glucose supplemented with 1.0 % sunflower oil in fermentor studies. Lycopene productions in the presence of sunflower and corn oils in the fermentor were 12.2 and 11.1 times higher, respectively, then without oil from 4 % glucose in a shake flask. Lycopene production from orange peel was two times higher in the fermentor than in the shake flask. Zygospores of *B. trispora* are the morphological forms, which are responsible for the production of the lycopene. The highest level of zygospores was correlated with the highest amount of intracellular lycopene in the total biomass dry weight. The media containing only orange powder (1%) gave a 4.9 mg L^{-1} lycopene production in a fermentor. The biosynthesis of lycopene has been started in most cases simultaneously in the early growth phase even in trace amounts. Maximum lycopene concentration was obtained when the medium was supplied with sunflower and corn oils. There is an indirect relationship between biomass and lycopene concentration.

Keywords: lycopene; *Blakeslea trispora*; fermentation; vegetable oil; orange powder

1. Introduction

Lycopene is an important naturally occurring intermediate metabolite in the mevalonate metabolic pathway of microorganisms and can be transformed into β-carotene by lycopene cyclase. Thus, in order to enhance lycopene accumulation, lycopene cyclase activity should be inhibited by adding lycopene cyclase inhibitors into the fermentation medium. Lycopene has important physiological functions to prevent chronic diseases, including osteoporosis, certain types of cancer, cataract formation and cardiovascular diseases; enhance immune responses; and other biological effects in humans and animals [1,2]. In the last few years, demand on lycopene has increased due to its use in the food, pharmaceutical, cosmetic and animal feed industries [3]. Moreover, lycopene is used as an antioxidant to reduce cellular or tissue damage, and as a coloring agent for food products [4]. These make lycopene very attractive in the food and feed industries, and in medicine and cosmetic formulation. Lycopene used industrially is manufactured from plant extraction and chemical synthesis. Market needs for lycopene are not met using plant extraction due to the restricted number of plant sources and high cost. Chemical synthesis also has disadvantages including low yields, product instability, low product quality and high production cost. Due to decreased natural production of lycopene and its increased worldwide demand, there is the potential for lycopene to be produced using fermentation. Various algae and fungi produce intracellular carotenoids, including β-carotene, lycopene and astaxanthin.

Blakeslea trispora, *Mucor circinelloides*, *Candida utilis* and *Phycomyces blakesleeanus* have the ability to produce lycopene [5]. *B. trispora* has an advantage in that it does not need any specific fermentation conditions for growth. Mating type of (+) and (−) *B. trispora* strains together can increase production of lycopene [6].

There is much interest in biotechnological production of lycopene due to consumer demand for high quality and "natural" food additives. Efforts have been made to increase the lycopene yield and reduce process costs, by using low-cost agro-food media rich in organic compounds (such as carbon, nitrogen, mineral and other sources). The amount of lycopene production depends on microorganism, the culture medium, substrates and the fermentation conditions (temperature, pH, aeration rate etc.). Most of the research has been aimed at optimizing the culture conditions that directly affect the growth of the microorganism. The main research is focused on optimization of the medium, extraction of lycopene from *B. trispora* and fermentation conditions [4–9].

An industrial mold over-producing lycopene is *B. trispora* which accumulates all-trans-carotene, as a secondary metabolite [10]. *B. trispora* is a saprophyte and performs vegetative cycle of spores and filamentous mycelia [6]. There has been a lot of effort to use food wastes in the production of lycopene mitigation [11]. At present, there are no research on the use of orange powder and sunflower oil in the production of lycopene. The transport cost, sales problems, low quality and susceptibility to spoilage of the food-wastes by microorganisms have led to alternative utilization approaches. Agro-food wastes (fruits and vegetables: cabbage residues, watermelon husk and peach powders) have been used in the production of carotenes by *B. trispora* [12,13].

Optimization of fermentation conditions can also be required in the production of lycopene from different nutrient sources. This report was focused on the effect of a series of media containing various substrates (glucose, refined vegetable oils and orange powder) in the accumulation of lycopene in submerged shake flasks and fermentor studies. Morphological, biomass and pH changes occurring during fermentations were also studied.

2. Materials and Methods

2.1. Microorganism and Chemicals

Blakeslea trispora mating strains ATCC 14,271 (+) and ATCC 14,272 (−) were obtained from the American Type Culture Collection (ATCC; Rockville, MA, USA). Lyophilized cultures were rehydrated with malt extract broth (MEB; Darmstadt, Germany) by incubation at 35 °C for 3 days and were used in the stock culture preparation. Stock cultures of *B. trispora* were prepared on potato dextrose agar (PDA; Darmstadt, Germany) slant. Yeast extract, glucose, agar, asparagine, starch, lycopene, nicotine, $KHPO_4$, $MgSO_4$, HPLC grade petroleum ether, methanol, acetonitrile and dichloromethane were obtained from Sigma-Aldrich (Interlab Company, Adana, Turkey).

2.2. Preparation of B. Trispora Cultures

B. trispora (+) and (−) cultures were prepared for fermentation studies using a yeast phosphate soluble starch (YpSS) agar medium. The composition of YpSS agar medium (g L^{-1}) was: Yeast extract 4.0, K_2HPO_4 1.0, $MgSO_4$ 0.5, starch 15.0 and agar 20.0. The pH of the medium was adjusted to 6.5. Each of the *B. trispora* strains from stock culture was inoculated separately onto YpSS agar plates and incubated at 28 °C for 5 days. After sporulation of cultures, 10 mL of sterile distilled water was added onto the cultures in the Petri plates and the spores were collected by scraping off the medium surface using a sterile cotton swab. The spore suspension containing 3.9–8.5 × 10^6 spores ml^{-1} was used to inoculate the fermentation media. Strains were inoculated into the fermentation medium with 2.5 and 7.5 mL of spore suspension (+) and (−) strains, respectively, to provide 1:3 ratio of inoculation.

2.3. *Preparation of Fermentation Media*

The basal fermentation medium (BFM) had the following composition (g L^{-1}): Yeast extract 1.0, asparagine 2.0, K_2HPO_4 1.5 and $MgSO_4$ 0.5. BFM was supplemented with different concentrations of ingredients as given in Table 1: Refined vegetable oils (sunflower and corn oils), glucose and milled orange peel (powder). Samples of orange (*Citrus sinensis*) peel were dried at 40 °C to reach a final moisture lower than 10%, milled to a particle size (250 μm) using a laboratory grinder (Roller type lab mill RM 1300, Erkaya, Ataşehir, İstanbul, Turkey), homogenized in a single lot to avoid any variation in composition, and stored at 4 °C in a cold chamber until use. Fermentation media were prepared at two different pH: 6.5 and 5.5. Fermentation media (50 mL) in Erlenmeyer flasks (250 mL) were sterilized at 121 °C for 15 min in autoclave. Fermentation media for fermentor studies were sterilized in a 7 L Bioflow 410 sterilizable-in-place benchtop fermentor (New Brunswick Scientific BioFlo 410 SIP Fermentor, Eppendorf, New York, MA, USA).

Table 1. Medium composition.

Medium Number	Composition			
	Glucose (g L^{-1})	Sunflower Oil (ml L^{-1})	Corn Oil (ml L^{-1})	Orange Powder (g L^{-1})
		In shake flask studies		
1	40	-	-	-
2	60	-	-	-
3	40	10	-	-
4	40	30	-	-
6	40	-	10	-
7	40	-	30	-
8	-	-	-	10
9	-	-	-	20
		In fermentor studies		
10	40 [a,b]	-	-	-
11	60 [a]	-	-	-
12	40 [a]	10	-	-
13	40 [a]	-	10	-
14	-	-	-	10 [a]

[a] At 3 L min^{-1} aeration and 500 rpm agitation. [b] At 12 L min^{-1} aeration and 750 rpm agitation.

2.4. *Shake Flask Fermentation Process*

Fermentation media (50 mL) in Erlenmeyer flasks (250 mL) were inoculated with 10 mL *B. trispora* strains ATCC 14,271 (+) and 14,272 (−) by 1:3 ratio from spore stock culture. The lycopene cyclase inhibitor of nicotine (5 mM) was added on the second day of fermentation. Fermentation media (total volume 60 mL) were incubated at 28 °C for 7 days on a bench type water bath shaker ST-402 (NÜVE; Sanayi Malzemeleri Imalat ve Ticaret A. Ş., İstanbul, Turkey) with wrist shaking at 120 rpm.

2.5. *Fermentation Process in Fermentor*

All fermentations were performed in the Bioflow 410 fermentor with a working volume of 5.0 L. Sterilization sequences in this fermentor are fully automatic and heat-up and cool down in under 30 min. All easily initiated using the advanced touch-screen controller. The fermenter was equipped with a pH probe, dissolved oxygen probes, automatic sampler, temperature probe, inoculation port, sparger, exhaust condenser, agitation, vessel light, level sensor and BioCommand SCADA Software (RS-232; New Brunswick Scientific BioFlow 410 SIP Fermentor, Eppendorf, New York, MA, USA).

Four liter of fermentation media (from BFM) were prepared in the fermentor. The initial pH of fermentation was adjusted to 6.5. The fermentation with 4% glucose media was also performed at two aerations and agitations. The fermentor was incubated at 28 °C. The inoculation ratio of two strains (+/−) into the fermentation medium from plate cultures was the same as those in the shake flask. The lycopene cyclase inhibitor of nicotine (5 mM) was added on the second day of fermentation. Dissolved oxygen tension was not controlled during fermentation.

2.6. *Sampling*

Fermented samples were aseptically removed from the shake flask and fermentor through automatic sampler after 2, 3, 4, 6 and 7 days of fermentation. Initial samples were also removed at the beginning of fermentation. At every sampling interval, 5 mL of sample was taken from the fermentation media under aseptic conditions and the contents were analyzed for lycopene, pH and biomass changes. Two ml of the sample was used in lycopene analysis and 3 mL was used in pH and biomass analysis. At each sampling time and after the first day, 0.4 mL of the sample was also removed for morphological analysis.

Two samples were removed and two parallel analyses were performed from each sample. All experiments were repeated three times.

2.7. *Analysis*

2.7.1. Lycopene Analysis

Samples were analyzed for lycopene by a High-Performance Liquid Chromatography (HPLC) method [1]. Two ml of a 5 mL sample was mixed with 15 mL of petroleum ether. The mixture was subjected to ultrasound (Soniprep 150 Ultrasonic Disintegrator, MSE, London, UK) for 30 s and then, the sample was centrifuged using a table-type centrifuge (Hettich eba III) at 6000 rpm for 15 min. The supernatant was passed through 4 μm filter paper. About 2.5 mL of liquid was added into a 3 mL vial and the sample was analyzed by HPLC immediately. The presence of lycopene was detected by HPLC using a fluorescence detector. The flow rate was 1 mL min^{-1} and the column was nukleosil C18 (250 × 4.6 mm ID). Temperature was 28 °C. Lycopene was detected at 450 nm and 20 μL sample was injected to HPLC automatically. The result was read for 40 min. The mobile phase was acetonitrile-methanol-water-dichloromethane (7:1.5:0.5:1, v:v:v:v). The mobile phase was filtered through a disposable filter unit (0.45 μm) and degassed in a degasser (Bransonic 2200, 41 Eagle Road Danbury, Connecticut, 06810-1961, CT, USA). The peaks in a chromatogram were evaluated according to the lycopene standard curve.

Analytical Method Validation: Linearity was determined between 0.1 to 0.0001 g ml^{-1} using five levels of calibration in triplicate. The Mandel's fitting test was used to evaluate the linearity of the straight-line regression model [14].

Limit of detection (LOD) and limit of quantification (LOQ) were determined according to the method described by Cucu et al. [15]. For this, standards of 0.1 to 0.0001 g lycopene ml^{-1} were prepared and injected three times each. The mean of the slopes (S) and standard deviation of the intercepts (σ) were calculated from the three calibration curves. The LOD and the LOQ were calculated according to the formulas below [15]:

$$LOD = (3.3 * \sigma)/S$$
$$LOQ = (10 * \sigma)/S$$

For the assessment of the matrix effect, calibration curves were prepared in the petroleum ether and analyzed in triplicates. The calibration curve of lycopene was the equations: y = ((area+intercept)/slope).

2.7.2. pH, Biomass and Morphological Analysis

In biomass analysis, Whatman No. 41 filter paper was dried at 105 °C to constant weight, cooled in a desiccator and weighed before use. Three ml of the remaining sample was filtered through the filter paper. The filter cake on paper was washed three times with distilled water. The filter paper was placed into an incubator at 105 °C, dried until constant weight and then weighed to calculate the biomass (g L^{-1}). The medium with %10 orange powder was used as a control; in biomass detection, this was subtracted from biomass.

In pH analysis, a filtered solution was filled to 10 mL with distilled water and pH was detected using a pH meter (EMAF EM78X model, Interlab Company, Adana, Turkey) equipped with a glass electrode.

In image analysis, the morphological changes of *B. trispora* during the fermentation was analyzed using an image analysis system consisting of a light microscope (Olympus BX51; Olympus Corporation, Shinjuku Monolith, 3-1, Nishi Shinjuku 2-chome, Shinjuku-ku, Tokyo, Japan) equipped with a Pixera PVC 100C camera. Samples for image analysis were prepared by mixing 0.4 mL of fermentation broth with 0.1 mL of lactophenol blue. One drop of the mixed sample was pipetted on to a microscope slide, covered by a cover slip so that no air gap or bubbles were trapped between the sample and the coverslip and observed immediately with 20X objective by taking 5 different images. The morphological parameters measured were the area of zygospores and zygospores (% of total area of mycelium), the diameter of zygospores (mm), freely dispersed hyphae and clumps (aggregates) of different sizes on the basis of their projected area, and the hyphae length (mm). The microscope eyepiece is equipped with a scale micrometer that is used to measure the morphological parameters of mold. For each sample, the process was repeated at least 5 times using new positions on the same slide, and the morphological parameters were expressed as the mean values of each sample [16].

2.8. Statistical Analysis

All data were analyzed by SPSS 16 software (SPSS Inc., Chicago, IL, USA). Statistical differences between fermentation time (days) and between substrates used in the fermentations were tested by one-way analysis of variance following Duncan's multiple-range test. A probability of 0.05 was used to determine statistical significance.

3. Results

The fermentations were carried out at 28 °C for 7 days using different carbon sources and ingredients in the shake flask and fermentor.

The initial pH is one of the important parameters in the production of lycopene by *B. trispora*. The pH of the fermentation media changed during the fermentation time. The pH of the fermentation media was decreased during the first 2 days then increased during the remaining 7 days. At 2 days, the pH reduced to approximately 5.0, and then the pH increased over 6.0. The pH drop would be due to trisporic acid or/and other unidentified acidic formations in the lycopene production [17]. According to Nanou et al. [18], the pH of the media decreased slightly during the first 2 days of the fermentation from 7.6 to 5.3 and then increased slowly up to 7.0 at the end of the fermentation. The pH of the fermentation media was probably increased by ammonia liberation during degradation of proteins in the media by *B. trispora*. This would be indicative of amine metabolic product being released as a consequence of cell death and subsequent lysis occurring after that time.

3.1. Shake Flask Studies

Lycopene production of two glucose concentrations (4 and 6%) were investigated at two initial pH values (6.5 and 5.5). Figures 1 and 2 show the effect of glucose concentrations on lycopene production at the initial pH 6.5 and 5.5 respectively. Lycopene production at pH 6.5 with both glucose concentrations was higher than at pH 5.5. The amount of lycopene production was 77.7 and 28.1 mg L^{-1} with 4 and 6% glucose, respectively, after 7 days fermentation at pH 6.5. The biomass dry weight (DW) increased with the increase in glucose concentration from 4 to 6%. The lowest amount of lycopene content (0.3 mg g^{-1} DW) was obtained at pH 5.5 with glucose concentration 6%. In this research, 4% glucose yielded better lycopene than 6% while the biomass is better produced in 6% glucose. Since, there is an indirect relationship between biomass and lycopene concentration. Subsequently, increasing the glucose concentration to 6% resulted in a decrease in lycopene production by 36.2%. The decreased concentration of lycopene encountered with the highest concentration of glucose was probably due to osmotic effects. It has been reported that above a critical substrate concentration, the decreased water activity and the onset of plasmolysis combine to cause a decrease in the rates of fermentation and product formation [19]. In all cases, the biomass DW increased during the first two days of the fermentation and then remained constant until the maximum concentration of the lycopene was obtained. The maximum lycopene content was 2.4 and 0.6 mg g^{-1} DW with 4 and 6% glucose, respectively, at pH 6.5 after 7 days while they were 0.7 and 0.1 mg g^{-1} DW after 4 days, respectively. There are significant differences ($p < 0.05$) in lycopene production during fermentation. There are also significant differences ($p < 0.05$) in lycopene production between 4 and 6% glucose concentrations, and pH 6.5 and 5.5 at both glucose concentrations.

Figures 3 and 4 show the effect of sunflower and corn oils, respectively, on the production of lycopene in 4 % glucose medium at initial pH 6.5. The maximum lycopene was produced 795.1 and 714.2 mg L^{-1} with 1 % sunflower and corn oils respectively. The highest amount of lycopene (335.4 mg L^{-1}) was produced with 3 % sunflower oil rather 3 % corn oil (275.3 mg L^{-1}). Lycopene content was 131.4 and 115.0 mg g^{-1} DW at the end of fermentation for 1% sunflower and corn oils respectively. There are significant differences ($p < 0.05$) in lycopene production during the 7 days of fermentation. There are also significant differences ($p < 0.05$) in lycopene production with and without oil, and between both oil types.

Lycopene productions with 1 and 2% orange powder during 7 days of shake flask fermentation were given in Figure 5. Lycopene productions after 7 days were 2.9 and 1.7 mg L^{-1} with 1 and 2% orange powder respectively. Biomasses formations were 8.6 and 11.6 g L^{-1} for orange powder respectively. Lycopene content was 0.3 and 0.1 mg g^{-1} DW respectively at the end of fermentation. There were significant differences ($p < 0.05$) in lycopene production during the 7 days of fermentation for 1 and 2% orange powder, between the two orange powder concentrations.

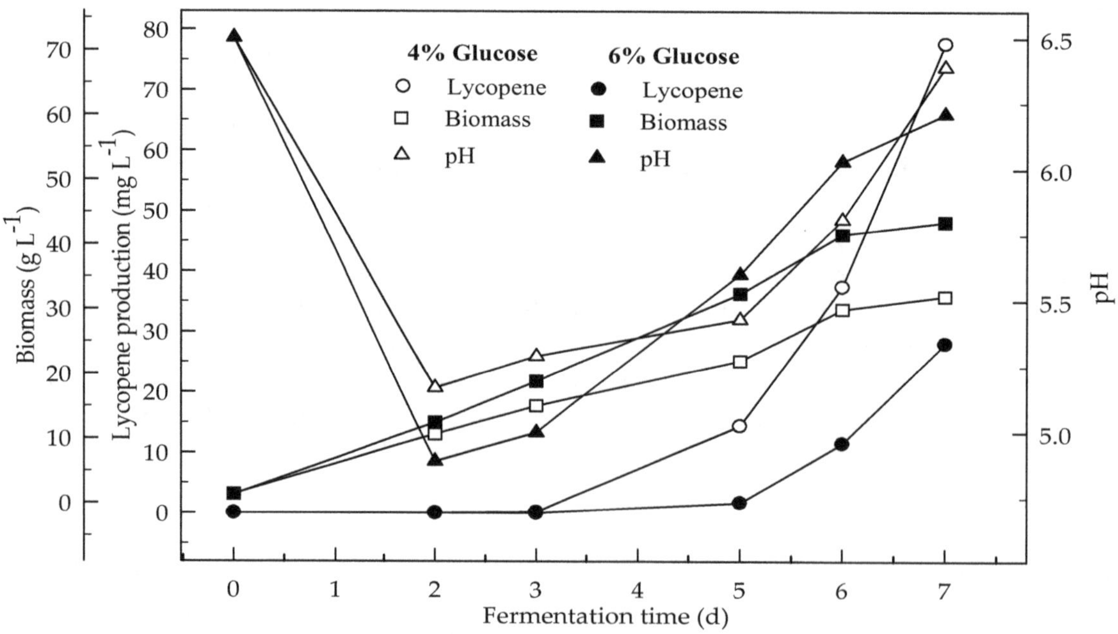

Figure 1. Changes in lycopene production, biomass formation and pH with initial pH 6.5 in a medium containing 4 and 6% glucose.

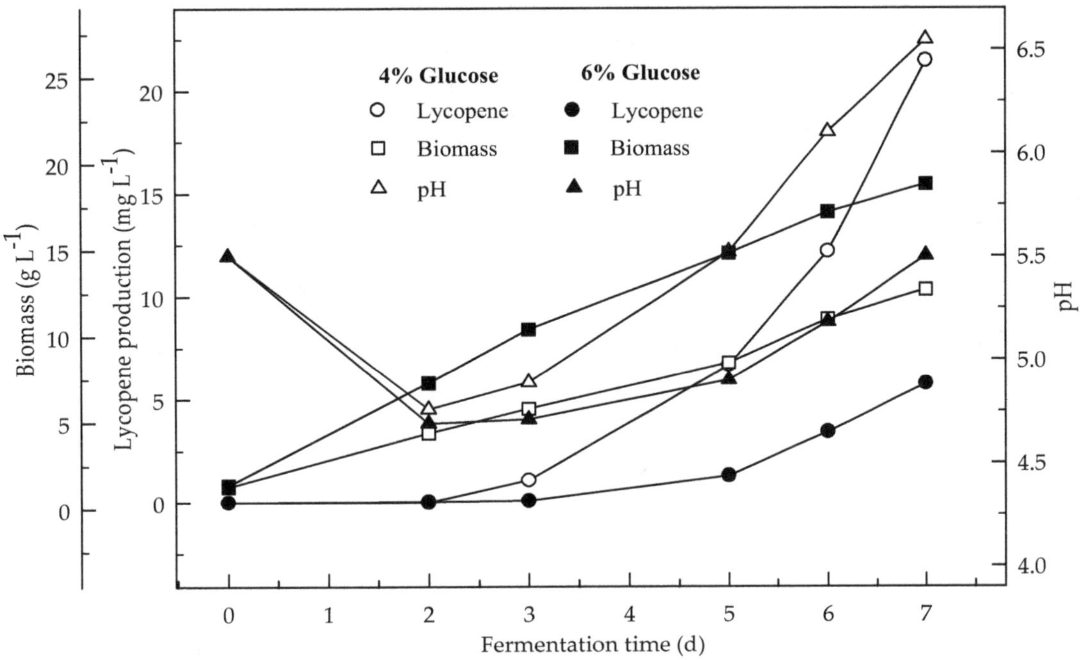

Figure 2. Changes in lycopene production, biomass formation and pH with initial pH 5.5 in a medium containing 4 and 6% glucose.

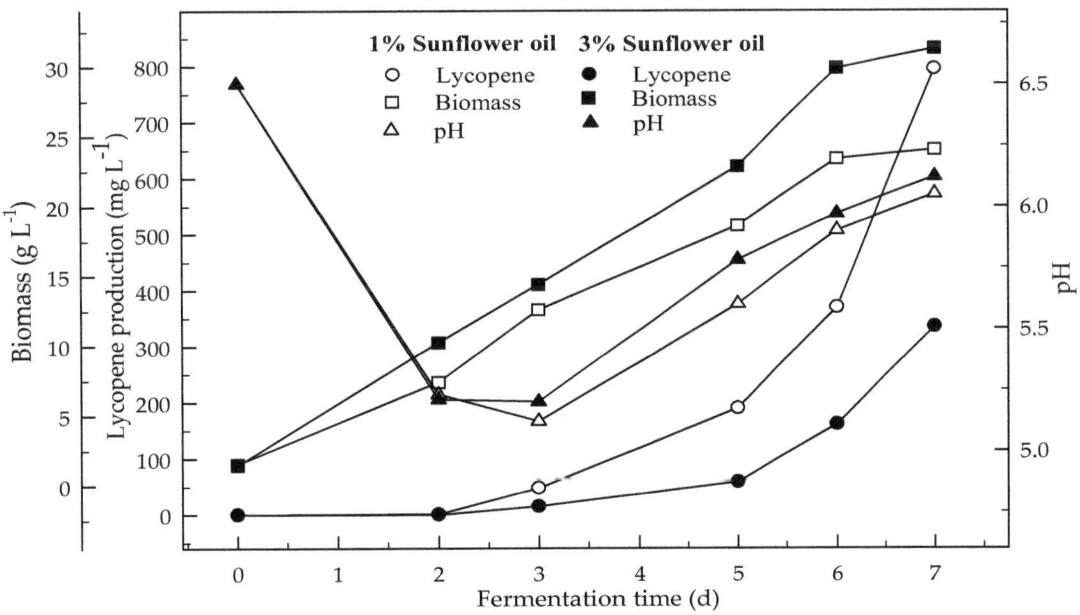

Figure 3. Changes in lycopene production, biomass formation and pH in fermentation with an initial pH 6.5 in a 4% glucose medium containing 1 and 3% sunflower oil.

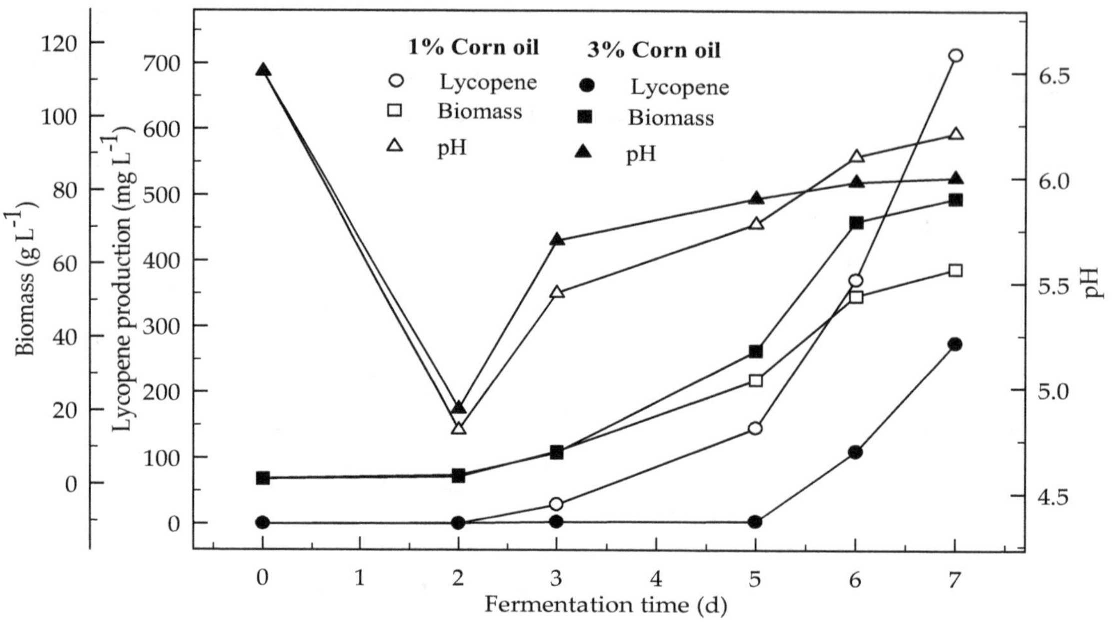

Figure 4. Changes in lycopene production, biomass formation and pH in fermentation with an initial pH 6.5 in a 4% glucose medium containing 1 and 3% corn oil.

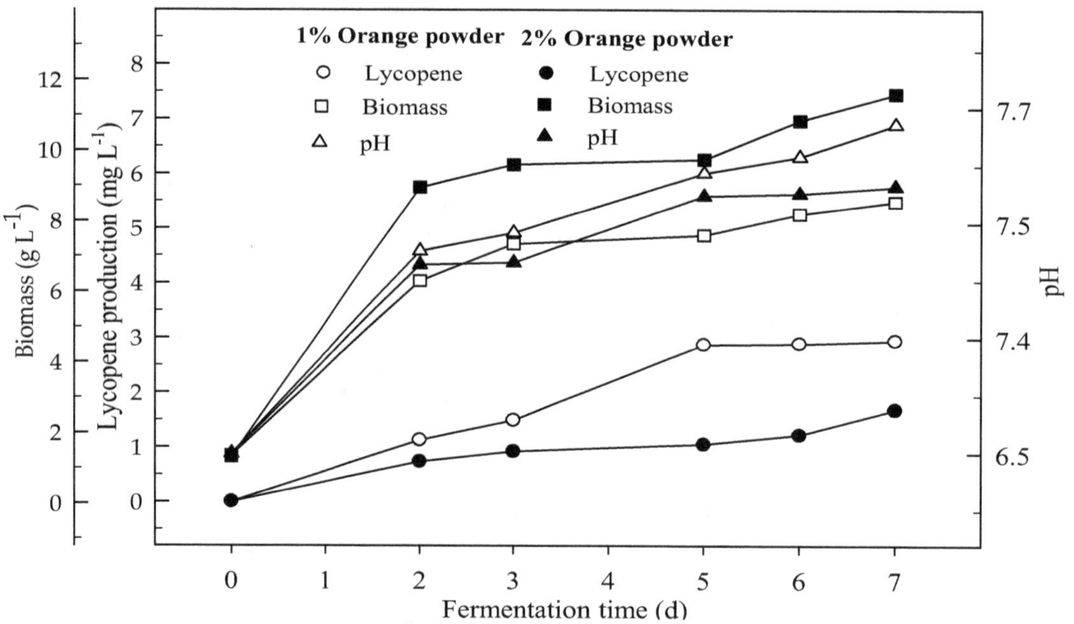

Figure 5. Changes in lycopene production, biomass formation and pH in a shake-flask fermentation with an initial pH 6.5 in a medium containing 1 and 2% orange powder.

3.2. Fermentor Studies

Effects of 4 and 6% glucose concentration (pH 6.5) on the production of lycopene were studied at 3 L min^{-1} aeration with 500 rpm agitation (Figure 6). The highest amount of lycopene was produced (92.3 mg L^{-1}) with 4% glucose concentration rather than 6% glucose (57.8 mg L^{-1}). Biomass DW formations after 7 days of fermentation were 154.9 and 196.7 mg L^{-1} with 4 and 6% glucose concentration respectively. Lycopene content was 3.8 and 1.9 mg g^{-1} DW at the end of fermentation for 4 and 6% glucose concentrations respectively. There is an indirect relationship between biomass and lycopene formation similar to the shake flask. The production of lycopene in the fermentor was higher than in the shake-flask from glucose. This would be due to the better aeration of the medium in the fermentor. There were significant differences ($p < 0.05$) in lycopene production during the 7 days of fermentation. There were also significant differences ($p < 0.05$) in lycopene production between 4 and 6% glucose concentrations.

The effect of high level of aeration (12 L min^{-1}) and agitation (750 rpm) on the production of lycopene in a 4% glucose medium during the 7 days of fermentation is given in Figure 7. The highest amount of lycopene was produced at low level of aeration (3 L min^{-1}) and agitation (500 rpm) rather than at the high levels (12 L min^{-1} and 750 rpm). The highest amount of biomass was formed at the higher aeration (12 L min^{-1}) and agitation (750 rpm) rather than at the lower levels. Lycopene content of DW (3.8 mg L^{-1}) was higher at 3 L min^{-1} aeration and 500 rpm agitation rather than 12 L min^{-1} at 750 rpm (1.8 mg L^{-1}). Generally, the results showed that the biomass increased with increasing aeration and agitation. This was due to the better air supply to the cells. This is especially important for high biomass concentrations. *B. trispora* is a strictly aerobic microorganism. Thus, moderate aeration rates in combination with high impeller agitation improved the growth of mold. There are significant differences ($p < 0.05$) in lycopene production during the 7 days of fermentation and between the two fermentation conditions (3 and 12 L min^{-1} aeration).

Figure 8 shows the effect of 1% sunflower and corn oils on the lycopene production in the fermentor. Lycopene production was 944.8 and 859.8 mg L^{-1} respectively. Biomass formations were 29.5 and 19.6 g L^{-1}. Lycopene content was 65.0 and 48.9 mg g^{-1} DW. Lycopene production in the presence of sunflower and corn oils in the fermentor was 12.2 and 11.1 times higher, respectively, then without oil from 4% glucose in a shake flask. This would be due to retaining higher amount of oxygen in the media. Since oil slightly increases the density of the fermentation media. There are significant differences ($p < 0.05$) in lycopene production during fermentation periods. There are also significant differences ($p < 0.05$) in lycopene production with and without oil, and between sunflower and corn oils.

Lycopene production was studied from different concentrations of orange peel in 4 L fermentation media with aeration 3 L min^{-1} and agitation 500 rpm (Figure 9). Lycopene was produced 4.9 mg L^{-1} with 1% orange peel. Biomass was 9.7 g L^{-1} and lycopene content was 0.05 mg g^{-1} DW at the end of fermentation. Lycopene production from orange peel was two times higher in the fermentor than in the shake flask. There are significant ($p < 0.05$) differences in lycopene production during the 7 days of fermentation.

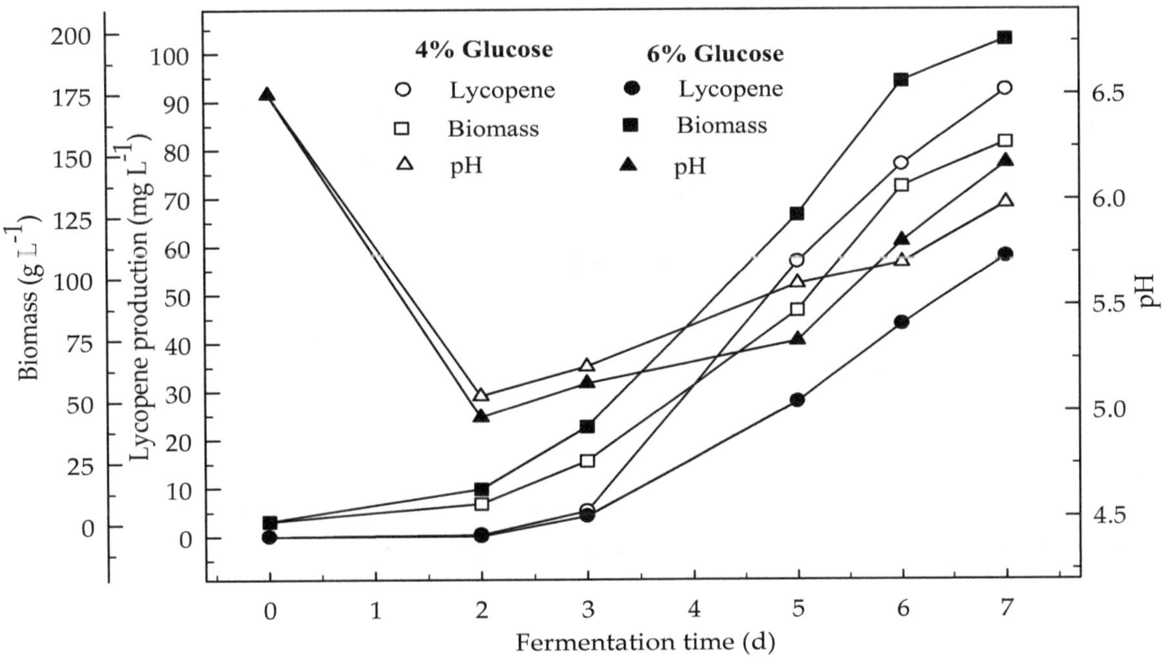

Figure 6. Changes in lycopene production, biomass formation and pH in a fermentor with an initial pH 6.5 in a 4 and 6% glucose medium at 3 L min^{-1} aeration and 500 rpm agitation.

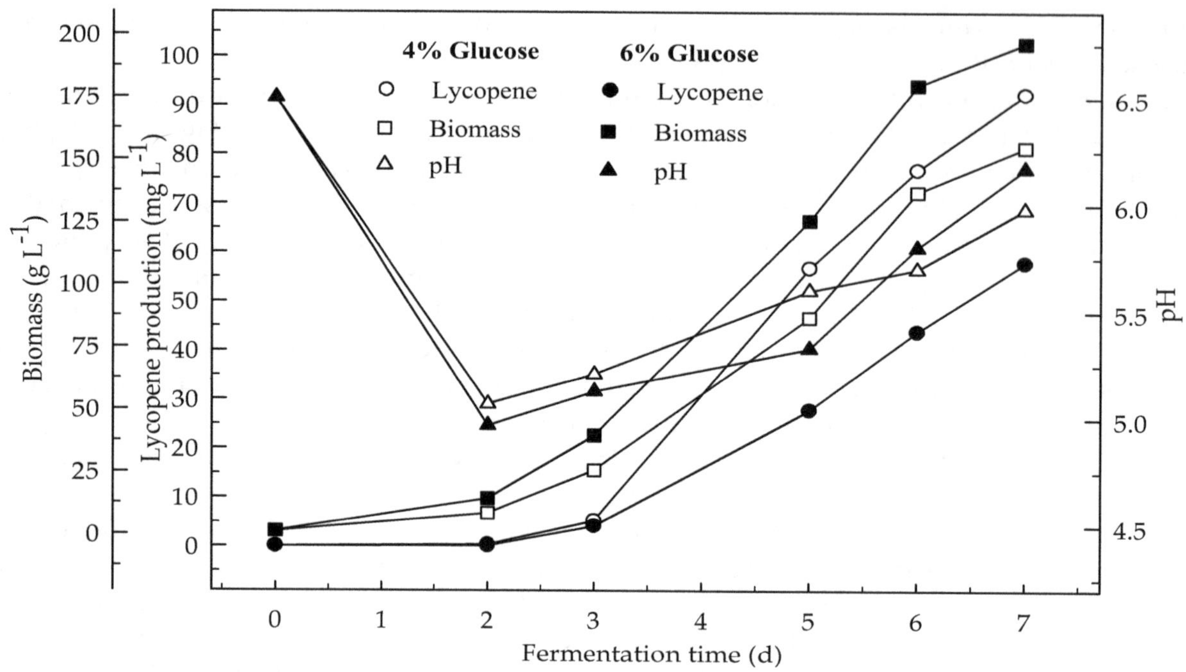

Figure 7. Changes in lycopene production, biomass formation and pH in a fermentor with an initial pH 6.5 in a 4 and 6% glucose medium at 12 L min^{-1} aeration and 750 rpm agitation.

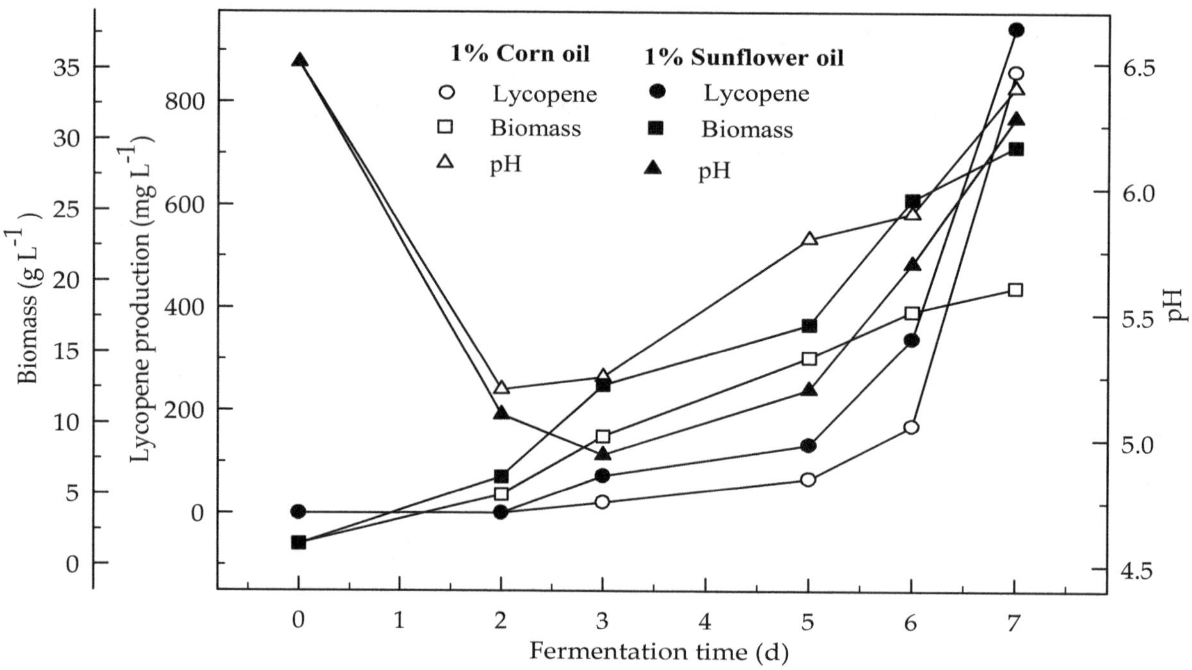

Figure 8. Changes in lycopene production, biomass formation and pH in a fermentor with an initial pH 6.5 in a 4% glucose fermentation medium 1% corn and sunflower oils (at aeration 3 L min^{-1} with 500 rpm agitation).

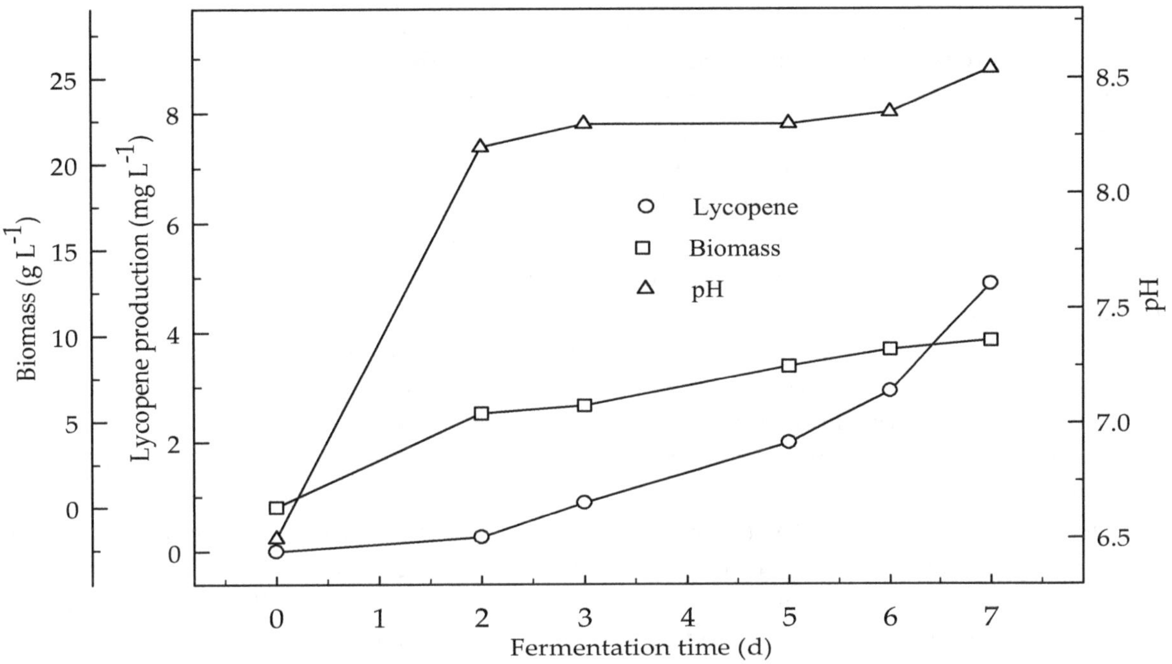

Figure 9. Changes in lycopene production, biomass formation and pH in a fermentor with an initial pH 6.5 from a 1% orange powder in a fermentor with aeration 3 L min^{-1} at agitation 500 rpm.

3.3. Morphological Analysis

The morphology of *B. trispora* was studied in the shake-flask and fermentor studies (3 L min^{-1} aeration and 500 rpm agitation) in only 4% glucose medium containing 1% sunflower oil using an image analysis system. During the first day of fermentation, microscopic examination showed that *B. trispora* formed a great amount of mycelium in the fermentation broth. After one day of fermentation, two opposite mating types of *B. trispora* produced zygospores which grew towards each other and produced pro-gametangia at their tips. Septation in the pro-gametangia led to the production of terminal gametangia, which fused to form the zygospores. The area of zygospores to the total area of mycelium remained almost constant up to 4 days of fermentation and then decreased significantly ($p < 0.05$) and disappeared on the 7th days of fermentation. On the other hand, the area of zygospores to the total area of mycelium increased significantly ($p < 0.05$) with the increase of fermentation time from 4 to 7 days. The hyphae length increased from the first day of fermentation up to 4 days and then slightly increased until the end of the fermentation. The diameter of zygospores increased from the first 2 days of incubation up to 4 days and then decreased slightly. Generally, morphological measurements using image analysis showed that *B. trispora* formed zygophores, zygospores and mycelium in which the hyphae appeared as a homogeneous dispersed suspension through the fermentation medium.

4. Discussion

Various concentration of carbon sources and refined natural vegetable oils as co-substrates were used in the production of lycopene. The concentration of carbon sources and vegetable oils greatly affected the final amount of lycopene. Furthermore, the use of orange powder components gives a first indication that *B. trispora* is able to metabolize and produce lycopene.

The highest concentration of lycopene was produced from a low concentration of glucose (4%) rather than at the high concentration (6%) in both the shake flask and fermentor studies. High concentrations of glucose may cause inhibition of the activity of mevalonate kinase [20], which is one of the key enzymes of the lycopene biosynthesis pathway. The carbon source can act as a major constituent for the building of cellular material and as an important energy source during the microbial fermentations [21]. Lycopene production in all fermentation conditions was lower than 1.0 mg L^{-1} during the first 2 days of fermentation and continuously increased during the next 5 days. It reached maximum concentration after 7 days. Sugar metabolism was slightly enhanced at the beginning of fermentation and increased during next fermentation period. This increase may provide more lycopene production [22]. On the other hand, biomass formation increased continuously during the 6 days of fermentation and it slowed on last day. When lycopene production increased, biomass formation decreased. Dry weight increased continuously up to 6 days and then slowed down. But lycopene production rate was higher on the last day. The maximum lycopene content in cells occurred after 7 days of fermentation when compared with 6 days in all fermentation conditions. This indicates that lycopene and biomass formations are inversely proportional. The biomass rapidly increased after 2 days of fermentation and this continued up to 6 days of fermentation. Nanou et al. [18] reported that the concentration of residual sugars fell rapidly during the first 4 days of the fermentation after which it decreased slowly and this was accompanied by a rapid increase of biomass concentration.

The refined vegetable oils stimulate different biosynthetic pathways in *B. trispora*. In this study, about 944.7 mg L^{-1} of lycopene was produced in fermentor studies from 4% glucose supplemented with 1 % sunflower oil. With 1% corn oil, about 859.8 mg L^{-1} of lycopene was produced in a 4% glucose medium. These results indicate that sunflower oil has a greater influence on lycopene production than corn oil due to a higher amount of vitamin E and linoleic acid in sunflower oil [23,24]. Similar results were demonstrated by Mantzouridou et al. [7] that corn steep liquor, olive oil, soybean oil, cottonseed oil and linoleic acids significantly increased the β-carotene production. Mantzouridou et al. [24] was also indicated that the addition of 10 g oil L^{-1} of substrate stimulated β-carotene production. Beside triacylglycerol, the main component of oils can be used in the lipid biosynthesis (involving acetyl-CoA formation resulting from β-oxidation of fatty acids) of the mold mycelium. Oils can be hydrolyzed to fatty acids and glycerol by mold exolipases [23]. When the concentration of natural oils increases (from 1 to 3%), the production of the lycopene decreases while the biomass dry weight increases significantly. This may be related to the consumed amount of the oils converted to biomass instead of lycopene. The production of lycopene without oils in the medium was lower while biomass formation was higher.

Two different aerations (3 and 12 L min^{-1}) and agitations (500 and 750 rpm) were studied in a 7 L fermentor (pH 6.5). The highest amount of lycopene 944.8 mg L^{-1} was produced with 3 L min^{-1} aeration and 500 rpm agitation in 4% glucose medium containing 1% sunflower oil. The positive impact of oils in the production of lycopene has been confirmed in other reports, such as those based on the use of crude olive or soybean olive [7,24] or waste cooked oil [25]. Supplementation of the medium with industrial glycerol, obtained either from soap manufacturing or biodiesel production industries, allows up to a tenfold increase in β-carotene levels [26]. Very promising results have been also obtained using agro-food wastes rich in carbohydrates and mineral salts, as beet molasses [27], cheese whey [28]. The concentration of lycopene was higher in fermentor studies than in the shake flask. Aeration could be beneficial to the growth and performance of aerobic *B. trispora*. Agitation of the fermentation medium creates shear forces which affect microorganisms in several ways: causing morphological changes, variation in their growth and product formation, and damaging the cell structure [19].

Orange powder was used as a raw material for production of lycopene in a shake flask and fermentor. The highest amount of lycopene (4.8 mg L^{-1}) was produced in the fermentor with 1% orange powder rather than in the shake flask (2.9 mg L^{-1}). Citrus peels are rich in cellulose, hemicelluloses, proteins and pectin, but the fat content is low. Pourbafrani et al. [21] reported that more than 95% of the peel oil is D-limonene which is extremely toxic to fermenting microorganisms. The addition of tomato sauce as a waste into the fermentation medium enhanced the production of lycopene and its production was 3.52 mg/100 g cell DW [29].

B. trispora is a micro-fungus with a life-cycle involving hyphae, zygophores and zygospores in submerged fermentation. The zygophores are the precursors of zygospores, which are responsible for the production of lycopene. [19]. The highest percentage of zygospores in an observed microscope field was correlated with the highest percentage of intracellular lycopene in the total biomass dry weight after the 7 days of fermentation. High percentages of vacuolated hyphae, evacuated cells and degenerated hyphae of *B. trispora* were observed at higher aeration (12 L min^{-1}). The percentage of the vacuolated hyphae, evacuated cells and the degenerated hyphae formed during the first 2 days of fermentation were higher than the remaining fermentation time. The growing mycelium was composed primarily of intact hyphae (such as 96.8% of the biomass dry weight), and zygospores on the 2nd day of fermentation, whereas on the next day the concentration of the intact hyphae was reduced to 67.9 of the biomass dry weight and the concentration of the zygospores was about 8.3%. On the 7th day of fermentation, the mycelium was composed mainly of evacuated cells. The addition of 1% oils to the fermentation medium increased the concentration of the intracellular lycopene during fermentation and reached to maximum level after 7 days, whereas the percentage of zygospores to the biomass dry weight increased significantly ($p < 0.05$). The highest concentration of lycopene correlated with the highest percentage of zygospores in the biomass DW. When the natural oils were used in the medium with 4% glucose in the fermentor, a great increase in the amount of lycopene occurred after the days 7 of fermentation, while the concentration of evacuated cells and the number of zygospores increased significantly ($p < 0.05$).

The effect of aeration rate and agitation speed on culture morphology was also observed. At an aeration rate of 3 L min^{-1} with 500 rpm agitation, the area of zygospores increased significantly and then remained constant. On the other hand, at aeration rates of 12 L min^{-1} with 750 rpm agitation, the area of zygospores decreased and then remained constant. The maximum concentration of lycopene was observed in the same conditions where a large number of zygospores were observed. This means that the zygospores were responsible for the synthesis of lycopene.

5. Conclusions

In this study, various substrates are compared with lycopene production in the shake flask and fermentor. The amount of lycopene production is based on the concentration of carbon sources and natural oil content. The amount of orange powder used in the fermentation as carbon sources affected the formation of lycopene. The use of natural oil is important for stimulation of the biosynthetic pathway in *B. trispora.* The medium with natural oil led to more lycopene than only carbon source in the medium. The oils degraded into acetyl-CoA, which is the precursor of lycopene derived from mevalonic acid. The mated fermentation process for lycopene production may be useful and a reference to the other fermentation. Also, lycopene production from *B. trispora* is better than other alternative plant extracts which is one of the other methods of lycopene production. For the future, this study is provided to contribute to the development in the lycopene production industry from this method. Oils improved lycopene production and enhanced vacuolation and evacuation of the hyphae. The morphological characteristics of the hyphae and the proportion of zygospores to the biomass DW were changed significantly ($p < 0.05$) within the medium composition and fermentation conditions. Moreover, there was a parallel relationship between the area of zygospores and production of lycopene. Generally, the results showed that *B. trispora* is a micro-mold that produces lycopene with a life-cycle involving hyphae, zygophores and zygospores. The hyphae do not play a role in the biosynthesis of lycopene. The zygphpores are the precursors of zygospores, which are responsible for the production of the lycopene. Maximum lycopene concentration was obtained when the medium was supplied with sunflower and corn oils.

Author Contributions: Examined the literature, methodology, original draft, writing-review and editing, supervision: O.E.; Performed the analysis, investigation, literature survey: A.S.

Acknowledgments: The author acknowledges the support received from the Gaziantep University.

References

1. Shi, Y.; Xin, X.; Yuan, Q. Improved lycopene production by *Blakeslea trispora* with isopentenyl compounds and metabolic precursors. *Biotechnol. Lett.* **2002**, *34*, 849–852. [CrossRef] [PubMed]

2. Liu, X.-J.; Liu, R.-S.; Li, H.M.; Tang, Y.-J. Lycopene production from synthetic medium by *Blakeslea trispora* NRRL 2895 (+) and 2896 (−) in a stirred-tank fermenter. *Biopro. Biosyst. Eng.* **2012**, *35*, 739–749.
3. Valduga, E.; Valério, A.; Treichel, H.; Júnior, A.F.; Di Luccio, M. Kinetic and stoichiometric parameters in the production of carotenoids by *Sporidiobolus salmonicolor* (CBS 2636) in synthetic and agroindustrial media. *Appl. Biochem. Biotechnol.* **2009**, *157*, 61–69. [PubMed]
4. Wang, J.F.; Liu, X.J.; Liu, R.S.; Li, H.M.; Tang, Y.J. Optimization of the mated fermentation process for the production of lycopene by *Blakeslea trispora* NRRL 2895 (+) and NRRL 2896 (−). *Biopro. Biosys. Eng.* **2012**, *35*, 553–564. [CrossRef] [PubMed]
5. Mehta, B.J.; Obraztsova, I.N.; Cerdá-Olmedo, E. Mutants and intersexual heterokaryons of *Blakeslea trispora* for production of beta-carotene and lycopene. *Appl. Env. Microbiol.* **2003**, *69*, 4043–4048. [CrossRef]
6. Tereshina, V.M.; Memorskaya, A.S.; Feovilova, E.P. Dormant cells in the development cycle of *Blakeslea trispora*: Distinct patterns of the lipid and carbohydrate composition. *Microbiology* **2002**, *71*, 684–689. [CrossRef]
7. Mantzouridou, F.; Roukas, T.; Kotzekidou, P.; Liakopoulou, M. Optimization of beta-carotene production from synthetic medium by *Blakeslea trispora*: A mathematical modeling. *Appl. Biochem. Biotechnol.* **2002**, *101*, 153–175. [CrossRef]
8. Tereshina, V.M.; Memorskaya, A.S.; Feovilova, E.P. Zygote formation in *Blakeslea trispora*: Morphological peculiarities and relationship with carotenoid synthesis. *Microbiology* **2003**, *72*, 448–454. [CrossRef]
9. Lopez-Nieto, M.J.; Costa, J.; Peiro, E.; Mendez, E.; Rodriguez-Saiz, M.; de la Fuente, J.L.; Cabri, W.; Barredo, J.L. Biotechnological lycopene production by mated fermentation of *Blakesiea trispora*. *Appl. Microbiol. Biotechnol.* **2004**, *66*, 153–159. [CrossRef]
10. Jeong, J.C.; Lee, J.; Park, Y.H. A unique pattern of mycelial elongation of *Blakeslea trispora* and its effect on morphological characteristics and beta-carotene synthesis. *Curr. Microbiol.* **2001**, *42*, 225–228. [CrossRef]
11. Stabnikova, O.; Wang, J.Y.; Ding, H.B.; Tay, J.H. Biotransformation of vegetable and fruit processing wastes into yeast biomass enriched with selenium. *Biores. Technol.* **2005**, *96*, 747–751. [CrossRef]
12. Bendini, A.; Lecce, G.D.; Valli, E.; Barbieri, S.; Tesini, F.; Toschi, T.G. Olive oil enriched in lycopene from tomato by-product through a co-milling process. *Int. J. Food Sci. Nutr.* **2015**, *66*, 371–377. [CrossRef] [PubMed]
13. Hernandez-Almanza, A.; Montanez, J.; Martínez, G.; Aguilar-Jiménezc, A.; Contreras-Esquivel, J.C.; Aguilar, C.N. Lycopene: Progress in microbial production. *Trend Food Sci. Technol.* **2016**, *56*, 142–148. [CrossRef]
14. Loco, J.V.; Js Elskens, M.; Croux, C.; Beernaert, H. Linearity of calibration curves: Use and misuse of the correlation coefficient. *Accred. Qual. Assur.* **2002**, *7*, 281–285.
15. Cucu, T.; Huvaere, K.; Bergh, M.-A.V.D.; Vinkx, C.; Loco, J.V. A simple and fast HPLC method to determine lycopene in foods. *Food Anal. Met.* **2012**, *5*, 1221–1228. [CrossRef]
16. Paul, G.C.; Thomas, C.R. Characterization of mycelial morphology using image analysis. *Adv. Biochem. Eng. Biotechnol.* **1998**, *60*, 1–59. [PubMed]
17. Papaioannou, E.H.; Liakopoulou-Kyriakides, M. Substrate contribution on carotenoids production in *Blakeslea trispora* cultivations. *Food Bioprod. Process.* **2010**, *88*, 305–311. [CrossRef]
18. Nanou, K.; Roukas, T.; Papadakis, E. Improved production of carotenes from synthetic medium by *Blakeslea trispora* in a bubble column reactor. *Biochem. Eng. J.* **2012**, *67*, 203–207. [CrossRef]
19. Mantzouridou, F.; Roukas, T.; Kotzekidou, P. Effect of the aeration rate and agitation speed on β-carotene production and morphology of *Blakeslea trispora* in a stirred tank reactor: Mathematical modeling. *Biochem. Eng. J.* **2002**, *10*, 123–135. [CrossRef]
20. Mantzouridou, F.; Roukas, T.; Kotzekidou, P. Production of beta-carotene from synthetic medium by *Blakeslea trispora* in fed-batch culture. *Food. Biotechnol.* **2004**, *18*, 343–361. [CrossRef]
21. Pourbafrani, M.; Talebnia, F.; Niklasson, C.; Taherzadeh, M.J. Effect of encapsulation in fermentation of limonene-containing media and orange-peel hydrolysate. *Inter. J. Molec. Sci.* **2007**, *8*, 777–787. [CrossRef]
22. Wang, H.-B.; Xu, R.-G.; Yu, L.-J.; Lu, J.; Zhang, L.-W.; Huang, X.-Y.; Zou, W.-A.; Zhao, Q.; Lu, M.-B. Improved β-carotene and lycopene production by *Blakeslea trispora* with ultrasonic treatment in submerged fermentation. *Z. Naturforsch. C* **2014**, *69*, 237–244. [CrossRef]
23. Vereschagin, O.A.; Memorskaya, A.S.; Tereshina, V.M. The role of exogenous lipids in lycopene synthesis in the Mucoraceous fungus *Blakeslea trispora* *Microbiology* **2010** *79*, 593–601. [CrossRef]
24. Mantzouridou, F.; Tsimidou, M.Z.; Roukas, T. Performance of crude olive pomace oil and soybean oil

during carotenoid production by *Blakeslea trispora* in submerged fermentation. *J. Agric. Food Chem.* **2006**, *54*, 2575–2581. [CrossRef]
25. Nanou, K.; Roukas, T. Waste cooking oil: A new substrate for carotene production by *Blakeslea trispora* in submerged fermentation. *Biores. Technol.* **2016**, *203*, 198–203. [CrossRef]
26. Mantzouridou, F.; Naziri, E.; Tsimidou, M.Z. Industrial glycerol as a supplementary carbon source in the production of β-carotene by *Blakeslea trispora*. *J. Agric. Food Chem.* **2008**, *56*, 2668–2675. [CrossRef]
27. Goksungur, Y.; Mantzouridou, F.; Roukas, T.; Kotzekidou, P. Production of beta-carotene from beet molasses by *Blakeslea trispora* in stirred-tank and bubble column reactors: Development of a mathematical modeling. *Appl. Biochem. Biotechnol.* **2004**, *112*, 37–54. [CrossRef]
28. Papaioannou, E.H.; Liakopoulou-Kyriakides, M. Agro-food wastes utilization by *Blakeslea trispora* for carotenoids production. *Acta Biochim. Pol.* **2012**, *59*, 151–153. [CrossRef]
29. Radu, G.L.; Litescu, S.C.; Albu, C.; Truica, G. Beta-carotene and lycopene determination in new enriched bakery products by HPLC-DAD method. *Rom. Biotechnol. Lett.* **2012**, *17*, 7005–7012.

11

Protective Effect of Selenium-Enriched Ricegrass Juice against Cadmium-Induced Toxicity and DNA Damage in HEK293 Kidney Cells

Rattanamanee Chomchan [1], Sunisa Siripongvutikorn [2], Pattaravan Maliyam [3], Bandhita Saibandith [1] and Panupong Puttarak [3,4,*]

[1] Interdisciplinary Graduate School of Nutraceutical and Functional Food, Prince of Songkla University, Hat-Yai, Songkhla 90112, Thailand; pui_galz@hotmail.com (R.C.); bandhita.s@psu.ac.th (B.S.)

[2] Department of Food Technology, Faculty of Agro-Industry, Prince of Songkla University, Hat-Yai, Songkhla 90112, Thailand; sunisa.s@psu.ac.th

[3] Department of Pharmacognosy and Pharmaceutical Botany, Faculty of Pharmaceutical Sciences, Prince of Songkla University, Hat-Yai, Songkhla 90112, Thailand; Tak_kypoko@hotmail.com

[4] Phytomedicine and Pharmaceutical Biotechnology Excellence Center (PPBEC), Prince of Songkla University, Hat-Yai, Songkhla 90112, Thailand

* Correspondence: panupong.p@psu.ac.th

Abstract: Cadmium (Cd) contamination in food is a problem endangering human health. Cd detoxication is an interesting topic particularly using food which provides no side effects. Ricegrass juice is a squeezed juice from young rice leaves which is introduced as a functional drink rich in polyphenol components. Se-enrichment into ricegrass is initiated to provide extra advantages of their functional properties. The protective role of ricegrass juice (RG) and Se-enriched ricegrass juice (Se-RG) against Cd toxicity during pre-, co- and post-treatment on HEK293 kidney cells were investigated. Results confirmed that RG and Se-RG had very low toxicity for kidney cells. Both extracts showed a protective role during pre-treatment and co-treatment against Cd toxicity by exerting a reduction in malondialdehyde (MDA) content and the percentage of DNA damage in tail and tail length of the comets over the Cd-treated cells. However, the Se-RG indicated additional benefits in all properties over RG. High Se content in Se-RG resulted in more protective effects of the regular ricegrass juice. In summary, this study provides clear evidence that Se-enriched ricegrass juice has potential to be developed as a functional food to protect the human body from Cd contamination via the reduction of oxidative stress and DNA damage.

Keywords: anti-cadmium toxicity; comet assay; DNA protective; HEK293 cells; ricegrass juice; selenium enrichment

---

1. Introduction

Currently, daily food consumption could lead to the unexpected exposure of contaminated compounds in the human body. Heavy metals, known as harmful agents, enter the food chain excessively via industrial operations, mining, sewage sludge and waste disposal from households into agricultural lands and water resources [1]. Accumulation of heavy metals in the environment has been reported as increasing substantially over the past decades [2]. Due to the highly soluble ability of cadmium (Cd) compounds as compared to other metals, Cd is readily taken up by plants resulting in food and feed accumulation. Cd contamination from the environment is a subject of serious health complications affecting cellular organelles and components such as cell membrane, mitochondrial, lysosome as well as genetic DNA [3]. The kidney is a critical target organ where Cd is predominantly bioaccumulated. The exposed level of Cd can cause chronic difficulties, thus leading to damage of kidney filtering mechanisms, kidney dysfunction, liver damage as well as damage to skeletal, reproductive and respiratory systems [4,5]. The mechanism of Cd toxicity is related to its interaction with carboxyl and thiol groups of protein which generate the production of reactive oxygen species (ROS) such as superoxide ions, hydrogen peroxides, and hydroxyl radicals, and therefore inducing oxidative stress and DNA damage by initiation of lipid peroxidation [6].

Recently, several studies have been reported that antioxidant molecules have protective effects against renal and hepatic cadmium toxicity via a function of free radical scavenging [7]. Plants are the foremost source of natural antioxidant molecules such as vitamin C, vitamin E, polyphenols and some minerals like Se and Zn [8], thus they can be hypothesized as effective anti-cadmium toxicity materials. The discovery of functional plant food rich in antioxidant compounds is now being considered. Sprouts or young plants of cereals, grains or legumes are currently of interest since plants at the beginning of the growing stage are associated with large amounts of quality bioactive compounds and antioxidant molecules like polyphenols. Ricegrass is a brand-new sprout which was recently introduced as a substitute for wheatgrass, particularly in tropical areas, as a low-cost ingredient. It is rich in polyphenol compounds and has been previously investigated for its ability to scavenge free radicals in vitro effectively [9].

It was proposed that the human body attempts to reduce heavy metals toxicity via some antioxidant mechanisms such as metal chelation or degradation of free radicals [10]. Selenium (Se) has been stated as a cofactor of antioxidant enzymes and can be used as antidote agent for mercury (Hg), cadmium (Cd) and silver (Ag) [11]. The enrichment of Se into plants has been studied worldwide to increase the level of Se content and may possibly propose an extra role for the biological properties in plant foods, although concern must be given to appropriate forms and concentrations of Se [12]. Therefore, the objective of this study was to identify the specific phenolic types of polyphenol in ricegrass juice extract (RG) and Se-rich ricegrass juice extract (Se-RG) and to investigate the effect of them on in vitro anti-cadmium toxicity in HEK293 (human embryonic kidney cells kidney cells), lipid peroxidation and DNA protective properties.

2. Materials and Methods

2.1. Reagents

Di-sodium ethylenediaminetetraacetic acid (EDTA-Na_2), malondialdehyde (MDA), 2-thiobarbituric acid (TBA) and 3-(4,5-dimethylthiazol-2-yl)-2,5-diphenyltetrazolium bromide (MTT) were acquired from Sigma Aldrich Co. (St. Louis, MO, USA). SYBR gold nucleic acid stain and trichloroacetic acid (TCA) were purchased from Thermo Fisher Scientific Co. (San Jose, CA, USA). Reagents and media for the cell line included a trypan blue dye, trypsin-EDTA, fetal bovine serum (FBS), penicillin-streptomycin and Dulbecco's Modified Eagle Medium (DMEM) were purchased from Gibco BRL, Life Technologies Inc. (Rockville, MD, USA). Low melting point agarose (LMA), dimethyl sulfoxide (DMSO) and Triton-X was purchased from Amresco Inc. (Solon, OH, USA).

2.2. Plant Materials

Oryza sativa L. cv. Chainat 1 obtained from the Phatthalung Rice Research Center, Phatthalung, Thailand was used in this study. Se in the form of sodium selenite at range 40 mg Se/L was used to produce Se rich ricegrass as the best enrichment condition according to previous work [13]. Regular young ricegrass and Se-rich ricegrass was grown for 8 d. After harvesting, both grasses were aqueous extracted and the juices were lyophilized into powder. Ricegrass juice extract (RG) and Se-enriched ricegrass juice extract (Se-RG) were determined for the total Se content using induced coupled plasma optical emission spectroscopy (ICP-OES) and the contents were reported as 1.3 and 59.8 μg/g of extract, respectively.

2.3. Polyphenols Identification

RG and Se-RG were investigated for the major compounds using the reversed-phase ultra-high-performance liquid chromatography–electron spray ionization–mass detector (UHPLC–ESI–MS) since only restricted data has been stated earlier on the specific types of polyphenols found in the aqueous extract of young ricegrass. Polyphenols in RG and Se-RG were identified using a Thermo Scientific (Dionex Softron GmbH., Germering, Germany) Ultimate 3000 UHPLC system equipped with diode array absorbance detector, electron spray ionization and linear ion trap (LTQ XL) mass detector (DAD-ESI-MS). 10 mg/mL of extracts were dissolved in HPLC water and filtered with a sterile syringe filter of 0.45 μm. Purosper STAR (250 mm × 4.6 mm) with LiChrocart, Reverse Phase-18 column end-capped with 5 μm diameter particles (Merck, Darmstadt, Germany) was used as the stationary phase. H_2O containing 0.5% formic acid (solvent A) and acetonitrile (solvent B) were selected as the mobile phase. The gradient condition was run according to Table 1 and followed by washing with 100% methanol for 15 min and re-equilibration. The flow rate was 0.8 mL/min, column temperature was 40 °C with the injection volume of 20 μL. The MS parameters were as follows for both the negative and positive mode: heater temperature: 250 °C; capillary temperature: 330 °C; sheath gas flow: 50 arbitrary units; auxiliary gas flow: 10 arbitrary units. The mass data for the molecular ions were processed with Thermo XcaliburTM software version 2.2.44 (Thermo Scientific., Hemel Hempstead, UK). The peaks were examined based on the ultraviolet (UV) spectra and mass ion compared to the existing literature.

Table 1. The gradient condition of ultra-high-performance liquid chromatography–diode array absorbance detector–electron spray ionization–mass detector (UHPLC–DAD–ESI–MS).

Time (min)	% Solvent B
0.00–10.00	0.00–10.00
10.01–15.00	10.00
15.01–20.00	10.00–15.00
20.01–30.00	15.00–25.00
30.01–35.00	25.00
35.01–45.00	25.00–100.00

2.4. Cell Culture Model

HEK293, human embryonic kidney cells, were purchased from the American Type Culture Collection (Manassas, VA, USA). Dulbecco's Modified Eagle Medium (DMEM) supplemented with 1.5% sodium bicarbonate, 10% fetal bovine serum (FBS), 1% penicillin-streptomycin was used for the maintenance of cells at 37 °C, 5% CO_2, in a fully humidified incubator. Phosphate buffer saline (PBS) at pH 7.2 was used to wash the cells through the experiment.

2.5. Cell Viability Assay

Functional food products which can be claimed as safe need to be confirmed on their viability effect of mammalian cells. The experiment was operated on human embryonic kidney cells, HEK293, to define the dose of extracts indicated as safe to the cells to be used for the anti-cadmium toxicity test. The MTT assay was used to determine the cell viability. Cells grown at 80–90% confluent were harvested with 0.25% trypsin–EDTA and suspended in a fresh medium. Cell counts were measured using a standard haemocytometer based trypan blue cell counting technique [14]. HEK293 cells at the density of 1×10^6 cells/mL were seeded in 96-well tissue culture plates and allowed to adhere for 24 h. After the cells were washed with PBS (pH 7.2), the media was mixed with a various concentration of the extracts (250–10,000 μg/mL), then applied to the cells followed by 24 h incubation. After 24 h, the cell viability was evaluated by adding 20 μL of MTT solution and 2 h incubation. Afterward, the MTT solution was removed, and 100 μL of 0.04 N HCl in isopropanol was added to dissolve the formazan crystals. Absorbances were recorded at 570 nm using a microplate reader. The percentage of cell viability was calculated with Equation (1);

$$\% \text{ Cell viability} = (\text{Absorbance of sample}/\text{Absorbance of control}) \times 100 \quad (1)$$

2.6. Anti-Cadmium Toxicity Properties

To examine the anti-cadmium toxicity properties of RG and Se-RG in HEK293 cells, initially, the half maximal cytotoxicity concentration (CC_{50}) of $CdCl_2$ was investigated to be used as the established dose to induce toxicity to the cells. After seeding HEK293 cells into 96-well plates at a density of 1×10^6 cells/mL, the cells were left to attach for 24 h before being treated with either $CdCl_2$ or extracts. The experiment was divided into three groups separated by different time order for treating the cells with extracts. The first treatment group was the extracts' pre-treatment; the ideal substances that can reduce toxicity from this treatment could represent the role of the protective substances. Secondly, the group of co-treatment was examined to check if the extracts could provide a protective role to cells while it directly reacted to Cd. Lastly, the post-treatment group was designed to indicate the role of the extracts as therapeutic agents. The detail of each group is briefly indicated in Table 2. The extract was fixed to have a contact time of 24 h on cells in all treatments. The percentage of cell viability was detected by MTT cytotoxicity assay and calculated as Equation (1). The morphology of the cells in each treatment was also observed and captured using a microscope.

Table 2. The experimental treatment group on anti-cadmium toxicity and DNA protective properties.

	Control		**Negative Control**		**Sample**	
Time	24 h + 24 h		24 h + 24 h		24 h + 24 h	
Pre-incubation	Media	Media	Media	$CdCl_2$ *	Extracts **	$CdCl_2$
Co-incubation	Media	-	Media + $CdCl_2$	-	Extracts + $CdCl_2$	-
Post-incubation	Media	Media	$CdCl_2$	Media	$CdCl_2$	Extracts

* $CdCl_2$ at CC_{50} level was used. ** Extracts from RG and Se-RG at 10,000 μg/mL were used.

2.7. Determination of Lipid Peroxidation

TBARS (thiobarbituric acid reactive substances) assay was used to determine the level of lipid peroxidation. The endogenous cellular fluid was extracted according to the modified method of Du, et al. [15]. Cells were harvested with 0.25% trypsin-EDTA and followed by centrifugation at 1000× *g* for 10 min. Cell pellets were washed with cold PBS until clean and re-suspended in 1 mL of cold PBS. Cells were lysed using a probe-type sonicator (Vibra-Cell, Sonics and Materials Inc., Newtown, CT, USA) by pulsing at 15 s on and 10 s off for 5 cycles on ice. The cell extracts were centrifuged at 10,000× *g* (4 °C) to discard the cell debris while supernatants were used for the determination of MDA content and protein levels. Protein content was examined using bovine serum albumin (BSA) as standard [16]. The modified method of Chen, et al. [17] was used to determine the MDA content. 1 mL of cellular extracts were mixed with 4 mL of 20% TCA containing 0.8% of TBA (*w*/*v*). The mixtures were heated at 95 °C for 60 min, then cooled in ice and centrifuged at 3000× *g* for 10 min. The absorbance was measured at 532 nm. The amount of MDA–TBA red complexes were compared to an external standard of MDA. The amount of TBARS was expressed as nmol MDA/mg protein.

2.8. DNA Protective Properties Using Comet Assay

DNA damage can be induced by exogenous agents such as heavy metals, polycyclic aromatic hydrocarbon from pollution, endogenous chemical genotoxic agents such as reactive oxygen species

(ROS) and natural chemical reactions [18]. The damage to the cellular genome can generate errors in the transcription of DNA and protein translation which impair signaling and the cellular function and could result in the development of diseases [19]. The alkaline single cell gel electrophoresis assay or comet assay was used to evaluate the DNA damage [20]. The DNA protective properties of the RG and Se-RG extracts on HEK293 cells towards the exposure to $CdCl_2$ were investigated. Briefly, HEK293 cells were seeded at 1×10^6 cells/mL in 12-well plates and incubated at 37 °C for 24 h. The cells were treated with the following condition stated above (Table 2). Then, cells were harvested and fixed into slides which had been covered with 150 µL of 1.5% LMA as the first layer. After solidification, 20 µL of freshly prepared cell suspension with 180 µL of 0.5% LMA (ratio 1:10) was rapidly mixed by pipetting, and 80 µL of the mixture was loaded as the second layer. Then, 70 µL of 1% LMA was added on to the cell layer as the third layer. Once the gel was solidified, the slides were placed in a chilled lysis buffer containing 2.5 M NaCl, 100 mM EDTA, 100 mM Tris–HCl at pH 10 and 1% DMSO, 1% Triton X-100 for at least 2 h at 4 °C. The slides were then removed and placed in a comet assay tank (Model CSL-COM20, Cleaver Scientific, Rugby, Warwickshire, UK) filled with freshly prepared alkaline buffer at 4 °C (300 mM NaOH, 1 mM Na_2EDTA, pH $\geq$ 13) for 15 min to unwind the DNA, and electrophoresis was carried out at 25 V and 300 mA for 45 min. Afterward, the slides were rinsed with deionized water and neutralized gently with 0.4 M Tris–HCl buffer, pH 7.5 for 5 min. Finally, the slides were soaked in ethanol for 5 min and left at room temperature until they were completely dried. The cellular DNA was stained using SYBR gold nucleic acid stain in the dark for 20 min and visualized using a fluorescent microscope (Eclipse 80i, Nikon, Tokyo, Japan). The comet images (45–60 cells/slide) were captured and analyzed. The quantification of the DNA strand breaks was done using CometScore 2.0.0.38 software (Tritek Corp., Sumerduck, VA, USA). The % DNA in tail and tail length were obtained.

2.9. *Statistical Analysis*

Completely randomized design (CRD) was used throughout the study. All experimental data were presented as the mean ± standard deviation (SD) of three replications. Means were analyzed using analysis of variance (ANOVA). The significant differences among means were determined by Tukey's test ($p < 0.05$) using SPSS for Windows (SPSS Inc, Chicago, IL, USA).

3. Results and Discussion

3.1. *Polyphenols Identification Using Ultra High-Performance Liquid Chromatography–Electron Spray Ionization–Mass Detector (UHPLC–ESI–MS)*

Results of polyphenols identification showed that RG and Se-RG contain similar types of identified compounds. Six major compounds comprising more than 70% of relative content were tentatively identified (Table 3) where the molecular weight and electrospray ionization mass spectrometry of detected compounds were reported. Phenolic glycoside was detected and defined as 1-*O*-sinapoyl-β-D-glucose. The ion found with the m/z of 367 was defined as 3-*O*-feruloyl quinic acid due to the presence of a ferulic acid fragment at m/z 193. The largest compounds in RG were identified as a group of flavone glycosides including chrysoeriol arabinosyl arabinoside, tricin, swertisin and tricin-7-*O*-β-D-glucopyranoside which has been earlier reported as having been found in the leaves of *Oryza sativa* and *Triticum aestivum* (wheat) [21,22].

Table 3. Tentative identification of phenolic compounds in ricegrass juice extract (RG) and Se-rich ricegrass juice extract (Se-RG) analyzed by UHPLC–ESI–MS.

Tentative Compounds	MW *	$[M - H]^+$ (m/z)	References
Tricin	330	329	[22,23]
1-*O*-Sinapoyl-β-D-glucose	386	385	[22]
3-*O*-Feruloylquinic acid	368	367	[22,24]
Chrysoeriol arabinosyl arabinoside	564	563	[22,24]
Swertisin	446	445	[22]
Tricin-7-*O*-β-D-glucopyranoside	492	491	[25]

* MW: Molecular weight.

3.2. Cytotoxicity of Ricegrass Juice Extract (RG) and Se-Rich Ricegrass Juice Extract (Se-RG)

The dose of extracts indicated as safe to cells was used for the anti-cadmium toxicity test. Figure 1 revealed that the cell number of HEK293 slightly decreases while treated with both RG and Se-RG and remained constant while the concentration of the extracts was increased up to the dose of 10,000 μg/mL. Se-RG extracts displayed no significantly different effect on the reduction of cell numbers compared to the RG ($p < 0.05$). There was a minor reduction in cell number, however, the cells remained higher than 80% of the control which was indicated as the acceptable range classified as safe [26]. Although the alteration of cell morphology after treatment with the extracts has been detected, it was regarded as a result of the sensitivity of cells when they had encountered the foreign matter and attempted to adapt to the new environment. Therefore, from this result it can be assumed that both extracts had no or low toxicity to the kidney cells and the dose of both extracts at the highest concentration (10,000 μg/mL) could be used for the next experiment.

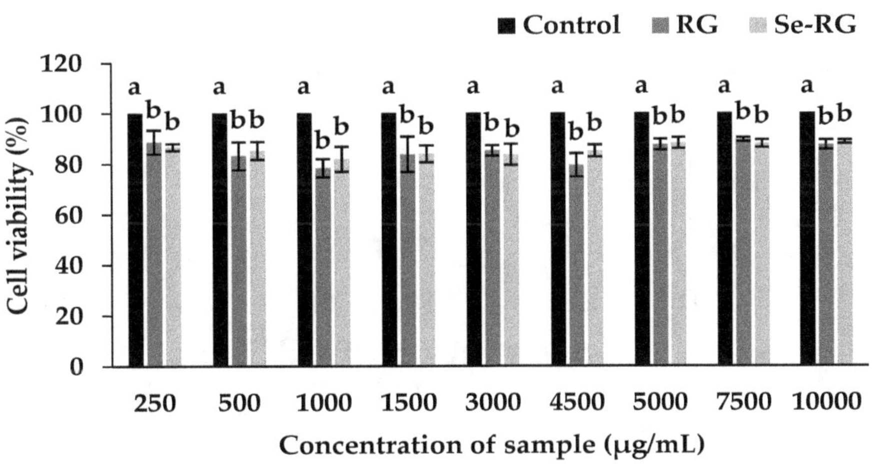

Figure 1. Effect of different concentrations of RG and Se-RG on the cell viability of HEK293 kidney cells. Data are means ± standard deviation (SD). Different letters indicated significant differences between treatment in the similar concentration of extracts ($p < 0.05$) in Tukey's significant differences test.

3.3. *Anti-Cd Toxicity of RG and Se-RG and Effect on Lipid Peroxidation*

The kidney is the critical organ affected by chronic Cd exposure and toxicity. Cd accumulates in the kidney because of its preferential uptake by the receptor in the renal proximal tubule and accumulates in the human kidney for a relatively long time, from 20 to 30 years [27]. The exposed level of Cd can cause chronic difficulties, thus leading to damage of kidney filtering mechanisms and kidney dysfunction [4]. HEK293 cells, human embryonic kidney cells, were used as a demonstrative model to examine the effect of $CdCl_2$ toxicity and the protective role of extracts against $CdCl_2$. The level of $CdCl_2$ which could be used to induce the cytotoxicity was examined. Figure 2 showed that the viability of HEK293 cells was significantly decreased ($p < 0.05$) while exposed to higher level of $CdCl_2$. Cd is not able to generate radical itself but the toxicity was related to the generation of reactive oxygen species (ROS) such as superoxide ions, hydrogen peroxides and hydroxyls radicals and therefore induced oxidative stress and DNA damage by initiation of the lipid peroxidation [6].The estimated half maximal concentration (CC_{50}) dose of $CdCl_2$ in HEK293 was indicated as 68.5 μmol/L and this level could be used as a suitable dose for the evaluation of anti-cadmium toxicity properties of the RG and Se-RG.

The experiment on anti-cadmium toxicity properties was designed to assess the effect of RG and Se-RG against $CdCl_2$ exposure on the cell viability and lipid peroxidation at different time orders, as each substance may alleviate the toxicity from Cd induction differently [10]. Results reveal that RG and Se-RG significantly increased ($p < 0.05$) the percentage of cell viability during pre-treatment and co-treatment but not during post-treatment with Cd compared to the cells treated with Cd at CC_{50} level alone (Figure 3).

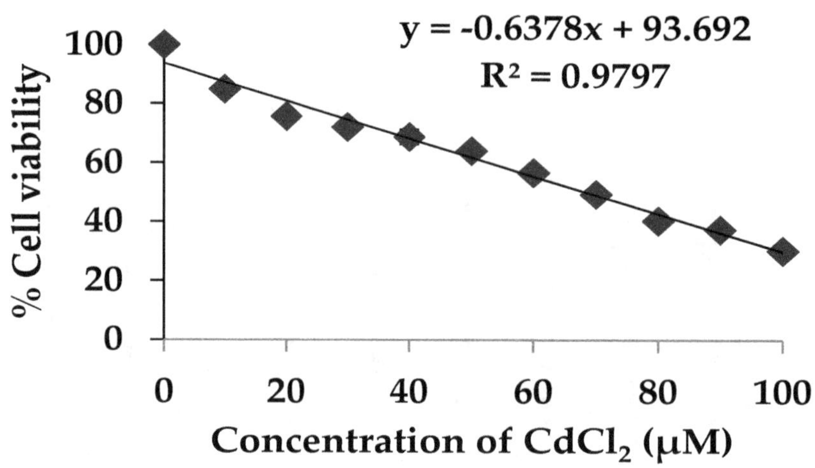

Figure 2. Effect of different concentrations of $CdCl_2$ on the cell viability of HEK293 kidney cells. Data are means ± standard deviation (SD).

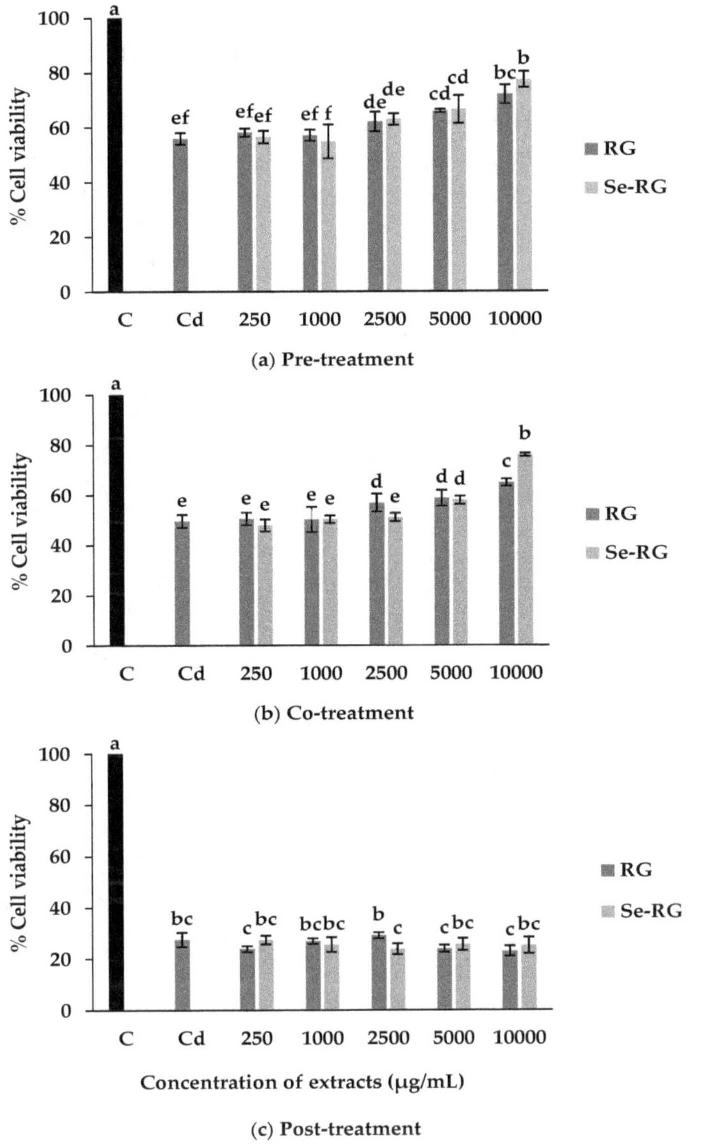

Figure 3. Anti-Cd toxicity properties of RG and Se-RG on HEK293 kidney cells while exposed to $CdCl_2$ at different time orders of treating the extracts compared to the control and Cd-treated (**a**) pre-incubation (**b**) co-incubation (**c**) post-incubation. C means control; Cd means $CdCl_2$ at CC_{50} level (68.50 μg/mL). The cell viability was expressed as a percentage of control. Data are means ± standard deviation (SD). Different letters indicated significant differences ($p < 0.05$) in Tukey's significant differences test.

The highest concentration of both extracts (10,000 μg/mL) exerted the highest ability to protect HEK293 cells against Cd toxicity. Thus, the pathological evaluation of cell morphology treated with the extracts at this concentration was observed as shown in Figure 4. The morphological changes while treating the cells with Cd were detected. A majority of the cells were broken and floated into the media while the rest were weakened and lost their cell structure. Although the cells in the condition of extracts pre-treatment illustrated some lost and unusual cells morphology, the cells remained strengthened in their frame similarly to web shape. The changes of cells in co-treatment conditions were also detected as they were swollen and changed to a circle-like shape, but they preserved their structure. These data suggested that pre-treatment and co-treatment of RG and Se-RG with Cd could improve the Cd-induced pathological damage of kidney cells better than the Cd-treated and can potentially protect against kidney cell damage. Living organisms contain lipid as the main structure of cellular membranes. Cd could induce the damaging effects to the cells from the lipid peroxidation process [28].

Therefore, the extent of lipid peroxidation by-products produced like malondialdehyde (MDA) can imitate the extent of cells oxidative damage initiated by Cd [29]. TBARS assay is a well-established method use as an index of lipid peroxidation and lipid hydroperoxides. When the cells exposed to Cd, the MDA content was markedly increased, thus suggesting the increased in oxidative stress of kidney cells (Figure 5). However, outcomes indicated that during pre-treatment and co-treatment of both RG and Se-RG, the level of MDA in HEK293 was significantly reduced compared to Cd-treated cells ($p < 0.05$).

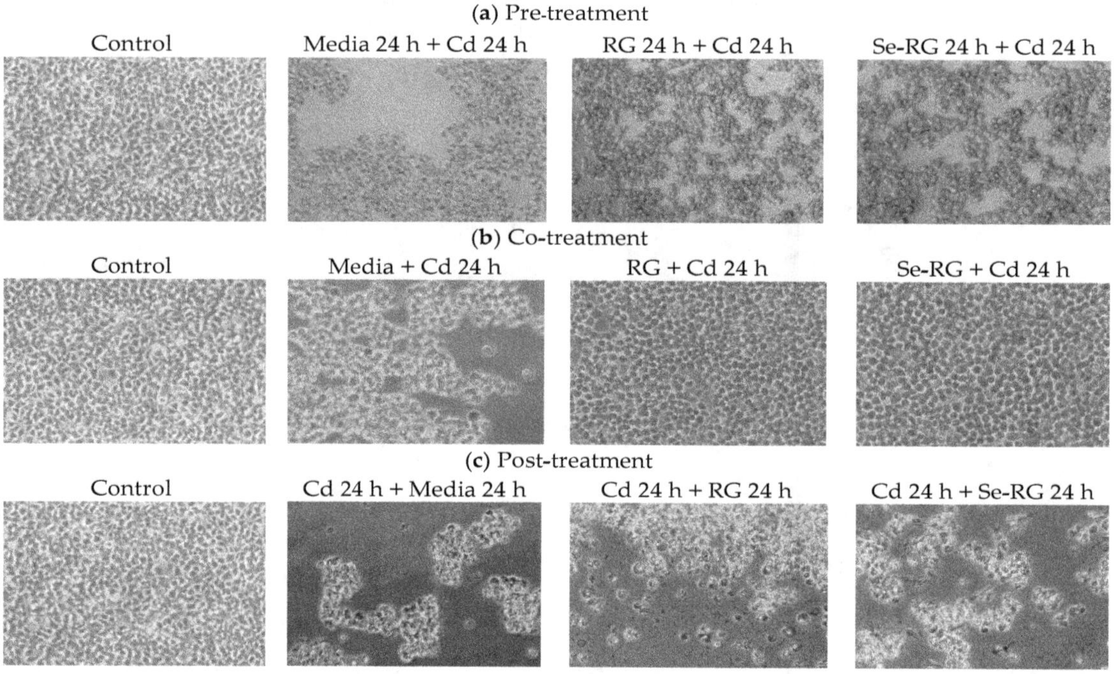

Figure 4. Morphology of cells of HEK293 kidney cells while incubated the cells with RG/Se-RG and $CdCl_2$ at different time order of treating the extracts (**a**) pre-incubation (**b**) co-incubation and (**c**) post-incubation. C means control; Cd means $CdCl_2$ at CC_{50} level (68.50 μg/mL).

The role of phenolic compounds in the extracts was considered as having the major effects on the protective role against Cd-induced damage. It could be explained that the extracts rich in polyphenols compounds possess the inhibition of lipid peroxidation chain reaction by stabilizing the hydroxyl radicals and lipid peroxyl radicals, thereby lowering the extent of oxidative damage to the lipid cell membrane and lower level of MDA [30,31]. Moreover, phenolic compounds as antioxidant molecules could propose the role of upregulating the antioxidant protection system by stimulating the production of antioxidant enzymes including super oxide dismutase (SOD), catalase (CAT), and glutathione peroxidase (GPx). As a result, strengthening the immunity and lowering the damage caused by Cd during pre-treatment and co-treatment to the cells [10]. RG and Se-RG contained abundant polyphenols such as flavone glycosides. Therefore, the protective role of the extracts could be related mainly to these groups of compounds. Similar results also indicated the protective effect of bioflavonoids, for example, quercetin against Cd-induced oxidative stress-related renal dysfunction in rats by attenuating the Cd-induced biochemical alterations in serum, urine and tissue pathological changes via a decrease in lipid peroxidation rate [32]. Flavonoid, namely catechin from green tea, has also been proved to protect against bone metabolic disorders in cadmium-poisoned rats [33]. While focusing on the effect of high Se, Se-RG extracts revealed marginally higher protective properties against Cd toxicity over the RG in pre-treatment and co-treatment conditions. Se was used as antidote agent to a range of heavy metal toxicities including Cd, Hg, and Ag [11]. Generally, studies have indicated the beneficial effect of Se on antioxidant status and lipid peroxidation when pre-exposed and co-exposed to Cd [34–36]. Lipid peroxidation occurred because of Cd exposure; moreover, a significant decrease in the antioxidant composition factors, such as glutathione (GSH) levels, the activities of glutathione peroxidase (GPx) and thioredoxin reductase (TrxR), was also stated [34]. Se compounds have been generally known as a major cofactor of GPx and TrxR, thus, Se could logically promote the greater level of these antioxidant enzymes activity and play a role in managing the radicals occurring in the cells. Se could also present protective effects on mitochondria dysfunction by blocking the ROS generation, a possible inhibition of Cd-induced mitochondrial membrane collapse [37].

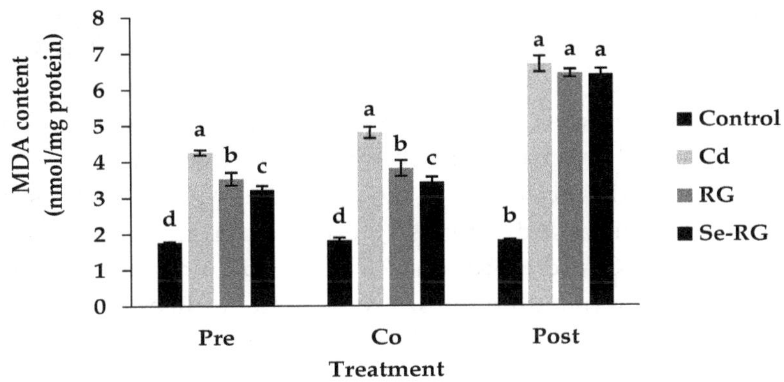

Figure 5. Level of malondialdehyde (MDA) in HEK293 cells treated with RG and Se-RG at the level 10,000 μg/mL compared to the control and Cd-treated ones. Data are means ± standard deviation (SD). Different letters indicated significant differences in the similar group of treatment ($p < 0.05$) in Tukey's significant differences test.

3.4. DNA Protective Properties

Comet assay or single cell gel electrophoresis is a standard rapid method for detecting DNA damage in individual cells. The percentage of DNA in tail and tail length was analyzed as the measure of primary DNA damage [24]. Therefore, comet assay is useful for this study to evaluate the DNA protective role of RG and Se-RG extracts against Cd. The highest concentration of both was used (10,000 μg/mL) as they protect the highest number of percent cell viability. Figure 6 illustrates the capture of comet cells of each treatment during pre-treatment, co-treatment, and post-treatment of RG and Se-RG compared to the Cd-treated and control. Figure 7 shows the parameters of the comet cells included % DNA in tail and tail length.

Comet cells of the control of every treatment displayed a circle-like shape in which the whole nuclei and DNA were beautifully stained with the fluorescent color. The condition of Cd-treated cells indicated the presence of a clouded comet tail in which the % DNA in tail and tail length were increased significantly ($p < 0.05$) because of Cd-induced the oxidative damage to cells. In both of pre-treatment and co-treatment conditions, the RG and Se-RG treated cells significantly exhibited the reduction in the % DNA in tail and tail length compared to the Cd-treated group (negative control), and thus illustrated a DNA protective effect. The results on comet assay parameters of each treatment were correlated to the content of MDA production.

The damaging of DNA could be a subsequent effect on the production of high ROS and lipid radicals induced by Cd. The role of flavone glycosides as a natural antioxidant in the RG and Se-RG may influence the protective property by possibly up-regulating the level of the antioxidant defense system and abolishing oxidative DNA damage via the donation of electrons to reactive metabolites and rendering them inactive to prevent the interaction to the DNA. The experiment on the protective role of flavonoid compounds as an excellent radical scavenger to reduce the DNA damage in human blood lymphocyte is also consistent with this result [38]. Se-RG showed higher ability on the reduction in the tail length and % DNA in the tail of the comets compared to the RG. This indicated that Se in combination with the polyphenols could provide an extra protection and promote a protective role for the kidney cells. Se as the cofactor of various endogenous enzymes works in the antioxidant system could support the activity on the destructive of ROS. Fischer, et al. [39] suggested another possible role of Se, especially in the organic form, of protecting DNA damage via induction of p53 DNA repair pathway and transactivation of p53-regulated effector genes.

In the post-treatment condition, although the addition of the RG and Se-RG showed no significant effect on an improvement in cell viability of HEK293 cells, a minor role of DNA protection can visibly be seen. In the Cd-treated condition, most DNA in cells were broken down as indicated by the size of the comet head being obviously decreased from the control. DNA fragments were spread into the surrounding area as detected from the blurred green background. However, the addition of the extracts could not save the cell viability from Cd exposure, and the intensive black background remained to be observed. This might indicate a slight reduction in the number of DNA fragments in the surrounding area as both RG and Se-RG indicated a reduction in % DNA in the tail of comets compared to Cd-treated cells. Moreover, the addition of Se-RG indicated significant reduction in the tail length ($p < 0.05$), and thus showed better DNA protective properties.

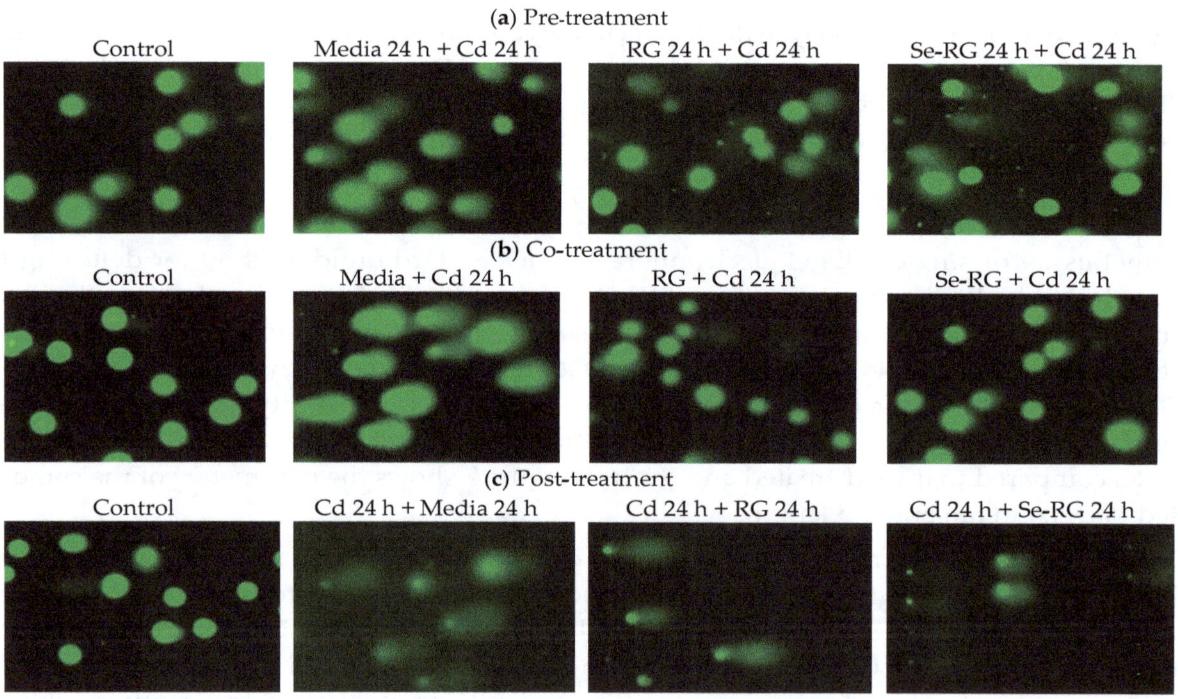

Figure 6. DNA protective effect of RG and Se-RG against $CdCl_2$ induced DNA break in HEK293 kidney cells while incubated the cells with RG/Se-RG and $CdCl_2$ at different time order of treating the extracts evaluated by comet assay (**a**) pre-incubation (**b**) co-incubation and (**c**) post-incubation. C means blank control; Cd means $CdCl_2$ at CC_{50} level (68.50 μg/mL).

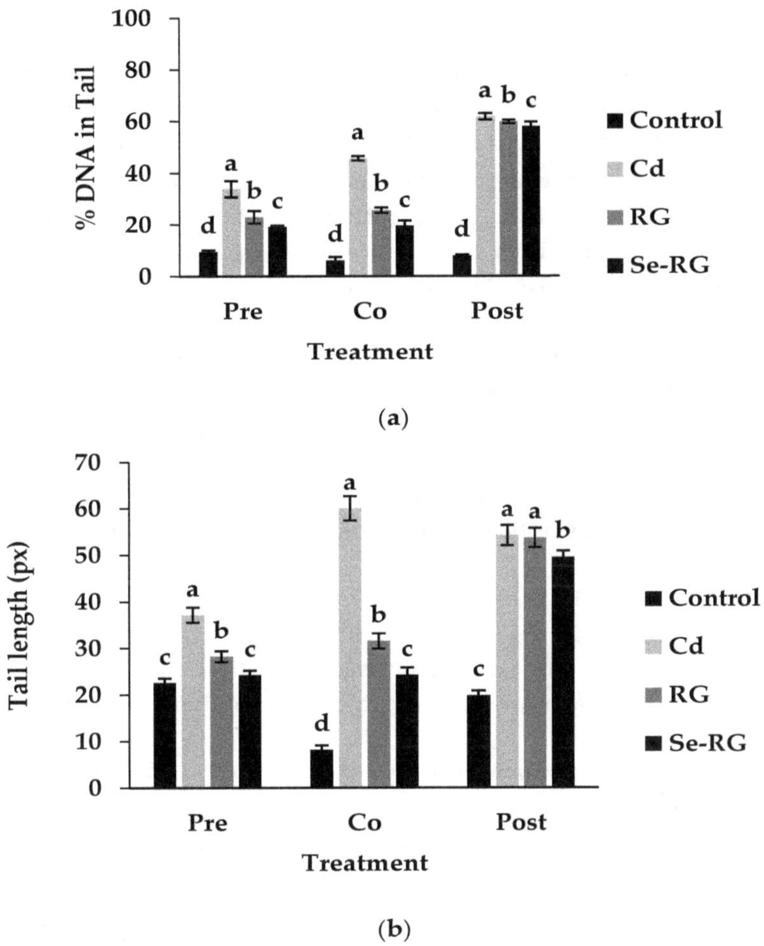

Figure 7. Assessment of DNA damage parameters in HEK293 cells treated with RG and Se-RG at the level 10,000 μg/mL compared to the control and Cd-treated ones evaluated using the CometScore software. (**a**) changes in % DNA in tail; (**b**) changes in tail length. Data are means ± standard deviation (SD). Different letters indicated significant differences ($p < 0.05$) in Tukey's significant differences test.

4. Conclusions

In conclusion, our results showed the protective effect of RG and Se-RG in counteracting Cd-induced damage in HEK293 kidney cells during pre-treatment and co-treatment with Cd. The results could support the hypothesis that polyphenols in combination with Se compounds may help in the reduction of oxidative stress, lipid peroxidation rate, morphological impairments and DNA damage to kidney cells. Flavone glycosides as the major polyphenols in the extracts should contribute to these beneficial effects. Se-enrichment to ricegrass could promote additional benefits over typical ricegrass through the upregulation of the GPx enzyme. Se-RG should have potential to be produced and consumed as a functional food to protect the human body from Cd contamination.

Author Contributions: R.C., P.P., and S.S. conceived and designed the experiments; R.C. performed the experiments with the assistance of P.M. and B.S.; R.C. analyzed the data and wrote the paper which was reviewed, edited and approved by all the authors.

Acknowledgments: The authors would like to acknowledge the guidance of comet assay techniques from Pasika Niamrit, Mahidol University and English copy editing from Maria Mullet.

References

1. Tchounwou, P.B.; Yedjou, C.G.; Patlolla, A.K.; Sutton, D.J. Heavy metal toxicity and the environment. In *Molecular, Clinical and Environmental Toxicology, Experientia Supplementum*; Luch, A., Ed.; Springer: Basel, Switzerland, 2012; Volume 101, pp. 133–164. ISBN 978-3-7643-8339-8.
2. Elinder, C.G.; Järup, L. Cadmium exposure and health risks: Recent findings. *Ambio* **1996**, *25*, 370–373.
3. Wang, X.Q.; Xu, D.; Lü, M.K.; Yuan, D.R.; Yin, X.; Zhang, G.H.; Xu, S.X.; Lu, G.W.; Song, C.F.; Guo, S.Y. Crystal growth and physical properties of UV nonlinear optical crystal zinc cadmium thiocyanate, $ZnCd(SCN)_4$. *Chem. Phys. Lett.* **2001**, *346*, 393–406. [CrossRef]
4. Järup, L. Hazards of heavy metal contamination. *Br. Med. Bull.* **2003**, *68*, 167–182. [CrossRef] [PubMed]
5. Rahimzadeh, M.R.; Rahimzadeh, M.R.; Kazemi, S.; Moghadamnia, A.A. Cadmium toxicity and treatment: An update. *Casp. J. Intern. Med.* **2017**, *8*, 135–145.
6. Liu, J.; Qu, W.; Kadiiska, M.B. Role of oxidative stress in cadmium toxicity and carcinogenesis. *Toxicol. Appl. Pharmacol.* **2009**, *238*, 209–214. [CrossRef] [PubMed]
7. Shaikh, Z.A.; Vu, T.T.; Zaman, K. Oxidative stress as a mechanism of chronic cadmium-induced hepatotoxicity and renal toxicity and protection by antioxidants. *Toxicol. Appl. Pharmacol.* **1999**, *154*, 256–263. [CrossRef] [PubMed]
8. Nahak, G.; Suar, M.; Sahu, R.K. Antioxidant Potential and Nutritional Values of Vegetables: A Review. *Res. J. Med. Plant* **2014**, *8*, 50–81. [CrossRef]
9. Chomchan, R.; Siripongvutikorn, S.; Puttarak, P.; Rattanapon, R. Investigation of phytochemical constituents, phenolic profiles and antioxidant activities of ricegrass juice compared to wheatgrass juice. *Funct. Foods Health Dis.* **2016**, *6*, 822–835.
10. Sandbichler, A.M.; Höckner, M. Cadmium protection strategies—A hidden trade-off? *Int. J. Mol. Sci.* **2016**, *17*, 139. [CrossRef] [PubMed]
11. Mukherjee, A.; Sharma, A. Effects of cadmium and selenium on cell division and chromosomal aberrations in *Allium sativum* L. *Water Air Soil Pollut.* **1988**, *37*, 433–438. [CrossRef]
12. Chomchan, R.; Siripongvutikorn, S.; Puttarak, P. Selenium bio-fortification: An alternative to improve phytochemicals and bioactivities of plant foods. *Funct. Foods. Health Dis.* **2017**, *7*, 263–279.
13. Chomchan, R.; Siripongvutikorn, S.; Puttarak, P.; Rattanapon, R. Influence of selenium bio-fortification on nutritional compositions, bioactive compounds content and anti-oxidative properties of young ricegrass (*Oryza sativa* L.). *Funct. Food Health. Dis.* **2017**, *7*, 195–209.
14. Louis, K.S.; Siegel, A.C. Cell viability analysis using trypan blue: Manual and automated methods. In *Mammalian Cell Viability. Methods in Molecular Biology (Methods and Protocols)*; Stoddart, M., Ed.; Humana Press: New York, NY, USA, 2011; Volume 740, pp. 7–12. ISBN 978-1-61779-107-9.
15. Du, Y.; Esfandi, R.; Willmore, W.G.; Tsopmo, A. Antioxidant activity of oat proteins derived peptides in stressed hepatic HepG2 cells. *Antioxidants* **2016**, *5*, 39. [CrossRef] [PubMed]
16. Bradford, M.M. A rapid and sensitive method for the quantitation of microgram quantities of protein utilizing the principle of protein-dye binding. *Anal. Biochem.* **1976**, *72*, 248–254. [CrossRef]
17. Chen, L.; Yang, X.; Jiao, H.; Zhao, B. Tea catechins protect against lead-induced cytotoxicity, lipid peroxidation, and membrane fluidity in HepG2 cells. *Toxicol. Sci.* **2002**, *69*, 149–156. [CrossRef] [PubMed]
18. Ercal, N.; Gurer-Orhan, H.; Aykin-Burns, N. Toxic metals and oxidative stress part I: Mechanisms involved in metal-induced oxidative damage. *Curr. Top. Med. Chem.* **2001**, *1*, 529–539. [CrossRef] [PubMed]
19. Lindahl, T.; Barnes, D. Repair of endogenous DNA damage. *Cold Spring Harb. Symp. Quant. Biol.* **2000**, *65*, 127–134. [CrossRef] [PubMed]
20. Singh, N.P. Microgels for estimation of DNA strand breaks, DNA protein crosslinks and apoptosis. *Mutat. Res.* **2000**, *455*, 111–127. [CrossRef]
21. Besson, E.; Dellamonica, G.; Chopin, J.; Markham, K.R.; Kim, M.; Koh, H.-S.; Fukami, H. C-glycosylflavones from *Oryza sativa*. *Phytochemisty* **1985**, *24*, 1061–1064. [CrossRef]
22. Yang, Z.; Nakabayashi, R.; Okazaki, Y.; Mori, T.; Takamatsu, S.; Kitanaka, S.; Kikuchi, J.; Saito, K. Toward better annotation in plant metabolomics: Isolation and structure elucidation of 36 specialized metabolites from *Oryza sativa* (rice) by using MS/MS and NMR analyses. *Metabolomics* **2014**, *10*, 543–555. [CrossRef] [PubMed]

23. Kim, J.H.; Cheon, Y.M.; Kim, B.G.; Ahn, J.H. Analysis of flavonoids and characterization of the *OsFNS* gene involved in flavone biosynthesis in rice. *J. Plant Biol.* **2008**, *51*, 97–101. [CrossRef]
24. Pourrut, B.; Pinelli, E.; Celiz Mendiola, V.; Silvestre, J.; Douay, F. Recommendations for increasing alkaline comet assay reliability in plants. *Mutagenesis* **2015**, *30*, 37–43. [CrossRef] [PubMed]
25. Henkler, F.; Brinkmann, J.; Luch, A. The role of oxidative stress in carcinogenesis induced by metals and xenobiotics. *Cancers* **2010**, *2*, 376–396. [CrossRef] [PubMed]
26. Langdon, S.R.; Mulgrew, J.; Paolini, G.V.; van Hoorn, W.P. Predicting cytotoxicity from heterogeneous data sources with Bayesian learning. *J. Cheminform.* **2010**, *2*, 11. [CrossRef] [PubMed]
27. Johri, N.; Jacquillet, G.; Unwin, R. Heavy metal poisoning: The effects of cadmium on the kidney. *Biometals* **2010**, *23*, 783–792. [CrossRef] [PubMed]
28. Eneman, J.; Potts, R.; Osier, M.; Shukla, G.; Lee, C.; Chiu, J.; Hart, B. Suppressed oxidant-induced apoptosis in cadmium adapted alveolar epithelial cells and its potential involvement in cadmium carcinogenesis. *Toxicology* **2000**, *147*, 215–228. [CrossRef]
29. Ayala, A.; Muñoz, M.F.; Argüelles, S. Lipid peroxidation: Production, metabolism, and signaling mechanisms of malondialdehyde and 4-hydroxy-2-nonenal. *Oxid. Med. Cell. Longev.* **2014**, *2014*, 1–31. [CrossRef] [PubMed]
30. Cai, Q.; Rahn, R.O.; Zhang, R. Dietary flavonoids, quercetin, luteolin and genistein, reduce oxidative DNA damage and lipid peroxidation and quench free radicals. *Cancer Lett.* **1997**, *119*, 99–107. [CrossRef]
31. Ding, Y.; Wang, S.Y.; Yang, D.J.; Chang, M.H.; Chen, Y.C. Alleviative effects of litchi (*Litchi chinensis Sonn.*) flower on lipid peroxidation and protein degradation in emulsified pork meatballs. *J. Food Drug Anal.* **2015**, *23*, 501–508. [CrossRef] [PubMed]
32. Renugadevi, J.; Prabu, S.M. Quercetin protects against oxidative stress-related renal dysfunction by cadmium in rats. *Exp. Toxicol. Pathol.* **2010**, *62*, 471–481. [CrossRef] [PubMed]
33. Choi, J.H.; Rhee, I.K.; Park, K.Y.; Park, K.Y.; Kim, J.K.; Rhee, S.J. Action of green tea catechin on bone metabolic disorder in chronic cadmium-poisoned rats. *Life Sci.* **2003**, *73*, 1479–1489. [CrossRef]
34. El-Sharaky, A.; Newairy, A.; Badreldeen, M.; Eweda, S.; Sheweita, S. Protective role of selenium against renal toxicity induced by cadmium in rats. *Toxicology* **2007**, *235*, 185–193. [CrossRef] [PubMed]
35. Liu, L.; Yang, B.; Cheng, Y.; Lin, H. Ameliorative effects of selenium on cadmium-induced oxidative stress and endoplasmic reticulum stress in the chicken kidney. *Biol. Trace Elem. Res.* **2015**, *167*, 308–319. [CrossRef] [PubMed]
36. Ognjanovic, B.; Markovic, S.; Pavlovic, S.; Zikic, R.; Stajn, A.; Saicic, Z. Effect of chronic cadmium exposure on antioxidant defense system in some tissues of rats: Protective effect of selenium. *Physiol. Res.* **2008**, *57*, 403–411. [PubMed]
37. Zhou, Y.J.; Zhang, S.P.; Liu, C.W.; Cai, Y.Q. The protection of selenium on ROS mediated-apoptosis by mitochondria dysfunction in cadmium-induced LLC-PK1 cells. *Toxicol. In Vitro* **2009**, *23*, 288–294. [CrossRef] [PubMed]
38. Devipriya, N.; Sudheer, A.R.; Srinivasan, M.; Menon, V.P. Quercetin ameliorates gamma radiation-induced DNA damage and biochemical changes in human peripheral blood lymphocytes. *Mutat. Res.* **2008**, *654*, 1–7. [CrossRef] [PubMed]
39. Fischer, J.L.; Lancia, J.K.; Mathur, A.; Smith, M.L. Selenium protection from DNA damage involves a Ref1/p53/Brca1 protein complex. *Anticancer Res.* **2006**, *26*, 899–904. [PubMed]

12

Betaine in Cereal Grains and Grain-Based Products

Bojana Filipčev *, Jovana Kojić, Jelena Krulj, Marija Bodroža-Solarov and Nebojša Ilić

Institute of Food Technology, University of Novi Sad, 21000 Novi Sad, Serbia; jovana.kojic@fins.uns.ac.rs (J.Ko.); jelena.krulj@fins.uns.ac.rs (J.Kr.); marija.bodroza@fins.uns.ac.rs (M.B.-S.); nebojsa.ilic@fins.uns.ac.rs (N.I.)

* Correspondence: bojana.filipcev@fins.uns.ac.rs

Abstract: Betaine is a non-essential nutrient which performs several important physiological functions in organisms. Abundant data exist to suggest that betaine has a potential for prevention of chronic diseases and that its dietary intake may contribute to overall health enhancement. Several studies have pointed out that the betaine status of the general population is inadequate and have suggested nutritional strategies to improve dietary intake of betaine. Cereal-based food has been implicated as the major source of betaine in the Western diet. This review summarizes the results on the betaine content in various cereals and related products. Attention has been given to the betaine content in gluten-free grains and products. It also discusses the stability of betaine during processing (cooking, baking, extrusion) and possibilities to increase betaine content by fortification.

Keywords: betaine; cereals; pseudocereals; gluten-free; stability; cooking; baking; extrusion

1. Introduction

Betaine (*N,N,N*-trimethylglycine, glycine betaine) is an organic nitrogenous compound, found for the first time in sugar beet juice (*Beta vulgaris*).

Betaine is a zwitterion of quaternary ammonium which is still named trimethylglycine and glycine betaine (Figure 1). It is a methyl derivative of the amino acid glycine ($(CH_3)_3N^+CH_2COO^-$ and molecular weight 117.2). It is characterized as methylamine due to its three free methyl groups [1].

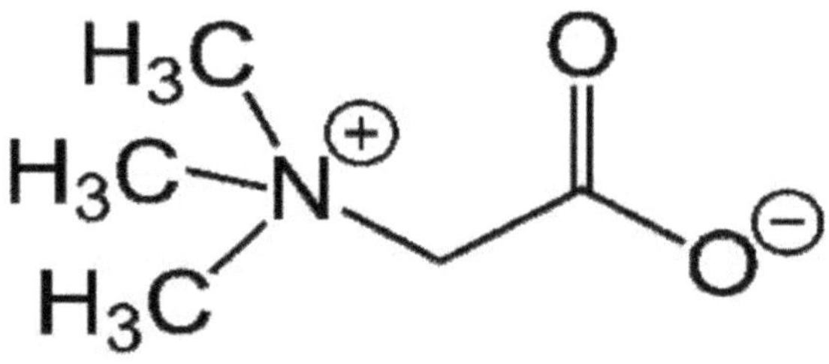

Figure 1. Betaine chemical structure.

Various analogues of glycine betaine exist in plants: proline betaine (stachydrine), trigonelline, arsenobetaine, betonicine, butirobetaine, ergothionine, propionobetaine, and sulfur analogues. The sulfur analogues are several in type: β-alaninebetaine, dimethylsulfonioacetate, and dimethylsulfoniopropionate (DMSP). The food survey study by de Zwart et al. [2] showed that only some betaine analogues were present in food at appreciable levels (>10 μg/g)—glycine betaine, proline betaine, trigonelline, and DMSP. Slow et al. [3] indicated glycine betaine as dominant in grain products, proline betaine in citruses, and trigonelline in coffee. Most recently, some rare forms of betaine were identified in the grains of most common cereals: pipercolic acid betaine in rye flour and valine betaine and glutamine betaine in flours of barley, rye, oat, durum, and winter wheat [4].

The content of betaine analogues was found to be vastly variable in grains; higher betaine levels seem to be induced by plant growth under stress conditions (drought, salt stress, cold, freezing, hypoxia, etc.) [2,3]. Since the potential health effects of betaine analogues, particularly trigonelline and proline, have not yet been fully resolved, currently only glycine betaine has dietary relevance.

Betaine represents a bioactive compound that has significant physiological functions in the human organism as an osmolite and donor of methyl groups for many biochemical processes. As such, it is indispensable to preserve the health of kidneys, liver, and heart [5]. This compound has an important role in preventing and treating many chronic diseases, among which lowering of plasma homocysteine levels has gained the most attention [5–7]. High serum homocysteine levels have been associated with increased risk for cardiovascular diseases (stroke, heart attack, atherosclerosis), cancer, peripheral neuropathy, etc. Moreover, betaine has been shown to improve athletic performance by enhancing muscle endurance [7,8].

Although betaine is not an essential nutrient, it cannot be synthesized in adequate quantities by the human body. Humans may obtain betaine from foods rich in betaine or choline or by oral supplements contained with pure preparations. The main sources of betaine in human nutrition are wheat bran, wheat germ, and spinach [9,10]. Several studies denoted cereal foods as major contributors of betaine [3,11–13]. The betaine intake from foods was estimated in a few food surveys (overviewed by Ross et al. [11]) which differ in methodologies used to collect food consumption data, and used different food databases to calculate the betaine intake. Wide gender, national, and international variations were observed [11]. The overall mean betaine intake estimated from these surveys was 131 mg/day [11]. Daily supply of betaine should reach 1500 mg [14] for the manifestation of health effects, so, obviously, the dietary betaine intakes of general populations can be considered to be on the low side. Elderly population (aged over 50 years) or other vulnerable groups (diabetic and homocystinuria patients) may be at a higher risk of inadequate intake. Therefore, many nutritionists advocate for betaine supplementation. Research by Olthof et al. [6] inferred that betaine delivery via food and oral administration of betaine supplement has a similar health effect, where a diet rich in betaine (betaine intake of about 2000 mg/day) had a higher effect on lowering homocysteine than a betaine poor diet (500 mg/day of betaine). It was reported that a betaine-rich meal providing ≈800 mg/day betaine exerted similar acute health effects (increased circulating betaine concentrations and lessened post-methionine load rise in homocysteine) as did the ≈1 g/day supplement [15]. This supports the idea of dietary adjustments to improve the betaine status of general population. These adjustments may span from an effort to include betaine-rich ingredients in the daily individual diet or to imply strategies of food fortification with betaine.

In the US, betaine is recognized as the Generally Recognized as Safe (GRAS) ingredient while in Europe it has been approved by the European Commission for use in food. In 2012, the European Union Regulatory Authority (Commission Regulation (EU) No. 432/2012) [14] permitted the declaration of a health claim on foods containing at least 500 mg betaine per serving, indicating that health effects may be expected if 1500 mg of betaine is administered daily. The medical statement reads: "Betaine contributes to the normal metabolism of homocysteine". However, this claim should be accompanied with a restriction due to risks associated with excessive intake of betaine: "In order to bear the claim information shall be given to the consumer that a daily intake in excess of 4 g may significantly increase blood cholesterol levels" [14].This work aims to summarize the current findings on the levels of betaine found in cereals and pseudocereals as well as in related products.

2. Experimental Methods used in the Analysis of Betaine

In order to determine the content of betaine in food, different methods have been developed. The most common is the liquid chromatography method, but there is no universal method that can be applied to all food matrices. Saarinen et al. [16] analyzed the content of betaine in the chicken liver using a cation exchange column Ca^{2+} and a refractometric detector, although quantification was limited due to poor sensitivity of the detector. Considering physical-chemical properties of betaine, it cannot be analyzed by conventional reversed phase liquid chromatography. Also, betaine has less absorption in the UV–visible spectrum and cannot be detected by a UV detector without derivatization and therefore it is necessary to use reagents for derivatization. De Zwart et al. [2] derivatized a wide range of foods and analyzed betaine with liquid chromatography and UV detector using various columns. Slow et al. [3] have extracted betaine from various foods by using water and dichloromethane, and by derivatization of betaine with 2-naphthacyl trifluoromethanesulphonate. Hefni et al. [17] developed a simple HPLC-UV method in several different food matrices such as spinach, whole grain wheat flour, wheat, and sugar beet, with the help of derivatization on the cation exchange column. More recently, the same group has used the same method to analyze 14 cereal samples, representing different genera and cultivars [18]. Bruce et al. [19] and Ross et al. [11] performed the betaine analysis using LC-MS/MS (liquid chromatography with mass spectrometry) and HILIC (hydrophilic interactions liquid chromatography) column. Bruce et al. [19] developed the LC-MS/MS method for the analysis of 47 blood samples, 32 grains of cereals and cereal fractions, and 51 cereal products. Additionally, Ross et al. [11] analyzed betaine with LC-MS/MS in a wide range of commercially available cereals and cereal fractions. Also, recently Servillo et al. [4] have used LC-ESI-MS/MS for determination of different betaines present in commercial flours of cereals and pseudocereals. Instead of a conventional UV detector for the quantitative determination of betaine in order to avoid derivatization, the evaporative light scattering detector (ELSD) detector is used more recently and as a universal detector that provides a stable base line even in a gradient mode that can detect the majority non-volatile analytes. Shin et al. [20] have proposed a HILIC column in combination with an ELSD detector for betaine analysis. HILIC is an alternative to reverse phase chromatography, namely a type of normal phase chromatography, in which the stationary phase is polar but larger amounts of organic solvents can be used as a mobile phase as opposed to ordinary normal phase chromatography. Kojić et al. have used the HPLC-ELSD system using the HILIC column with isocratic mode of operation [21].

3. Cereal Grains as a Source of Betaine

Data on the distribution of betaine in various cereals and pseudocereals are scarce and there is definitely a lack of detailed study. Most data come from various studies that were focused on estimation of betaine dietary intake. Nevertheless, available studies report on wide variations in betaine content in cereals. Different types of cereals may have different amounts of betaine [22]. The following ranges were found by de Zwart et al. [2]: 270–1110 μg/g (dry solids) in wheat flour, and 200–1000 μg/g in oats. More detailed overview of betaine levels in various cereals and pseudocereals from different studies is displayed in Table 1. The displayed data showed that betaine content spanned in wide ranges within the studied grains. According to Corol et al. [22], betaine content in cereals varies depending on multiple factors including genotype and environmental differences such as geographical and/or year-to-year variations and their interactions with genotype. This study revealed a three-fold difference in glycine betaine content within bread wheat genotypes and a 3.8-fold difference across six environments. The highest glycine betaine levels were found in Hungarian wheat grains whereas the lowest in those grown in the UK [22]. Slow et al. [3] and de Zwart et al. [2] indicated that the level of betaine depends on the level of stress under which the crop grows. This is due to osmoprotectant and cryoprotectant function of betaine. For example, growth under drought can cause higher levels of betaine compared to well-watered crops.

Table 1. Betaine content in different samples of cereals and pseudocereals.

Cereals and Pseudocereals	Betaine (μg/g Dry Weight)	References
Wheat (*Triticum aestivum*)		
raw grain	1150–1320	[18]
	490–574	[23]
bran	5047–5383	[23]
	2717	[21]
	2300–7200	[3]
aleurone	4538–6242	[11]
germ	3414	[11]
wholegrain flour	792	[11]
	730 *	[24]
	604	[19]
	540	[23]
refined flour	718 *	[25]
	700 *	[24]
	415–593	[21,23]
	398	[11]
	180 *	[4]
	141.2	[19]
flour (not specified by origin)	270–1110	[2]
Wheat Emmer (*T. dicoccum*)		
raw grain	830–940	[18]
refined flour	195 *	[4]
Wheat Einkorn (*T. monococcum*)		
refined flour	367.3 *	[4]
Durum wheat (*T. durum*)		
semolina	1227	[23]
	483	[21]
	683	[11]
refined flour	253–303	[23]
	310	[21]
wholegrain flour	713	[11]
	245 *	[4]
Spelt wheat (*T. aestivum* ssp. spelta)		
raw grain	973–2723	[23]
	565–714	[21]
wholegrain flour	1296–1442	[23]
	1370–1430	[18]
refined flour	978	[11]
	522–593	[23]
	410	[21]
Kamut wheat, Khorasan (*T. turgidum* ssp. turanicum)		
raw grains	1100	[24]
Triticale (xTriticosecale)		
raw grain	986–1030	[23]
Rye		
raw grain	2213	[23]
	1530–1760	[18]
	444	[21]
bran	1651	[19]
refined flour	310 *	[4]
wholegrain flour	1500 *	[24]
	1182	[23]
	986	[21]
Barley		
raw grain	460	[18]
raw grain from naked var.	980	[18]
wholegrain flour	776–1023	[23]
	779	[21]
refined flour	250 *	[4]
flour from naked var	424	[21]
	574	[23]
pearled grain	274	[21]

Table 1. *Cont.*

Cereals and Pseudocereals	Betaine (µg/g Dry Weight)	References
Oats		
raw grain	280	[18]
	388	[21]
raw grain from naked var.	440	[18]
wholegrain flour	310 *	[24]
flour	404–688	[23]
	53 *	[4]
bran	200 *	[24]
	190	[11]
Maize		
raw grain	107–304	[23]
	175	[21]
wholegrain meal	120 *	[24]
degermed meal	4 *	[24]
semolina	3–22	[11]
refined corn grits	37	[11]
flour, enriched	20 *	[24]
refined flour	2.1 *	[4]
bran	184	[21]
	104	[23]
	46 *	[24]
flakes	103–120	[23]
	7–9	[11]
	n.d.	[21]
starch	n.d.	[21]
popped	19	[11]
	n.d.	[21]
Rice		
grain	1–5	[11]
	n.d.	[21]
refined flour	8.4 *	[4]
expanded	n.d.	[21]
starch	n.d.	[21]
Amaranth (*Amaranthus cruentus*)		
raw grain	7420	[23]
	680 *	[24]
	646	[11]
expanded grain	669	[23]
	607	[21]
flour	895–1225	[23]
	871	[21]
Proso millet		
sample type not specified	95–112	[11]
dehulled grain	281	[23]
refined flour	1320 *	[4]
Buckwheat		
wholegrain flour	108	[23]
	7–20	[11]
refined flour	n.d.	[21]
groats, roasted	10 *	[4]
	26 *	[24]
Sorghum		
refined flour	425 *	[4]
Quinoa		
	6300 *	[24]
grains	3042–4428	[11]
	610.8 *	[4]

n.d. not detected; * result expressed on wet weight.

Among glutinous cereals, the highest content of betaine was found in the bran fraction of wheat grain (2300–7200 µg/g) and in the germ (3414 µg/g) (Table 1). In spelt wheat, higher upper betaine levels were detected in comparison to common wheat. Wholegrain spelt flour was much higher in betaine than the wholegrain flour of common wheat (Table 1). Wholegrain flours were mainly higher in betaine when compared to refined flours. Ross et al. [11] estimated that wholegrain flours and products were two to four times higher in betaine in comparison to the refined counterparts. Similar betaine content was found in flour from durum wheat and conventional wheat. In contrast, Ross et al. [11] reported higher levels of betaine in durum semolina in comparison to common, non-refined wheat.

The most abundant source of betaine was amaranth, a pseudocereal. Raw amaranth grains contained 7420 µg/g betaine which was the highest value determined in a single sample [23]. According to Ross et al. [11] and USDA database [24], quinoa can also be listed as an outstanding source of betaine, having been reported to contain 3930 µg/g and 6300 µg/g betaine, respectively.

4. Betaine Content in Cereal-Based Products

The betaine content in cereal products depends on the processing method. Two to four times lower betaine content were found in refined grain products compared to equivalent whole grain products [11]. Betaine content is notably dependent on the loss of bran fraction during processing. The higher the abrasion of aleurone layer, the lower the betaine content in the product. Outstanding betaine levels were determined in wheat bran, up to 7200 µg/g (Table 1). Likes et al. [25] analyzed the betaine contents in different milling streams and reported the lowest betaine level in the cleanest milling fractions. In the study of de Zwart et al. [2], a wide range of different foods was analyzed for betaine content and flour was denoted as an item high in betaine (730 µg/g), however it was not specified the type of flour, except that it was available from retail markets. Betaine ranges in bread, pasta, breakfast cereals and snacks are given in Table 2. As it can be seen, the variation within each product category is high due to versatility of ingredients in product formulations. In each product category, the highest betaine content was reported for wholegrain products or products containing bran or germ. Among breads, rye, spelt, and wholemeal breads were abundant in betaine. Moderate to high betaine contents were reported for pasta products, but it must be noted that mainly uncooked samples were analyzed (Table 2). Breakfast cereals are a mixture of cereal and non-cereal ingredients and the betaine content will depend on the contribution of each ingredient. In the study of Filipčev et al. [23], two samples of commercially available breakfast cereals were analyzed, one of which contained no detectable levels of betaine whereas the other had 471 µg/g (on dry solids). A similar concluded was made by Ross et al. [11] for muesli and muesli bars which were found to contain only low-to-moderate betaine levels. These products were mainly based on oats and contained other low-betaine ingredients such as dried fruits. In contrast to Ross et al. [11], the USDA data [24] report on much wider span of betaine in breakfast cereals, from 7 µg/greaching to as much as 3600 µg/g (on wet weight) betaine.

Table 2. Betaine content in various grain-based products.

Product	Betaine Content (µg/g Dry Weight)	References
Bread		
rye bread	855–1377	[11]
wholegrain spelt	913	[11]
wholemeal	670–790	[3]
wholegrain	499–781	[11]
	560–620	[3]
multigrain	247–678	[11]
white (refined)	360–520	[3]
	174–287	[11]
various (white, sourdough)	310–590 *	[24]
	380 *	[24]
	579	[19]
wheat tortilla	311	[11]

Table 2. *Cont.*

Product	Betaine Content (µg/g Dry Weight)	References
Pasta		
wholegrain wheat pasta	710–1286	[11]
	375	[19]
pasta, not specified	480–1350	[2]
refined wheat pasta	628–706	[11]
refined wheat (*T. aestivum*) pasta, uncooked	253	[21]
durum wheat pasta, uncooked	188	[21]
one–egg spelt pasta	243–516	[11]
barley pasta	211	[11]
noodles with egg, enriched, uncooked	1300 *	[24]
noodles with egg, enriched, cooked	190 *	[24]
refined couscous	691	[11]
bulghur	1311	[11]
cooked bulghur	830 *	[24]
Breakfast cereals		
ready-to-eat wheat germ, toasted, plain	4100 *	[24]
ready-to-eat wheat bran, toasted	3200 *	[24]
wholegrain rye flakes	1640	[11]
wholegrain wheat-based cereals	732–915	[11]
wholegrain oat and wheat-based muesli	310	[11]
wholegrain oat-based muesli	117–226	[11]
breakfast cereals, not specified	180–300	[21]
muesli bar	171	[11]
wholegrain porridge oats	128–167	[11]
extruded whole grain oat cereals	73–91	[11]
cereal bar	74–75	[11]
various ready-to-eat cereals	7–3600 *	[24]
Snacks, cookies, crackers, crispbread, cakes, pastry		
wholegrain rye crispbread	1428–1527	[11]
frozen, read-to-eat pancakes	690–720 *	[24]
wholegrain wheat crackers	293–649	[11]
crackers, classic, saltines, cheese	340–580 *	[24]
wholegrain wheat rusks	556–564	[11]
wholegrain wheat muffin	437–501	[11]
various commercial cakes	190–480 *	[24]
wholegrain wheat biscuit	425	[21]
Graham cookies	390 *	[24]
doughnuts	270–380 *	[24]
English muffins	220–360 *	[24]
extruded spelt	308	[21]
refined wheat crackers	258–332	[11]
digestive biscuit	271–309	[11]
apple pie, commercial	160 *	[24]
biscuit	4–144	[11]
Danish pastry, fruit enriched	140 *	[24]
plain Danish pastry	81 *	[24]

* Result expressed on wet weight.

5. Betaine Content in Gluten-Free Cereal Products

Gluten-free products have been generally recognized to be low in betaine content [11,19]. In the majority of commercially available gluten-free products, a very low level of betaine (<50 µg/g) was observed [11]. Table 3 lists the betaine levels reported for commercial gluten-free products from several studies. In the bread and biscuits category, betaine levels ranged from non-detectable to 107 µg/g. Similar findings were reported by Kojić et al. [21], who also found that gluten-free samples (starch, corn extrudates, pasta, cornflakes, and rice) contained no detectable levels of betaine. Gluten-free cereals contained much lower amounts of betaine in comparison to glutenous cereals: corn had

107–304 μg/g betaine [23]; teff and millet between 50–150 μg/g [11], proso millet 280 μg/g [23]. Buckwheat is a frequent ingredient in gluten-free products. According to Ross et al. [11], buckwheat was among those ingredients low in betaine (<20 μg/g) although as high as 390 μg/g betaine was found in buckwheat uncooked pasta (Table 3).

As mentioned earlier, gluten-free ingredients with appreciable amounts of betaine are amaranth and quinoa. Amaranth grain was reported to contain 646–680 μg/g betaine and a remarkable figure of 7420 μg/g betaine in a single sample of raw grains (Table 1). Processed amaranth contained 817–1225 μg/g of betaine (flour) and 669 μg/g (expandate) (Table 1).

In order to increase betaine levels in gluten-free products and consequently improve dietary intake of betaine among people adhereing to gluten-free and vegan diets, the incorporation of amaranth, quinoa, proso millet, and buckwheat as base ingredients into gluten-free products as well as their enrichment with sugar beet molasses was proposed [11]. Sugar beet molasses can remarkably increase betaine content in some baked products, even when used at fortification levels that do not compromise the sensory properties [26]. It was reported a 43× increase in betaine content of molasses-enriched plain biscuits in comparison to the control biscuit (without molasses) [23]. In gluten-free cookies enriched with molasses at 30% (flour basis), the betaine level was raised ≈64 times [26].

When considering fortification of products with betaine, the challenge is to achieve sufficient delivery of betaine for the claim for lowering blood homocysteine (500 mg/portion). A trial to incorporate betaine in the range from 0.5% to 3% (flour basis) into the formulation of gluten-free biscuits revealed that they were capable of providing from 280 to 1370 mg of betaine per 100 g [27]. The highest fortification level (3%) significantly increased the biscuit spread and contributed to perceiving a weak aftertaste described as burning-like sensations of the tongue and palate which might be due to weak acid reaction of betaine [27]. Rising betaine doses improved color vividness in the biscuits [27]. Similar results were observed in the case of fortifying plain wheat cookies with betaine [28].

Table 3. Betaine content in gluten-free products.

Product	Betaine Content (μg/g Dry Weight)	References
Bread and biscuits		
gluten-free crispbread	9–107	[11]
savory biscuits	n.d.–104	[23]
wholegrain gluten-free bread	12–68	[11]
oatmeal biscuits	3	[11]
gluten-free flour enriched with fibers	1	[11]
sweet biscuits	n.d.	[21]
flour mixture for gluten-free bread	n.d.	[21]
gluten-free cookies with almonds, crackers, salty sticks	n.d.	[21]
expanded maize	n.d.	[21]
Pasta		
buckwheat pasta, uncooked	390	[23]
	382	[11]
	175	[21]
maize-based pasta	2–20	[11]
maize and rice-based pasta, uncooked	n.d.	[21]
rice-based pasta, uncooked	n.d.	[21]
Breakfast cereals and related products		
soy bran	182	[21]
unseasoned popcorn	19	[11]
cornflakes	14	[11]
buckwheat flakes	10	[11]
rice-based breakfast cereals	4–5	[11]
expanded rice	n.d.	[21]

n.d. not detected.

6. Stability of Betaine in Grain-Based Products

Betaine is known to be a thermostable compound which survives the severe treatment during sugar beet processing (extracting with water, treatment with $CaOH_2$ and CO_2, concentration, crystallization) and almost quantitatively accumulates in molasses [29]. Pure anhydrous betaine decomposes at > 245 °C. Since food processing practices do not employ such high temperatures, betaine losses caused by food thermal treatments were initially not expected [30]. However, some data suggest that certain cooking and baking losses of betaine may exist in spite of its thermostability in the pure form. Being a water soluble compound with a small molecule, it is not unlikely that some betaine losses will occur, depending on the type of food processing and cooking.

Only few studies exist that deal with the stability of betaine in food during processing. De Zwart et al. [2] compared the average betaine content in various food, before and after cooking. They concluded that the level of betaine varied widely, depending on the food and cooking method. The lowest losses (10–14%) were observed with microwave cooking of vegetables (frozen peas, silverbeet) and the highest losses with boiling (43–73%) [2]. In the case of cereal-based food, high betaine losses (76–84%) were detected during pasta boiling which could be attributed to dissolution of betaine in cooking water and its removal upon water draining [2]. Betaine reduction of ≈85% between uncooked and cooked noodles was reported in the USDA database [24] (Table 2). Similar results were confirmed by Ross et al. [11] in cooked pasta and noodles. During baking of scones, de Zwart et al. [2] determined a 17% betaine loss. Similar betaine losses were found after baking gluten-free biscuits fortified with betaine at a 0.5–3.0% level [27]. Somewhat higher baking losses in betaine were reported by Filipčev et al. [28] ranging from 17% to 28.6% in wheat biscuits fortified with betaine at 0.5–3.0% level. Very high betaine losses (>90%) were observed after baking betaine-enriched bread [31]. It was assumed that this loss could be partly due to betaine consumption by baker's yeast throughout dough fermentation since yeast can use betaine as a source of nitrogen.

During the preparation of extruded snack products enriched with betaine, the influence of extrusion cooking parameters like screw speed, feed flow rate, and feed moisture on the betaine content was analyzed [32]. The most significant influences on betaine content were feed rate and feed moisture content. Under the most extreme conditions applied during the extrusion process betaine losses were from 50–60% [32].

In some cases, an increase in betaine could be observed after thermal treatment as reported for fried and baked falafel [2] and for oatmeal cooked in a microwave oven [11]. The increases were 9, 14, and 31%, respectively. Ross et al. [11] suggested that a plausible explanation of this phenomenon could be the liberation of betaine from food matrix or betaine synthesis throughout heating. So far, it has not been reported that betaine is capable of forming any bonds with matrix components.

7. Conclusions

Comparison of betaine levels in cereals from different studies showed that cereals are good sources of betaine. Wheat bran and germs were the most abundant wheat fractions. There were large differences in the betaine contents of different cereals. The wholegrain flours from spelt, rye, and barley showed higher betaine levels in comparison to that of common wheat. Non-glutinous cereals are generally moderately to very low in betaine. The best gluten-free sources of betaine are amaranth and quinoa.

Cereal grain processing may lead to lowering of betaine content, especially if removal of aleurone layers is included. Thermal treatment of cereal products also provokes certain loss of betaine, in spite of its thermal stability on food processing temperatures. Losses are very high if processing involves water removal after cooking or boiling, since betaine is soluble in water. Very high losses were observed during baking of betaine-enriched bread, implying that fermentation by baker's yeast may be one of the causes but future research is needed to understand the possible mechanisms.

Fortification of grain-based food with sugar beet molasses even at low or moderate levels considerably raises their betaine content and may be considered as a possible way to increase the functionality of the products.

Acknowledgments: The authors declare the financial support from the Ministry of Education, Science and Technological Development, Serbia, grant III 46005. No funds were received to cover publication costs.

Author Contributions: Nebojša Ilić and Marija Bodroža-Solarov conceived and reviewed the manuscript; Jovana Kojić contributed to data collection, analysis, interpretation, and to writing the paragraph dealing with methods for betaine analysis; Jelena Krulj contributed to data collection, analysis, and interpretation; Bojana Filipčev performed the background research and wrote the manuscript.

References

1. Yancey, P.H.; Clark, M.E.; Hand, S.C.; Bowlus, R.D.; Somero, G.N. Living with stress: Evolution of osmolyte systems. *Science* **1982**, *217*, 1214–1222. [CrossRef] [PubMed]
2. De Zwart, F.J.; Slow, S.; Payne, R.J.; Lever, M.; George, P.M.; Gerrard, J.A.; Chambers, S.T. Glycine betaine and glycine betaine analogues in common foods. *Food Chem.* **2003**, *83*, 197–204. [CrossRef]
3. Slow, S.; Donaggio, M.; Cressey, P.J.; Lever, M.; George, P.M.; Chambers, S.T. The betaine content of New Zealand foods and estimated intake in the New Zealand diet. *J. Food Compos. Anal.* **2005**, *18*, 473–485. [CrossRef]
4. Servillo, L.; D'Onofrio, N.; Giovane, A.; Casale, R.; Cautela, D.; Ferrari, G.; Castaldo, D.; Balestrieri, M.L. The betaine profile of cereal flours unveils new and uncommon betaines. *Food Chem.* **2018**, *239*, 234–241. [CrossRef] [PubMed]
5. Craig, S.A. Betaine in human nutrition. *Am. J. Clin. Nutr.* **2004**, *80*, 539–548. [CrossRef] [PubMed]
6. Olthof, M.R.; Van Vliet, T.; Boelsma, E.; Verhoef, P. Low dose betaine supplementation leads to immediate and long term lowering of plasma homocysteine in health men and women. *J. Nutr.* **2003**, *133*, 4135–4138. [CrossRef] [PubMed]
7. Steenge, G.R.; Verhoef, P.; Katan, M.B. Betaine supplementation lowers plasma homocysteine in healthy men and women. *J. Nutr.* **2003**, *133*, 1291–1295. [CrossRef] [PubMed]
8. Hoffman, J.R.; Ratamess, N.A.; Kang, J.; Rashti, S.L.; Faigenbaum, A.D. Effect of betaine supplementation on power performance and fatigue. *J. Int. Soc. Sports Nutr.* **2009**, *6*, 7–17. [CrossRef] [PubMed]
9. Melnyk, S.; Fuchs, G.J.; Schulz, E.; Lopez, M.; Kahler, S.G.; Fussell, J.J.; Bellando, J.; Pavliv, O.; Rose, S.; Seidel, L.; et al. Metabolic imbalance associated with methylation dysregulation and oxidative damage in children with autism. *J. Autism Dev. Disord.* **2012**, *42*, 367–377. [CrossRef] [PubMed]
10. Jill James, S.; Melnyk, S.; Jernigan, S.; Cleves, M.A.; Halsted, C.H.; Wong, D.H.; Cutler, P.; Bock, K.; Boris, M.; Bradstreet, J.J.; et al. Metabolic endophenotype and related genotypes are associated with oxidative stress in children with autism. *Am. J. Med. Genet.* **2006**, *141B*, 947–956. [CrossRef] [PubMed]
11. Ross, A.B.; Zangger, A.; Guiraud, S.P. Cereal foods are the major source of betaine in the Western diet—Analysis of betaine and free choline in cereal foods and updated assessments of betaine intake. *Food Chem.* **2014**, *145*, 859–865. [CrossRef] [PubMed]
12. Chu, D.M.; Wahlgvist, M.L.; Chang, H.Y.; Yeh, N.H.; Lee, M.S. Choline and betaine food sources and intakes in Taiwanese. *Asia Pac. J. Clin. Nutr.* **2012**, *21*, 547–557. [PubMed]
13. Konstantinova, S.V.; Tell, G.S.; Vollset, S.E.; Ulvik, A.; Drevon, C.A.; Ueland, P.M. Dietary patterns, food groups, and nutrients as predictors of plasma choline and betaine in middle-aged and elderly men and women. *Am. J. Clin. Nutr.* **2008**, *88*, 1663–1669. [CrossRef] [PubMed]
14. European Commission (EC). Commission Regulation (EU) No. 432/2012 of 16 May2012 establishing a list of permitted health claims made on foods, other than those referring to the reduction of disease risk and to children's development and health. *Off. J. Eur. Union* **2012**, *136*, 1–40. Available online: https://www.fsai.ie/uploadedFiles/Reg432_2012.pdf (accessed on 15 August 2015).
15. Atkinson, W.; Slow, S.; Elmslie, J.; Lever, M.; Chambers, S.; George, P. Dietary and supplementary betaine: Effects on betaine and homocysteine concentrations in males. *NMCD* **2009**, *19*, 767–773. [CrossRef] [PubMed]
16. Saarinen, M.T.; Kettunen, H.; Pulliainen, K.; Peuranen, S.; Tiihonen, K.; Remus, J. A novel method to analyze betaine in chicken liver: Effect of dietarymbetaine and choline supplementation on the hepatic betaine concentration in broiler chicks. *J. Agric. Food Chem.* **2001**, *49*, 559–563. [CrossRef] [PubMed]

17. Hefni, M.; McEntyre, C.; Lever, M.; Slow, S. Validation of HPLC-UV methods for the quantification of betaine in foods by comparison with LC-MS. *Food Anal. Methods* **2016**, *9*, 292–299. [CrossRef]
18. Hefni, E.M.; Schaller, F.; Witthöft, M.C. Betaine, choline and folate content in different cereal genotypes. *J. Cereal Sci.* **2018**, *80*, 72–79. [CrossRef]
19. Bruce, S.J.; Guy, P.A.; Rezzi, S.; Ross, A.B. Quantitative measurement of betaine and free choline in plasma, cereals and cereal products by isotope dilution LC-MS/MS. *J. Agric. Food Chem.* **2010**, *58*, 2055–2061. [CrossRef] [PubMed]
20. Shin, H.D.; Suh, J.H.; Kim, J.H.; Lee, H.Y.; Eom, H.Y.; Kim, U.Y.; Youm, J.R. Determination of betaine in Fructus Lycii using hydrophilic interaction liquid chromatography with evaporative light scattering detection. *Bull. Korean Chem. Soc.* **2012**, *33*, 553–558. [CrossRef]
21. Kojić, J.; Krulj, J.; Ilić, N.; Lončar, E.; Pezo, L.; Mandić, A.; Bodroža-Solarov, M. Analysis of betaine levels in cereals, pseudocereals and their products. *J. Funct. Foods* **2017**, *37*, 157–163. [CrossRef]
22. Corol, D.I.; Ravel, C.; Raksegi, M.; Bedo, Z.; Charmet, G.; Beale, M.H.; Ward, J.L. Effects of genotype and environment on the contents of betaine, choline, and trigonelline in cereal grains. *J. Agric. Food Chem.* **2012**, *60*, 5471–5481. [CrossRef] [PubMed]
23. Filipčev, B.V.; Brkljača, J.S.; Krulj, J.A.; Bodroža-Solarov, M.I. The betaine content in common cereal-based and gluten-free food from local origin. *Food Feed Res.* **2015**, *42*, 129–137. [CrossRef]
24. Patterson, K.Y.; Bhagwat, S.A.; Williams, J.R.; Howe, J.C.; Holden, J.M. USDA Database for the Choline Content of Common Foods—Release 2. Available online: http://www.ars.usda.gov/SP2UserFiles/Place/12354500/Data/Choline/Choln02.pdf (accessed on 5 January 2018).
25. Likes, R.; Madl, R.L.; Zeisel, S.H.; Craig, S.A.S. The betaine and choline content of a whole wheat flour compared to other mill streams. *J. Cereal Sci.* **2007**, *46*, 93–95. [CrossRef] [PubMed]
26. Filipčev, B.; Mišan, A.; Šarić, B.; Šimurina, O. Sugar beet molasses as an ingredient to enhance the nutritional and functional properties of gluten-free cookies. *Int. J. Food Sci. Nutr.* **2016**, *67*, 249–256. [CrossRef] [PubMed]
27. Filipčev, B.; Krulj, J.; Brkljača, J.; Šimurina, O.; Jambrec, D.; Bodroža-Solarov, M. Fortification of gluten-free biscuits with betaine. In Proceedings of the 8th International Congress FLOUR-BREAD'15 and 10th Croatian Congress of Cereal Technologists, Opatija, Croatia, 29–30 October 2015; Koceva-Komlenić, D., Ed.; Faculty of Food Technology Osijek, University of Osijek: Osijek, Croatia, 2016; pp. 92–98. Available online: http://www.ptfos.unios.hr/joomla/znanost/flour-bread/images/PDF/proceedings_FB15_web.pdf (accessed on 16 October 2016).
28. Filipčev, B.; Krulj, J.; Kojić, J.; Šimurina, O.; Bodroža Solarov, M.; Pestorić, M. Quality attributes of cookies enriched with betaine. In Proceedings of the III International Congress "Food Technology, Quality and Safety-FOODTECH", Novi Sad, Serbia, 25–27 October 2016; Đuragić, O., Ed.; Institute of Food Technology, University of Novi Sad: Novi Sad, Serbia; pp. 46–51.
29. Šušić, S.; Sinobad, V. Ispitivanja u cilju unapređenja industrije šećeraJugoslavije. *Hem. Ind.* **1989**, *43* (Suppl. 1–2), 10–21.
30. The Scientific Panel on Dietetic Products, Nutrition and Alergies. Opinion on the scientific panel on dietetic products, nutrition and allergies on a request from the Commission related to an application concerning the use of betaine as a novel food in the EU. *EFSA J.* **2005**, *191*, 1–17.
31. Filipčev, B.; Šimurina, O.; Brkljača, J.; Krulj, J.; Bodroža-Solarov, M.; Popov, S. Nutritional quality and baking performance of bread enriched with betaine. In Proceedings of the 11th Symposium "Novel Technologies and Economic Development", Leskovac, Serbia, 23–24 October 2015; Lazić, M., Ed.; Faculty of Technology in Leskovac, University of Niš: Leskovac, Serbia; pp. 83–88.
32. Kojić, J.S.; Ilić, N.M.; Kojić, P.S.; Pezo, L.L.; Banjac, V.V.; Krulj, J.A.; Bodroža-Solarov, M.I. Twin-Screw Extrusion of Spelt Flour Enriched with Betaine—Multi-Objective Optimization Approach. In preparation.

13

Use of Selected Lactobacilli to Increase γ-Aminobutyric Acid (GABA) Content in Sourdough Bread Enriched with Amaranth Flour

Manuel Venturi [1], Viola Galli [2,*], Niccolò Pini [2], Simona Guerrini [1] and Lisa Granchi [2]

1 FoodMicroTeam s.r.l., Via di Santo Spirito, 14, 50125 Florence, Italy; manuel@foodmicroteam.it (M.V.); simona@foodmicroteam.it (S.G.)
2 Department of Agriculture, Food, Environment and Forestry (DAGRI), University of Florence, Piazzale delle Cascine, 18, 50144 Florence, Italy; niccolo.pini@unifi.it (N.P.); lisa.granchi@unifi.it (L.G.)
* Correspondence: viola.galli@unifi.it

Abstract: γ-Aminobutyric acid (GABA) is the primary inhibitory neurotransmitter of the central nervous system and possesses various physiological functions. GABA production can be obtained thanks to lactic acid bacteria activity in different foods such as sourdoughs. Recently, breads made from blends of pseudocereals and wheat flours have attracted much attention. Amaranth is especially interesting because of its high nutritional value, having a high protein content and containing different antioxidant compounds. Therefore, this study aimed to obtain sourdough breads enriched with GABA thanks to bacterial activity and to investigate the effect of amaranth flour addition on the antioxidant and sensorial properties of bread. Eighteen lactobacilli strains were assayed for GABA production in amaranth and wheat flour liquid sourdoughs. Two strains, *Lactobacillus brevis* A7 and *Lactobacillus farciminis* A11, demonstrated high GABA producing capability; hence, they were used to prepare breads containing 20% amaranth flour. The results confirmed the capability of the two strains to increase GABA concentrations (up to 39 mg/kg) in breads. Samples with amaranth addition showed a significantly higher total phenolic content compared to the control bread (more than 15 mg GAE 100 g^{-1} dwb); sensory analysis showed that breads with amaranth were moderately acceptable. Nevertheless, their general liking evaluation was significantly lower compared to the control bread. The addition of pseudocereal to traditional wheat sourdough and selection of lactobacilli allowed the production of baked goods with enhanced GABA content and antioxidant capacity, but recipes have to be developed to increase the organoleptic acceptability of the final products.

Keywords: sourdough; γ-aminobutyric acid GABA; amaranth flour; lactobacilli; bioactive compounds

1. Introduction

Sourdough fermentation represents a traditional biotechnology able to improve and enhance the overall quality of leavened bakery goods obtained using a wide variety of flours [1]. Due to the activity of the occurring microbiota (lactic acid bacteria and yeasts) and the long fermentation times, sourdough positively influences the final products, improving flavour, texture, shelf-life, and above all the nutritional and functional features of the final product [2–4]. Particularly, the metabolic capability of lactic acid bacteria (LAB) is fundamental to obtain these distinctive characteristics. For instance, microbial activities toward cereal proteins, such as decarboxylation, deamination, transamination, and side chain modification, may lead to the production of several compounds which have an impact both on the nutritional quality and the flavour of bakery products [5–9]. In this context, the production of bioactive compounds, such as γ-aminobutyric acid (GABA), by LAB during sourdough fermentation could be particularly attractive [10,11]. γ-aminobutyric acid, a non-protein aminoacid, has several physiological functions in humans: Diuretic and hypotensive activity, a tranquillizing effect, and it acts as an inhibitory neurotransmitter in sympathetic brain function [10,12–15]. In fact, foods fortified with GABA are efficient in the regulation of sleeplessness, autonomic disorders, and depression [10,16]. GABA is produced from the irreversible α-decarboxylation of L-glutamic acid, catalysed by a specific enzyme, glutamic acid decarboxylase (GAD), found in bacteria, plants and animals [5,10,17]. Some works have already shown the presence of GAD activity in LAB [18–20]. In this regard, fermented foods represent an excellent source of dietary GABA [5]. Furthermore, as a stable part of diet worldwide, cereal-based products enriched with GABA are of particular interest. GABA enrichment of baked goods by exploiting selected LAB, belonging to various species, has been obtained using different flours [10,11,18,19,21]. Diana et al. [11] used a strain of *Lactobacillus brevis*, isolated from cheese, for the manufacture of wheat bread with a final GABA content of 24.2 mg/100 g. Strains of *Lactococcus lactis* and *Lactobacillus plantarum* isolated from cheese were used for the production of a bread GABA enriched, using a mixture of pseudocereals and leguminous flours [18]. The selection of peculiar cereals or pseudocereals, based on their nutritional potential, may be very useful to improve the technological and functional features of baked goods [22]. Indeed, the successful replacing of standard wheat flour with unconventional flours pseudocereal or legume flours has been demonstrated [22,23]. Whole pseudocereal grains such as quinoa, amaranth, and buckwheat have abundant content of different compounds, i.e., vitamins, fatty acids, flavonoids and phenolic acids, with a known positive impact on human health [24–27]. For these reasons, an increment of these cereals' consumption in the daily human diet has been recommended [24,28–30]. Among the pseudocereal group, amaranth is of particular interest because of its high nutritional value, having a high protein content, a high concentration of essential aminoacids [31], and containing different antioxidant compounds. Hence, the potential of sourdough fermentation, combined with amaranth supplement, could be a tool to develop new healthy baked products. Nevertheless, the sensory quality of the final products has to be taken into account since it is strongly influenced by the addition of amaranth flour [32]. Therefore, this study aimed to screen GABA-producing lactobacilli in order to obtain naturally GABA-enriched sourdough breads, and concurrently to investigate the effect of 20% addition of amaranth flour on the antioxidant properties of the final products. The sensory quality of the breads was also evaluated to determine the contribution of lactobacilli fermentation and amaranth flour addition on the organoleptic characteristics.

2. Materials and Methods

2.1. Lactobacilli Strains and Culture Conditions

Eighteen lactobacilli strains of five species (*L. brevis*, *L. farciminis*, *L. plantarum*, *L. rossiae* and *L. sanfranciscensis*), previously isolated from six Italian sourdoughs and belonging to the culture collection of the Department of Agriculture, Food, Environment and Forestry (DAGRI) of the University of Florence, were used in this study (Table 1).

Table 1. Lactobacilli strains and the isolation source.

Lactobacilli Strains	Italian Sourdough
L. brevis A7; *L. farciminis* A11	*Schiacciata* (flat, salty bread)
L. brevis B1; *L. sanfranciscensis* B3; *L. farciminis* B5; *L. farciminis* B7; *L. rossiae* B6; *L. farciminis* B8	Bread
L. plantarum C2	Tuscan bread
L. brevis Ga1; *L. rossiae* Ga11; *L. rossiae* Ga12; *L. rossiae* Ga14; *L. sanfranciscensis* Gd44; *L. rossiae* Gd63	*Lagaccio* biscuit
L. farciminis H3	Ancient grain bread
L. rossiae O1; *L. plantarum* O4	*Panettone* cake

2.2. Liquid Sourdough Fermentations

The lactobacilli strains, grown overnight in MR3i broth [33], were singly inoculated (9.0 log CFU/mL) into wheat and amaranth flour doughs. The sourdoughs were prepared by mixing water and flour to obtain a dough yield (DY), i.e., the percent ratio of the weight of the dough to the weight of the flour, of 333 and 667, for wheat and amaranth liquid sourdoughs, respectively. The samples were incubated for 6 h at 30 °C under stirring conditions (ca. 100 rpm). Control and acid control doughs (acidified to pH 3.5 by lactic acid addition) without bacterial inoculum were prepared and incubated under the same conditions. At the end of the fermentation time, sourdough samples were taken in order to perform analysis of GABA content and select the highest-GABA-producing lactobacilli strains.

2.3. Sourdough Fermentation and Bread Making

Six breads were prepared according to the recipes reported in Table 2. For each bread, a prefermented dough was prepared. Four doughs were inoculated with only baker's yeast (termed as PFC W, PFAC W, PFC Am and PFAC Am) and two with the inoculum of baker's yeast and the selected lactobacilli strains: *Lactobacillus brevis* A7 and *Lactobacillus farciminis* A11 (termed PFSD A7 and PFSD A11, respectively) (Table 2).

Table 2. Recipes for pre-fermented dough manufacture and bread making and related dough yield (dough weight × 100/flour weight). PF—prefermented; C—control; AC—acid control; SD—sourdough; W—wheat flour; Am—Amaranth flour; A7—*L. brevis* A7 strain; A11—*L. farciminis* A11 strain.

	Prefermented Dough					
Ingredients (% on Total Flour)	**PFC W**	**PFAC W**	**PFC Am**	**PFAC Am**	**PFSD A7**	**PFSD A11**
Wheat flour	100	100	80	80	80	80
Amaranth flour	–	–	20	20	20	20
Water	58	58	58	58	58	58
Baker's yeast	1	1	1	1	1	1
L. brevis A7 (log (CFU/g))	–	–	–	–	9	–
L. farciminis A11 (log (CFU/g))	–	–	–	–	–	9
	Bread					
Ingredients (% on total flour)	**C W**	**AC W**	**C Am**	**AC Am**	**SD-A7**	**SD-A11**
Prefermented dough	50	50	50	50	50	50
Wheat flour	100	100	80	80	80	80
Amaranth flour	–	–	20	20	20	20
Water	58	58	58	58	58	58
Dough yield	158	158	158	158	158	158

Amaranth flour was added as 20% of the total flour in four doughs; acid control doughs were acidified by lactic acid to 3.5. The prefermented doughs were fermented for 18 h at 30 °C and then added to the final mixtures. In the final dough (Table 2) the ingredients were added at the same time and mixed for 10 min in a twin arms mixer (model RS12, Bernardi, Italy). The doughs were placed in the trays at 30 °C with 88–90% relative humidity for 3 h. Samples were taken at the beginning and at the end of the leavening time. Finally, doughs were baked at 180 °C for 15 min.

2.4. Monitoring of Selected Lactobacilli Strains in Sourdough Fermentations

A Randomly Amplified Polymorphic DNA (RAPD) analysis was performed according to Venturi et al. [34] to assess the occurrence of the selected lactobacilli in liquid and firm sourdoughs and final doughs. DNA was amplified using the following primers: OPL-05 (50 ACGCAGGCA 30), designed by Seseña et al. [35], and MV1 (50 GGACGCTTCTG 30) designed by Venturi et al. [34]. The random primer MV1 was used separately, while OPL-05 was used along with the primer RD1 (5′ GCTTAAGGAGGTGATCCAGCC 3′). DNA amplification was performed as described by Reguant and Bordons [36]. Amplification products were separated (at 100 V for 2.5 h) on 1.4% (*w*/*v*) agarose gel (Lonza Group Ltd, Basel, Switzerland); containing ethidium bromide (Sigma e Aldrich, St Louis, MI, USA) and TEB buffer (1 M Tris, 10 mM EDTA, 0.9 M boric acid, pH 8.3). The resulting profiles were captured as images after UV transillumination, and compared to those previously obtained for each bacterial strain.

2.5. Determination of pH, Total Titratable Acidity, Volume Increase, and Enumeration of Cultivable Bacteria and Yeasts

Ten grams of dough sample were transferred into 90 mL of sterile physiological solution, homogenized for 2 min in a Stomacher Lab Blender 400 (Seward Ltd, Worthing, West Sussex, UK). After decimal dilutions, 100 μL of these suspensions were plated for cell enumeration using MR3i medium for the lactobacilli and MYPG for the baker's yeast using the pour plate method. Lactobacilli were counted after incubation for 48–72 h at 30 °C under anaerobic conditions. Yeasts, plated on MYPG agar containing sodium propionate (2 g/L), were counted after incubation for 48 h at 30 °C under aerobic conditions. Plate counts were performed in duplicate. The pH values were determined by a pH-meter (Metrohm Italiana Srl, Varese, Italy). Total titratable acidity (TTA) was measured on 10 g of dough samples, which were homogenized with 90 mL of distilled water for 3 min and expressed as the amount (mL) of 0.1 N NaOH to achieve a pH of 8.5. To assess sourdough increase of volume, 100 g of each dough were placed in a graduated cylinder (0.5 L). The volume of the doughs (in mL) was recorded immediately (t_0) and after 3 h of fermentation at 30 °C. The leavening was calculated using the following formula: $((V_3 - V_0)/V_0) \times 100$, where V_3 was the volume after the 3 h fermentation and V_0 was the initial volume.

2.6. Determination of Lactic Acid by HPLC

Bread samples were diluted ten times with distilled water and then filtered by Amicon® Ultra-4 Centrifugal Filters (3000 Da NMWL) (Merck Millipore) before the injection for lactic acid determination by high-performance liquid chromatography (HPLC) analysis (Varian Inc., Palo Alto, CA, USA) connected to a refractive index detector (Knauer K-2301, Knauer GmbH, Berlin, Germany) and UV detector (λ = 210). Elution was performed at 65 °C with 0.01 N H_2SO_4 eluent at a flow rate of 0.6 mL/min. Data were collected and analysed by using the Galaxie software (Varian Inc., Palo Alto, CA, USA). Quantitative analysis was carried out by a standard curve.

2.7. Total Phenols Assay by Folin–Ciocalteau Reagent

Total phenols content of bread samples was determined according to Alvarez-Jubete et al. [37], with some modifications. Bread samples were dried for 24 h at 60 °C and ground. 1.25 g were weighted and added to 25 mL methanol. Samples were vortexed and left in horizontal shaking for 24 h, then centrifuged for 10 min at 2000× *g*. The final extracts were obtained by filtering 10 mL of the supernatant through 0.22 μm PTFE syringe filters (Whatman) and they were stored at −20 °C until analysis. The reaction mixture consisted of 100 μL of methanolic bread extract, 100 μL of methanol, 100 μL of Folin–Ciocalteu reagent and 700 μL of Na_2CO_3. The samples were vortexed immediately, and the tubes were incubated in the dark for 20 min at room temperature. After incubation, all samples were centrifuged at 11,300× *g* for 3 min. The absorbance of the supernatant was then measured at 735 nm in 1 mL plastic cuvette using a spectrophotometer (Cary 50 Scan, Varian Inc., Palo Alto, CA, USA). Gallic acid was used as a standard and a calibration curve was prepared with a range of concentrations from 10−200 mg/L. The results are expressed in mg of gallic acid equivalent per 100 g of dry-weight basis (mg GAE 100 g^{-1} dwb).

2.8. Antioxidant Capacity by DPPH Assay

The free radical scavenging capacity of methanolic bread extracts was determined using the stable 2,2-diphenyl-1-picrylhydrazyl radical (DPPH). The scavenging effect was measured according to the method of Alvarez-Jubete et al. [37]. Also, 500 μL of extracts were added to 500 μL of DPPH methanolic solution (0.05 mg/mL). After vortexing, the mixture was left for 40 min at room temperature, and the absorbance of the resulting solution was read at 517 nm. The absorbance measured after 40 min was used for the calculation of the antioxidant capacity according to the following formula: DPPH radical-scavenging activity (%): ((blank absorbance − sample absorbance)/blank absorbance) × 100. Butylated hydroxytoluene (BHT) was also assayed as antioxidant references.

2.9. HPLC Determination of GABA Content

GABA content was determined on the water-soluble extracts of liquid doughs and breads. The extracts were obtained by extracting the samples with sterile distilled water (1:3 *w*/*v*), held at 4 °C for 1 h and vortexed at 15-min intervals. Samples were finally centrifuged at 14,000× *g* for 20 min. The supernatants, containing the water-soluble fraction, were used for GABA quantification. Before the injection, the samples were prepared according to Tuberoso et al. [38]. The reaction mixture consisted of 100 μL of sample extracts, 5 μL of 100 mg/L eptilammine (internal standard, IS), 200 μL of dansyl chloride solution (derivatization agent) and 0.2 M $Na_2B_4O_7 \cdot 10H_2O$ (pH 9.3) solution up to a final volume of 1000 μL. The mixture was incubated for 30 min at 40 °C in a Termoblok and centrifuged at 11,300× *g* for 10 min. The supernatant was recovered and diluted with MeOH (1:1 *v*/*v*) for HPLC analysis. Separation was obtained with a Phenomenex Gemini C18 110A column (150 4.60 mm, 3 lm; Chemtek Analitica, Anzola Emilia, Bologna, Italy) connected to fluorimetric detector (Jasco Europe, Cremella, LC, Italy) with wavelengths set at 293 nm (Ex) and 492 nm (Em) under the following conditions: Mobile phases buffer acetate/CH_3CN (pH 4.1) and acetonitrile, flow rate 0.8 mL/min, column temperature 25 °C. The quantitative analysis was performed using calibration graphs constructed according to the internal standard method.

2.10. Sensory Evaluation

Sensory evaluation of lactobacilli inoculated breads and non-acidified control breads was carried out by 46 panellists (15 male and 31 female) aged 21–65 years old. Breads were cut into pieces of 3 cm × 3 cm and randomly codified before serving. Colour, aroma, consistency, and general liking were evaluated using the hedonic 9-point scale (from "1-dislike extremely" to "9-like extremely") [39]. Panellists have also optionally chosen among 13 attributes for the taste of breads: Salty, vapid, sweet, earthy, strange taste, sour, delicate, tasty, astringent, not to eat, gummy, interesting, and persistent [24].

2.11. Statistical Analysis

Chemical and microbiological determinations, performed in duplicate, were elaborated according to *t*-Test procedures or nonparametric one-way ANOVA followed by Tukey's Test (Statistica 7.0 software package, Stat Software Inc., Tulsa, OK, USA). Differences were reported at a significance level of $p \leq 0.05$.

3. Results and Discussion

3.1. Selection of GABA-Producing Lactobacilli Strains

Eighteen lactobacilli strains were singly inoculated in liquid doughs made with either wheat or amaranth flour and incubated at 30 °C for 6 h in order to evaluate the GABA production. All the strains were able to acidify the doughs although some differences were registered. The final pH values ranged from ca 3.50–4.10 with an average decrease of 2.35 ± 0.13 in wheat sourdoughs. Due to the lower flour content (DY = 667) and a different buffering capacity, the final pH of amaranth sourdoughs resulted higher, in a range from 4.10–5.10, with an average pH decrease of 1.74 ± 0.41. The most acidifying strains, both in wheat and amaranth flour, were *L. brevis* A7, *L. farciminis* A11, *L. farciminis* B7 and *L. rossiae* Ga12. The values of pH of the non-inoculated doughs (C) were 5.96 ± 0.05 and 6.20 ± 0.11 for wheat and amaranth dough, respectively. After 6 h of fermentation GABA concentrations were determined.

Results showed a variability ($p \leq 0.05$) among the tested strains in both the flours, even if GABA concentrations were generally higher in wheat sourdoughs (Figure 1). Differences in GABA concentration in sourdoughs produced by the two flours could be due to higher glutamic acid content in wheat flour, since it is the substrate for glutamic acid decarboxylase enzyme (GAD). In agreement with the literature, the GABA producing activity was not related to the species, resulting in strain dependency [40]. In wheat sourdoughs, six lactobacilli strains displayed GABA concentrations significantly higher than the control and the acidified control, whereas in amaranth sourdoughs this trend was observed only for one strain (*L. rossiae* Gd63). Particularly, the highest ($p \leq 0.05$) GABA concentration in wheat sourdoughs was found in the dough inoculated with *L. brevis* A7 (136.62 ± 4.00 mg/kg of flour), followed by *L. plantarum* O4, *L. brevis* Ga1, *L. farciminis* H3, *L. rossiae* O1, *L. farciminis* A11. The strain *L. rossiae* Gd63 displayed the highest GABA production in amaranth sourdough fermentation (47.6 ± 14.3 mg/kg of flour), although other six lactobacilli strains (*L. plantarum* C2, *L. brevis* A7, *L. sanfranciscensis* Gd44, *L. brevis* B1, *L. rossiae* Ga14 and *L. farciminis* A11) did not show statistical differences from the GABA amounts produced by the best performing strain. Hence, based on the reported results concerning GABA production and acidification ability, *L. farciminis* A11 and *L. brevis* A7 were selected to prepare firm sourdoughs and breads.

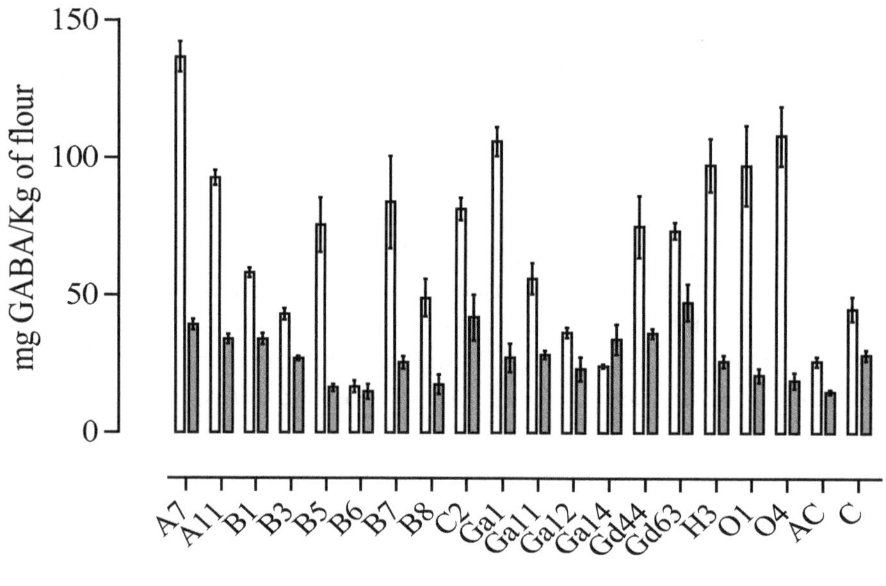

Figure 1. Production of GABA after 6 h fermentation in wheat (white bar) and amaranth (grey bar) sourdoughs obtained with 18 lactobacilli strains singly inoculated (data are expressed as mean ± coefficient of variation %). C—control; AC—acid control.

3.2. Sourdough Bread Fermentation with Selected Lactobacilli Strains

Breads were prepared with the addition of 20% of amaranth flour. This percentage was chosen because it is considered appropriate by various authors in order to maintain product structural quality [41], preserve the principal nutritional benefit of this ingredient [42], and meet sensory approval [43]. Table 3 shows the main technological and microbiological characteristics at the end of fermentation of the sourdoughs prepared with the inoculum of *L. brevis* A7 (SD-A7) and *L. farciminis* A11 (SD-A11). The occurrence of the two inoculated strains throughout the process was confirmed by molecular analysis. In particular, all the lactobacilli isolates from sourdoughs displayed solely the genotypic patterns of *L. brevis* A7 or *L. farciminis* A11.

Table 3. Values (mean ± standard deviation) of pH, Total Titratable Acidity (TTA; mL NaOH), lactic acid (g/kg), volume increase (%), and microorganism (lactobacilli and baker's yeast) concentrations (log (CFU/g)) after sourdough fermentations carried out by *L. brevis* A7 (SD-A7) and *L. farciminis* A11 (SD-A11).

Dough	Final pH	ΔpH	Final TTA	ΔTTA	Lactic acid	ΔV/V0 × 100	Lactobacilli	Yeasts
SD-A7	4.35 ± 0.03 [a]	0.95 ± 0.39 [a]	6.90 ± 0.14 [b]	2.80 ± 0.66 [a]	4.60 ± 0.63 [b]	105 ± 7.07 [a]	8.50 ± 0.72 [a]	7.35 ± 0.64 [a]
SD-A11	4.60 ± 0.18 [b]	0.82 ± 0.10 [a]	6.45 ± 0.07 [a]	2.95 ± 0.78 [a]	3.20 ± 0.56 [a]	105 ± 21.2 [a]	8.59 ± 0.73 [a]	7.40 ± 0.62 [a]

ΔV = difference between the final and the initial value; V_0—initial volume. Values in the same column with different letters (**a**,**b**) are significantly different ($p \leq 0.05$).

The 20% amaranth incorporation did not affect the considered features. At the end of leavening time, both the sourdough pH decreased of about 0.88, reaching a value of 4.35 ± 0.03 for SD-A7 and 4.60 ± 0.18 for SD-A11, statistically different from each other and showing proper acidification [44,45]. SD-A11 final total titratable acidity was lower compared to SD-A7, while the TTA increase did not point out any significant differences. Regarding organic acids production, the highest content of lactic acid was found in SD-A7 dough (4.60 ± 0.63 g/kg). Both the samples doubled their volume, indicating an adequate leavening process. Microbiological analyses did not show any significant differences in the microorganism concentrations at the end of the fermentation. *L. farciminis* A11 and *L. brevis* A7 reached a concentration of about 8.55 log CFU/g, which is a typical value in sourdough [46], and *S. cerevisiae* reached a concentration of 7.37 log CFU/g.

3.3. Phenolic Content and Antioxidant Capacity of Breads

The results of the total phenolic content, determined on the methanolic extracts of all the breads, are shown in Figure 2.

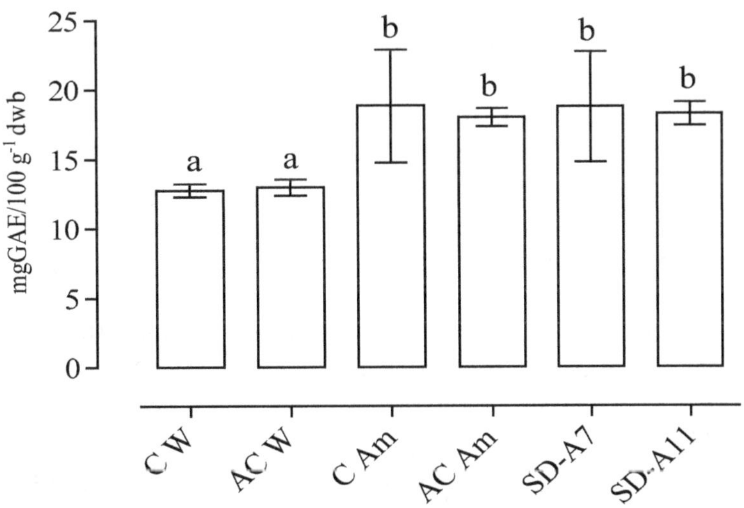

Figure 2. Total phenolic content (expressed as mg of gallic acid equivalents GAE100 g^{-1} dwb) of the breads (data are expressed as mean ± coefficient of variation %). C W—wheat control bread; AC W—wheat acid control bread; C Am—amaranth control bread; AC Am—amaranth acid control bread; SD-A7—*L. brevis* A7 bread; SD-A11—*L. farciminis* A11 bread. Different letters (**a**,**b**) indicate significant differences ($p \leq 0.05$).

Results indicated that amaranth flour addition significantly increased the phenolic content of breads. Indeed, whole pseudocereal grains are rich in this class of minor components, therefore their use as a supplement can increase the nutritional value of baked goods. Data showed that samples integrated with 20% of amaranth flour displayed a phenolic content of more than 15 mg GAE 100 g^{-1} dwb, which was significantly higher than the control breads, C W and AC W, made only with wheat flour ($p \leq 0.05$). These results are in agreement with those reported by Chlopicka et al. [24], which showed a higher content of phenolic compounds in breads enriched with amaranth flour, compared to a control bread without this pseudocereal addition.

The radical-scavenging capacity of the breads was tested by the DPPH method (Figure 3).

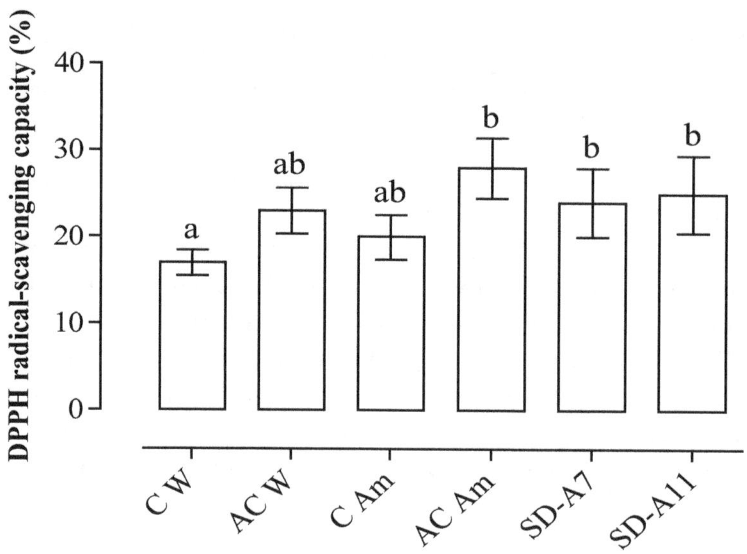

Figure 3. Radical-scavenging capacity (%) of the breads (data are expressed as mean ± coefficient of variation %). C W—wheat control bread; AC W—wheat acid control bread; C Am—amaranth control bread; AC Am—amaranth acid control bread; SD-A7—*L. brevis* A7 bread; SD-A11—*L. farciminis* A11 bread. Different letters (**a**,**b**) indicate significant differences ($p \leq 0.05$).

The antioxidant capacity of control bread made with only wheat flour result was the lowest among the samples (less than 17%), while AC Am, SD-A7 and SD-A11 showed the highest values ($p \leq 0.05$), up to 28%. According to Vollmannova et al. [47], total phenolic content was partially correlated to the antioxidant capacity; indeed, AC Am, SD-A7 and SD-A11 showed the highest values for both these parameters. Amaranth addition only slightly increased the antioxidant capacity, on the contrary, the acidification seems to have a higher role in increasing this activity. In fact, both the chemically acidified controls showed higher values than the controls. Hence, the combination of amaranth addition and acidification might be responsible of the observed phenomenon. In this context, it was demonstrated that acidification, as a consequence of microbial fermentation, can increase the levels of easily-extractable phenolic compounds and their bioavailability [4,48,49].

3.4. GABA Content of Breads

GABA concentrations in the breads prepared by lactobacilli inoculated sourdoughs and in the control breads are reported in Figure 4.

GABA content in the breads ranged from 8.0–39.0 mg/kg. Sourdough breads showed the highest concentration with values of 26.9 ± 1.53 and 39.0 ± 1.53 mg/kg for SD-A7 and SD-A11, respectively, confirming the capability of LAB to produce GABA. The lowest content was detected in the control breads with 100% of wheat flour, less than 10 mg/kg. Compared to the control wheat breads, the GABA increase of SD-A11 was of about 350%. Other studies exploited high GABA producing biotype of *Lactobacillus plantarum* and *Lactococcus lactis* in order to obtain a bread with improved nutritional features [10,18,19]. The ability of *L. brevis* strains to synthetize GABA was reported in various food matrices such as cheese [40], yoghurt [50], black raspberry juice [51], and wheat sourdough [11], while this capability was observed only in a strain of *L. farciminis* isolated from Myanmar traditional fermented fishery products with boiled rice [52]. To the best of our knowledge, this was the first time in which GABA production by a strains of *L. farciminis* was exploited in a bakery product.

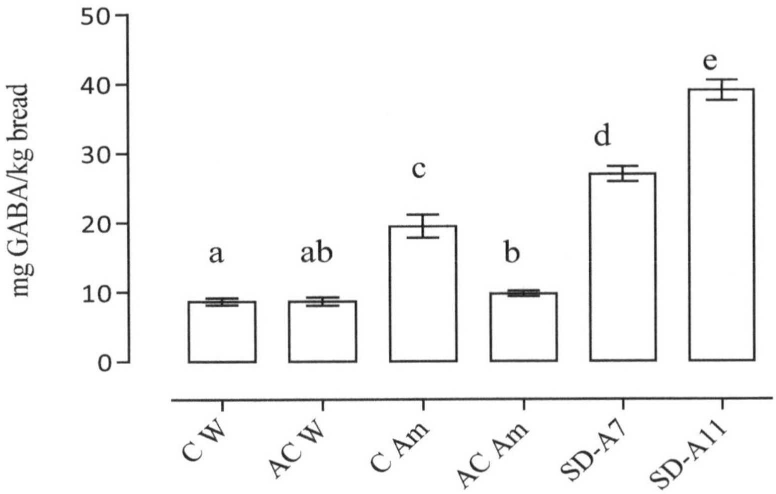

Figure 4. GABA concentration (mg/kg) in the breads (data are expressed as mean ± standard deviation). C W—wheat control bread; AC W—wheat acid control bread; C Am—amaranth control bread; AC Am—amaranth acid control bread; SD-A7—*L. brevis* A7 bread; SD-A11—*L. farciminis* A11 bread. Different letters (**a**–**c**) indicate significant differences ($p \leq 0.05$).

3.5. Sensory Evaluation

To evaluate the contribution of amaranth flour and lactobacilli fermentation on organoleptic characteristics of breads, a sensory evaluation was carried out with a panel of 46 members. Table 4 shows the results of a 9-point hedonic scale analysis of colour, odour, consistency, and general liking.

Table 4. Sensory evaluation of breads (mean ± standard deviation). Values were determined with a 9-point scale (extremely disliked = 1, neither like, nor dislike = 5, extremely liked = 9). C W—wheat control bread; C Am—amaranth control bread; SD-A7—*L. brevis* A7 bread; SD-A11—*L. farciminis* A11 bread.

	C W	C Am	SD-A7	SD-A11
Colour	6.7 ± 1.3 ^{a}	6.2 ± 1.2 ^{a}	6.1 ± 1.2 ^{a}	6.0 ± 1.5 ^{a}
Aroma	6.1 ± 1.5 ^{a}	5.6 ± 1.6 ^{a}	5.6 ± 1.5 ^{a}	5.3 ± 2.0 ^{a}
Consistency	6.3 ± 1.4 ^{b}	5.8 ± 1.6 ^{ab}	5.1 ± 1.6 ^{a}	5.2 ± 1.5 ^{a}
General liking	6.3 ± 1.5 ^{b}	5.3 ± 1.6 ^{a}	4.9 ± 1.6 ^{a}	4.9 ± 1.8 ^{a}

Values in the same column with different letters (**a**,**b**) are significantly different ($p \leq 0.05$).

Values of colour and aroma were not significantly different among the breads, ranging from 6–6.7 and from 5.3–6.1, hence indicating a moderate appreciation. On the contrary, the consistency of bread was negatively affected by the addition of amaranth flour; in fact, the best value was registered for the control wheat bread (6.3 ± 1.4), statistically higher ($p \leq 0.05$) compared to the inoculated amaranth breads (5.1–5.2). General liking of the 100% wheat control bread showed a significantly higher value (6.3 ± 1.5) compared to bread with amaranth replacement; however, none of the breads were negatively evaluated by the panellists. These results pointed out that substituting 20% of wheat flour with amaranth flour in bread was not advantageous for bread sensory evaluation, even if the panellists gave a moderate appreciation. In addition, other authors [42] reported that, considering the better nutritional features, consumers would choose to consume amaranth bread instead of common wheat bread, even if the taste is different. Furthermore, the spider plot in Figure 5 shows the different attributes chosen by panellists to describe breads.

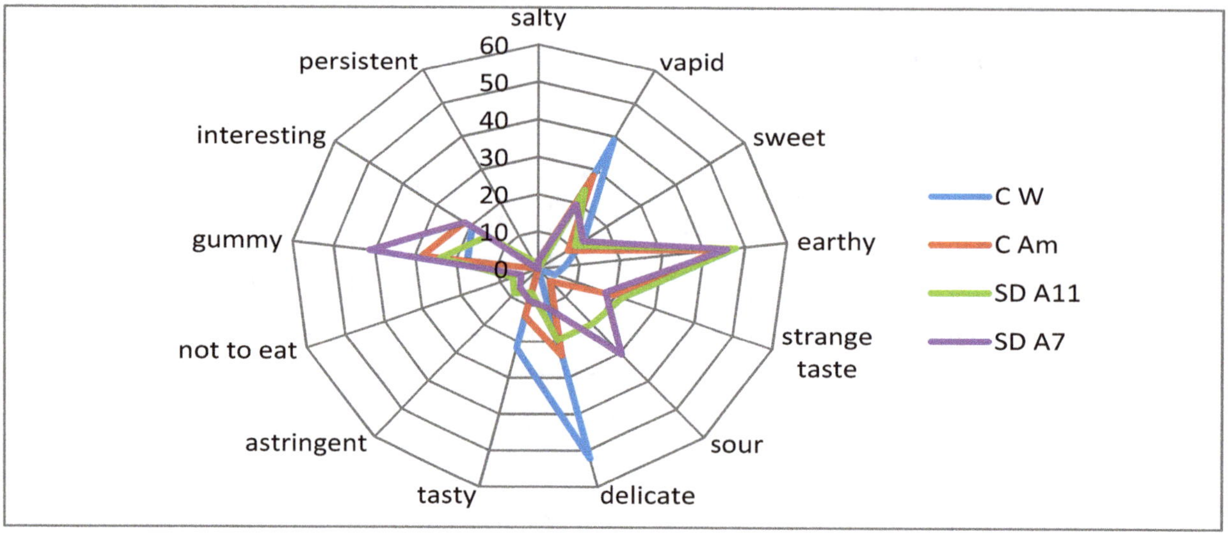

Figure 5. Spider plot of the sensory evaluation (%) of breads. Blue line: % of positive answers given to wheat control bread (C W); red line: % of positive answers given to amaranth control bread (C Am); green line: % of positive answers given to *L. farciminis* A11 sourdough bread (SD-A11); purple line: % of positive answers given to *L. brevis* A7 sourdough bread (SD-A7).

Amaranth clearly characterized bread for earthy taste (about 50% panellists for all the amaranth breads). More than 50% panellists defined the wheat control bread as delicate, even if 40% also defined breads as vapid with respect to 20–30% of the breads with amaranth. In particular, panellists declared that SD-A7 bread was sour (30%) and gummy (more than 40%). Nevertheless, about 20% of panellists described as interesting the taste of all the breads, and only a few testers (about 5%) declared SD amaranth breads "not to eat", in contrast with the 10–30% reported in other experiments [24]. Sensory analysis highlighted some differences between the two sourdough amaranth breads. SD-A7 bread taste was described as less delicate, gummier, and sourer, but also more interesting compared to SD-A11 bread. However, results showed that the 20% amaranth incorporation did not strongly reduce the breads' appreciation.

4. Conclusions

The screening of GABA-producing lactobacilli in liquid sourdoughs led to the selection of two strains belonging to *L. farciminis* and *L. brevis* species. These strains were able to increase GABA concentration (up to 350%) in breads enriched with 20% of amaranth flour, with a final content of 26.9 ± 1.53 and 39.0 ± 1.53 mg/kg respectively. The final products showed higher antioxidant activity and an increased content of total phenolic compounds compared to the wheat control bread. Sensory evaluation indicated moderate acceptability of breads with amaranth flour, mainly characterized by an earthy taste. Although organoleptic acceptability of the final products could be improved, the combination of selected lactobacilli and pseudocereal flours can be a suitable tool for the production of innovative baked goods with improved nutritional features.

Author Contributions: Conceptualization, M.V. and V.G.; methodology, M.V. and V.G.; formal analysis, M.V., V.G. and N.P.; investigation, M.V., V.G. and N.P.; data curation, M.V., V.G. and L.G.; writing—original draft preparation, M.V. and V.G; writing—review and editing, M.V., V.G., S.G. and L.G.; supervision, S.G. and L.G.

References

1. Chavan, R.S.; Chavan, S.R. Sourdough technology—A traditional way for wholesome foods: A review. *Compr. Rev. Food Sci. Food Saf.* **2011**, *10*, 169–182. [CrossRef]
2. Arendt, E.K.; Ryan, L.A.; Dal Bello, F. Impact of sourdough on the texture of bread. *Food Microbiol.* **2007**, *24*, 165–174. [CrossRef] [PubMed]
3. Hammes, W.P.; Gänzle, M.G. Sourdough breads and related products. In *Microbiology of Fermented Foods*, 2nd ed.; Woods, B.J.B., Ed.; Blackie Academic: London, UK, 1998; pp. 199–216.
4. Gobbetti, M.; De Angelis, M.; Di Cagno, R.; Calasso, M.; Archetti, G.; Rizzello, C.G. Novel insights on the functional/nutritional features of the sourdough fermentation. *Int. J. Food Microbiol.* **2018**. [CrossRef] [PubMed]
5. Diana, M.; Quílez, J.; Rafecas, M. Gamma-aminobutyric acid as a bioactive compound in foods: A review. *J. Funct. Foods* **2014**, *10*, 407–420. [CrossRef]
6. Di Cagno, R.; De Angelis, M.; Lavermicocca, P.; De Vincenzi, M.; Giovannini, C.; Faccia, M.; Gobbetti, M. Proteolysis by sourdough lactic acid bacteria: Effects on wheat flour protein fractions and gliadin peptides involved in human cereal intolerance. *Appl. Environ. Microbiol.* **2002**, *68*, 623–633. [CrossRef]
7. Gänzle, M.G.; Loponen, J.; Gobbetti, M. Proteolysis in sourdough fermentations: Mechanisms and potential for improved bread quality. *Trends Food Sci. Technol.* **2008**, *19*, 513–521. [CrossRef]
8. Gobbetti, M.; Rizzello, C.G.; Di Cagno, R.; De Angelis, M. How the sourdough may affect the functional features of leavened baked goods. *Food Microbiol.* **2014**, *37*, 30–40. [CrossRef]
9. Paterson, A.; Piggott, J.R. Flavour in sourdough breads: A review. *Trends Food Sci. Technol.* **2006**, *17*, 557–566. [CrossRef]
10. Bhanwar, S.; Bamnia, M.; Ghosh, M.; Ganguli, A. Use of *Lactococcus lactis* to enrich sourdough bread with γ-aminobutyric acid. *Int. J. Food Sci. Nutr.* **2013**, *64*, 77–81. [CrossRef]
11. Diana, M.; Rafecas, M.; Quílez, J. Free amino acids, acrylamide and biogenic amines in gamma-aminobutyric acid enriched sourdough and commercial breads. *J. Cereal Sci.* **2014**, *60*, 639–644. [CrossRef]
12. Huang, J.; Mei, L.H.; Wu, H.; Lin, D.Q. Biosynthesis of γ-aminobutyric acid (GABA) using immobilized whole cells of *Lactobacillus brevis*. *World J. Microbiol. Biot.* **2007**, *23*, 865–871. [CrossRef]
13. Komatsuzaki, N.; Shima, J.; Kawamoto, S.; Momose, H.; Kimura, T. Production of γ-aminobutyric acid (GABA) by *Lactobacillus paracasei* isolated from traditional fermented foods. *Food Microbiol.* **2005**, *22*, 497–504. [CrossRef]
14. Komatsuzaki, N.; Tsukahara, K.; Toyoshima, H.; Suzuki, T.; Shimizu, N.; Kimura, T. Effect of soaking and gaseous treatment on GABA content in germinated brown rice. *J. Food Eng.* **2007**, *78*, 556–560. [CrossRef]
15. Su, Y.C.; Wang, J.J.; Lin, T.T.; Pan, T.M. Production of the secondary metabolites γ-aminobutyric acid and monacolin K by *Monascus*. *J. Ind. Microbiol. Biot.* **2003**, *30*, 41–46. [CrossRef] [PubMed]
16. Okada, T.; Sugishita, T.; Murakami, T.; Murai, H.; Saikusa, T.; Horino, T.; Onoda, A.; Kajimoto, O.; Takahashi, R.; Takahashi, T. Effect of the defatted rice germ enriched with GABA for sleeplessness, depression, autonomic disorder by oral administration. *J. Jpn. Soc. Food Sci.* **2000**, *47*, 596–603. [CrossRef]
17. Ueno, H. Enzymatic and structural aspects on glutamate decarboxylase. *J. Mol. Catal. B-Enzym.* **2000**, *10*, 67–79. [CrossRef]
18. Coda, R.; Rizzello, C.G.; Gobbetti, M. Use of sourdough fermentation and pseudo-cereals and leguminous flours for the making of a functional bread enriched of γ-aminobutyric acid (GABA). *Int. J. Food Microbiol.* **2010**, *137*, 236–245. [CrossRef] [PubMed]
19. Rizzello, C.G.; Cassone, A.; Di Cagno, R.; Gobbetti, M. Synthesis of angiotensin I-converting enzyme (ACE)-inhibitory peptides and γ-aminobutyric acid (GABA) during sourdough fermentation by selected lactic acid bacteria. *J. Agric. Food Chem.* **2008**, *56*, 6936–6943. [CrossRef]
20. Villegas, J.M.; Brown, L.; de Giori, G.S.; Hebert, E.M. Optimization of batch culture conditions for GABA production by *Lactobacillus brevis* CRL 1942, isolated from quinoa sourdough. *LWT-Food Sci. Technol.* **2016**, *67*, 22–26. [CrossRef]
21. Lamberts, L.; Joye, I.J.; Beliën, T.; Delcour, J.A. Dynamics of γ-aminobutyric acid in wheat flour bread making. *Food Chem.* **2012**, *130*, 896–901. [CrossRef]
22. Coda, R.; Di Cagno, R.; Gobbetti, M.; Rizzello, C.G. Sourdough lactic acid bacteria: Exploration of non-wheat cereal-based fermentation. *Food Microbiol.* **2014**, *37*, 51–58. [CrossRef] [PubMed]

23. Schoenlechner, R.; Siebenhandl, S.; Berghofer, E. Pseudocereals. In *Gluten-Free Cereal Products and Beverages*, 1st ed.; Arendt, E.K., Dal Bello, F., Eds.; Academic Press: New York, NY, USA, 2008; p. 149-VI.
24. Chlopicka, J.; Pasko, P.; Gorinstein, S.; Jedryas, A.; Zagrodzki, P. Total phenolic and total flavonoid content, antioxidant activity and sensory evaluation of pseudocereal breads. *LWT-Food Sci. Technol.* **2012**, *46*, 548–555. [CrossRef]
25. Gorinstein, S.; Vargas, O.J.M.; Jaramillo, N.O.; Salas, I.A.; Ayala, A.L.M.; Arancibia-Avila, P.; Toledo, F.; Katrich, E.; Trakhtenberg, S. The total polyphenols and the antioxidant potentials of some selected cereals and pseudocereals. *Eur. Food Res. Technol.* **2007**, *225*, 321–328. [CrossRef]
26. Kalinova, J.; Dadakova, E. Rutin and total quercetin content in amaranth (*Amaranthus* spp.). *Plant. Food. Hum. Nutr.* **2009**, *64*, 68. [CrossRef]
27. Li, S.Q.; Zhang, Q.H. Advances in the development of functional foods from buckwheat. *Crit. Rev. Food Sci.* **2001**, *41*, 451–464. [CrossRef]
28. Lin, L.Y.; Liu, H.M.; Yu, Y.W.; Lin, S.D.; Mau, J.L. Quality and antioxidant property of buckwheat enhanced wheat bread. *Food Chem.* **2009**, *112*, 987–991. [CrossRef]
29. Paśko, P.; Sajewicz, M.; Gorinstein, S.; Zachwieja, Z. Analysis of selected phenolic acids and flavonoids in *Amaranthus cruentus* and *Chenopodium quinoa* seeds and sprouts by HPLC. *Acta Chromatogr.* **2008**, *20*, 661–672. [CrossRef]
30. Richardson, D.P. Wholegrain health claims in Europe. *Proc. Nutr. Soc.* **2003**, *62*, 161–169. [CrossRef]
31. Nimbalkar, M.S.; Pai, S.R.; Pawar, N.V.; Oulkar, D.; Dixit, G.B. Free amino acid profiling in grain Amaranth using LC–MS/MS. *Food Chem.* **2012**, *134*, 2565–2569. [CrossRef]
32. Jekle, M.; Houben, A.; Mitzscherling, M.; Becker, T. Effects of selected lactic acid bacteria on the characteristics of amaranth sourdough. *J. Sci. Food Agric.* **2010**, *90*, 2326–2332. [CrossRef]
33. Galli, V.; Venturi, M.; Pini, N.; Guerrini, S.; Granchi, L.; Vincenzini, M. Liquid and firm sourdough fermentation: Microbial robustness and interactions during consecutive backsloppings. *LWT-Food Sci. Technol.* **2019**, *105*, 9–15. [CrossRef]
34. Venturi, M.; Guerrini, S.; Granchi, L.; Vincenzini, M. Typing of *Lactobacillus sanfranciscensis* isolates from traditional sourdoughs by combining conventional and multiplex RAPD–PCR profiles. *Int. J. Food Microbiol.* **2012**, *156*, 122–126. [CrossRef] [PubMed]
35. Seseña, S.; Sánchez, I.; Palop, L. Characterization of *Lactobacillus* strains and monitoring by RAPD-PCR in controlled fermentations of "*Almagro*" eggplants. *Int. J. Food Microbiol.* **2005**, *104*, 325–335. [CrossRef]
36. Reguant, C.; Bordons, A. Typification of *Oenococcus oeni* strains by multiplex RAPD-PCR and study of population dynamics during malolactic fermentation. *J. Appl. Microbiol.* **2003**, *95*, 344–353. [CrossRef] [PubMed]
37. Alvarez-Jubete, L.; Wijngaard, H.; Arendt, E.K.; Gallagher, E. Polyphenol composition and in vitro antioxidant activity of amaranth, quinoa buckwheat and wheat as affected by sprouting and baking. *Food Chem.* **2010**, *119*, 770–778. [CrossRef]
38. Tuberoso, C.I.G.; Congiu, F.; Serreli, G.; Mameli, S. Determination of dansylated amino acids and biogenic amines in *Cannonau* and *Vermentino* wines by HPLC-FLD. *Food Chem.* **2015**, *175*, 29–35. [CrossRef] [PubMed]
39. Corona, O.; Alfonzo, A.; Ventimiglia, G.; Nasca, A.; Francesca, N.; Martorana, A.; Moschetti, G.; Settanni, L. Industrial application of selected lactic acid bacteria isolated from local semolinas for typical sourdough bread production. *Food Microbial.* **2016**, *59*, 43–56. [CrossRef]
40. Siragusa, S.; De Angelis, M.; Di Cagno, R.; Rizzello, C.G.; Coda, R.; Gobbetti, M. Synthesis of γ-aminobutyric acid by lactic acid bacteria isolated from a variety of Italian cheeses. *Appl. Environ. Microbiol.* **2007**, *73*, 7283–7290. [CrossRef]
41. Ayo, J.A. The effect of amaranth grain flour on the quality of bread. *Int. J. Food Prop.* **2001**, *4*, 341–351. [CrossRef]
42. Sanz-Penella, J.M.; Wronkowska, M.; Soral-Smietana, M.; Haros, M. Effect of whole amaranth flour on bread properties and nutritive value. *LWT-Food Sci. Technol.* **2013**, *50*, 679–685. [CrossRef]
43. Sindhuja, A.; Sudha, M.L.; Rahim, A. Effect of incorporation of amaranth flour on the quality of cookies. *Eur. Food Res. Technol.* **2005**, *221*, 597. [CrossRef]
44. Minervini, F.; Lattanzi, A.; De Angelis, M.; Di Cagno, R.; Gobbetti, M. Influence of artisan bakery-or laboratory-propagated sourdoughs on the diversity of lactic acid bacterium and yeast microbiotas. *Appl. Environ. Microbiol.* **2012**, *78*, 5328–5340. [CrossRef] [PubMed]

45. Ventimiglia, G.; Alfonzo, A.; Galluzzo, P.; Corona, O.; Francesca, N.; Caracappa, S.; Moschetti, G.; Settanni, L. Codominance of *Lactobacillus plantarum* and obligate heterofermentative lactic acid bacteria during sourdough fermentation. *Food Microbiol.* **2015**, *51*, 57–68. [CrossRef] [PubMed]
46. Lattanzi, A.; Minervini, F.; Di Cagno, R.; Diviccaro, A.; Antonielli, L.; Cardinali, G.; Cappelle, S.; De Angelis, M.; Gobbetti, M. The lactic acid bacteria and yeast microbiota of eighteen sourdoughs used for the manufacture of traditional Italian sweet leavened baked goods. *Int. J. Food Microbiol.* **2013**, *163*, 71–79. [CrossRef] [PubMed]
47. Vollmannova, A.; Margitanova, E.; Tóth, T.; Timoracka, M.; Urminska, D.; Bojňanská, T.; Čičová, I. Cultivar influence on total polyphenol and rutin contents and total antioxidant capacity in buckwheat, amaranth, and quinoa seeds. *Czech J. Food Sci.* **2013**, *31*, 589–595. [CrossRef]
48. Liukkonen, K.H.; Katina, K.; Wilhelmsson, A.; Myllymaki, O.; Lampi, A.M.; Kariluoto, S.; Piironen, V.; Heinonen, S.M.; Nurmi, T.; Adlercreutz, H.; et al. Process-induced changes on bioactive compounds in whole grain rye. *Proc. Nutr. Soc.* **2003**, *62*, 117–122. [CrossRef] [PubMed]
49. Poutanen, K.; Flander, L.; Katina, K. Sourdough and cereal fermentation in a nutritional perspective. *Food Microbiol.* **2009**, *26*, 693–699. [CrossRef]
50. Park, K.B.; Oh, S.H. Production of yogurt with enhanced levels of gamma-aminobutyric acid and valuable nutrients using lactic acid bacteria and germinated soybean extract. *Bioresour. Technol.* **2007**, *98*, 1675–1679. [CrossRef]
51. Kim, J.Y.; Lee, M.Y.; Ji, G.E.; Lee, Y.S.; Hwang, K.T. Production of γ-aminobutyric acid in black raspberry juice during fermentation by *Lactobacillus brevis* GABA100. *Int. J. Food Microbiol.* **2009**, *130*, 12–16. [CrossRef]
52. Thwe, S.M.; Kobayashi, T.; Luan, T.; Shirai, T.; Onodera, M.; Hamada-Sato, N.; Imada, C. Isolation, characterization, and utilization of γ-aminobutyric acid (GABA)-producing lactic acid bacteria from Myanmar fishery products fermented with boiled rice. *Fish. Sci.* **2011**, *77*, 279–288. [CrossRef]

14

Nanoparticles and Controlled Delivery for Bioactive Compounds: Outlining Challenges for New "Smart-Foods" for Health

MCarment Martínez-Ballesta [1], Ángel Gil-Izquierdo [2], Cristina García-Viguera [2] and Raúl Domínguez-Perles [2,*]

1 Department of Plant Nutrition, Centro de Edafología y Biología Aplicada del Segura-Spanish Council for Scientific Research (CEBAS-CSIC), Campus de Espinardo 25, 30100 Espinardo, Murcia, Spain; mballesta@cebas.csic.es

2 Research Group on Quality, Safety and Bioactivity of Plant Foods, Department of Food Science and Technology, Centro de Edafología y Biología Aplicada del Segura-Spanish Council for Scientific Research (CEBAS-CSIC), Campus de Espinardo 25, 30100 Espinardo, Murcia, Spain; angelgil@cebas.csic.es (A.G.-I.); cgviguera@cebas.csic.es (C.G.-V.)

* Correspondence: rdperles@cebas.csic.com or rdperles@cebas.csic.es

Abstract: Nanotechnology is a field of research that has been stressed as a very valuable approach for the prevention and treatment of different human health disorders. This has been stressed as a delivery system for the therapeutic fight against an array of pathophysiological situations. Actually, industry has applied this technology in the search for new oral delivery alternatives obtained upon the modification of the solubility properties of bioactive compounds. Significant works have been made in the last years for testing the input that nanomaterials and nanoparticles provide for an array of pathophysiological situations. In this frame, this review addresses general questions concerning the extent to which nanoparticles offer alternatives that improve therapeutic value, while avoid toxicity, by releasing bioactive compounds specifically to target tissues affected by specific chemical and pathophysiological settings. In this regard, to date, the contribution of nanoparticles to protect encapsulated bioactive compounds from degradation as a result of gastrointestinal digestion and cellular metabolism, to enable their release in a controlled manner, enhancing biodistribution of bioactive compounds, and to allow them to target those tissues affected by biological disturbances has been demonstrated.

Keywords: phytochemicals; nanoparticles; controlled release; improved functionality; health; smart-formulations

1. Introduction

In the late 1980s, Dr. Stephen De Felice first coined the term "nutraceuticals" that was defined as "as foods, food ingredients, or dietary supplements with demonstrated specific health or medical benefits, including the prevention and treatment of disease beyond basic nutritional functions" [1]. Nutraceuticals, in general, have been strongly suggested as candidates for the development of chemo-preventive agents, regarding several pathophysiological situations based in the experimental results retrieved from a range of studies [2]. Hence, upon the extensive research developed so far, some of their mechanisms of action that involve competencies to modulate multiple molecular pathways, without eliciting toxic side effects, have been demonstrated [1].

In recent years, and in close connection with the application of the promising chemo-preventive agents, technological advancements have allowed describing nano-biotechnology as a powerful tool to create and enhance the utility of nano-size materials [3], especially concerning the administration of bioactive phytochemicals in the frame of medical treatments [4]. In this respect, diverse types of nanoparticles have been tested for various uses. For instance, nano-silver has been widely used aimed to take advantage of its toxicity against a broad spectrum of microbes responsible, for instance, for superficial skin and nail infections in humans [5], in addition to oral and vulvovaginal corruptions [6]. Based on the recently gathered knowledge, one of the most relevant advantages of implementing this technology is to control the delivery of bioactive compounds, providing new and valuable responses to the current challenges for new "smart-foods", able to promote human health and wellbeing. In this regard, this work reviews critically the recent advances on nanotechnology-related administration of bioactive compounds and its socio-economic implications.

Societal Impact of Nanobased Technological Innovations for Food and Health

In recent years, nanotechnology has been noticed as one of the most important fields with clear socio-economic impact in several fields of activity. In this aspect, it has been estimated that the private sector has invested around 150 billion US dollars in the development of nanotechnology and application models during 2015. Regarding this, the number of products that incorporate nanoparticles in their formulations has enhanced, accounting for more than 1800 products containing nanomaterials, produced by 622 companies [7]. This new application alternative has been possible due to the 3.7 billion US dollars investment by USA, upon the National Nanotechnology Initiative, followed by the European Union and Japan, which have invested up to 1.2 billion and 750 million dollars, respectively, per year. If this evolution continues, in 2020, the worldwide economy could be supported by nanotechnologies, with an input of 3 trillion US dollars [8].

Nowadays, and regarding the Science and Technology of Foods, the application by the industry of the knowledge generated regarding nanotechnology is mainly focused on agriculture, foodstuffs transformation, packaging, and storage, and the production of dietary supplements [9]. Indeed, during food processing, the advances achieved so far have focused on nutrient delivery, considering distinct issues that deserve to be depth studied, such as the preservation of the physico-chemical features of foods (taste and color), and their safety, stability, bioavailability, and bioactivity. Regarding this, the use of new nanosystems might result in great interest to achieve additional application for the currently most widely characterized bio-functional compounds. Indeed, nanoencapsulation is a very valuable approach that could allow controlling bioactives' release and their pathophysiological relevance, as well as their preservation after oral ingestion, with relevant applications for human health. As an example of such applications, structural lipids have been explored as carriers of healthy component applied for the inhibition of cholesterol transport from the digestive system to the bloodstream [10]. Thus, resorting to the research results, colloids, emulsions, biopolymers, liposomes, solid–lipid nanoparticles, and nanofibers have demonstrated an indubitable utility as vehicles of functional compounds [11].

Nonetheless, despite the increasing use of nanomaterials and the high number of derived commercial applications, nowadays, there are some concerns regarding the potential risk for human health derived from their use, as well as on the extent in which the inclusion of nanomaterials in foods formulation could compromise foods safety. Indeed, in this concern, one of the main matters of debate nowadays is focused on unravelling the extent to which nanoparticles and the bioactive compounds carried by them are competent to access to tissues naturally protected by biological barriers such as the blood–brain barrier [12,13], as well as the toxicological effects that this transportation could cause that have not been properly addressed so far.

Depending on the nature of nanoparticles, as well as the surrounding environment, the materials currently used can be aggregated, modifying their chemical properties, size, and shape [14]. These changes could result in an altered nanomaterial form and, in this sense, some reports have been focused on the evaluation of nanomaterials toxicity when they form part of a particular matrix [15]. To date, the gap in information existing in these concerns entails a lack of consensus about toxicity and direct/indirect consequences on health. As a result, the legislation governing the use of nanoparticles does not elucidate clearly this situation, being almost limited to the requirement of labeling food products containing nanomaterials. In 2009, the European Food Safety Authority published "The Potential Risks Arising from Nanoscience and Nanotechnologies on Food and Feed Safety" as an official document, while the European Union legislation differs depending if intended use of a specific nanocarrier is as a primary ingredient or constitutes a food additive [16]. However, the soft demand of the industry for incorporating this technology to production chains has prompted to a lack of a regulatory frame for the use of nanotechnologies in foods. In any event, to extend the utilization of this promising technology with industrial purposes, the advance of the desirable features of nanoparticles in diverse food matrixes constitutes an important challenge that deserves to be explored towards an enhanced use of such materials, according to their specific properties, at the time that contribute to preserve safety and bioactivity.

2. Biocompatible and Biodegradable Nanoparticles: Looking for the Best Option

2.1. *Solid Nanoparticles as Attractive Drug Vehicles: Composition and Properties*

A variety of nutrients and non-nutrients has been identified, regarding their biological activity once ingested by diet, being responsible for a diversity of biological activities, closely related with the promotion of human health. However, bioactive compounds from nutrients such as lipid derivatives (plant and mammals oxylipins), bioactive peptides, minerals and vitamins, as well as non-nutrients (phytochemicals), can be degraded as a result of the gastrointestinal digestion. Moreover, diverse barriers must be crossed by these compounds, which route towards the bloodstream, and the final distribution to cells and tissues, including their absorption at gastric or intestinal levels. During last decades, the search for effective carriers for bioactive compounds and drugs has been based on the identification of new alternatives for oral administration with health-promoting purposes, avoiding their early inactivation [17,18], because these factors limit the bioavailability of actives or drugs [19]. According to the results retrieved in recent years, nanoencapsulation developed using particles with diameters ranging from 1 to 100 nm enables augmented concentrations of bioactive compounds in cells and tissues, enhancing also shelf-life (reducing the metabolization and excretion of bioactive compounds) through a slowdown delivery [20]. Given these advantages, and aimed to optimize the benefits for health derived from nutraceutical formulations, regarding antioxidant, antiradical, and antitumor abilities, among others, the industry has boosted the research on this technology.

Upon evaluating the profits of implementing nanotechnology in agro-food industries, it has been noticed that nanoparticles have some advantages that deserve to be further explored. For instance, specific high surface zone of nanomaterials has been related to an enhanced number of functional groups, available for chemical reactions, relative to free functional compounds [14]. In addition, the class of relationships between nanocarriers and bioactive nutrients and non-nutrients, and the high area/volume ratios, contribute in some cases to suitable formulations, in which the adhesive properties of the nanocapsules led to prolonged transits of functional compounds through the gastrointestinal tract. This situation lets them reach unaltered specific areas, where their liberation provides enhanced benefits. Consequently, an augmentation of its absorption and bioavailability is achieved [21–23]. Moreover, additional constraints associated to the inclusion of bioactive compounds in the food matrix, such as the effect of light, temperature or oxygen, which compromise their stability and, thus, the bioactivity of the compounds of interest, can be attenuated using nanoparticles [24,25].

Among the nanometric size delivery systems, there are different types of encapsulation, which are classified depending not only on their nature, but also on the production method, properties of the system, the system free energy, the interaction force in the system, etc. [14]. To date, the most suitable nanoparticles with marked potential, regarding distribution of bioactive compounds, are lipid-based delivery systems, which may comprise solid–lipid nanoparticles, liposomes, and micelles, as well as protein- and polysaccharides-based biopolymeric nanoparticles. Specific structural properties of these nanosystems, as well as their low cost and non-toxic nature, make them suitable carriers in food delivery compared to others, such as synthetic polymeric nanoparticles [26]. In addition to nanoparticles, another nanotechnology application for the administration of bioactive compounds are nanoemulsion droplets, formed by dispersion or high-energy and low-energy emulsification methods. Although the main application of nanoemulsions is the preparation where droplets work as nanoreactors, nowadays new specific applications are being envisaged concerning controlled drug delivery and targeting [27].

2.1.1. Lipid Nanoparticles

In the frame of nanotechnology, lipid-based systems are mainly represented by solid–lipid nanoparticles and nanostructured lipid carriers that have been commercially introduced as nanocarriers of functional compounds, in the last years, mainly due to their natural composition and biocompatibility. They can be made of different lipids, including fatty acids, steroids, and waxes to monoglycerides, diglycerides, and triglycerides [28]. A typical percentage ratio fat/aqueous medium of 0.1:30.0 (*w*/*w*) has been considered for developing solid–lipid nanoparticles [29] that feature spherical morphology and can be visualized, for instance, by transmission electron microscopy [30]. Particle size and stability can be affected by their lipid composition and the surfactant properties.

Within lipid nanoparticles, there are advantages associated to the use of liposomes that constitute nanosize artificial vesicles suitable to be obtained from phospholipids and cholesterol. In this concern, recently, the role of these vesicles as immunological adjuvants and drug carriers has been revealed [30, 31]. Thus, it seems evident that several advantages can be obtained from using liposomes as carriers of bioactive compounds, including their capacity to encapsulate diverse bioactive compounds featured by a range of polarities, which are included into the aqueous core of the phospholipid vesicle or at the bilayer interface, and their structural versatility [32]. Besides, an interesting characteristic of liposomes is that they are obtained from natural lipids, being thus biodegradable, biologically inactive, and without antigenic, pyrogenic, or intrinsic toxicity [33,34]. the compounds within these nanoparticles are preserved from the deleterious activity of external factors, especially concerning enzymes and inhibitors present in the gastrointestinal tract [35]. Based on these benefits, liposomes are increasingly used by the pharmaceutical industry to control the release of several compounds of interest, because of their biological activity (drugs, vaccines, and enzymes) in the prevention of a range of pathological situations [32,36–38]. Nonetheless, liposomes are not absolutely free of drawbacks, as nanocarriers, due to their instability in plasma [39]. In this regard, nowadays, it is required to develop an evasion system to enhance the circulation time of these nanoparticles that would results in an augmented concentration in vascularized tissues [40], especially in cases involving active neoangiogenesis.

Apart from liposomes, micelles are very slim spherical additional lipid molecules of 10 to 100 nm formed in aqueous solutions [41]. These nanoparticles have been revealed as a valuable alternative to improve bioavailability and retention of bioactive phytochemicals, since they provide appropriate protection to these compounds against inactivation reactions by surrounding factors, and constitute an alternative featured by even higher loading capacity and improved stability [41,42]. the release of bioactive compounds from micelles is conditioned by an array of factors, including micelle stability, rate of bioactive compounds diffusion, the partition coefficient, the rate of copolymer biodegradation, the drug concentration within the micelles, the molecular weight, and the physicochemical features of the bioactive phytochemical and its location within the micelles [43,44]. Interestingly, release from micelles can also be enhanced in the targeted area by certain stimuli, such as pH, temperature, ultrasound, and light [45]. Thus, besides providing innovative solution to the solubility and long circulation of bioactive nutrients and non-nutrients, micelles contribute to a more efficient internalization and the proper localization within the separate cell compartments, where the biological activity of the compounds carried is required. This is extremely important because it helps take the highest advantage of the specific mechanism of action from the entrapped bioactive compounds [46], also contributing to higher concentrations at the organic site affected by pathological situations, thus decreasing side effects relatively to systemic administration [47].

Additionally, niosomes are microscopic lamellar structures formed upon non-ionic surfactant of alkyl or dialkyl polyglycerol ether class and cholesterol [48]. These lipid-based nanoparticles are structurally similar to liposomes, constituting an effective alternative to these carriers. Indeed, given their features as non-ionic particles, they seem to be less toxic, while providing an improved therapeutic index for bioactive compounds [49]. Moreover, the niosome vesicles are osmotically active and stable, and, thus, may act as a storage system, providing the controlled delivery of bioactive compounds. Thus, they augment oral bioavailability of compounds with limited absorption, allowing to envisage different therapeutic applications [50–53] and use as diagnostic imaging agents [49].

Solid–lipid nanoparticles share some features with nanoemulsions, such as low cost, good release profile, stability, scalable for industrial production, and food safety [54]. As described for nanoemulsions, when considering solid–lipid nanoparticles, the bioactive compounds are situated in the core of particle; however, higher stability and ability to withhold phytochemicals in the nanosystem complex has been described in relation to emulsions or liposomes [55].

Despite the promising features of solid–lipid nanoparticles, some potential disadvantages have been associated to these nanocarriers [55,56]. Regarding this, the loading capacity is one of the major constraints described so far. This seems to be a consequence of the crystallization or transformation of lipids. Hence, the use of nanostructured lipid carriers could be an alternative to overcome this constraint. Indeed, in nanostructured lipid carriers, although the lipid particles are also solid, the use of specific lipids, such as isopropyl myristate or hydroxyl octacosanyl, avoids crystallization at low temperatures [54].

2.1.2. Polysaccharide Nanoparticles

In respect to biocompound delivery systems based on biocompatible materials, it is remarkable that those developed resorting to polysaccharides have been stressed as a valuable alternative to achieve controlled and prolonged release of bioactive phytochemicals [57]. In this aspect, the application of this type of compounds is reinforced by their amphiphilic nature that allows self-assembly in aqueous environments and helps to form specific structures [58,59]. Besides, polysaccharides feature a high affinity to mucosal cell layers in the respiratory and gastrointestinal tracts [60] that turns nanoparticles developed using these compounds into very valuable alternatives to enhance the bioavailability of the bioactive compounds of interest.

Based on the intrinsic charge of polysaccharide materials, they are classified into polyelectrolytes that include cationic, anionic and neutral subtypes, and non-polyelectrolytes [61]. Besides the intrinsic advantages noticed for this type of biocompatible material, it has recently been demonstrated that coat materials, applied on nanoparticles developed using polysaccharides, can interact with specific receptors in cells and tissues. the description of this interaction has allowed envisaging active and site-specific controlled targeting for compounds carried in polysaccharide nanoparticles [60].

Concerning cationic polyelectrolytes, chitosan, which is composed of repeated units of D-glucosamine, has been described as a non-toxic, biodegradable, and bioadhesive material that provides the advantages of control of release of encapsulated agents, complexation with negative charged macromolecules, avoidance of toxic solvents during preparation, and prolonged residence time at the site of absorption due to its mucoadhesive nature [62]. Indeed, the latter is one of the major advantages for the administration of compounds of interests against nasal, oral, ocular, and dermal disorders [63]. Several factors condition the preparation, conformation, and loading of chitosan nanoparticles, affecting their ability to delivery compounds [62]. In addition, chitosan nanoparticles are suitable to be modified by adding specific ligands that contribute to a more rapid and efficient interaction with cells membranes, and thus, to an enhanced delivery of bioactive compounds [64].

In respect to anionic polysaccharide nanoparticles alginate, heparin, pectin, and hyaluronic acid are important to mention [62]. An overview of the interest of these nanoparticles indicates that alginate features biocompatibility, biodegradability, non-antigenicity, and mucoadhesive features [65–67], which make it an interesting candidate for controlled delivery of bioactive compounds [62]. Regarding the mechanism of release, the electrostatic interaction between carboxyl groups and divalent ions mediates the formation of cross-linked gels, with a close relationship with the release of bioactive compounds [62], thus the data reported in the literature indicate these nanoparticles are a valuable alternative delivery system suitable for incorporating positively charged compounds. Interestingly, a combination of alginate and chitosan has been pointed out as an alternative system for the controlled delivery of bioactive compounds that could contribute to extend the circulation time, relatively to alginate and/or chitosan alone [62].

Apart from alginate, hyaluronic acid nanoparticles feature high aqueous solubility and stability, and are non-toxic and non-immunogenic, which have given rise to a reduced number of systems with potential on passive tumor targeting [68], since they exhibit affinity to hyaluronan receptors with a high expression pattern in tumor cells and, therefore, with high potential to carry bioactive compounds, specifically identified concerning anti-tumor activity, that could release in the precise site, contributing to increase their bioactivity.

Finally, in respect to neutral compounds, represented by dextran, pullulan, and pectin [62], the presence of hydroxyl groups modulates the incorporation of bioactive molecules in the base skeleton. Within this class of nanoparticles, dextran, for instance, has been used to design delivery systems able to escape the reticuloendothelial system, thus enhancing the circulation time of the bioactive compound of interest [62].

2.1.3. Protein Nanoparticles

To date, diverse arguments have been proposed supporting the use of protein nanoparticles: (1) simple manufacturing by just heating protein solutions; (2) absence of requirement of emulsification performance; and (3) compatibility with the high pressure emulsification process. Moreover, protein nanoparticles feature high freeze–thaw stability, since the particles at the interface provide good stearic stabilization [69]. To date, different types of nanoparticles have been described, which are synthesized resorting to diverse classes of molecules. Actually, protein nanoparticles can be obtained with a plethora of lab approaches, each of them with its advantages and constraints. However, when compared with additional compounds suggested as nanoparticles for carrying bioactive compounds, protein-based nanoparticles have various advantages, namely the abundance of proteins in nature, their suitability to be transformed, and the absence of deleterious effects concerning the biological systems in which they are applied.

the first classification of protein-based nanoparticles refers to their origin (animal or plant proteins). the diverse types are associated to benefits and constraints, mainly regarding toxicity and/or infections associated to their application (animal proteins), while plant proteins provide the advantage of their hydrophobic characteristics because, which is associated with a lack of toxicity and a lower economic cost [70]. Besides, the surface features of protein-based nanoparticles are susceptible to be modified due to the occurrence of functional groups, which is of crucial relevance for obtained desired biodistribution, biocompatibility, molecules carrying capacity, and stability [70]. In addition, the surface amino groups, characteristics of proteins, allow the addition of hydrophilic polymers, such as polyethylene glycol that augment the circulation time [71]. the loading efficiency of protein-based nanoparticles is closely related to the isoelectric point. When assessing the compounds loading to the protein nanoparticles, it is noticed that the total amount of bioactive compounds is determined by monitoring (ultraviolet (UV)-spectrophotometry, fluorescence spectrophotometry or high performance liquid chromatography (HPLC)) the non-entrapped compounds present in the supernatants. This constitutes critical information for setting up the correct administration of the bioactive compounds. Additional features that should be considered regarding protein-based nanoparticles are the delivery of the compounds carried and the biodegradation of the nanoparticles, being both interdependent reactions [69].

2.1.4. Nanoemulsions

As mentioned before, the application of nanoemulsion droplets, to the controlled delivery of bioactive compounds, is a recent approach in the field of Food Science and Technology, thus still has much further to go [27]. To date, nanoemulsions have been mainly applied to the design of new functional foods, since this technology allows regulating the release of bioactive nutrients and non-nutrients featured by poor water solubility [72,73]. For the preparation of nanoemulsions, aqueous solutions of lipid droplets (size approximately 100 nm) are prepared using different methodologies. the most common technology applied is high pressure homogenization [74,75] that avoids particle aggregation and compounds separation by gravitation in comparison with normal emulsions [76]. In fact, in nanoemulsions, the functional compounds are protected from reacting with the food matrix, which helps to preserve organoleptic properties, while enhancing the bioavailability of the bioactive compounds of interest, because of favoring passive transport through biological membranes [77,78]. Afterwards, during digestion, it has been reported that nanoencapsulation increases solubility of bioactive nutrients and non-nutrients, as well as their presence suiting aborbtion at the gastric and intestinal levels. Moreover, the application of these compounds using nanoemulsions provides enhanced protection, reducing their metabolism and lowering the activity of efflux transporters [79,80].

Currently, there is an extensive literature on the encapsulation of functional compounds, such as curcumin and resveratrol [73,81–83], using nanoemulsions to protect these compounds from digestion. Indeed, despite the evidence retrieved through the last decades from the array of in vivo and in vitro characterizations, developed on the benefits for human health of bioactive phytochemicals, their current use is still limited due to poor bioavailability [84]. Regarding this constraint, an adequate formulation of nanoemulsifier has been demonstrated as a valuable alternative to improve the protection of these compounds from chemical and enzymatic aggressions in the intestinal lumen, and thus provide an enhanced absorption and bioavailability. In this sense, combinations of lipophilic and hydrophilic emulsifiers, specifically nanoemulsions composed by lecithin, are competent to entrap resveratrol in the nanoparticle core by hydrophobic forces, enhancing not only the shelf-life of the bioactive molecules, but also their bioavailability by increasing the intestinal absorption and cellular uptake [85].

In addition to the specificity of the nanoemulsions for the diverse bioactive compounds, their stability is also a critical issue that has been deeply evaluated in recent years. Hence, the stability during storage is conditioned by an array of factors, namely pH, temperature, and ion strength, but also on some intrinsic properties of the formulation as the emulsifier concentration or the use of additives that should be adjusted carefully to guarantee the appropriate functionality of nanoemulsions [75,86].

Another factor that has to be considered to achieve the best outcomes from nanoemulsions, as carriers of bioactive compounds, is the nanoparticles size. the right nanosize of emulsions could be reached using co-adjuvants, since droplets prepared from low viscosity oils have been shown to be able to reach the nanoscale. An example of this is the addition of butanol to sodium caseinate that presents a nanoscale after the addition of the alcohol [87]. Polyethylene glycol and ethylene glycol have also been used to achieve the desired nanomagnitude.

From the technological point of view, in the beverage industry, an additional quality of nanoemulsions, i.e. the high optical clarity, provides advantages during manufacturing that have advised on the challenge of prioritizing this technology in the design of new added-value products [88]. However, it is required to state that each protein has the capacity to encapsulate specific compounds according to their hydrophobicity or hydrophilic features.

2.2. Nanotechnology for Medical and Nutrition Research

As mentioned above, dietary supplements are useful for the prevention or reduction of different pathophysiological situations and diseases, supported by their antioxidant, anti-inflammatory, and antitumoral properties, among others [89]. Encouraged by the extensive bibliography on these biological activities, many supplements have included phytochemicals in their composition. Given diverse troubles reported regarding bioavailability (that is closely linked to their biological activity in vivo), to take advantage of their biological potential, research efforts have been addressed to explore the diverse encapsulation modes that would enhance bioavailability. Although this approach has allowed developing new nanoencapsulated products addressed to be administrated via ocular, transdermal, and intravenous [90,91], their application in the design of functional foods, because of the specific chemical and enzymatic conditions in the gastro-intestinal compartments, with a direct impact on their release from the food matrix after oral ingestion, integrity, and functionality, needs to be further explored [92].

As an example of these applications, nanoemulsions have been successfully used for curcumin (diferuloylmethane) and dibenzoylmethane (a structural analog of curcumin) encapsulation [93]. These compounds have demonstrated valuable therapeutic potential, while exerting reduced toxicity, in phase I human clinical trials [94]. Upon the studies developed to improve their bioavailability and bioactivity, it has been found that using a mix of triacylglycerol (as oil) and Tween-20 (as emulsifier) could be enhanced the cellular uptake of curcumin and, consequently, an amended anti-inflammatory activity [93,95]. Hence, although other encapsulation alternatives have been considered for curcumin, such as hydrophobic starch [96], albumin [97], β-lactoglobulin [98] or chitosan [99], the poor water-solubility of these compounds limited their application, remaining nanoemulsions as the most suitable and efficient encapsulation alternative.

Other polyphenols of interest have been nanoencapsulated in emulsions for experimentation, such as tannin, stilbenes, and flavonoids [100]. This reinforces the idea of nanoemulsions as a valuable choice for these types of bioactive compounds. However, the emulsion composition has been reported as a decisive factor for the final bioactivity. Thus, epigallocatechin gallate, a hydrophilic flavonol, featured by similar and low bioactivity as antioxidant, in mice tissues, when formulated in two esterified emulsions or in an aqueous phase, while the selection of a third emulsion composition results in an increased antioxidant activity in mice plasma [101].

Essential oils are other important plant derived bioactive compounds with interesting benefits, regarding the prevention of chronic pathologies or infectious diseases. Indeed, based on this evidence, these compounds have been applied as analgesic, sedative, anti-inflammatory, spasmolytic, and local anesthetic treatments [102]. Thus, although a great variability in micro encapsulation methods has been described for these compounds, such as polysaccharides, spray-dried powders or Ca-alginate [103,104], these encapsulation alternatives provide protection to essential oils but seem to be no competent to enhance their antimicrobial activity. However, the nanoscale promoted a slower delivery and higher cell permeability, especially in the skin layers, increasing the activity of essential oils [105].

According to the information referred above, lipid-based nanocarriers are noticed as valuable alternatives to entrap essential oils in the core of the nanostructure and thus, reach different type of cells. In this regard, these nanoparticles have been applied in microbial infections due to their higher cell penetrability [106]; however, in some cases, antimicrobial capacity was reduced when compares with microencapsulation forms [24].

Efficient nanoencapsulation of other compounds, such as ferulic acid and tocopherol in solid–lipid nanoparticles, has been also reported recently [107]. Thus, in nanoemulsions, bioactive lipids were protected against autoxidation [108,109] and carotenoids [110], increasing their bioaccesibility.

Another functional compounds used in the formulation of health foods are probiotics, microorganisms, that improve intestinal microflora. Regarding probiotics, targeting specific regions in gastrointestinal tract after nanoencapsulation has been achieved [111]. Nanoemulsions were used to protect lactic acid bacteria [112] and, thus, to fine-tune the microbiota in the diverse intestinal conditions.

the micelle delivery system, for instance, is widely accepted as valuable carriers of antitumor drugs, and has been evaluated in the frame of clinical trials [43]. In this regard, hydrophobic drugs, for instance, can only be administered intravenously after their conditioning with solubilizing adjuvants, which has been associated with the appearance of toxic symptoms [113]. However, the addition of these drugs into nanocarrier-like micelles allows the replacement of the toxic adjuvants and contributes to minimize toxic effects [114]. Furthermore, as an additional advantage, the unimolecular micelles exhibit a maintained distribution jointly with a controlled pH-sensitive drug release. Likewise, it has been demonstrated that rapamycin could be loaded efficiently in mixed micelles up to a concentration of 1.8 mg/mL by using a hot-shock protocol. Upon these characterization, the release kinetic of obtained for rapamycin indicates that this micellar system could be triggered by varied pH environments under physiological conditions [115]. Matsumura et al. demonstrated that a paclitaxel micellar formulation consisting of polyethylene glycol and modified polyaspartate as hydrophobic block features cytotoxicity in a range of human tumor cell lines compared with the administration of the bioactive compound alone [116].

3. Phytochemicals Loaded Nanoparticles: Diving into Nanosized Drug Delivery Systems

3.1. Bioavailability Advantages of Nanoencapsulated Phytochemicals

Phytochemicals feature a diversity of chemical structures, represented by phenolic acids, indoles, alkaloids, isothiocyanates, phytosterols, saponins, and phytoprostanes/furanes [117,118]. These compounds have received growing attention boosted by their benefits for human health [119,120], upon a plethora of mechanisms including free radicals scavenging, inhibition of the assembly of microtubule and microfilament, metal chelation, and/or protease inhibition, among others [121]. Hence, the assessment of these compounds, from their in vivo metabolization point of view, has revealed that, after oral intake, phytochemicals are recognized and processed as xenobiotics and degraded as a consequence of the different digestion chemical, enzymatic, and microbial phases in mouth, stomach, and small and large intestine; then absorbed, distributed, and metabolized in cells and tissues; and finally excreted via renal, biliary or pulmonary [122]. Meanwhile, the maximum bioaccessibility and bioavailability of phytochemicals give rise to their actual capacity to exert biological effects in vivo (bioefficacy). the bioactivity of the bioactive nutrients and non-nutrients is demonstrated by short-term changes in the expression of biomarkers of liver function, plasma lipid profiles, blood pressure, plasma glucose, and plasma antioxidant activity [123]. In this sense, bioefficacy is influenced by the chemical nature of these compounds and their metabolic derivatives.

the innumerous articles published to date on the bioavailability of phytochemicals thereafter their oral intake have demonstrated that these compounds or their metabolites may fall in the nano/picomolar range in cells and tissues, which may result in insufficient dose to achieve the biological efficacy, demonstrated upon in vitro characterizations [124].

the dispersion and absorption, of these compounds, is closely dependent on their polarity. Once absorbed, small intestinal enterocytes are responsible for the cellular uptake, efflux pumping, and phase I and II metabolism, while the results of these processes are responsible for the amount of bioaccessible phytochemicals [122]. Moreover, transformations occurring in the frame of phase I and II reactions in hepatocytes give rise to active formats from inactive precursors that are the actual responsible of their biological value [125]. In addition, unabsorbed phytochemicals reach the large intestine, where are further metabolized by the local microbiota. This additional modification also affects their bioefficacy, providing new bioactive compounds that contribute to the final biological interest of a given plant matrix [122].

To prevent the deleterious effect of metabolization on the occurrence of truly bioactive compounds in cells and tissues, at operative concentrations, it has been pointed out that edible nanoencapsulation vehicles could be a valuable alternative. Regarding this, nanoencapsulation technology has been implemented, based on the information retrieved from an array of in vitro and in vivo characterizations, set up aimed at assessing the capability of different tissues and cell types to uptake the bioactive compounds at operative concentrations, according to an array of pathophysiological situations.

Diverse safe ingredients including lipids, polysaccharides, proteins, and biodegradable polymers are currently applied towards the development of edible nanoparticles featured by well-characterized size, surface properties, matrix materials, and compartment structure. These nanoparticles are developed foreseen to obtain improved strategies to enhance the release of the compounds of interest in target cells and tissues, as well as an increased bioefficiency [126,127]. the diverse types of nanoparticles suitable to be used as carriers of bioactive phytochemicals, in the frame of oral administrations, display a variety of structural features, such as is exemplified by nanoliposome, micelle, nanoemulsion, solid–lipid nanoparticles, polymeric nanoparticles (nanospheres and nanocapsules), protein–polysaccharide complex coacervation, cyclodextrin inclusion, and polymeric nanogel. Indeed, these alternative nanoparticles provide a range of features, including the process of loading phytochemical compounds, encapsulation efficiency, stability during gastrointestinal digestion, the releasing mechanisms and, therefore, their capacity to enhance the bioefficacy of the carried phytochemicals [122].

This situation has been recently illustrated by the evaluation of neuroblastoma cells (SH-SY5Y cell line), on their ability to uptake nanoparticles that provide promising results. In fact, the results retrieved from this work revealed that nanoparticles contribute to reach efficient concentrations of the bioactive compounds in the nervous system, especially when applying anionic charged nanoparticles, that exert a higher capacity to successfully go-through the blood–brain barrier, in comparison with cationic nanoparticles [128]. In addition, when using this type of nanoparticles, given the repulsion among the high negatively charged nanoparticles, it is possible to achieve extra stability for the bioactive compounds in cells and tissues, in vivo [129].

A careful revision of the literature gives a close relationship between the capacity of nanoparticles to enhance phytochemicals' bioefficacy with particle size (the most relevant feature), surface properties, matrix materials, and compartment structure [130]. Actually, these features affect bioefficacy, influencing dispersion and gastrointestinal stability, as well as the release rate and the delivery site, the efficacy of the transportation through the endothelial cell layer, the systemic spread, and their capacity to control the impact of the microbiota metabolism [122]. Besides, when targeting the improvement of cellular uptake, it is essential to notice that particle size, jointly with the use of polymeric nanoparticles, solid–lipid nanoparticles, or nanoemulsions, contribute to the stability by affecting to the repulsion facts and/or interfacial-tension-decreasing compounds [131,132], which contributes to augment cellular uptake.

Based on these advantages, loading phytochemicals within such edible nanoparticles enhances the dispersion of initially water-insoluble phytochemicals in aqueous media [133], while the physical barrier provided by nanoparticles protects bioactive compounds against oxidation under acidic and alkaline degradative conditions, in stomach and small intestine, respectively [134,135].

In the literature the bioactivity of phytochemicals in their native state has been frequently reported, while, in vivo, as mentioned before, the delivery of bioactive nutrients and non-nutrients are critically affected by their solubility, which affects stability and penetration under gastrointestinal conditions. To overwhelm this conflict is a basic objective of nanotechnology in the field of Science and Technology of Foods, specifically regarding the development of functional foods and nutraceuticals. Hence, encapsulation of phytochemicals constitutes valuable alternatives to release bioactive compounds in specific tissues, affected by pathophysiological situations. In this sense, carrying bioactive compounds on nanoparticle limits their degradation under the chemical and enzymatic conditions of the gastrointestinal tract, as well as their general metabolism. In this regard, the physico-chemical features of the materials used to develop nanoparticles, as well as the digestibility of nanoparticles in the gastric or intestinal sections, are key issues that should be addressed, firstly, when designing a nanoparticles-based strategy to the oral administration of phytochemicals [122].

Some examples illustrate this situation: while starch-based nanoparticles are digested at oral level by the activity of α-amylase, additional polysaccharide nanoparticles are degraded in the small intestine and protein−polysaccharide nanoparticles can be due to variations of pH and salt concentrations, such as those occurring in the gastrointestinal lumen during the separate stages of digestion [135]. Lipid nanovesicles release phytochemicals in the small intestine simultaneously to the digestion of triglycerides [122].

In addition to the nature of the nanoparticle, the loading method has been revealed to be critical for the final release of phytochemicals and, thus, for their bioavailability and bioactivity. Regarding this, the drug-loading method strongly influences the loading efficiency, and it has been described that nanoencapsulated compounds release to a lower extent relative to nanosphere-based delivery, even if both formulations have similar efficiency [90].

Recently, a new type of compounds has emerged, plant oxylipins, such as phytoprostanes and phytofurans, which are formed by non-enzymatic oxidation of α-linolenic acid. Bioavailability and biological activity of such compounds have been suggested based on their structural analogy with human eicosanoids [118,136]. These lipid phytochemicals are compounds of special features as they migrate into fatty acids-based micelles, which contribute to their solubility and subsequent cellular transportation [122].

Apart from the control of phytochemicals release, nanoparticles also influence the transport of bioactive compounds through enterocytes (by transcellular endocytosis for particles between 20 and 1000 nm), by modulating residence time, transportation efficiency, and pathways, as well as the metabolic reactions undergone by such compounds within endothelial cells. Hence, for instance, chitosan derivatives have been related to mucoadhesive features and their capacity to open tight junctions, improving paracellular transport [137–139]. Moreover, the nanoparticle's charge also influences the formation of hydrogen bonds with the mucosal surface, contributing to a momentary retention [140]. Another feature of nanoparticles that influences their role as carriers of bioactive compounds is the incorporation of cell-penetrating ligands that could contribute to enhance transmembrane transport efficiency [122].

Once absorbed from the intestinal lumen, nanoparticles loaded with bioactive phytochemicals move through endothelial layer to migrate to tissues into bloodstream. At this stage, nanoparticles have already been included in endosomes and undergone oxidation, reduction, and hydrolysis reactions, among others, as well as conjugations by diverse metabolization routes upon phase II metabolism. However, unlike metabolism of free phytochemicals, when carried on nanoparticles, the bioactive compounds are protected from such reactions, by modulating the exposition to metabolizing enzymes in enterocytes [141].

Highly lipophilic phytochemicals featured by specific features, regarding the logarithm of the oil—water partition coefficient and a long-chain triglyceride solubility (e.g., phytoprostanes and phytofurans), may go through enterocytes and form chylomicrons with enterocyte lipoproteins [142]. These reach the bloodstream via mesenteric lymph and thoracic ducts, avoiding hepatic first-pass metabolism. This route of absorption has been imitated using nanoparticles incorporating a lipid phase (for instance, emulsions, liposomes, and solid–lipid nanoparticles), which enhance the participation of the lymphatic absorption at the time that augment the rate of transcellular absorption [143]. Given the interest of integrating lipid phase in nanoparticles as modulators of the absorption rate, the extent to which the phospholipid composition and concentration of emulsifiers are competent to fine-tune biodistribution by modifying the lipophylicity and plasma-binding properties of phytochemicals has been investigated [144].

Additional approaches that have been explored, as valuable modes to control release and bioavailability of bioactive nutrients and non-nutrients administered, using nanoparticles as carriers are represented by the use of magnetic nanoparticles, the alteration of the surface chemical properties, and the inclusion of ligands facilitating the cellular uptake [122]. However, for some types of compounds, such as stilbenes, flavonols, and anthocyanins, which are metabolized by the intestinal microbiota towards even more powerful bioactive compounds, could be interesting for avoiding their digestion and absorption at gastric and small intestine levels. With this objective, the best option lies in the use of nanoparticles manufactured with materials or multilayer structures, resistant to gastric and small intestine conditions in terms of pH, osmotic conditions, and enzymatic activities. In addition, to achieve this objective, it is required to design release mechanisms that allow the delivery of bioactive phytochemicals under the osmotic and pH conditions of the large intestine, in which the microbiota responsible for its transformation is present [122]. On the other hand, once this objective is achieved, the challenge of reaching highly bioavailable compounds, derived from the microbiota metabolism, constitutes an additional constraint, due to the low colonic absorption at the conditions of luminal fluid volume, viscosity, and neutral pH of colon [145,146].

Once absorbed and circulating in blood stream, diverse strategies have been suggested and explored to control the length of circulation, such as using hydrophilic coating. Polyethylene glycol has been demonstrated as reliable to enhance circulation time, by acting as a steric barrier and thus protecting nanoparticles from opsonization [147].

One of the most widely used material for the development of nanoparticles is poly-(lactic-coglycolic acid) that represents a successfully used biodegradable polymer due to the production of the metabolite monomers lactic acid and glycolic acid during their physiological hydrolysis, that are easily processed via the Krebs cycle. Due to this rapid metabolization, low systemic toxicity has been described associated to the application of this biomaterial for the control of the bioactives compounds release [148]. However, it is crucial to develop surface modifications using nontoxic and blood compatible material, that allow their uptake by macrophages and the augment of the length of blood circulation, which contribute to the sustained delivery of the bioactive compounds carried in this nanosystem [149,150]. In this connection, poly(ethylene-glycol) is used as hydrophilic nontoxic segment in combination with hydrophobic biodegradable aliphatic polyesters, because this provides the capacity to resist against opsonizing and the ulterior phagocytosis, contributing to enlarged shelf life in the bloodstream and tissues [151–153].

3.2. Nanotechnology for Bioactives Delivery

In recent years, nanotechnology has emerged as a valuable alternative to control drugs delivery and tissue engineering [31], because of the chance provided by this to design and develop new strategies that could enhance the efficacy of natural bioactive molecules, currently used in a very limited extent, as therapeutic compounds for the treatment of different pathophysiological situations [32]. Indeed, nanotechnology is an alternative to traditional formulation, which could contribute to improve general bioavailability and site-specific release, simultaneously to toxicity reduction [33–35]. According to these aims, several epidemiological studies have been developed, during the last years, aiming to take higher advantages of the influence of dietary habits on the incidence of an array of pathophysiological situations, that have focused the assessment of several plant foods. From such work, multiple compounds that display potential health benefits in vitro have been identified [154,155]. However, when evaluating the activity of those compounds upon in vivo studies, many of them were not competent to translate the activities previously demonstrated in vitro, appearing as unstable in the intestinal environments and, thus, exhibiting poor bioavailability. Thus, to achieve the required bioavailability rates to take advantage of their biological activities, as a first approach, higher doses were tested, which showed efficacy but resulted in systemic toxicity [95].

the major outcomes from these studies have allowed to notice that several factors are involved in bioavailability, viz. chemical structure, solubility, stability against gastric and colonic pH, metabolism by gut microflora, absorption across the intestinal wall, active efflux mechanism, and first-pass metabolic effects [147]. However, when reviewing the data reported on the bioavailability of phytochemicals, it is revealed that many of them are only partially absorbed/metabolized by the intestinal epithelium, a cellular type responsible for systemic occurrence by their uptake using efflux transporters (mainly P-glycoprotein) [156]. the efflux transporter proteins mediate the active extrusion of compounds back into the intestinal lumen [157] that, in turn, limit the bioavailability of the bioactive phytochemicals of interest to nanomolar concentrations in blood, even if the ions have been detected the intestinal section, where they are absorbed, in high concentrations [158]. Indeed, this situation demonstrates that it is difficult to assess the bioavailability of chemical agents based solely on their physicochemical properties.

This is not just a general concept related to the biological activity of a given phytochemical compound, the bioavailability of the compound itself, at the target site, is a major issue that has not be appropriately addressed in the last years [159]. In this regard, understanding the concerns enclosed to the bioavailability of an individual compound is essential to draw strategies that might help to overwhelm these limitations. In this sense, the emergence of new technologies that allow the advance towards efficient and safe administration of newly identified bioactive compounds, has increased the interest in new "smart" delivery systems that contributes to improve the pharmacological properties of the administrated compounds [147]. Hence, a promising approach to avoid low bioavailability and systemic toxicity, associated in some extent to the use of xenoparticles as carriers of the bioactive compounds of interest, is the application of nanoparticles manufactured using materials of demonstrated safety, such as polymeric nanoparticles, liposomes, dendrimers, and micelles [160,161]. Actually, the use of these types of carriers is associated to innumerous advantages relatively to the traditional systemic administration, since this approach constitutes a powerful tool to modulate the pharmacokinetics and to improve delivery of bioactive agents to target sites [147].

Indeed, nanoparticles may enhance the oral bioavailability of poorly soluble compounds, as well as the tissue uptake after parenteral administration, supplying enhanced adherence capacity to the capillary wall during the initial diffusion phases (tethering, rolling, adhesion, and transmigration). Moreover, the selection of the most appropriate options between the currently developed could also allow augmenting the delivery across membranes and biological barriers [162]. In this regard, the size limitation to go through diverse biological barriers is closely related to target location and the chemical features of the tissue [163].

In recent years, stimuli-responsive polymer-based nanocarriers have focused the attention of researchers, working on the evaluation of bioactive phytochemicals in vivo. Regarding this, such nanoparticles are exposed to modification of their physical and chemical properties when exposed to the specific conditions (pH, temperature, light, magnetic field or glucose levels) in the intestinal tract or the diverse tissues after distribution [163,164]. This dependency could be of significant interest, as they provide the chance to set up valuable relationships between the release of bioactive compounds and specific niches or pathological state [132]. This situation is exemplified by paclitaxel delivery once loaded on pH-responsive nanoparticles, which has evidenced its utility upon in vitro and in vivo antitumoral determinations [165,166].

Anthocyanins have been highlighted, for several years, as model phytochemical to assess the potential of competence of polymeric nanoparticles to encapsulate hydrophilic compounds. the final objective of these studies is to establish the contribution of these approaches to the bioavailability and controlled release and release kinetics in vitro. In the case of anthocyanin, these features have been evaluated on polyethylene glycol moieties. Hence, in these works, anthocyanins were encapsulated with 60% efficiency in biodegradable nanoparticle formulation based on polylactide-*co*-glycolide, which were stabilizer resorting to the use of polyethylene glycol. These nanoparticles evidenced a biphasic release profile, in vitro. In addition, all the polyethileneglicosylated nanoparticles present a similar delivery pattern, characterized by an initial abrupt release followed by a continued supply [167]. Hence, this work described that bioactive compounds may be adsorbed on the surface of nanoparticles as a burst release that is not maintained in time, while the sustained release is due to the liberation of compounds encapsulated in the core domains of the nanoparticle [168].

3.3. Nanoparticles towards Targeted Bioactivity

A further step of what has been discussed above is the exploration of the advantages provided by nanotechnology concerning the release bioactive compounds carried in nanoparticles in specific tissues or cell types affected by pathophysiological events that needs to be treated. In the last decades, it has been boosted the application of bioactive phytochemicals as promising compounds capable to prevent health disturbance by modulating molecular pathways in cells. These compounds feature strong radical scavenging, anti-inflammatory, and neuroprotective activities, among others. Nonetheless, most bioactive nutrients and non-nutrients are unstable and rapidly transformed into other compounds with different biological attributions, which jointly with their fast degradation and excretion, limits the actual benefits that could be retrieved from such healthy compounds [169]. For instance, during digestion, the hydroxyl radicals of phenolics (for instance, anthocyanins) are oxidized into quinones, reducing the biological power of these molecules [170]. Traditionally, these constraints have been overwhelmed by therapeutic alternatives outlined for several diseases, which include invasive in situ administration of bioactive drugs, as a way to guarantee high tissue concentrations of the functional molecules of interest. Nevertheless, these administration alternatives are characterized by reduced patient compliance, because of the distress associated with frequent administrations, generally related to an array of side effects [171,172]. Alternatively, substitutive application forms of bioactive phytochemicals have been associated to augmented costs, particularly when repeated administrations are required to complete the treatment for a specific pathophysiological situation [173].

Apart from the side-impacts of the traditional administration of bioactive compounds, a loss of bioactivity during storage, due to the xenobiotics metabolism in mammals, has recently been reported, which could prevent them from reaching the target tissues and cells in which their activity is desired [174–176].

To date, diverse works have been developed aimed to identify alternatives that allow to overcome these problems; for instance, by using high dose or multiple treatments of bioactive compounds. However, this has been associated with dangerous side effects related to overdoses due to nonspecific toxicity of such compounds [174]. As a result, it has been identified an urgency to develop biocompatible and biodegradable systems for packaging phytochemicals, based on carrier systems constituted, for example, by oil-in-water emulsions and liposomes [177]. These alternatives have been demonstrated useful to provide sustained release of therapeutics in target tissues and, in addition, to reduce biological disturbances in cells and tissues, no compromising the stability and functionality of macromolecules [178]. Hence, this provides stability that in turn is responsible for a higher bioavailability and long term circulation [178], due to the protection supplied against outer stresses in vivo [179]. the research on controlled delivery options in respect to tissue, concentration, and pathophysiological modifications, has given rise to the description of biodegradable polymers and formulations specific for diverse types of bioactive compounds, with interesting biological activities, which have focused the preparation of phytochemicals-encapsulated nanoparticles [180]. Based on these applications, this technology has been noticed as highly useful for controlled delivery of bioactive compounds in target sites.

Moreover, the structural features of the nanoencapsulations pointed out so far, have a direct impact on the release profile [90,181]. This is specifically referred to as core–shell nanoparticles, double-emulsions, gelled networks, multiple coating systems, and "prodrug delivery systems". Actually, when these systems are conjugated with azo- or glucuronic acid-including polymers, it is possible to control the bioactive compounds carried by enzymatic hydrolysis, which can contribute to retard the speed of phytochemicals release, as well as a noticeable change of their physical dispersion state [123].

This is of special relevance regarding compounds that develop their biological functions in tissues with high protection against xenobiotics by biological barriers, such as the blood–brain barrier. In this frame, anthocyanins contribute to improve brain functionality and to reduce oxidative stress associated to normal cells metabolism, resorting to their radical scavenging, anti-inflammatory, and anti-neurodegenerative capacity [168,170], thus preventing memory losses in estrogen-deficient rats [182]. the polymer-based nanoparticles used for characterization in this model were featured by a biphasic release profile, providing enhanced neuroprotective power of anthocyanins against Alzheimer's dementia. Besides, the efficiency of the anthocyanins administered associated to nanoparticles has been further demonstrated by monitoring the capacity to attenuate the expression of clinical (amyloid precursor protein and beta-site amyloid precursor protein cleaving enzyme-1), inflammatory (p-nuclear factor kappa-B, Tumor Necrosis Factor-alpha, and nitric oxide synthase), and apoptotic (B-cell lymphoma-2 (BCL2), BCL2 associated X (Bax), and caspase-3 protein) markers [170]. Using this model, it was evidenced that anthocyanins loaded nanoparticles reduced significantly the level of protein markers and were also more efficient in modulating the P38/JNK pathway, according to reduced expression of various inflammatory markers, cytotoxic compounds, and proinflammatory cytokines [168]. In respect to oxidative stress, non-conjugated anthocyanins or molecules associated to nanoparticles significantly upregulate endogenous antioxidant genes, such as nuclear respiratory factor-2 and HO-1 proteins, which has been related with the prevention of oxidative stress and consequently, with an attenuation of the clinical symptoms of the Alzheimer's dementia [183].

An additional functionality demonstrated for anthocyanins loaded nanoparticles is related with their capacity to revert the augmented and decreased expression of pro-apoptotic (caspase-3 and Bax) and anti-apoptotic proteins (BCL2), respectively, thus reducing DNA damage in a higher extent than native non-conjugated anthocyanin. All these findings together prompted Amin et al. [168] to suggest a neuroprotection activity of anthocyanins loaded nanoparticles that surpassed significantly the biological potential, enclosed to free anthocyanin. This enhanced activity, when combined with polysaccharides, seems to be related to an increased stability and prolonged degradation time [170].

4. In Situ Bioactive Compounds Delivery Control: Drawbacks and Breakthrough Advantages

According to the constraints outlined before, in the last decades, growing attention and resources have been devoted to the development of carrier systems that allow local delivery of therapeutic agents, for instance, by using organic materials. Regarding this, control delivery has been identified as a key stage of bioactive compounds administration, foreseen as a way to set up the timing, tissue/cell, and pathophysiological conditions, under which therapeutic agents are released. Indeed, achieving this objective would allow reaching higher local concentration near to the operative levels demonstrated in vitro, while reducing the overall administered dose (and consequently systemic toxicity associated). According to this objective, as a result of the research efforts developed in the last years, a diversity of internal and external factors can control the specific release of bioactive phytochemicals, according to a range of factors, including pH, the activity of local, temperature, ultrasound, magnetic field, and/or light incidence [184].

Moreover, recently, the nanoencapsulation of compounds identified as potential therapeutic agents has raised growing interest, due to the augment of the range of biomaterials with valuable applications in this field [163,185]. Thus, polymeric nanocarriers can increase the bioavailability, improve solubility, and prolong the shelf-life of potential compounds which, to date, have been difficult to deliver in a controlled way. For instance, oil-cored nanocapsules improve originally the administration of bioactive compounds, allowing targeted delivery and controlled, long-term, release that contribute to decrease the dosage and frequency of administration giving rise to an increased patient compliance [184]. Due to this, the layer-by-layer self-assembly of pH-sensitive building blocks has been explored as a promising approach to obtain biomaterials with customized properties [186] and, thus, with interesting applications as stimuli-responsive nanocarriers for controlled release of phytochemical compounds, which could also provide transport capacity through diverse biological barriers [187]. Moreover, the use of appropriate pH-dependent biocompatible polyelectrolyte for nanocapsule shell formation can provide the tools required to design non-toxic nanocarriers, with shell permeability [184].

Loading bioactive phytochemicals in nanoparticles turns bioactive compounds into more effective and contributes to achieve site-specific delivery. Once into the cells, some nanoparticles release the bioactive phytochemicals slowly, contributing to sustained therapeutic effects, which constitutes an additional advantage [188]. This capacity was demonstrated recently by using rhodamine-loaded polyethylene glycol-nanoparticles. Upon this characterization, after the application of rhodamine labeled nanoparticles to SH-SY5Y neuroblastoma cells, red fluorescence is visualized in the cytoplasm, suggesting that nanoparticles are internalized via endocytosis [189], saving the phospholipidic barrier that the cell membrane represent for hydrophilic compounds. An additional demonstration of these advantages was obtained on prostate cancer DU145 cells with similar positive results [190].

In addition, in relation with the administration of bioactive compounds, pursuing the development of activity at neural tissues and in the frame of deficits or overexpression of neurotrophins, responsible for neurodegenerative diseases and psychiatric disorders, to date, the research has demonstrated a delivery system competent to control of neurotrophin dosage in the brain. In fact, the major outcomes obtained in this issue have suggested that carrying bioactive compounds in nanoparticles might favor targeted delivery in specific brain areas, minimizing biodistribution to the systemic circulation and, consequently, toxic side-effects. Indeed, this approach provides valuable benefits concerning neuroregeneration [191].

In addition to oral administration, polymeric microspheres, scaffolds, and conduits have been used as sustained-release systems for neurotrophic proteins [192,193] that even provide enhanced neuroregeneeration, relatively to the implantation of polymeric scaffolds resorting to invasive surgery techniques into the central nervous system [191]. Indeed, this situation is exemplified by a slow release achieved of glial cell line-derived neurotrophic factor, by-using micro-reservoirs created by biodegradable poly-(lactic-*co*-glycolic acid) microspheres or by Poly(lactic-*co*-glycolic acid) microparticles [194,195].

Although the actual significance and advantages of the abrupt release of bioactive compounds, when using controlled delivery systems, has not been entirely ignored over the last years, to date, no plenary successful theories have explained completely the phenomenon. In addition, it has to be considered that the negative effects, associated to burst release, are pharmacologically dangerous and economically inefficient [196]. To overwhelm this inconvenience, new nanoformulations composed of thermo-sensitive gelling copolymer has been successfully formulated and characterized. the negligible amount of bioactive compounds released, when using these systems, prevent the toxicity enclosed to peaks and valleys of concentration in target tissues. Therefore, the delivery systems developed resorting to the application of this copolymer can minimize the side effects associated with frequent injections for the administration of therapeutics of interest, without reducing the efficiency of the bioactive compound, serving as a promising platform for avoiding pathophysiological complications [173]. However, the demonstration of such advantages is based on in vitro evidence, and remains to be further elucidated upon in vivo evaluations.

Studies on nanoencapsulation and controlled release from nanostructured carriers have demonstrated the safety of these systems and their contribution to achieve operative concentrations in target cells and tissues, when applying polymer- and lipid-based nanostructured systems [191]. Due to this and according to previous reports, on the capacity of such carriers to protect instable therapeutic proteins, e.g., from enzymatic degradation and other environmental stress factors [191], similar approaches could be applied to the administration of bioactive phytochemicals and take advantage of their biological potential, preventing their metabolization in vivo. In this frame, the research on the beneficial effects of anthocyanins loaded nanoparticles against neurotoxicity in vitro, has been focused on the evaluation of the cytotoxic profile of nanoparticles in the human neuroblastoma model (SH-SY5Y cell line). Upon this study, different concentrations of both free-anthocyanins and anthocyanins loaded in poly(lactide-*co*-clycolide) nanoparticles allowed discarding significant cytotoxic effects, while the joint application of anthocyanins loaded nanoparticles increased the viability of treated cells, by protecting them from neurotoxic events [168]. Thus, poly(lactide-*co*-clycolide) nanoparticles might constitute promising phytochemical carriers with negligible cytotoxicity events. Additionally, the administration of the mentioned nanoparticles provides the advantage of avoiding the need of removing an eventual implant placed as a local source of the bioactive compounds, and thus, no surgery would be required [197,198].

5. Toxicity Facts Associated to the Administration of Biodegradable Nanoparticles

In respect to the toxicity associated to the administration of biodegradable nanocarrier systems for bioactive compounds, as far as we are aware, there is no evidence on deleterious effects, although the risks to human health that could be associated to the long term use, remain under explored [148]. the mechanisms responsible for the deleterious effects of nanoparticles in the frame of complex biological systems are associated to increased productions of Reactive Oxygen Species (ROS) and free radicals, that could give rise to oxidative stress, inflammation, and consequently to several disabling pathophysiological situations, associated with solvent residues and polymers toxicity [199]. To shed some light on the actual toxicity of nanoparticles, it is required to evaluate the separate trials independently, paying attention to interactions between nanocarriers and biological systems. This way of processing the available information on the toxicity, associated to nanoparticles, is crucial to establish the reliability of the delivery systems. Actually, to translate successfully nanoformulations from the experimental level to their practical clinical application, it is essential to establish their safety profiles, including the evaluation of immunotoxicity. In this concern, special attention should be paid to the linkage between the physico-chemical and functional properties of nanoparticles (surface charge, size, modulate uptake and interactions with cells, control over surface modification and biodegradation of nanovectors), and the extent in which, these features, contribute to achieve the functional potential envisaged and to minimize potential health risks [200].

Hence, toxicological facts associated to nanocarrier systems involve several physiological, physicochemical and molecular considerations. However, despite the evident interest of understanding the toxicity of these delivery systems, to date, it has not been deeply explored, possibly because the industrial use of this technology is in its infancy. From the information available in the literature regarding this, it is noticed that toxicological facts associated to nanocarriers is closely linked to their size and shape, biomaterials, as well as to their capacity to cross biological barriers [201]. Regarding the molecular mechanisms, behind the toxicological effects, associated to treatments with bioactive compounds carried on biodegradable nanoparticles, it has been noticed the formation of pro-oxidants after their administration, disrupting the balance between their production and the detoxification capacity of cells. This fact also entails augmented inflammation reactions due to the level of redox-sensitive transcription factors [202,203].

In relation with the use of nanoparticles to carry bioactive compounds addressed to be ingested in foods, water or drug delivery devices, the interest of biodegradable nanoparticles and the constraints associated to their toxicity, following oral ingestion, has been associated to the occurrence of deleterious effects on liver, kidney and spleen. In addition, even if the mechanisms responsible for triggering the immune response induced by nanoparticles (especially concerning non-protein-based carriers) are not clear, there is a growing attention on possible allergic reaction [202]. To gain a further insight in this issue, further studies of the immunogenicity of nanocarriers are required to understand under which conditions they are identified by the immune system, deserving the generation of a specific immune responses [202]. Polyethylene glycol (PEG)-grafted liposome infusion has been described to trigger non-IgE-mediated signs of hypersensitivity [204]. On the other hand, advantages can be obtained from the immunogenic characteristics of nanoparticles, as these features suggest them as valuable adjuvants, for instance, for the development of vaccines.

6. Future Perspectives for Targeting and Controlled Delivery

In the coming years, the research trends in the application of edible nanoparticles to the administration of bioactive phytochemicals will be closely linked to new manufacturing strategies that combine multiple structural designs, more specific for the diverse types of bioactive compounds. Achieving this objective is foreseen to strengthen the property of nanoparticles and to combine the benefits identified on two or more types of biomaterials. This strategy would contribute to maximize the benefits of loading bioactive compounds on nanoparticles, in terms of effectivity, extended release, and in situ delivery control. Among the desired features, target delivery has not been completely developed yet, remaining an issue with future prospects for implementation. In this sense, materials and fabrication strategies would allow the creation of edible nanoparticles with improved properties is constantly ongoing. Once improved, the specificity and versatility of available nanoparticles, the administration of bioactive compounds orally, by using edible nanoparticles, will constitute a valuable approach that would allow to take advantage from the actual potential of phytochemicals to prevent and treat specific pathophysiological status, due to accurate tissue-targeted delivery.

One of the major constraints enclosed to the administration of bioactive compounds, even when using nanotechnology products, lies in the degradation of these compounds in the gastrointestinal lumen before being absorbed. Thus, although in vitro the works, available in the literature, reveal promising potential of the use of nanoparticles for the administration of phytochemicals loaded nanoparticles, nowadays it is required to complete the determination of the impact of gastrointestinal digestion, by informative in vitro simulation models, as cost-efficient tools for forecasting the oral bioavailability [167,205]. With this aim, in addition to implementing a model mimicking the salivary, gastric, and intestinal fluids concerning salt and enzyme concentrations, it is required to avoid an excessive simplification of the models, by including appropriate simulators of gastrointestinal dynamics, structure, and mechanical issues.

the consideration of gut metabolism, on the actual biological activity of compounds ingested by oral administration, requires a review of the current definition of "bioaccessibility" and "bioavailability", emphasizing the value of the absorption in the upper gastrointestinal tract. Indeed, information on the features of this physiological process, according to the chemical properties of the bioactive compounds of interest, and the derivatives that can be formed during the gastrointestinal digestion, is crucial for the rational design of the specific nanoparticle system. With this objective, the selection of the type of nanoparticles, to improve the absorption at the gastric and small intestine (duodenum) level, may not serve as a gold standard anymore, because, for some phytochemicals, high bioefficacy is associated with the additional compounds synthesized, for instance in the large intestine, as a result of the metabolism of the local microbiota, turning into undesirable their absorption in the upper gastrointestinal.

Besides, when evaluating the effects of nanoparticles and/or nanovesicles on the bioefficacy of phytochemicals, special attention should be paid to eventual changes in the nanoparticle structure as a result of the digestive conditions. Indeed, this modification of the nanoparticles structure could entail changes in their functionality as carriers of bioactive nutrients and non-nutrients and, consequently, induce misunderstanding results. Thus, considering that, when mixed with digestion fluids, the dilution would have a crucial effect on the stability of micelles, liposomes, and nanoemulsions, is required. This deserves to be considered because the surfactant concentration should be maintained in a slim range. Moreover, pH and ions environments in the gastrointestinal fluids, as well as the enzymatic activity in these compartments could also compromise the stability of nanoparticles and the successful development of their role as carriers of bioactive compounds [122]. According to these constraints, it is necessary to evaluate the behavior of nanoparticles in complex matrices and biological systems that will provide actual information on their practical significance.

An additional situation, that needs to be addressed, is the extent in which nanoparticles modify the pharmacokinetics of bioactive phytochemicals, which would contribute to draw new applications, for instance as boosters of the internalization speed. Clarifying this situation is essential for the proper design of the sampling timing to determine pharmacokinetics bioavailability and bioactivity of bioactive compounds subject of study. Overall, encapsulated phytochemicals within appropriate nanoparticles enhance the bioavailability by protecting them from degradation during storage and gastrointestinal digestion, improving solubility in aqueous media, augmenting contact time with the intestinal wall, increasing of the mucus penetration and intestinal permeation, facilitating cellular uptake, prolonging residence time within the body circulation, controlling release rate and site, and altering, according to the envisaged results, the microbiota metabolism. In addition, it should be considered that loading bioactive compounds in nanoparticles, somehow, could be an interesting strategy to prevent their metabolic conversion, while to date, little is known about how the modification of cellular signaling routes differs between free and nanoparticles-linked phytochemicals. In this regard, seems evident that the interaction between phytochemicals and matrix material, or molecules in complex biological systems (for instance in mammals), deserves to be further explored concerning metabolism and bioefficacy [122]. Hence, the information retrieved from studies, focused on the correlation between the application of bioactive compounds carried by nanoparticles with the metabolic profile, biodistribution and bioactivity, will be very useful as a guide for future evaluation of the bioefficacy and predictable in vivo properties.

Concerning the final intestinal stage, the interactions between phytochemicals and drugs with gut microbiota, as well as the consequences of these interactions on bioefficacy, remain underexplored, even if it seems evident that they constitute additional challenges. Indeed, the application of the gathered knowledge on the use of nanoparticles, as carriers of bioactive phytochemicals, would provide the opportunity to decode and take advantage of the reciprocal interactions between phytochemicals and gut microbiota.

Despite the rational utility of the nanotechnology to enhance the bioavailability and bioactivity of bioactive compounds, nanoparticles are synthesized by physical and chemical methods, by using expensive and hazardous chemicals, especially concerning metallic biomaterials, which could limit their actual application in vivo. These constraints are also enclosed to the environmental impact derived of the residues, generated from the nanoparticles synthesis, being required green technologies using no toxic reagents to prepare metal nanoparticles. In this regard, the synthesis of nanoparticles using eco-friendly and biocompatible reagents could contribute to minimize the side effect of these processes.

7. Conclusions

Nutraceuticals' potential benefits have been demonstrated, but increasing applications in the near future, for the prevention of diseases onset and severity, are highly demanded. To take maximum advantages of bioactive compounds (nutrients and non-nutrients), responsible for the functionality of nutraceuticals, promising applications have been suggested based on combinations of individual, well characterized, bioactive phytochemicals. This approach would allow synergic situations that would help to reduce dosages and, thus, eventual toxic side effects, while becoming instrumental in the prevention of an array of pathophysiological situations.

To improve the bioavailability of phytochemicals identified as valuable bioactive compounds, in the frame of a specific clinical entity of health disorders, nanoparticles have been investigated as promising delivery systems that could contribute to control release and to fine-tune pharmacokinetics, bioavailability, and bioefficacy. Indeed, nanotechnology would contribute to improve stability of encapsulated bioactive nutrients and non-nutrients against environmental changes (in the diverse in vivo environments) and to release control. Therefore, it should be assumed that nanoparticles have great potential as phytochemical carriers, as, at the dosages monitored, they are not cytotoxic. However, critical aspects and potential for application of nanotechnology in Food Science and Technology field, should be noticed, especially regarding the implementation of green technology for their development and their use in the studies of additional issues, such as the crucial role of the intestinal microbiota for obtaining additional bioactive metabolites, contributing to the health benefits attributed to plant foods and nutraceuticals.

Author Contributions: M.M.-B. and R.D.-P. conceived the focus of this review and drafted the manuscript. A.G.-I. and C. G.-V. supervised the project and contributed to the final version of the manuscript upon critical revision of the texts.

Acknowledgments: This work was partially funded by the Spanish Ministry of Science and Innovation (MICINN) through the Research Projects AGL2016-75332-C2-1-R, AGL2016-80247-C2-1-R, and AGL2017-83386-R. In addition, this work is included in the framework of the collaboration between the Spanish Research Council (CEBAS-CSIC) and CNRS by "Projets Internationaux de Cooperation Scientifique" (PICS-2015-261141). R.D.-P. was sponsored by a Postdoctoral Contract (Juan de la Cierva de Incorporación ICJI-2015-25373) from the Ministry of Economy, Industry, and Competitiveness of Spain.

References

1. Pitchaiah, G.; Akula, A.; Parvathaneni, M. Anticancer potential of nutraceutical formulation through antioxidant, anti-inflammatory, and antiproliferative mechanisms in N-methyl-N-nitrosourea-induced mammary cancer. *Int. J. Green Pharm.* **2017**, *11*, 230–235.
2. Henrotin, Y.; Lambert, C.; Couchourel, D.; Ripoll, C.; Chiotelli, E. Nutraceuticals: Do they represent a new era in the management of osteoarthritis?—A narrative review from the lessons taken with five products. *Osteoarthritis Cartil.* **2011**, *19*, 1–21. [CrossRef] [PubMed]
3. Ahmad, A.; Wei, Y.; Syed, F.; Tahir, K.; Taj, R.; Khan, A.U.; Hameed, M.U.; Yuan, Q. Amphotericin B-conjugated biogenic silver nanoparticles as an innovative strategy for fungal infections. *Microb. Pathog.* **2016**, *99*, 271–281. [CrossRef] [PubMed]
4. Mittal, A.K.; Chisti, Y.; Banerjee, U.C. Synthesis of metallic nanoparticles using plant extracts. *Biotechnol. Adv.* **2013**, *31*, 346–356. [CrossRef] [PubMed]
5. Havlickova, B.; Czaika, V.A.; Friedrich, M. Epidemiological trends in skin mycoses worldwide. *Mycoses* **2008**, *51*, 2–15. [CrossRef] [PubMed]
6. Sobel, J.D. Vulvovaginal candidosis. *Lancet* **2007**, *369*, 1961–1971. [CrossRef]
7. Vance, M.E.; Kuiken, T.; Vejerano, E.P.; McGinnis, S.P.; Hochella, M.F., Jr.; Rejeski, D.; Hull, M.S. Nanotechnology in the real world: Redeveloping the nanomaterial consumer products inventory. *Beilstein J. Nanotechnol.* **2015**, *6*, 1769–1780. [CrossRef] [PubMed]
8. Roco, M.C.; Harthorn, B.; Guston, D.; Shapira, P. Innovative and responsible governance of nanotechnology for societal development. In *Nanotechnology Research Directions for Societal Needs in 2020*; Roco, M.C., Mirkin, C.A., Hersam, M.C., Eds.; Springer: Dordrecht, the Netherlands, 2011; pp. 561–617.
9. López-Lorente, A.I.; Mizaikoff, B. Recent advances on the characterization of nanoparticles using infrared spectroscopy. *TrAC Trends Anal. Chem.* **2016**, *84*, 97–106. [CrossRef]
10. Dingman, J. Nanotechnology its impact on food safety. *J. Environ. Health* **2008**, *70*, 47–50. [PubMed]
11. Abbas, K.A.; Saleh, A.M.; Mohamed, A.; MohdAzhan, N. the recent advances in the nanotechnology and its applications in food processing: A review. *J. Food Agric. Environ.* **2009**, *7*, 14–17.
12. Oberdörster, G.; Maynard, A.; Donaldson, K.; Castranova, V.; Fitzpatrick, J.; Ausman, K.; Carter, J.; Karn, B.; Kreyling, W.; Lai, D.; et al. Review Principles for characterizing the potential human health effectsfrom exposure to nanomaterials: Elements of a screening strategy. *Part. Fibre Toxicol.* **2005**, *2*, 8. [CrossRef] [PubMed]
13. Nel, A.; Xia, T.; Mädler, L.; Li, N. Review Toxic Potential of Materials at the Nanolevel. *Science* **2006**, *311*, 622–627. [CrossRef] [PubMed]
14. Khan, I.; Saeed, K.; Khan, I. Nanoparticles: Properties, applications and toxicities. *Arab. J. Chem.* **2017**. [CrossRef]
15. Linsinger, T.P.J.; Chaudhry, Q.; Dehalu, V.; Delahaut, P.; Dudkiewicz, A.; Grombe, R.; von der Kammer, F.; Larsen, E.H.; Legros, S.; Loeschner, K.; et al. Validation of methods for the detection and quantification of engineered nanoparticles in food. *Food Chem.* **2013**, *138*, 1959–1966. [CrossRef] [PubMed]
16. Gallocchio, F.; Bellucoa, S.; Ricci, A. Nanotechnology and food: Brief overview of the current scenario. *Procedia Food Sci.* **2015**, *5*, 85–88. [CrossRef]
17. Rahimnejad, M.; Mokhtarian, N.; Ghasemi, M. Production of protein nanoparticles for food and drug delivery system. *Afr. J. Biotechnol.* **2009**, *8*, 4738–4743.
18. Singh, T.; Shukla, S.; Kumar, P.; Wahla, V.; Bajpai, V.K.; Rather, I.A. Application of Nanotechnology in Food Science: Perception and Overview. *Front. Microbiol.* **2017**, *8*, 1501–1506. [CrossRef] [PubMed]
19. Sant, S.; Tao, S.L.; Fisher, O.Z.; Xu, Q.; Peppas, N.A.; Khademhoseini, A. Microfabrication technologies for oral drug delivery. *Adv. Drug Deliv. Rev.* **2012**, *64*, 496–507. [CrossRef] [PubMed]
20. Momin, J.K.; Jayakumar, C.; Prajapati, J.B. Potential of nanotechnology in functional foods. *Emir. J. Food Agric.* **2013**, *25*, 10–19. [CrossRef]
21. Bengoechea, C.; Jones, O.G.; Guerrero, A.; McClements, D.J. Formation and characterization of lactoferrin/pectin electrostatic complexes: Impact of composition, pH and thermal treatment. *Food Hydrocoll.*

2011, *25*, 1227–1232. [CrossRef]

22. Berton-Carabin, C.C.; Coupland, J.N.; Elias, R.J. Effect of the lipophilicity of model ingredients on their location and reactivity in emulsions and solid lipid nanoparticles. *Colloids Surf. A Physicochem. Eng. Asp.* **2013**, *431*, 9–17. [CrossRef]
23. Cerqueira, M.A.; Pinheiro, A.C.; Silva, H.D.; Ramos, P.E.; Azevedo, M.A.; Flores-López, M.L.; Rivera, M.C.; Bourbon, A.I.; Ramos, O.L.; Vicente, A.A. Design of bio-nanosystems for oral delivery of functional compounds. *Food Eng. Rev.* **2014**, *6*, 1–19. [CrossRef]
24. Weiss, J.; Takhistov, P.; McClements, D.J. Functional materials in food nanotechnology. *J. Food Sci.* **2006**, *71*, R107–R116. [CrossRef]
25. Neethirajan, S.; Jayas, D.S. Nanotechnology for the food and bioprocessing industries. *Food Bioprocess Technol.* **2011**, *4*, 39–47. [CrossRef]
26. Harde, H.; Das, M.; Jain, S. Solid lipid nanoparticles: An oral bioavailability enhancer vehicle. *Expert Opin. Drug Deliv.* **2011**, *8*, 1407–1424. [CrossRef] [PubMed]
27. Solans, C.; Izquierdo, P.; Nolla, J.; Azemar, N.; Garcia-Celma, M.J. Nano-emulsions. *Curr. Opin. Colloid Interface Sci.* **2005**, *10*, 102–110. [CrossRef]
28. Blasi, P.; Giovagnoli, S.; Schoubben, A.; Ricci, M.; Rossi, C. Solid lipid nanoparticles for targeted brain drug delivery. *Adv. Drug Deliv. Rev.* **2007**, *59*, 454–477. [CrossRef] [PubMed]
29. Thatipamula, R.; Palem, C.; Gannu, R.; Mudragada, S.; Yamsani, M. Formulation and in vitro characterization of domperidone loaded solid lipid nanoparticles and nanostructured lipid carriers. *Daru* **2011**, *19*, 23–32. [PubMed]
30. Gregoriadis, G. Immunological adjuvants: A role for liposomes. *Immunol. Today* **1990**, *11*, 89–97. [CrossRef]
31. Alving, C.R. Liposomes as carriers of antigens and adjuvants. *J. Immunol. Methods* **1991**, *140*, 1–13. [CrossRef]
32. Sharma, A.; Sharma, U.S. Liposomes in drug delivery: Progress and limitations. *Int. J. Pharm.* **1997**, *154*, 123–140. [CrossRef]
33. Vanrooijen, N.; Vannieuwmegen, R. Liposomes in immunology–multilamellar phosphatidylcholine liposomes as a simple, biodegradable and harmless adjuvant without any immunogenic activity of its own. *Immunol. Commun.* **1980**, *9*, 243–256. [CrossRef]
34. Campbell, P.I. Toxicity of some charged lipids used in liposome preparations. *Cytobios* **1983**, *37*, 21–26. [PubMed]
35. Chaize, B.; Colletier, J.P.; Winterhalter, M.; Fournier, D. Encapsulation of enzymes in liposomes: High encapsulation efficiency and control of substrate permeability. *Artif. Cell Blood* **2004**, *32*, 67–75. [CrossRef]
36. Zhou, F.; Neutra, M.R. Antigen delivery to mucosa-associated lymphoid tissues using liposomes as a carrier. *Biosci. Rep.* **2002**, *22*, 355–369. [CrossRef]
37. Matteucci, M.L.; Thrall, D.E. the role of liposomes in drug delivery and diagnostic imaging: A review. *Vet. Radiol. Ultrasound* **2000**, *41*, 100–107. [CrossRef] [PubMed]
38. Mady, M.M.; Ghannam, M.M.; Khalil, W.A.; Repp, R.; Markus, M.; Rascher, W.; Muller, R.; Fahr, A. Efficient gene delivery with serum into human cancer cells using targeted anionic liposomes. *J. Drug Target.* **2004**, *12*, 11–18. [CrossRef] [PubMed]
39. Koo, O.M.; Rubinstein, I.; Onyuksel, H. Role of nanotechnology in targeted drug delivery and imaging: A concise review. *Nanomed. Nanotechnol. Biol. Med.* **2005**, *1*, 193–212. [CrossRef] [PubMed]
40. Jain, R.K. Delivery of molecular and cellular medicine to solid tumors. *J. Control. Release* **1998**, *53*, 49–67. [CrossRef]
41. Kataoka, K.; Harada, A.; Nagasaki, Y. Block copolymer micelles for drug delivery: Design, characterization and biological significance. *Adv. Drug Deliv. Rev.* **2001**, *47*, 113–131. [CrossRef]
42. Gong, J.; Chen, M.; Zheng, Y.; Wang, S.; Wang, Y. Polymeric micelles drug delivery system in oncology. *J. Control. Release* **2012**, *159*, 312–323. [CrossRef] [PubMed]
43. Kwon, G.S.; Okano, T. Polymeric micelles as new drug carriers. *Adv. Drug Deliv. Rev.* **1996**, *21*, 107–116. [CrossRef]
44. Teng, Y.; Morrison, M.E.; Munk, P.; Webber, S.E.; Prochazka, K. Release kinetics studies of aromatic molecules into water from block polymer micelles. *Macromolecules* **1998**, *31*, 3578–3587. [CrossRef]
45. Rapoport, N. Physical stimuli-responsive polymeric micelles for anti-cancer drug delivery. *Prog. Polym. Sci.* **2007**, *32*, 962–990. [CrossRef]
46. Zia, Q.; Farzuddin, M.; Ansari, M.A.; Alam, M.; Ali, A.; Ahmad, A.; Owais, M. Novel drug delivery systems

for antifungal compounds. In *Combating Fungal Infections*; Ahmad, I., Owais, M., Shahid, M., Aqil, F., Eds.; Springer: Berlin/Heidelberg, Germany, 2010; pp. 485–528.

47. Mikhail, A.S.; Allen, C. Block copolymer micelles for delivery of cancer therapy: Transport at the whole body, tissue and cellular levels. *J. Control. Release* **2009**, *138*, 214–223. [CrossRef] [PubMed]
48. Malhotra, M.; Jain, N.K. Niosomes as drug carriers. *Indian Drugs* **1994**, *31*, 81–86.
49. Uchegbu, I.F.; Vyas, S.P. Non-ionic surfactant based vesicles (niosomes) in drug delivery. *Int. J. Pharm.* **1998**, *176*, 139–172. [CrossRef]
50. Jain, S.; Singh, P.; Mishra, V.; Vyas, S.P. Mannosylated niosomes as adjuvantcarrier system for oral genetic immunization against Hepatitis B. *Immunol. Lett.* **2005**, *101*, 41–49. [CrossRef] [PubMed]
51. Balasubramaniam, A.; Kumar, V.A.; Pillai, K.S. Formulation and in vivo evaluation of niosome-encapsulated daunorubicin hydrochloride. *Drug Dev. Ind. Pharm.* **2002**, *28*, 1181–1193. [CrossRef] [PubMed]
52. Gude, R.P.; Jadhav, M.G.; Rao, S.G.; Jagtap, A.G. Effects of niosomal cisplatin and combination of the same with theophylline and with activated macrophages in murine B16F10 melanoma model. *Cancer Biother. Radiopharm.* **2002**, *17*, 183–192. [CrossRef] [PubMed]
53. Shahiwala, A.; Misra, A. Studies in topical application of niosomally entrapped Nimesulide. *J. Pharm. Pharm. Sci.* **2002**, *5*, 220–225. [PubMed]
54. Pardeshi, C.; Rajput, P.; Belgamwar, V.; Tekade, A.; Patil, G.; Chaudhary, K.; Sonje, A. Solid lipid based nanocarriers: An overview. *Acta Pharm.* **2012**, *62*, 433–472. [CrossRef] [PubMed]
55. Mukherjee, S.; Ray, S.; Thakur, R.S. Solid Lipid Nanoparticles: A Modern Formulation Approach in Drug Delivery System. *Indian J. Pharm. Sci.* **2009**, *71*, 349–358. [CrossRef] [PubMed]
56. Naseri, N.; Valizadeh, H.; Zakeri-Milani, P. Solid lipid nanoparticles and nanostructured lipid carriers: Structure preparation and application. *Adv. Pharm. Bull.* **2015**, *5*, 305–313. [CrossRef] [PubMed]
57. Singh, R.; Lillard, J.W. Nanoparticle-based targeted drug delivery. *Exp. Mol. Pathol.* **2009**, *86*, 215–223. [CrossRef] [PubMed]
58. Nitta, S.; Numata, K. Biopolymer-based nanoparticles for drug/gene delivery and tissue engineering. *Int. J. Mol. Sci.* **2013**, *14*, 1629–1654. [CrossRef] [PubMed]
59. Fojan, P.; Schwach-Abdellaoui, K.; Tommeraas, K.; Gurevich, L.; Petersen, S.B. Polysaccharide based Nanoparticles and Nanoporous matrices. *Nano Sci. Technol. Inst.* **2006**, *2*, 79–82.
60. Lemarchand, C.; Gref, R.; Couvreur, P. Polysaccharide-decorated nanoparticles. *Eur. J. Pharm. Biopharm.* **2004**, *58*, 327–341. [CrossRef] [PubMed]
61. Liu, Z.; Jiao, Y.; Wang, Y.; Zhou, C.; Zhang, Z. Polysaccharides-based nanoparticles as drug delivery systems. *Adv. Drug Deliv. Rev.* **2008**, *60*, 1650–1662. [CrossRef] [PubMed]
62. Salatin, S.; Jelvehgarim, M. Natural Polysaccharide based Nanoparticles for Drug/Gene Delivery. *Pharm. Sci.* **2017**, *23*, 84–94. [CrossRef]
63. Amidi, M.; Mastrobattista, E.; Jiskoot, W.; Hennink, W.E. Chitosan-based delivery systems for protein therapeutics and antigens. *Adv. Drug Deliv. Rev.* **2010**, *62*, 59–82. [CrossRef] [PubMed]
64. Duceppe, N.; Tabrizian, M. Advances in using chitosan-based nanoparticles for in vitro and in vivo drug and gene delivery. *Expert Opin. Drug Deliv.* **2010**, *7*, 1191–1207. [CrossRef] [PubMed]
65. You, J.O.; Peng, C.A. Calcium-Alginate Nanoparticles Formed by Reverse Microemulsion as Gene Carriers. *Macromol. Symp.* **2005**, *219*, 147–153. [CrossRef]
66. Ojea-Jiménez, I.; Tort, O.; Lorenzo, J.; Puntes, V.F. Engineered nonviral nanocarriers for intracellular gene delivery applications. *Biomed. Mater.* **2012**, *7*, 1–6. [CrossRef] [PubMed]
67. Sun, J.; Tan, H. Alginate-based biomaterials for regenerative medicine applications. *Materials* **2013**, *6*, 1285–1309. [CrossRef] [PubMed]
68. Arpicco, S.; Milla, P.; Stella, B.; Dosio, F. Hyaluronic Acid Conjugates as Vectors for the Active Targeting of Drugs, Genes and Nanocomposites in Cancer Treatment. *Molecules* **2014**, *19*, 3193–3230. [CrossRef] [PubMed]
69. Zhu, S.F.; Zheng, J.; Liu, F.; Qiu, C.Y.; Lin, W.F.; Tang, C.H. the influence of ionic strength on the characteristics of heat-induced soy protein aggregate nanoparticles and the freeze–thaw stability of the resultant Pickering emulsions. *Food Funct.* **2017**, *8*, 2974–2981. [CrossRef] [PubMed]
70. Tarhini, M.; Greige-Gerges, H.; Elaissari, A. Protein-based nanoparticles: From preparation to encapsulation of active molecules. *Int. J. Pharm.* **2017**, *522*, 172–197. [CrossRef] [PubMed]
71. Kaul, G.; Amiji, M. Biodistribution and targeting potential of poly(ethylene glycol)-modified gelatin

nanoparticles in subcutaneous murine tumor model. *J. Drug Target.* **2004**, *12*, 585–591. [CrossRef] [PubMed]
72. Donsìa, F.; Sessaa, M.; Mediounic, H.; Mgaidic, A.; Ferrari, G. Encapsulation of bioactive compounds in nanoemulsionbased delivery systems. *Procedia Food Sci.* **2011**, *1*, 1666–1671. [CrossRef]
73. Ahmed, K.; Li, Y.; McClements, D.J.; Xiao, H. Nanoemulsion- and emulsion-based delivery systems for curcumin: Encapsulation and release properties. *Food Chem.* **2012**, *132*, 799–807. [CrossRef]
74. Schultz, S.; Wagner, G.; Urban, K.; Ulrich, J. High-pressure homogenization as a process for emulsion formation. *Chem. Eng. Technol.* **2004**, *27*, 361–368. [CrossRef]
75. McClements, D.J. *Food Emulsions: Principles, Practice and Techniques*; CRC Press: Boca Raton, FL, USA, 2005.
76. Montes de Oca-Ávalos, J.M.; Herrera, M.L. Nanoemulsions: Stability and physical properties. *Curr. Opin. Food Sci.* **2017**, *16*, 1–6. [CrossRef]
77. Aboalnaja, K.O.; Yaghmoor, S.; Kumosani, T.A.; McClements, D.J. Utilization of nanoemulsions to enhance bioactivity of pharmaceuticals, supplements, and nutraceuticals: Nanoemulsion delivery systems and nanoemulsion excipient systems. *Expert Opin. Drug Deliv.* **2016**, *13*, 1–10. [CrossRef] [PubMed]
78. Kumar, K.; Sarkar, P. Encapsulation of bioactive compounds using nanoemulsions. *Environ. Chem. Lett.* **2018**, *16*, 59–70. [CrossRef]
79. Li, M.; Cui, J.; Ngadi, M.O.; Ma, Y. Absorption mechanism of whey-protein-delivered curcumin using caco-2 cell monolayers. *Food Chem.* **2015**, *180*, 48–54. [CrossRef] [PubMed]
80. Yu, H.; Huang, Q. Investigation of the cytotoxicity of food-grade nanoemulsions in caco-2 cell monolayers and hepg2 cells. *Food Chem.* **2013**, *141*, 29–33. [CrossRef] [PubMed]
81. Sari, T.P.; Mann, B.; Kumar, R.; Singh, R.R.B.; Sharma, R.; Bhardwaj, M.; Athira, S. Preparation and characterization of nanoemulsion encapsulating curcumin. *Food Hydrocoll.* **2015**, *43*, 540–546. [CrossRef]
82. Sessa, M.; Tsao, R.; Liu, R.; Ferrari, G.; Donsì, F. Evaluation of the stability and antioxidant activity of nanoencapsulated resveratrol during in vitro digestion. *J. Agric. Food Chem.* **2011**, *59*, 12352–12360. [CrossRef] [PubMed]
83. Sessa, M.; Balestrieri, M.L.; Ferrari, G.; Servillo, L.; Castaldo, D.; D'Onofrio, N.; Donsì, F.; Tsao, R. Bioavailability of encapsulated resveratrol into nanoemulsion-based delivery systems. *Food Chem.* **2014**, *147*, 42–50. [CrossRef] [PubMed]
84. Wenzel, E.; Somoza, V. Metabolism and bioavailability of trans-resveratrol. *Mol. Nutr. Food Res.* **2005**, *49*, 472–481. [CrossRef] [PubMed]
85. Gupta, A.; Eral, H.B.B.; Hatton, T.A.; Doyle, P.S. Controlling and predicting droplet size of nanoemulsions: Scaling relations with experimental validation. *Soft Matter* **2016**, *12*, 1452–1458. [CrossRef] [PubMed]
86. Zeeb, B.; Herz, E.; McClements, D.J.; Weiss, J. Reprint of: Impact of alcohols on the formation and stability of protein-stabilized nanoemulsions. *J. Colloid Interface Sci.* **2015**, *449*, 13–20. [CrossRef] [PubMed]
87. Wang, T.; Soyama, S.; Luo, Y. Development of a novel functional drink from all natural ingredients using nanotechnology. *LWT Food Sci. Technol.* **2016**, *73*, 458–466. [CrossRef]
88. Pan, L.; Liu, J.; He, Q.; Shi, J. MSN-mediated sequencial valscular to-cell nuclear targeted drug delivery for efficient tumor regression. *Adv. Mater.* **2014**, *26*, 6742–6748. [CrossRef] [PubMed]
89. Sarkar, S.; Siddiqui, A.A.; Mazumder, S.; De, R.; Saha, S.J.; Banerjee, C.; Iqbal, M.S.; Adhikari, S.; Alam, A.; Roy, S.; et al. Elagic Acid, a Dietary Polyphenol, Unhibits Tautomerase Activity of Human Magrophage Migration Inhibitory Factor and Its Pro-Inflammatory Responses in Human Perfipheral Blood Mononuclear Cells. *J. Agric. Food Chem.* **2015**, *63*, 4988–4998. [CrossRef] [PubMed]
90. Ezhilarasi, P.N.; Karthik, P.; Chhanwal, N.; Anandharamakrishnan, C. Nanoencapsulation techniques for food bioactive components: A review. *Food Bioprocess Technol.* **2013**, *6*, 628–647. [CrossRef]
91. Fathi, M.; Martín, T.; McClements, D.J. Nanoencapsulation of food ingredients using acrobhidrate based delivery systems. *Trends Food Sci. Technol.* **2014**, *39*, 19–38. [CrossRef]
92. Shani-Levi, C.; Levi-Tal, S.; Lesmes, U. Comparative performance of mild proteins and their emulsions under dynamic in vitro adult and infant gastric digestion. *Food Hydrocoll.* **2013**, *32*, 349–357. [CrossRef]
93. Wang, X.; Jiang, Y.; Wang, Y.W.; Huang, M.T.; Ho, C.T.; Huang, Q. Enhancing anti-inflammation activity of curcumin through O/W nanoemulsions. *Food Chem.* **2008**, *108*, 419–424. [CrossRef] [PubMed]
94. Cheng, A.L.; Hsu, C.H.; Lin, J.K.; Hsu, M.M.; Ho, Y.F.; Shen, T.S.; Ko, J.Y.; Lin, J.T.; Lin, B.R.; Ming-Shiang, W.; et al. Phase I clinical trial of curcumin, a chemopreventive agent, in patients with high-risk or pre-malignant lesions. *Anticancer Res.* **2001**, *21*, 2895–2900. [PubMed]
95. Simion, V.; Stan, D.; Constantinescu, C.A.; Deleanu, M.; Dragan, E.; Tucureanu, M.M.; Gan, A.M.; Butoi, E.;

Constantin, A.M.; Maduteanu, I.; et al. Conjugation of curcumin-loaded lipid nanoemulsions with cell-penetrating peptides increases their cellular uptake and enhances the anti-inflammatory effects in endothelial cells. *J. Pharm. Pharmacol.* **2016**, *68*, 195–207. [CrossRef] [PubMed]

96. Yu, H.; Huang, Q. Enhanced in vitro anti-cancer activity of curcumin encapsulated in hydrophobically modified starch. *Food Chem.* **2010**, *119*, 669–674. [CrossRef]
97. Bourassa, P.; Kanakis, C.D.; Tarantilis, P.; Pollissiou, M.G.; Tajmir-Riahi, H.A. Resveratrol, genistein, and curcumin bind bovine serum albumin. *J. Phys. Chem. B* **2010**, *114*, 3348–3354. [CrossRef] [PubMed]
98. Mohammadi, F.; Bordbar, A.K.; Divsalar, A.; Mohammadi, K.; Saboury, A. Interaction of curcumin and acetylcurcumin with the lipocalin member beta-lactoglobulin. *Protein J.* **2009**, *28*, 117–123. [CrossRef] [PubMed]
99. Shelma, R.; Sharma, C.P. Acyl modified chitosan derivatives for oral delivery of insulin and curcumin. *J. Mater. Sci. Mater. Med.* **2010**, *21*, 2133–2140. [CrossRef] [PubMed]
100. Scalbert, A.; Williamson, G. Dietary intake and bioavailability of polyphenols. *J. Nutr.* **2000**, *130*, 2073S–2085S. [CrossRef] [PubMed]
101. Koutelidakis, A.E.; Argyri, K.; Sevastou, Z.; Lamprinaki, D.; Panagopoulou, E.; Paximada, E.; Sali, A.; Papalazarou, V.; Mallouchos, A.; Evageliou, V.; et al. Bioactivity of Epigallocatechin Gallate Nanoemulsions Evaluated in Mice Model. *J. Med. Food* **2017**, *20*, 923–931. [CrossRef] [PubMed]
102. Orafidiya, L.O.; Agbani, E.O.; Oyedele, A.O.; Babalola, O.O.; Onayemi, O. Preliminary clinical tests on topical preparations of *Ocimum gratissimum* linn leaf essential oil for the treatment of Acne vulgaris. *Clin. Drug Investig.* **2002**, *22*, 313–319. [CrossRef]
103. Baranauskiene, R.M.; Venskutonis, P.R.; Dewettinck, K.; Verhe, R. Properties of oregano (*Origanum vulgare* L.), citronella (*Cymbopogon nardus* G.) and marjoram (*Majorana hortensis* L.) flavors encapsulated into milk protein-based matrices. *Food Res. Int.* **2006**, *39*, 413–425. [CrossRef]
104. Wang, X.; Wang, Y.W.; Huang, Q. Enhancing stability and oral bioavailability of polyphenols using nanoemulsions. *ACS Symp. Ser.* **2009**, *1007*, 198–212.
105. Bilia, A.R.; Guccione, C.; Isacchi, B.; Righeschi, C.; Firenzuoli, F.; Bergonzi, M.C. Essential Oils Loaded in Nanosystems: A Developing Strategy for a Successful Therapeutic Approach. *Evid.-Based Complement. Altern. Med.* **2014**, *2014*, 1–14. [CrossRef] [PubMed]
106. Maryam, I.; Huzaifa, U.; Hindatu, H.; Zubaida, S. Nanoencapsulation of essential oils with enhanced antimicrobial activity: A new way of combating antimicrobial Resistance. *J. Pharmacogn. Phytochem.* **2015**, *4*, 165–170.
107. Oejhlke, K.; Behsnilian, D.; Mayer-Miebach, E.; Weidler, P.G.; Greiner, R. Edible solid lipid nanopartilces (SLN) as carrier systems for antioxidants of different lipophylicity. *PLoS ONE* **2017**, *12*, e0171662.
108. Jung, S.; Choi, C.H.; Lee, C.S.; Yi, H. Integrated fabrication–conjugation methods for polymeric and hybrid microparticles for programmable drug delivery and biosensing application. *Biotechnol. J.* **2016**, *11*, 1561–1571. [CrossRef] [PubMed]
109. González, M.J.; Medina, I.; Maldonado, O.S.; Lucas, R.; Morales, J.C. Antioxidant activity of alkyl gallates and glycosyl alkyl gallates in fish oil in water emulsions: Relevance of their surface active properties and of thetype of emulsifier. *Food Chem.* **2015**, *183*, 190–196. [CrossRef] [PubMed]
110. Nagao, A.; Kotake-Nara, E.; Hase, M. Effects of fats and oils on the bioaccessibility of carotenoids and vitamin E in vegetables. *Biosci. Biotechnol. Biochem.* **2013**, *77*, 776–785. [CrossRef] [PubMed]
111. Vidhyalakshmi, R.; Bhakyaraj, R.; Subhasree, R. Encapsulation "the future of probiotics"—A review. *Adv. Biol. Res.* **2009**, *3*, 96–103.
112. Hou, R.C.W.; Lin, M.Y.; Wang, M.M.C.; Tzen, J.T.C. Increase of viability of entrapped cells of *Lactobacillus delbrueckii* ssp. *bulgaricus in artificial sesame oils emulsions. J. Dairy Sci.* **2003**, *86*, 424–428. [PubMed]
113. Kloover, J.S.; den Bakker, M.A.; Gelderblom, H.; van Meerbeeck, J.P. Fatal outcome of a hypersensitivity reaction to paclitaxel: A critical review of premedication regimens. *Br. J. Cancer* **2004**, *90*, 304–305. [CrossRef] [PubMed]
114. Rijcken, C.J.F.; Soga, O.; Hennink, W.E.; van Nostrum, C.F. Triggered destabilisation of polymeric micelles and vesicles by changing polymers polarity: An attractive tool for drug delivery. *J. Control. Release* **2007**, *120*, 131–148. [CrossRef] [PubMed]
115. Chen, Y.C.; Lo, C.L.; Lin, Y.F.; Hsiue, G.H. Rapamycin encapsulated in dualresponsive micelles for cancer

therapy. *Biomaterials* **2013**, *34*, 1115–1127. [CrossRef] [PubMed]
116. Matsumura, Y.; Kataoka, K. Preclinical and clinical studies of anticancer agent-incorporating polymer micelles. *Cancer Sci.* **2009**, *100*, 572–579. [CrossRef] [PubMed]
117. Swamy, M.K.; Sinniah, U.R. A comprehensive review on the phytochemical constituents and pharmacological activities of pogostemon cablin benth: An aromatic medicinal plant of industrial importance. *Molecules* **2015**, *20*, 8521–8547. [CrossRef] [PubMed]
118. Pinciroli, M.; Domínguez-Perles, R.; Abellán, A.; Guy, A.; Durand, T.; Oger, C.; Galano, J.M.; Ferreres, F.; Gil-Izquierdo, A. Comparative study of the Phytoprostane and Phytofuran Content of indica and japonica Rice (*Oryza sativa* L.) Flours. *J. Agric. Food Chem.* **2017**, *65*, 8938–8947. [CrossRef] [PubMed]
119. Lu, B.Y.; Li, M.Q.; Yin, R. Phytochemical Content, Health benefits, and toxicology of common edible flowers: A review (2000–2015). *Crit. Rev. Food Sci. Nutr.* **2016**, *56*, S130–S148. [CrossRef] [PubMed]
120. Chang, S.K.; Alasalvar, C.; Shahidi, F. Review of dried fruits: Phytochemicals, antioxidant efficacies, and health benefits. *J. Funct. Foods* **2016**, *21*, 113–132. [CrossRef]
121. Son, Y.R.; Choi, E.H.; Kim, G.T.; Park, T.S.; Shim, S.M. Bioefficacy of graviola leaf extracts in scavenging free radicals and upregulating antioxidant genes. *Food Funct.* **2016**, *7*, 861–871. [CrossRef] [PubMed]
122. Xiao, J.; Cao, Y.; Huang, Q. Edible Nanoencapsulation Vehicles for Oral Delivery of Phytochemicals: A Perspective Paper. *J. Agric. Food Chem.* **2017**, *65*, 6727–6735. [CrossRef] [PubMed]
123. Medina, S.; Domínguez-Perles, R.; Gil, J.I.; Ferreres, F.; Gil-Izquierdo, A. Metabolomics and the Diagnosis of Human Diseases—A Guide to the Markers and Pathophysiological Pathways Affected. *Curr. Med. Chem.* **2014**, *21*, 823–848. [CrossRef] [PubMed]
124. Ting, Y.; Jiang, Y.; Ho, C.T.; Huang, Q. Common delivery systems for enhancing in vivo bioavailability and biological efficacy of nutraceuticals. *J. Funct. Foods* **2014**, *7*, 112–128. [CrossRef]
125. Melo-Filho, C.C.; Braga, R.C.; Andrade, C.H. Advances in methods for predicting phase I metabolism of polyphenols. *Curr. Drug Metab.* **2014**, *15*, 120–126. [CrossRef] [PubMed]
126. Huang, Q.R.; Yu, H.L.; Ru, Q.M. Bioavailability and delivery of nutraceuticals using nanotechnology. *J. Food Sci.* **2010**, *75*, R50–R57. [CrossRef] [PubMed]
127. Radhakrishnan, R.; Kulhari, H.; Pooja, D.; Gudem, S.; Bhargava, S.; Shukla, R.; Sistla, R. Encapsulation of biophenolic phytochemical EGCG within lipid nanoparticles enhances its stability and cytotoxicity against cancer. *Chem. Phys. Lipids* **2016**, *198*, 51–60. [CrossRef] [PubMed]
128. Lockman, P.R.; Koziara, J.M.; Mumper, R.J.; Allen, D.D. Nanoparticle surface charges alter blood-brain barrier integrity and permeability. *J. Drug Target.* **2004**, *12*, 635–641. [CrossRef] [PubMed]
129. Liu, Y.; Li, K.; Liu, B.; Feng, S.S. A strategy for precision engineering of nanoparticles of biodegradable copolymers for quantitative control of targeted drug delivery. *Biomaterials* **2010**, *31*, 9145–9155. [CrossRef] [PubMed]
130. Kumari, A.; Singla, R.; Guliani, A.; Yadav, S.K. Nanoencapsulation for drug delivery. *EXCLI J.* **2014**, *13*, 265–286. [PubMed]
131. Xiao, J.; Nian, S.; Huang, Q.R. Assembly of kafirin/carboxymethyl chitosan nanoparticles to enhance the cellular uptake of curcumin. *Food Hydrocoll.* **2015**, *51*, 166–175. [CrossRef]
132. Kumar, D.V.; Verma, P.R.P.; Singh, S.K. Development and evaluation of biodegradable polymeric nanoparticles for the effective delivery of quercetin using a quality by design approach. *LWT Food Sci. Technol.* **2015**, *61*, 330–338. [CrossRef]
133. Pan, K.; Zhong, Q.X.; Baek, S.J. Enhanced dispersibility and bioactivity of curcumin by encapsulation in casein nanocapsules. *J. Agric. Food Chem.* **2013**, *61*, 6036–6043. [CrossRef] [PubMed]
134. Hu, B.; Ting, Y.; Yang, X.; Tang, W.; Zeng, X.; Huang, Q. Nanochemoprevention by encapsulation of (−)-epigallocatechin-3gallate with bioactive peptides/chitosan nanoparticles for enhancement of its bioavailability. *Chem. Commun.* **2012**, *48*, 2421–2423. [CrossRef] [PubMed]
135. Zou, L.Q.; Zheng, B.J.; Zhang, R.J.; Zhang, Z.P.; Liu, W.; Liu, C.M.; Xiao, H.; McClements, D.J. Food-grade nanoparticles for encapsulation, protection and delivery of curcumin: Comparison of lipid, protein, and phospholipid nanoparticles under simulated gastrointestinal conditions. *RSC Adv.* **2016**, *6*, 3126–3136. [CrossRef]
136. Domínguez-Perles, R.; Abellán, A.; León, D.; Ferreres, F.; Guy, A.; Oger, C.; Galano, J.M.; Durand, T.; Gil-Izquierdo, A. sorting out the phytoprostane and phytofuran profile in vegetable oils. *Food Res. Int.* **2018**, *107*, 619–628. [CrossRef] [PubMed]

137. Xiao, J.; Li, C.; Huang, Q. Kafirin nanoparticles-stabilized Pickering emulsions as oral delivery vehicles: Physicochemical stability and in vitro digestion profile. *J. Agric. Food Chem.* **2015**, *63*, 10263–10270. [CrossRef] [PubMed]
138. Liu, M.; Zhang, J.; Zhu, X.; Shan, W.; Li, L.; Zhong, J.J.; Zhang, Z.R.; Huang, Y. Efficient mucus permeation and tight junction opening by dissociable "mucus-inert" agent coated trimethyl chitosan nanoparticles for oral insulin delivery. *J. Control. Release* **2016**, *222*, 67–77. [CrossRef] [PubMed]
139. Perez, Y.A.; Urista, C.M.; Martinez, J.I.; Nava, M.D.D.; Rodriguez, F.A.R. Functionalized polymers for enhance oral bioavailability of sensitive molecules. *Polymers* **2016**, *8*, 214. [CrossRef]
140. Barua, S.; Mitragotri, S. Challenges associated with penetration of nanoparticles across cell and tissue barriers: A review of current status and future prospects. *Nano Today* **2014**, *9*, 223–243. [CrossRef] [PubMed]
141. Johnson, B.M.; Charman, W.N.; Porter, C.J.H. the impact of P-glycoprotein efflux on enterocyte residence time and enterocytebased metabolism of verapamil. *J. Pharm. Pharmacol.* **2001**, *53*, 1611–1619. [CrossRef] [PubMed]
142. Charman, W.N.A.; Noguchi, T.; Stella, V.J. An experimental system designed to study the in situ intestinal lymphatic transport of lipophilic drugs in anesthetized rats. *Int. J. Pharm.* **1986**, *33*, 155–164. [CrossRef]
143. Kim, H.; Kim, Y.; Lee, J. Liposomal formulations for enhanced lymphatic drug delivery. *Asian J. Pharm. Sci.* **2013**, *8*, 96–103. [CrossRef]
144. Sha, X.; Yan, G.; Wu, Y.; Li, J.; Fang, X. Effect of selfmicroemulsifying drug delivery systems containing Labrasol on tight junctions in Caco-2 cells. *Eur. J. Pharm. Sci.* **2005**, *24*, 477–486. [CrossRef] [PubMed]
145. Xu, X.F.; Xu, P.P.; Ma, C.W.; Tang, J.; Zhang, X.W. Gut microbiota, host health, and polysaccharides. *Biotechnol. Adv.* **2013**, *31*, 318–337. [CrossRef] [PubMed]
146. Caesar, R.; Nygren, H.; Oresic, M.; Backhed, F. Interaction between dietary lipids and gut microbiota regulates hepatic cholesterol metabolism. *J. Lipid Res.* **2016**, *57*, 474–481. [CrossRef] [PubMed]
147. Aqil, F.; Munagala, R.; Jeyabalan, J.; Vadhanam, M.V. Bioavailability of phytochemicals and its enhancement by drug delivery systems. *Cancer Lett.* **2013**, *334*, 133–141. [CrossRef] [PubMed]
148. Kumari, A.; Yadav, S.K.; Yadav, S.C. Biodegradable polymeric nanoparticles based drug delivery systems. *Colloids Surf. B Biointerfaces* **2010**, *75*, 1–18. [CrossRef] [PubMed]
149. Boulle, F.; Kenis, G.; Cazorla, M.; Hamon, M.; Steinbusch, H.W.; Lanfumey, L.; van del Hove, D.L. TrkB inhibition as a therapeutic target for CNS-related disorders. *Prog. Neurobiol.* **2012**, *98*, 197–206. [CrossRef] [PubMed]
150. Huang, E.J.; Reichardt, L.F. Neurotrophins: Roles in neuronal development and function. *Annu. Rev. Neurosci.* **2001**, *24*, 677–736. [CrossRef] [PubMed]
151. Cowansage, K.K.; LeDoux, J.E.; Monfils, M.H. Brain-derived neurotrophic factor: A dynamic gatekeeper of neural plasticity. *Curr. Mol. Pharmacol.* **2010**, *3*, 12–29. [CrossRef] [PubMed]
152. Lindholm, P.; Voutilainen, M.H.; Laurén, J.; Peränen, J.; Leppänen, V.M.; Andressoo, J.O.; Lindahl, M.; Janhunen, S.; Kalkkinen, N.; Timmusk, T.; et al. Novel neurotrophic factor CDNF protects and rescues midbrain dopamine neurons in vivo. *Nature* **2007**, *448*, 73–77. [CrossRef] [PubMed]
153. Pattarawarapan, M.; Burgess, K. Molecular basis of neurotrophin-receptor interactions. *J. Med. Chem.* **2003**, *46*, 5277–5291. [CrossRef] [PubMed]
154. Gullett, N.P.; Ruhul Amin, A.R.; Bayraktar, S.; Pezzuto, J.M.; Shin, D.M.; Khuri, F.R.; Aggarwal, B.B.; Surh, Y.J.; Kucuk, O. Cancer prevention with natural compounds. *Semin. Oncol.* **2010**, *37*, 258–281. [CrossRef] [PubMed]
155. Naithani, R.; Huma, L.C.; Moriarty, R.M.; McCormick, D.L.; Mehta, R.G. Comprehensive review of cancer chemopreventive agents evaluated in experimental carcinogenesis models and clinical trials. *Curr. Med. Chem.* **2008**, *15*, 1044–1071. [CrossRef] [PubMed]
156. Zolk, O.; Fromm, M.F. Transporter-mediated drug uptake and efflux: Important determinants of adverse drug reactions. *Clin. Pharmacol. Ther.* **2011**, *89*, 798–805. [CrossRef] [PubMed]
157. Kusuhara, H.; Sugiyama, Y. Role of transporters in the tissue-selective distribution and elimination of drugs: Transporters in the liver, small intestine, brain and kidney. *J. Control. Release* **2002**, *78*, 43–54. [CrossRef]
158. Li, Y.; Paxton, J.W. Oral bioavailability and disposition of phytochemicals. In *Phytochemicals—Bioactivities and Impact on Health*; Rasooli, I., Ed.; InTech: Rijeka, Croatia, 2011; pp. 117–138.
159. Manach, C.; Scalbert, A.; Morand, C.; Remesy, C.; Jimenez, L. Polyphenols: Foodsources and bioavailability. *Am. J. Clin. Nutr.* **2004**, *79*, 727–747. [CrossRef] [PubMed]

160. Mishra, B.; Patel, B.B.; Tiwari, S. Colloidal nanocarriers: A review on formulation technology, types and applications toward targeted drug delivery. *Nanomed. Nanotechnol.* **2010**, *6*, 9–24. [CrossRef] [PubMed]
161. Oerlemans, C.; Bult, W.; Bos, M.; Storm, G.; Nijsen, J.F.W.; Hennink, W.E. Polymeric micelles in anticancer therapy: Targeting, imaging and triggered release. *Pharm. Res.* **2010**, *27*, 2569–2589. [CrossRef] [PubMed]
162. Davis, S.S. Biomedical applications of nanotechnology—Implications for drug targeting and gene therapy. *Trends Biotechnol.* **1997**, *15*, 217–224. [CrossRef]
163. Zhao, Y. Photocontrollable block copolymer micelles: What can we control? *J. Mater. Chem.* **2009**, *19*, 4887–4895. [CrossRef]
164. Gil, E.S.; Hudson, S.M. Stimuli-reponsive polymers and their bioconjugates. *Prog. Polym. Sci.* **2004**, *29*, 1173–1222. [CrossRef]
165. Shenoy, D.; Little, S.; Langer, R.; Amiji, M. Poly(ethylene oxide)-modified poly(beta-amino ester) nanoparticles as a pH-sensitive system for tumor targeted delivery of hydrophobic drugs: Part 2. In vivo distribution and tumor localization studies. *Pharm. Res.* **2005**, *22*, 2107–2114. [CrossRef] [PubMed]
166. Devalapally, H.; Shenoy, D.; Little, S.; Langer, R.; Amiji, M. Poly(ethylene oxide)-modified poly(beta-amino ester) nanoparticles as a pH-sensitive system for tumor-targeted delivery of hydrophobic drugs: Part 3. Therapeutic efficacy and safety studies in ovarian cancer xenograft model. *Cancer Chemother. Pharm.* **2007**, *59*, 477–484. [CrossRef] [PubMed]
167. Allen, C.; Maysinger, D.; Eisenberg, A. Nano-engineering block copolymer aggregates for drug delivery. *Colloids Surf. B Biointerfaces* **1999**, *16*, 3–27. [CrossRef]
168. Amin, F.U.; Shah, S.A.; Badshah, H.; Khan, M.; Kim, M.O. Anthocyanins encapsulated by PLGA@PEG nanoparticles potentially improved its free radical scavenging capabilities via p38/JNK pathway against Aβ1–42-induced oxidative stress. *J. Nanobiotechnol.* **2017**, *15*, 12–27. [CrossRef] [PubMed]
169. Torchilin, V.P.; Lukyanov, A.N. Peptide and protein drug delivery to and into tumors: Challenges and solutions. *Drug Discov. Today* **2003**, *8*, 259–266. [CrossRef]
170. Jiménez-Aguilar, D.M.; Ortega-Regules, A.E.; Lozada-Ramírez, J.D.; Pérez-Pérez, M.C.I.; Vernon-Cartere, E.J.; Welti-Chanesa, J. Color and chemical stability of spray-dried blueberry extract using mesquite gum as wall material. *J. Food Compos. Anal.* **2011**, *24*, 889–894. [CrossRef]
171. Sampat, K.M.; Garg, S.J. Complications of intravitreal injections. *Curr. Opin. Ophthalmol.* **2010**, *21*, 178–183. [CrossRef] [PubMed]
172. Thakur, S.S.; Barnett, N.L.; Donaldson, M.J.; Parekh, H.S. Intravitreal drug delivery in retinal disease: Are we out of our depth? *Expert Opin. Drug Deliv.* **2014**, *11*, 1575–1590. [CrossRef] [PubMed]
173. Agrahari, V.; Agrahari, V.; Hung, W.T.; Christenson, L.K.; Mitra, A.K. Composite Nanoformulation Therapeutics for Long-Term Ocular Delivery of Macromolecules. *Mol. Pharm.* **2016**, *13*, 2912–2922. [CrossRef] [PubMed]
174. Traka, M.H.; Mithen, R.F. Plant Science and Human Nutrition: Challenges in Assessing Health-Promoting Properties of Phytochemicals. *Plant Cell* **2011**, *23*, 2483–2497. [CrossRef] [PubMed]
175. Skrovankova, S.; Sumczynski, D.; Mlcek, J.; Jurikova, T.; Sochor, J. Bioactive Compounds and Antioxidant Activity in Different Types of Berries. *Int. J. Mol. Sci.* **2015**, *16*, 24673–24706. [CrossRef] [PubMed]
176. Sahoo, S.K.; Dilnawaz, F.; Krishnakumar, S. Nanotechnology in ocular drug delivery. *Drug Discov. Today* **2008**, *13*, 144–151. [CrossRef] [PubMed]
177. Bangham, A.D. Liposomes: the Babraham connection. *Chem. Phys. Lipids* **1993**, *64*, 275–285. [CrossRef]
178. Chiappetta, D.A.; Sosnik, A. Poly (ethylene oxide)-poly (propylene oxide) block copolymer micelles as drug delivery agents: Improved hydrosolubility, stability and bioavailability of drugs. *Eur. J. Pharm. Biopharm.* **2007**, *66*, 303–317. [CrossRef] [PubMed]
179. Labhasetwar, V.; Song, C.; Levy, R.J. Nanoparticle drug delivery system for restenosis. *Adv. Drug Deliv. Rev.* **1997**, *24*, 63–85. [CrossRef]
180. Pescina, S.; Sonvico, F.; Santi, P.; Nicoli, S. Therapeutics and carriers: the dual role of proteins in nanoparticles for ocular delivery. *Curr. Top. Med. Chem.* **2015**, *15*, 369–385. [CrossRef] [PubMed]
181. Oehlke, K.; Adamiuk, M.; Behsnilian, D.; Graf, V.; Mayer-Miebach, E.; Walz, E.; Greiner, R. Potential bioavailability enhancement of bioactive compounds using food-grade engineered nanomaterials: A review of the existing evidence. *Food Funct.* **2014**, *5*, 1341–1359. [CrossRef] [PubMed]
182. Varadinova, M.G.; Docheva-Drenska, D.I.; Boyadjieva, N.I. Effects of anthocyanins on learning and memory of ovariectomized rats. *Menopause* **2009** *16*, 345–349. [CrossRef] [PubMed]

183. Li, L.; Li, W.; Jung, S.W.; Lee, Y.W.; Kim, Y.H. Protective effects of decursin and decursinol angelate against amyloid β-protein-induced oxidative stress in the PC12 cell line: the role of Nrf2 and antioxidant enzymes. *Biosci. Biotechnol. Biochem.* **2011**, *75*, 434–442. [CrossRef] [PubMed]
184. Fomina, N.; Sankaranarayanan, J.; Almutairi, A. Photochemical mechanisms of light-triggered release from nanocarriers. *Adv. Drug Deliv. Rev.* **2012**, *64*, 1005–1020. [CrossRef] [PubMed]
185. Alvarez-Lorenzo, C.; Bromberg, L.; Concheiro, A. Light-sensitive intelligent drug delivery systems. *Photochem. Photobiol.* **2009**, *85*, 848–860. [CrossRef] [PubMed]
186. Bisby, R.H.; Mead, C.; Morgan, C.G. Wavelength-programmed solute release from photosensitive liposomes. *Biochem. Biophys. Res. Commun.* **2000**, *276*, 169–173. [CrossRef] [PubMed]
187. Morgan, C.G.; Yianni, Y.P.; Sandhu, S.S.; Mitchell, A.C. Liposome fusion and lipid exchange on ultraviolet irradiation of liposomes containing a photochromic phospholipid. *Photochem. Photobiol.* **1995**, *62*, 24–29. [CrossRef] [PubMed]
188. Panyam, J.; Labhasetwar, V. Sustained cytoplasmic delivery of drugs with intracellular receptors using biodegradable nanoparticles. *Mol. Pharm.* **2004**, *1*, 77–84. [CrossRef] [PubMed]
189. Bareford, L.M.; Swaan, P.W. Endocytic mechanisms for targeted drug delivery. *Adv. Drug Deliv. Rev.* **2007**, *59*, 748–758. [CrossRef] [PubMed]
190. Sha, X.Y.; Guo, J.; Chen, Y.Z.; Fang, X.L. Effect of phospholipid composition on pharmacokinetics and biodistribution of epirubicin liposomes. *J. Liposome Res.* **2012**, *22*, 80–88. [CrossRef] [PubMed]
191. Angelova, A.; Angelov, B.; Drechsler, M.; Lesieur, S. Neurotrophin delivery using nanotechnology. *Drug Discov. Today* **2013**, *18*, 1263–1271. [CrossRef] [PubMed]
192. Bertram, J.P.; Rauch, M.F.; Chang, K.; Lavik, E.B. Using polymer chemistry to modulate the delivery of neurotrophic factors from degradable microspheres: Delivery of BDNF. *Pharm. Res.* **2010**, *27*, 82–91. [CrossRef] [PubMed]
193. Checa-Casalengua, P.; Jiang, C.; Bravo-Osuna, I.; Tucker, B.A.; Molina-Martínez, I.T.; Young, M.J.; Herrereo-Vanrell, R. Preservation of biological activity of glial cell line-derived neurotrophic factor (GDNF) after microencapsulation and sterilization by gamma irradiation. *Int. J. Pharm.* **2012**, *436*, 545–554. [CrossRef] [PubMed]
194. Garbayo, E.; Ansorena, E.; Lanciego, J.L.; Blanco-Prieto, M.J.; Aymerich, M.S. Long-term neuroprotection and neurorestoration by glial cell-derived neurotrophic factor microspheres for the treatment of Parkinson's disease. *Mov. Disord.* **2011**, *26*, 1943–1947. [CrossRef] [PubMed]
195. Lampe, K.J.; Kem, D.S.; Mahoney, M.J.; Bjugstad, K.B. the administration of BDNF and GDNF to the brain via PLGA microparticles patterned within a degradable PEG-based hydrogel: Protein distribution and the glial response. *J. Biomed. Mater. Res.* **2011**, *96*, 595–607. [CrossRef] [PubMed]
196. Huang, X.; Brazel, C.S. On the importance and mechanisms of burst release in matrix-controlled drug delivery systems. *J. Control. Release* **2001**, *73*, 121–136. [CrossRef]
197. Pridgen, E.M.; Langer, R.; Farokhzad, O.C. Biodegradable, polymeric nanoparticle delivery systems for cancer therapy. *Nanomedicine* **2007**, *2*, 669–680. [CrossRef] [PubMed]
198. Yamamoto, H.; Tahara, K.; Kawashima, Y. Nanomedical system for nucleic acid drugs created with the biodegradable nanoparticle platform. *J. Microencapsul.* **2012**, *29*, 54–62. [CrossRef] [PubMed]
199. Maurer-Jones, M.A.; Bantz, K.C.; Love, S.A.; Marquis, B.J.; Haynes, C.L. Toxicity of therapeutic nanoparticles. *Nanomedicine* **2009**, *4*, 219–241. [CrossRef] [PubMed]
200. Shvedova, A.A.; Kagan, V.E.; Fadeel, B. Close encounters of the small kind: Adverse effects of man-made materials interfacing with the nano-cosmos of biological systems. *Annu. Rev. Pharm. Toxicol.* **2010**, *50*, 63–88. [CrossRef] [PubMed]
201. Vega-Villa, K.R.; Takemoto, J.K.; Yáñez, J.A.; Remsberg, C.M.; Forrest, M.L.; Davies, N.M. Clinical toxicities of nanocarrier systems. *Adv. Drug Deliv. Rev.* **2008**, *60*, 929–938. [CrossRef] [PubMed]
202. Lanone, S.; Boczkowski, J. Biomedical applications and potential health risks of nanomaterials: Molecular mechanisms. *Curr. Mol. Med.* **2006**, *6*, 651–663. [CrossRef] [PubMed]
203. Curtis, J.; Greenberg, M.; Kester, J.; Phillips, S.; Krieger, G. Nanotechnology and nanotoxicology: A primer for clinicians. *Toxicol. Sci.* **2006**, *25*, 245–260. [CrossRef]

204. Moghimi, S.M.; Hunter, A.C.; Murray, J.C. Nanomedicine: Current status and future prospects. *FASEB J.* **2005**, *19*, 311–330. [CrossRef] [PubMed]

205. Minekus, M.; Alminger, M.; Alvito, P.; Ballance, S.; Bohn, T.; Bourlieu, C.; Carrière, F.; Boutrou, R.; Corredig, M.; Dupont, D.; et al. A standardised static in vitro digestion method suitable for food—An international consensus. *Food Funct.* **2014**, *5*, 1113–1124. [CrossRef] [PubMed]

15

Production and Refinement of Omega-3 Rich Oils from Processing By-Products of Farmed Fish Species

Vida Šimat [1,*], Jelena Vlahović [1,2,*], Barbara Soldo [3], Danijela Skroza [4], Ivica Ljubenkov [3] and Ivana Generalić Mekinić [4]

1 Department of Marine Studies, University of Split, Ruđera Boškovića 37, HR-21000 Split, Croatia
2 Sardina d.o.o., Ratac 1, HR-21410 Postira, Croatia
3 Department of Chemistry, Faculty of Science, University of Split, Ruđera Boškovića 33, HR-21000 Split, Croatia; barbara@pmfst.hr (B.S.); ivica.ljubenkov4@gmail.com (I.L.)
4 Department of Food Technology and Biotechnology, Faculty of Chemistry and Technology, University of Split, Ruđera Boškovića 35, HR-21000 Split, Croatia; danci@ktf-split.hr (D.S.); gene@ktf-split.hr (I.G.M.)
* Correspondence: vida@unist.hr (V.Š.); jelena.vlahovic@sardina.hr (J.V.)

Abstract: In this study, the effect of a four-stage chemical refining process (degumming, neutralization, bleaching, deodorization) on the quality parameters, fatty acid composition and volatile compounds of crude oils produced from processing by-products of farmed fish species (tuna, seabass and gilthead seabream) was evaluated. The quality of the oils was compared to commercially available cod liver oil on the basis of free fatty acid, peroxide value, *p*-anisidine, total oxidation (TOTOX), thiobarbituric acid reactive species (TBARS), oxidative stability at 80, 100 and 120 °C, tocopherol content, and volatile components, while the fatty acid profile and the proportion of polyunsaturated fatty acids (PUFAs) were used as an indicator of the nutritional values of fish oils. Quality parameters of the studied oils and oil oxidative stability were enhanced with refining and were within the limits recommended for fish oils without the loss of PUFAs. In tuna by-product refined oils, the proportion of PUFAs was over 40%, with 30% of eicosapentaenoic and docosahexaenoic fatty acids. The volatile compounds of the oils were quantified (in mg/kg) and major components were 2,4-heptadienal, pentadecane, 2,4-decadienal, 2,4-nonadienal and dodecane. The use of aquaculture by-products as an alternative source for fish oil production could contribute to a more sustainable and profitable aquaculture production, providing economic benefits for the producers and setting new standards for a fish by-product disposal strategy.

Keywords: *Thunnus thynnus*; *Dicentrarhus labrax*; *Sparus aurata*; by-products; fish oil; chemical refining; fatty acid profile; volatile components

---

1. Introduction

The total aquaculture production of finfish is estimated at 54.1 million tonnes with a moderate annual growth rate of 5.8% with 37 world countries producing more farmed than wild-caught fish [1]. The Mediterranean and Black Sea areas have 62% of unsustainable fished stocks, particulary, the whitefish species. With the intent of making fisheries more productive and sustainable, mariculture (marine aquaculture) of seabass (*Dicentrarhus labrax*) and gilthead seabream (*Sparus aurata*) has grown exponentially, with these two species almost entirely farmed in the Mediterranean. The species with the highest commercial value in the Mediterranean is the Atlantic bluefin tuna (*Thunnus thynnus*) with capture-based mariculture (capture of fish from the wild and their rearing in sea cages for periods ranging between 3 months to 2 years) [2]. The growth of aquaculture also reflects on the generation of aquaculture by-products. In some countries such as Norway or Iceland, a large share of by-products is utilized by many different industries [3], in contrast to the Mediterranean region where this is not the practice. To our knowledge there is no available data for utilization of farmed tuna or seabass and gilthead seabream by-products for fish oil production or any other purpose that would benefit the producers economically and could serve as a reference for a fish by-product disposal strategy.

The many benefits that marine lipids contribute to our overall health are well known and widely documented. High levels of nutritionally valuable long-chain polyunsaturated fatty acids (PUFAs), mainly eicosapentaenoic acid (EPA) and docosahexaenoic acid (DHA) along with their physicochemical properties, make fish lipids unique and a promising economically valuable product. Although the current situation with fish oil production is stable, future projections show that available wild marine resources are becoming increasingly limited while the demand for PUFA continues to rise. This not only suggests, but stresses the need for exploration and exploitation of alternative sources [4]. Rest raw materials of the fish processing industry, also known as by-products, vary within species and processing methods used, but generally include parts that remain after edible parts of the fish is removed: Heads, viscera, frames (bones with attached flesh), skins, fins, trimmings, blood and others not utilized for human consumption [5,6]. Rest raw materials should not be considered waste or less valuable than the main product [5]. The high nutritive value of fish by-products is related to the content of valuable minerals, vitamins, protein and lipid fractions thus they are used in wide range of purposes, from production of fish cakes, pies and nuggets, gelatin, sauces and other products for human consumption to production of biodiesel [7]. Bioactive components such as peptides, enzymes or collagens that are used by pharmaceutical, biomedical and biotechnological industries can also be extracted from fish by-products [1,6]. With the growing interest and scientific knowledge within the field of by-product utilization and properties of certain components such as protein and oil that can be extracted from fish by-products, the low-value products such as mince or fish meal have been replaced by products of higher value [5,8]. Different fish species have specific processing yields and consequently, generate different proportions of by-products. In addition, the quality and chemical composition of marine by-products vary between species, season and catching ground as well as post-capture handling and processing. Although not directly used for human consumption, ingredients from by-products are used as feed in terrestrial livestock industries and aquaculture farming and indirectly contribute to human food production. The possible limitations to by-product utilization are related to lower quality of the fish meal and fish oil in comparison to products obtained from whole fish and elevated enzymatic activity that makes them highly perishable. Several studies showed that oil from by-products can be successfully extracted and refined to remove some undesirable compounds (moisture, pigments, free fatty acids, phospholipids, minerals, off-flavours, etc.) which affect oil stability, overall quality and consumers' acceptability, without the loss of PUFAs which enables its further application [9–13].

The aim of this research was to: (i) Produce and characterize crude oils from processing by-products obtained from farmed fish (tuna, seabass, and seabream); (ii) investigate the changes in fish oil characteristics during a four-stage refining process (degumming, neutralization, bleaching, deodorization) and differences in PUFAs composition between crude and refined oils; (iii) compare oils extracted from whole waste generated during tuna harvesting and tuna liver; (iv) report the characteristics of oil extracted from by-products obtained after filleting of farmed seabream and seabass; (v) compare the quality parameters and fatty acid composition of the obtained crude and refined oils with commercial cod liver oil in order to investigate the potential recycling of fish wastes for conversion into products of higher value.

2. Materials and Methods

2.1. General

All the standards compounds, solvents and reagents used in the study were obtained from Sigma-Aldrich (St. Louis, MO, USA), Fluka (Neu-Ulm, Germany), Merck (Darmstadt, Germany) and Kemika (Zagreb, Croatia). Spectrophotometric measurements were performed on a SPECORD 200 Plus (Analytik Jena AG, Jena, Germany). The analyses of fatty acid methyl esters (FAMEs) and volatile compounds were carried out by gas chromatograph (GC, model 3900; Varian Inc., Lake Forest, CA, USA) with flame-ionization detection (FID). The oil oxidative stability was determined using Rancimat model 743 (Metrohm, Herisau, Switzerland). The α-tocopherol content was determined by high-performance liquid chromatography (HPLC, all components of Series 200; Perkin Elmer, Waltham, MA, USA).

2.2. *Raw Materials and Fish Oil Extraction*

Farmed bluefin tuna (*Thunnus thynnus*) by-products were collected throughout December 2016 and January 2017 during harvesting and the evisceration process (done on board of fishing boat). By-products were separated into two groups: (i) Over 2000 kg of by-products (gills and gut content) were used for tuna by-product crude oil production; (ii) approximately 100 kg of tuna livers were collected (about 930 g each) and used for tuna liver crude oil production. During farming, tunas were fed with small pelagic fish such as sardines and herring and the average weight at harvesting was around 67 kg. Additionally, the farmed fish by-product crude oil was produced from approximately 1000 kg of heads, gills and gut content from seabream (*Sparus aurata*) and seabass (*Dicentrarhus labrax*) recovered from a local filleting plant. The fish were farmed at the same farm and fed with dry pellets (Efico plus, BioMar SAS, Nersac, France). Samples were 400–600 g at harvesting. Each oil was produced in two batches. Special attention was given to temperature regime during raw material manipulation. The crude oils were produced by grinding the raw materials in an industrial grinder (MG 250; Scansteel, Slagelse, Denmark), cooking at 95 °C for 12 min (cooking chamber model C2; Alfa Laval, Søborg, Denmark), and then pressed in a screw expeller and centrifuged at 4200 rpm using a decanter centrifuge type AC0303 CentryFish 1000 (Alfa Laval) which automatically separates dry matter (fishmeal), water and oil. With the interest of retaining the quality of crude oils, they were stored at <4 °C in dark bottles and refined within two days. Commercially available cod liver oil (oleum jecoris aselli; Kemig d.o.o., Zagreb, Croatia) was purchased from the local pharmacy and used as the control oil.

2.3. *Oil Refinement Process*

The refinement process, involving four major stages: Degumming (to separate phospholipids), neutralizing (to decrease acidity), bleaching (to remove coloured materials) and deodorization (to remove unwanted odour compounds), described by Chakraborty and Joseph [14] with slight modifications [15] was used. Extracted crude oil (500 g) was mixed with phosphoric acid (5 mL). The mixture was stirred in water bath heated to 70 °C for 20 min. After the cooling, samples were centrifuged (20 min, 4000 rpm) in order to remove the precipitated gum (degumming). Afterward, neutralization was done by slowly adding (drop by drop) NaOH solution (1 M) to the degummed oil samples in combination with constant stirring and heating at 65 °C for 20 min. The neutralization process was conducted until a pH of 7.0 was attained, and samples were then heated to 70 °C for 20 min, cooled and centrifuged for 15 min at 4000 rpm. The oil thus obtained was washed with deionized water (3-times with 10 mL) by agitation (500 rpm) and heating at 50 °C under vacuum. Neutralized oil samples were separated by centrifugation (10 min, 2500 rpm). The oil obtained after neutralization was bleached with adsorbents (4 g/100 g of oil) containing 1.13 g of activated carbon and 22.5 g of Fuller's earth. The oil samples were stirred using a magnetic stirrer at 40 °C for 40 min under N_2. After cooling, oil samples were again separated by centrifugation (30 min, 3500 rpm). Deodorization of the bleached oil samples was carried out by distillation under vacuum conditions. The mixture of the oil obtained after bleaching and deionized water (20 mL) was heated to 95–97 °C under the vacuum for one hour, with continual stirring. The refining process was repeated three times for each batch of oil.

2.4. Analytical Methodologies

American Oil Chemist' Society [16] methodologies were followed for oils chemical characterization as follows: Acidic value (AV, Method no. Ca 5a-40) expressed as percent of oleic acid, peroxide value (PV, Method no. Cd 8-53) expressed as milliequivalents of O_2/kg of oil, and anisidine values (*p*-AV, Method no. Cd 18-90) calculated as described in Chakraborty and Joseph [13]. The total oxidation (TOTOX) values were calculated as TOTOX = (2 × PV) + *p*-AV, while thiobarbituric acid reactive substances (TBARS) values were determined by the spectrophotometric assay described by Ke and Woyewoda [17]. The analyses were repeated five times.

The resistance of fish oil to auto-oxidation was determined at three different temperatures (80, 100 and 120 °C) by Rancimat method [18]. The fish oil (3 g) oxidative stability was tested at three different temperatures (80, 100 and 120 °C), while the airflow in all experiments was constant (20 L/h). The results were expressed as induction periods (IPs) which are the measure of oil stability or shelf-life, defined as the time in hours required to reach the end-point of oxidation.

2.5. Tocopherol Content

The tocopherol content was analyzed using HPLC system equipped with an autosampler, vacuum degasser, binary pump, fluorescent detector and the column oven on the Ultra Silica column (150 × 4.6 mm, 5 μm; Restek, Bellefonte, PA, USA) by a method previously described by Šimat et al. [15]. In short, an aliquot of 20 μL was obtained after dissolving 0.5 g of fish oil in 5 mL of hexane and injected into the chromatographic system. The following gradient elution program was applied using solvent A (hexane) and solvent B (isopropanol) at a flow rate of 0.9 mL/min: 3% B for the first 15 min, followed by an increase in solvent B to 80% through 5 min, after which the solvent ratio was maintained for 8 min. Over the next minute, the solvents returned to the initial conditions and this ratio of solvent was maintained for another 11 min to ensure column stabilization. The temperature of the column was held at 30 °C and detection observed by a fluorescent detector (excitation 290 nm and emission 330 nm). The compound was identified according to the retention time and quantified through the calibration curve of the standard. The analyses were performed in duplicate.

2.6. Fatty Acid Profile

The fatty acid methyl esters (FAMEs), prepared by dissolving oil samples (0.1 g) in heptane (2 mL) and by the addition of 2 M KOH in methanol (0.2 mL), were analyzed by gas chromatography with flame-ionisation detection (GC-FID) using capillary column RTX 2560 (100 m × 0.25 mm i.d., coating thickness 0.25 μm; Restek) by a method previously described in Šimat et al. [15]. In short, 1 μL of the heptane layer was injected into the chromatograph with a split ratio 1:100, with the temperature of injector et at 225 °C and of the detector at 240 °C. At a constant flow rate of 3 mL/min, helium was used as the carrier gas. The initial oven temperature was 140 °C, held for 5 min, raised to 240 °C at a rate of 4 °C/min and held at 240 °C for 20 min. FAMEs were identified by comparing to with standards (Supelco 37 Component FAME Mix; Sigma-Aldrich). The analyses were performed in duplicates and the results are expressed as percentages of methyl esters of individual fatty acids.

2.7. Analysis of Volatiles

The volatile compounds of oils were analyzed using headspace solid phase microextraction (HS-SPME) coupled with GC-FID. The samples were prepared using 2-cm long fibres of divinylbenzene-carboxen-polydimethylsiloxane (DVB-CAR-PDMS, thickness 50/30 μm) obtained from Supelco (Bellefonte, PA, USA). A total of 2 g of oil was placed into a 20 mL head space vial and equilibrated at 40 °C for 5 min, inserting the fibre into the headspace for adsorption at 40 °C for 30 min, then transferring the fibre to the injector port for desorption at 250 °C for 1 min.

The quantitative analyses and separation of volatile compounds of major fish oil volatile components were performed by GC-FID and CP-WAX 57 CB column (50 m × 0.25 mm i.d., coating thickness 0.2 μm; Varian). At a constant flow rate of 2 mL/min, helium was used as the carrier gas. The GC oven temperature was programmed at an initial 40 °C for 4 min, raised to 190 °C at a rate of 5 °C/min and kept constant for 11 min. The temperature was then raised up to 200 °C applying the same rate of 5 °C/min. The detector temperature was maintained at 250 °C. The total analysis time for each sample was 67 min. The analyses were performed in duplicates.

The investigated compounds were identified by the retention time of the corresponding analytical standard, while the quantification was made by external calibration. As the applied method did not ensure adequate separation of 2,4-heptadienal and pentadecane, results for these two compounds are presented as their sum while their concentration was calculated using the calibration curve obtained for 2,4-heptadienal. GC Workstation Version 6.41 chromatographic software (Varian) was used for data collection and calculation [19].

2.8. Statistical Analysis

The obtained results are expressed as mean values ± standard deviation. The means of detected parameters were analyzed for significance by analysis of variance (one-way ANOVA) using Statgraphics Centurion (StatPoint Technologies Inc., Warrenton, VA, USA). Differences were considered to be significant at $p < 0.05$.

3. Results and Discussion

3.1. Chemical Characterization and Oxidative Stability of Fish Oils

The results of the chemical and compositional quality characterization of oils from tuna by-products, tuna liver, seabass and gilthead seabream by-products during four refining stages and their comparison to cod liver oil (control) are presented in Table 1. Despite the high temperature used during the oil production (cooking at 95 °C for 12 min) the temperature was found to have a poor influence on oil quality parameters. During preliminary studies we inspected quality parameters in oils extracted at different temperatures (from 65–95 °C) and compared it to Bligh and Dyer extracts [20] and found no significant difference in oxidative parameters [21]. It has been previously found that oil extraction temperature is weakly linked to the oxidative quality of produced oil, but strongly affected by omega-3 content of the raw material, providing confirmation of our finding [22]. To control the quality of fish oil properties, which is very labile to hydrolytic spoilage and oxidative deterioration, numerous standards with variable acceptable levels have been established [23]. The express lipolysis and oxidation of fish oils are the results of high autolytic activity and high content of PUFAs in fish tissues. It is expected that this process is even more susceptible for fish by-products. For this reason, fish oils usually have high free fatty acid (FFA) content. In this study, the results of FFA values of crude oils were low confirming that short cooking periods during the oil extraction, even at higher temperatures, did not cause significant hydrolysis. Only in tuna liver oil the FFA values were over 3. The refinement process ensured an additional decrease of FFA by 3.7, 32 and 47% in tuna by-product, tuna liver and seabass/seabream oil, respectively. Among the three studied oils, seabass and gilthead seabream by-product oil had the lowest FFA values, even lower than the control. The allowable limit of FFAs value for crude fish oil is in the range of 1–7% of oleic acid, usually 2–5% [24], but the general recommendation is that FFA values of edible oils should be ≤3.0%. This is important since FFAs have an impact on the oil organoleptic properties as well as oil compositional quality [25], can act as pro-oxidants which initiate the oxidation mechanism [26] and high FFA values are problematic during omega-3 extraction and biodiesel production [27].

Primary oxidation of oil used to monitor hydroperoxides formation is determined by PV and should be ≤5 meq O_2/kg for fish oils intended for human consumption [28,29]. Despite the increase of the PVs for studied oils after degumming step, final values obtained for the refined oils were below the limit of 5 meq O_2/kg (Table 1) which opens the possibility of using these oils for human consumption.

The influences of the refining steps on oil oxidation status and products expressed as *p*-AV, TOTOX and TBARS are presented in Table 1. Among crude oils, *p*-AV and TOTOX values for tuna by-product oil were the highest, followed by those for tuna liver oil and seabass and gilthead seabream by-product oil. The processing steps of degumming, neutralizing and bleaching caused reduction of *p*-AV and TOTOX while these parameters increased after the deodorization step. The highest *p*-AV value was detected for refined tuna by-product oil (19.5), while TOTOX values of refined tuna liver and seabass and gilthead seabream by-product oils were higher than those obtained for crude oils, 27.7 and 24.7, respectively. This suggests that used adsorbents (activated carbon and Fuller's earth) have the capacity to adsorb primary and secondary oxidation compounds [14]. The allowable limit of *p*-AV for acceptability of fish oil for human consumption is ≤20 [30].

Although the *p*-AV obtained for oils in this study were under this limit, they were significantly higher than the control, thus additionally influencing the higher TOTOX value. The TOTOX is a parameter used to determine the presence of compounds generated by degradation of PUFAs under pro-oxidant conditions including high temperatures, oxygen, metal compounds and light, and the TOTOX value ≤ 26 under is found to be allowable for fish oil [31]. Therefore, in association to the above mentioned PV and *p*-AV values, the TOTOX values of studied by-product oils were above the mentioned limit in crude and refined oils from tuna by-products and just under the limit in seabass and seabream by-product oil (Table 1). The *p*-AV value and TOTOX obtained for crude sardine oil were found to be 16 and 40, respectively [14]. In that study, authors applied the same 4-stage refining process which was more effective for sardine oil and reduced *p*-AV value and TOTOX values to 10 and 19, respectively. On the other hand, as reported in Table 1, TBARS assay detected low accumulation of secondary oxidation products. TBARS detects lipid oxidation when thiobarbituric acid and oxidation products from unsaturated FAs react involving several secondary oxidation products, however, the TBARS of by-product oils was lower that the control oil.

Table 1. Chemical and quality parameters of crude oils from tuna by-products, tuna liver, seabass and gilthead seabream by-products at different stages of the refining process, and cod liver oil (control).

Oil Samples	Refining Phase	Measured Parameter				
		FFA (% Oleic Acid)	PV (meq O_2/kg)	*p*-AV	TOTOX	TBARS (μM/g)
Tuna by-product oil	*Crude oil*	2.94 ± 0.12 ^{a}	2.31 ± 0.73 ^{a}	25.2 ± 0.08 ^{a}	29.7 ± 0.20 ^{a}	0.94 ± 0.33 ^{a}
	Degummed	3.51 ± 0.03 ^{b}	3.93 ± 0.18 ^{b}	19.2 ± 1.25 ^{b}	27.1 ± 0.79 ^{b}	1.02 ± 0.14 ^{a}
	Neutralized	3.13 ± 0.10 ^{b}	3.46 ± 0.39 ^{b}	16.9 ± 1.23 ^{c}	23.8 ± 1.06 ^{c}	2.02 ± 0.45 ^{b}
	Bleached	2.93 ± 0.04 ^{a}	2.88 ± 0.11 ^{ab}	14.4 ± 0.90 ^{d}	20.2 ± 1.34 ^{d}	1.88 ± 0.37 ^{b}
	Deodorized	2.83 ± 0.01^{a}	3.78 ± 0.22 ^{b*}	19.5 ± 0.94 ^{b}	27.1 ± 2.15 ^{b}	1.14 ± 0.11 ^{a}
Tuna liver oil	*Crude oil*	3.13 ± 0.00 ^{a}	2.68 ± 0.86 ^{a}	20.9 ± 1.34 ^{a}	26.0 ± 0.14 ^{a}	2.88 ± 0.73 ^{a}
	Degummed	2.52 ± 0.05 ^{b}	3.01 ± 0.05 ^{ab}	19.1 ± 2.47 ^{b}	25.2 ± 1.17 ^{a}	1.35 ± 0.02 ^{b}
	Neutralized	2.65 ± 0.11 ^{c}	2.89 ± 0.22 ^{ab}	17.0 ± 4.78 ^{c}	22.7 ±1.22 ^{b}	1.76 ± 0.03 ^{b}
	Bleached	2.17 ± 0.03 ^{b}	2.85 ± 0.53 ^{ab}	14.0 ± 0.65 ^{d}	19.7 ± 0.43 ^{c}	1.92 ± 0.35 ^{b}
	Deodorized	2.12 ± 0.16 ^{b}	4.25 ± 0.28 ^{c}	19.2 ± 2.22 ^{b}	27.7 ± 2.22 ^{a}	1.97 ± 0.53 ^{b}
Seabass and gilthead seabream by-product oil	*Crude oil*	2.41 ± 0.47 ^{a}	4.63 ± 1.07 ^{a}	18.1 ± 0.19 ^{ab}	19.3 ± 2.45 ^{a}	0.53 ± 0.05 ^{a}
	Degummed	1.66 ± 0.05 ^{b}	2.70 ± 0.18 ^{b}	15.7 ± 1.12 ^{c}	20.2 ± 0.12 ^{a}	3.46 ± 2.08 ^{b}
	Neutralized	1.43 ± 0.18 ^{b}	3.13 ± 0.31 ^{b}	12.7 ± 0.65 ^{a}	18.9 ± 0.26 ^{a}	2.24 ± 1.05 ^{bc}
	Bleached	1.40 ± 0.01 ^{b}	3.44 ± 0.25 ^{ab}	11.4 ± 0.19 ^{b}	18.4 ± 0.52 ^{a}	1.14 ± 0.10 ^{ac}
	Deodorized	1.28 ± 0.15 ^{b}	4.20 ± 0.15 ^{ab}	16.5 ± 0.39 ^{c}	24.7 ± 0.32 ^{b}	1.42 ± 0.53 ^{ac*}
Cod liver oil	*Control*	2.15 ± 0.08	3.85 ± 0.44	13.3 ± 1.11	21.0 ± 0.18	1.63 ± 0.07

$n = 30$; Different superscript letters (a–d) in the same column denote statistically significant difference ($p < 0.05$); * Measured parameters in deodorized oils marked with * do not differ statistically ($p < 0.05$) from the control sample.

The Rancimat method, an accelerated method that employs high temperatures and air-flow supply to estimate the oxidative stability and shelf life of oil-containing products in a relatively short time, was used to measure the oxidative stability of oils (Figure 1). According to the presented results it can be seen that tuna by-product oil was the most stabile sample among crude oils with IP of 1.54 h at 80 °C, 0.58 h at 100 °C and 0.15 h at 120 °C, while lower values were obtained for the other two oils. The refinement process prolonged the oil oxidative stability in all cases, but unlike for crude oils, refined tuna liver oil and seabass and seabream by-product oil showed higher IP values than tuna by-product oil (prolongation of 36% at 80 °C, 35% at 100 °C and 52 % at 120 °C). The oil resistance to the lipid oxidation is a result of differences between fatty acid profiles of investigated oils. From the Table 2 and Figure 2 it can be seen that crude tuna by product oil contain the highest content of PUFAs ($\sum$ of 37.65%), as well as EPA + DHA ($\sum$ of 30.85%). Furthermore, the *n-3/n-6* ratio in crude tuna waste oil was more than 3.5-fold higher than in crude tuna liver oil, and more than 9.5-fold higher than in crude seabass and seabream by-product oil. The refinement process reduced this parameter by half in tuna by-product oil, slight reduction was obtained in seabass and seabream by-product oil, while a higher value was detected in refined tuna liver oil. Although the referent cod liver oil showed the highest stability at 80 °C, at higher temperatures its stability was lower that of the investigated refined oils. As can be seen in Figure 3, significantly higher content of tocopherol in cod liver oil has been detected. This compound has been added during the production of the commercial oil sample in order to improve it stability, but it has been established that tocopherol degrades at higher temperatures [32] which is probably caused lower IP of the cod liver at 100 and 120 °C.

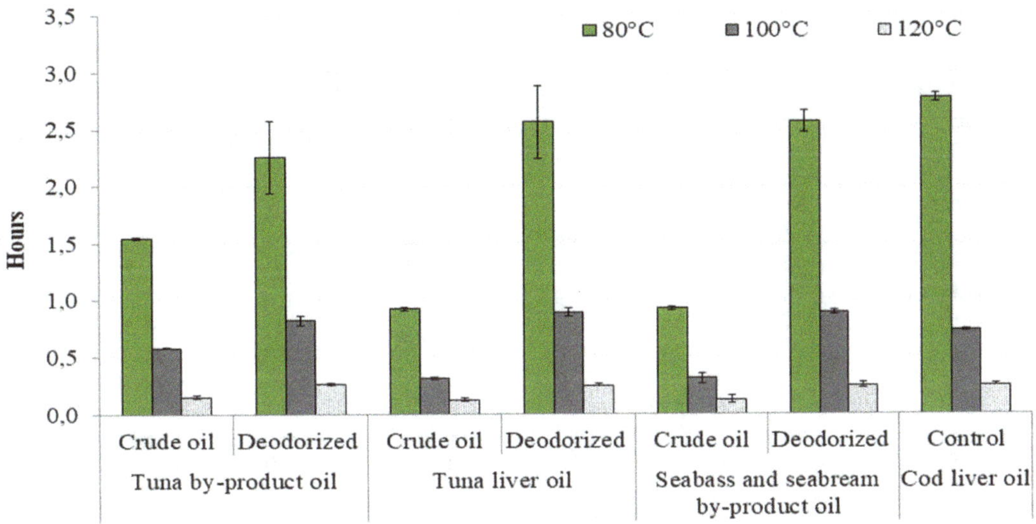

Figure 1. The oxidative stability (n = 18) of crude and deodorized (refined) oils from tuna by-products, tuna liver, seabass and gilthead seabream by-products, and cod liver oil (control).

3.2. Fatty Acid Profile of Oils

The results of the fatty acid profile of the crude oils and their changes after oil refinement are presented in Table 2 and in Figure 2A–D. The most dominant SFA contributing approximately 52–55% of total SFA, in all investigate oils was palmitic FA (C16:0). Its content was significantly higher in tuna oils in comparison to seabream/seabass oil and the control. Palmitic FA occurs naturally in fish, being a source of metabolic energy for their growth. The oleic acid (C18:1*n-9 cis*) was the major compound among MUFAs and in the studied oils amounted to approximately 14% in tuna oils, to 40% in seabass and gilthead seabream by-product refined oil. Among PUFAs, high concentrations of EPA (C20:5*n-3*) and even higher those of DHA (C22:6*n-3*) were found in all studied oils. The relative contents of EPA and DHA were expected to increase during the refining process [14,33], but in this study the minimal increase was observed after refinement only for DHA in tuna liver oil. However, in both crude and refined tuna by-product oils amounts of EPA and DHA were found to be extremely high. In tuna oils and the control oil, especially in tuna liver oil dihomo-γ-linolenic acid (20:3*n-6*), was found in higher amounts (7.32-9.89%), while in seabream/seabass oil its precursor, linoleic acid (C18:2*n-6*) was found significantly higher compared to other oils (17.32%). Erucic acid (22:1*n-9*) was found in small amounts in studied oils, with the highest content (1%) found in the control oil.

The crude oils from tuna by-products and liver contained significantly higher total amounts of saturated fatty acids (32.7 and 35.6%, Figure 2) in comparison to seabass and gilthead seabream by-product oil (23.6%). The SFA profile of the oils did not statistically change with the refining process and tuna oils had significantly higher SFA content than the control. The MUFAs content was the highest in seabass and gilthead seabream by-product oil (46%) and did not change after refining. Tuna by-product oil had slightly higher MUFA content then tuna liver oil. The PUFAs were significantly higher in tuna by-product and tuna liver crude oils (37.7 and 35.2%) and they increased to 40.2 and 39.6% in refined oils, respectively. The content of PUFA*n-3*, in the studied oils, ranged from 11.6–32.3% and was higher than that of PUFA*n-6* for 8.9-18.7% (Figure 2). A high percentage of PUFA indicates good nutritional values of the studied fish oils. The PUFA/SFA ratio of 0.4-0.5 is considered beneficial for human health [34], and it was significantly higher in the crude oils, while in refined oils it ranged from 1.1 to 1.2, significantly lower than in the control oil (Figure 2). In general, it is accepted that compared to wild caught fish, modern aquaculture products have lower *n-3* FAs, and higher levels of terrestrial plant-originating C18:2*n-6* as a result of feed composition [35]. Very high intake of *n-6* was recognized as undesirable and it reduces the nutritional quality of fish oil. The sum of n-6 was 18-19% higher in seabass and gilthead seabream by-product oils and along with the lowest sum of *n-3* and EPA+DHA.

Table 2. The changes in fatty acid profile (%) of crude and refined oils from tuna by-products, tuna liver, seabass and gilthead seabream by-products and comparison to cod liver oil (control).

Fatty Acid	Tuna By-Product Oil		Tuna Liver Oil		Seabass and Seabream By-Product Oil		Cod Liver Oil
	Crude Oil	*Refined*	*Crude Oil*	*Refined*	*Crude Oil*	*Refined*	*Control*
C12:0	n.d. [1]	0.06 ± 0.00	0.07 ± 0.00	0.06 ± 0.01	0.02 ± 0.01	0.03 ± 0.00	0.02 ± 0.02
C13:0	n.d.	0.06 ± 0.00	0.07 ± 0.00	0.07 ± 0.02	n.d.	0.02 ± 0.00	0.01 ± 0.01
C14:0	6.08 ± 0.98	6.05 ± 0.00	6.60 ± 0.49	6.50 ± 0.25	2.31 ± 0.02	2.57 ± 0.14	4.64 ± 0.02
C14:1	0.46 ± 0.65	0.04 ± 0.06	0.91 ± 0.06	n.d.	0.36 ± 0.00	0.40 ± 0.00	0.39 ± 0.03
C15:0	0.37 ± 0.52	0.82 ± 0.01	0.07 ± 0.00	0.88 ± 0.02	0.04 ± 0.01	0.05 ± 0.00	0.12 ± 0.01
C15:1	n.d.	0.01 ± 0.01	0.01 ± 0.00	n.d.	n.d.	n.d.	n.d.
C16:0	18.20 ± 2.12	18.09 ± 0.23	19.85 ± 1.54	18.97 ± 0.82	12.70 ± 0.02	13.87 ± 0.23	12.16 ± 0.18
C16:1	6.14 ± 0.74	6.09 ± 0.06	5.61 ± 0.43	5.40 ± 0.22	3.55 ± 0.09	3.88 ± 0.17	8.81 ± 0.01
C17:0	0.67 ± 0.07	0.65 ± 0.00	0.75 ± 0.06	0.71 ± 0.03	0.32 ± 0.02	0.34 ± 0.01	0.19 ± 0.02
C17:1	0.46 ± 0.10	0.44 ± 0.01	0.40 ± 0.04	0.35 ± 0.02	0.27 ± 0.01	0.29 ± 0.01	0.35 ± 0.02
C18:0	4.28 ± 0.36	4.23 ± 0.01	4.97 ± 0.36	4.66 ± 0.08	2.63 ± 0.01	0.17 ± 0.00	3.21 ± 0.34
C18:1n-9t	2.64 ± 0.41	0.16 ± 0.00	0.17 ± 0.02	0.16 ± 0.01	0.12 ± 0.00	0.15 ± 0.00	0.14 ± 0.00
C18:1n-9c	13.92 ± 1.14	13.73 ± 0.18	13.42 ± 1.09	13.05 ± 0.09	37.97 ± 0.08	40.52 ± 0.72	18.73 ± 0.01
C18:2n-6t	0.06 ± 0.08	0.05 ± 0.03	0.08 ± 0.09	0.13 ± 0.01	0.04 ± 0.00	0.04 ± 0.00	0.08 ± 0.00
C18:2n-6c	1.04 ± 1.47	2.18 ± 0.01	2.28 ± 0.18	2.13 ± 0.02	16.35 ± 0.02	17.32 ± 0.26	1.89 ± 0.02
C20:0	0.42 ± 0.03	0.42 ± 0.00	0.47 ± 0.04	0.43 ± 0.01	0.51 ± 0.00	0.39 ± 0.01	0.29 ± 0.01
C18:3n-6	0.39 ± 0.55	0.13 ± 0.00	0.12 ± 0.01	0.11 ± 0.02	0.19 ± 0.00	0.19 ± 0.00	0.15 ± 0.00
C20:1	5.07 ± 0.20	5.08 ± 0.02	6.50 ± 0.56	5.84 ± 0.04	2.47 ± 0.00	2.50 ± 0.05	12.67 ± 0.04
C18:3n-3	1.41 ± 0.12	n.d.	n.d.	0.65 ± 0.06	0.02 ± 0.02	0.18 ± 0.00	n.d.
C21:0	n.d.	1.44 ± 0.04	1.48 ± 0.13	0.67 ± 0.08	4.28 ± 0.01	4.46 ± 0.05	0.90 ± 0.02
C20:2	0.28 ± 0.01	0.27 ± 0.01	0.31 ± 0.03	0.11 ± 0.01	0.59 ± 0.01	0.58 ± 0.02	0.30 ± 0.02
C22:0	0.08 ± 0.11	0.15 ± 0.01	0.18 ± 0.02	0.17 ± 0.02	0.19 ± 0.02	0.17 ± 0.01	0.14 ± 0.00
C20:3n-6	3.54 ± 5.01	7.32 ± 0.02	10.25 ± 0.92	9.04 ± 0.17	1.04 ± 0.00	0.97 ± 0.01	9.89 ± 0.02
C22:1n-9	0.32 ± 0.01	0.30 ± 0.00	0.39 ± 0.03	0.37 ± 0.01	0.46 ± 0.03	0.43 ± 0.01	1.00 ± 0.02
C20:3n-3	n.d.	0.02 ± 0.00	0.05 ± 0.00	0.11 ± 0.11	0.03 ± 0.00	0.02 ± 0.00	n.d.
C20:4n-6	0.19 ± 0.13	0.18 ± 0.00	0.19 ± 0.01	0.09 ± 0.14	0.16 ± 0.00	0.16 ± 0.00	0.16 ± 0.01
C23:0	1.02 ± 0.08	0.97 ± 0.00	1.01 ± 0.07	1.92 ± 0.01	0.51 ± 0.01	0.48 ± 0.01	0.58 ± 0.01
C22:2	n.d.	0.03 ± 0.00	0.05 ± 0.01	0.36 ± 0.07	0.05 ± 0.01	0.05 ± 0.00	0.02 ± 0.01
C24:0	0.87 ± 0.04	0.02 ± 0.00	0.07 ± 0.01	0.40 ± 0.02	0.07 ± 0.00	0.05 ± 0.01	0.82 ± 0.04
C20:5n-3	9.56 ± 0.76	9.29 ± 0.04	8.81 ± 0.68	8.21 ± 0.03	3.33 ± 0.03	3.04 ± 0.00	9.58 ± 0.06
C24:1	0.60 ± 0.02	0.65 ± 0.00	0.90 ± 0.09	0.77 ± 0.14	0.45 ± 0.01	0.34 ± 0.04	0.48 ± 0.00
C22:6n-3	21.29 ± 1.09	20.75 ± 0.19	13.07 ± 7.00	18.66 ± 1.21	8.26 ± 0.24	6.37 ± 0.47	11.9 ± 0.26

[1] n.d.—not detected; $n = 12$.

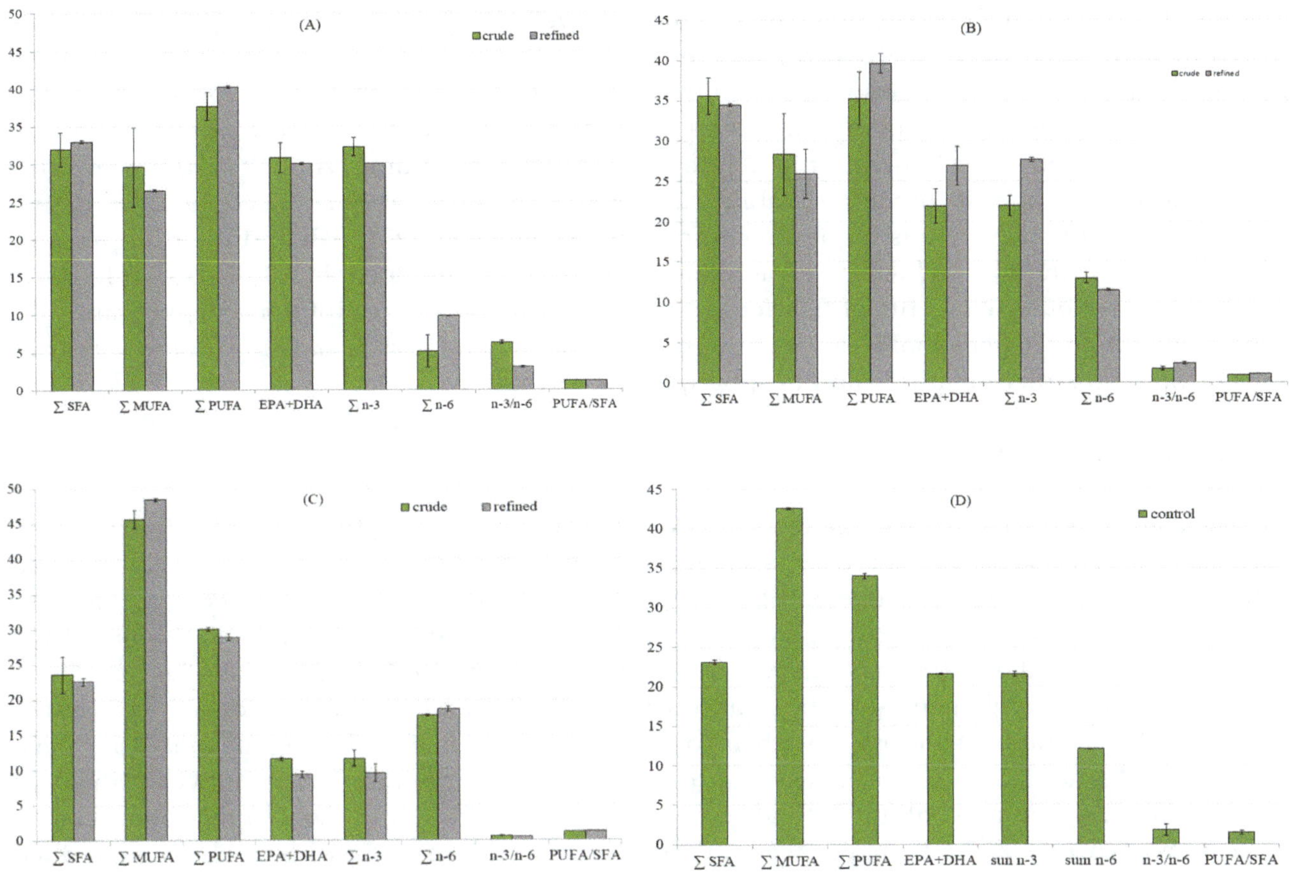

Figure 2. The sum of monounsaturated (∑MUFA) and polyunsaturated (∑PUFA) fatty acids, the sum of eicosapentaenoic and docosahexaenoic fatty acids (EPA + DHA), the sum of *n-3* and *n-6* content plus ratios between *n-6/n-3* and polyunsaturated fatty acids/saturated fatty acids (PUFA/SFA) in crude and refined oils from: (**A**) tuna by-products, (**B**) tuna liver, (**C**) seabass and gilthead seabream by-products and (**D**) cod liver oil (control).

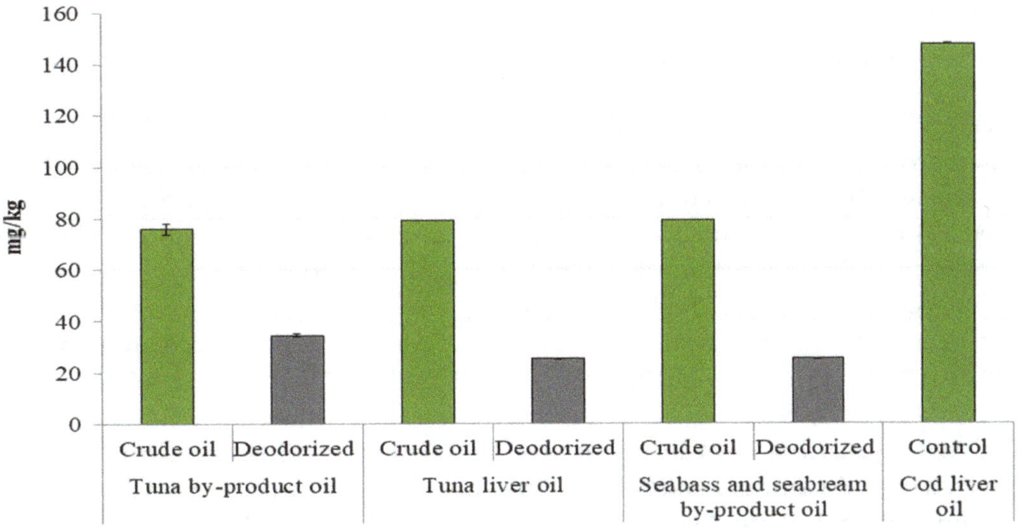

Figure 3. The tocopherol content ($n = 12$) in crude and deodorized (refined) oils from tuna by-products, tuna liver, seabass and gilthead seabream by-products and cod liver oil (control).

In tuna by-product oils the refining process resulted with a decrease share of MUFAs and the increase of PUFAs. This, as well as the content of antioxidant compounds such as tocopherol (Figure 3), can contribute to the oxidative stability of oils. Crude oils from farmed fish by-products had high tocopherol content which was significantly reduced by refining process in all oils (31–45%). At the same time, oxidative stability was prolonged by the refining process thus the role of tocopherol in oxidative stability appears to be smaller than the removal impurities which act as pro-oxidants [36]. This is confirmed on the control oil which had over 140 mg of tocopherol per kilogram (data from declaration sheet indicate a content of 1190 International Units of vitamin A per gram) however this content did not enhance its oxidative stability at elevated temperatures. The tocopherol content of oils from farmed fish species is higher in comparison to oils from wild fish and their by-products. For example, sardine by-product crude oil has approximately 30 mg tocopherol /kg [15]. It has been suggested that dietary elements of fish feed, such as vitamin E, do not influence significantly the amount of total lipids, phospholipids, polyunsaturated and general muscle fatty acid composition but protect from peroxide formation and phospholipid hydrolysis [35].

3.3. Volatile Profile of Oils

The composition and relative contents of volatile compounds of crude, bleached and deodorized oils from tuna by-products, tuna liver, seabass and gilthead seabream by-products and cod liver oil (control) are presented in Table 3. Sixteen volatile components were identified (one ester, six aldehydes, five alcohols and three hydrocarbons). In tuna by-product oil the most dominant was the sum of 2,4-heptadienal (from *n-3* fatty acids) and pentadecane, followed by (E,E)-2,4-decadienal, dodecane and 4-methylpenten-2-ol. The applied GC-FID method did not ensure adequate separation of 2,4-heptadienal and pentadecane, and their concentration was calculated using the calibration curve obtained for 2,4-heptadienal since it was considered more important in fish oil, however the exact amount of the 2,4-heptadienal in the total sum is unknown. Taking into account that other volatile compounds such as (E,Z)-2,6-nonadienal and (E,E)-2,4-decadienal (secondary lipid oxidation products) were found in low concentrations, low TBARs values (Table 1) and previous reports that suggest pentadecane as dominant component in fish oil samples [37,38], we can assume that pentadecane is the dominant compound in this mixture. Similar was observed for tuna liver oil with exception to high levels of 1-penten-3-ol. Among unsaturated alcohols responsible for the fishy odour of the oil, one of the most important components is 1-pentene-3-ol [39]. The content of this compound was significantly reduced in all studied oils and in refined oils, with the findings ranging from 0.01–1.03 mg/kg.

In seabass and gilthead seabream by-products oil aldehydes, (E,E)-2,4-decadienal and 2,4-nonadienal, were found to be higher than in tuna by-product oils and levels of 2,4-heptadienal+pentadecane were significantly lower. The amount of 2,4-decadienal (from the *n-6* fatty acids) increased after the distillation, especially in seabass and seabream oil. In comparison to studied oils, the control oil was characterized with high levels of tetradecene. The values of two fatty aldehydes, 2,4-heptadienal and 2,4-decadienal are of great importance due to their contribution to the characteristic unpleasant odour of the oil [14,39]. The composition and proportion of volatile compounds changed significantly during the refining process and only in tuna by-product oil the total sum of volatile compounds was reduced during refining. The aldehydes are known as essential indicators of the oxidation processes and are also responsible for oil fishy odour, same for ketones which usually have very low thresholds and are derived from autoxidation of PUFAs via hydroperoxides or lipid oxidative degradation. In order to remove undesirable favor components, such as oxidation products (aldehydes and ketone, residual free fatty acids, etc.) the deodorization step is generally carried out by conventional steam distillation at temperatures below 200 °C. The suggested procedure does not affect all volatile components equally. The effectiveness of this process is influenced by the applied pressure and volatility of components at high temperature. In this stage, it is also important to inhibit the degradation of the essential components by cyclization and polymerization of long chain PUFAs [26].

Table 3. The concentration of volatiles (mg/kg) in crude oils from tuna by-products, tuna liver, seabass and gilthead seabream by-products at different stages of the refining process, and cod liver oil (control).

	Volatile Compound	Tuna By-Product Oil			Tuna Liver Oil			Seabass and Seabream By-Product Oil			Cod Liver Oil
		Crude	*Bleached*	*Deodorized*	*Crude*	*Bleached*	*Deodorized*	*Crude*	*Bleached*	*Deodorized*	*Control*
Esters	Ethyl acetate	1.51 ± 0.14 ^{a}	1.45 ± 0.19 ^{a}	1.00 ± 0.02 ^{b*}	0.93 ± 0.28 ^{a}	1.03 ± 0.29 ^{a}	1.19 ± 0.01 ^{a*}	0.50 ± 0.03 ^{a}	1.69 ± 0.25 ^{b}	0.99 ± 0.07 ^{c*}	0.73 ± 0.07
Aldehydes	Pentanal	1.12 ± 0.14 ^{a}	1.55 ± 0.06 ^{a}	1.94 ± 0.32 ^{a*}	0.95 ± 0.20 ^{ab}	0.81 ± 0.05 ^{ab}	0.54 ± 0.01 ^{bc}	2.09 ± 0.05 ^{a}	1.53 ± 0.11 ^{b}	0.55 ± 0.04 ^{c}	1.22 ± 0.11
	E-2-hexenal	0.08 ± 0.01 ^{a}	0.05 ± 0.01 ^{a}	0.05 ± 0.02 ^{a}	0.04 ± 0.01 ^{a}	0.04 ± 0.01 ^{a}	0.02 ± 0.0 ^{a}	0.01 ± 0.0 ^{a}	0.01 ± 0.0 ^{a}	0.02 ± 0.0 ^{a}	0.51 ± 0.04
	Octanal	0.29 ± 0.25 ^{a}	0.53 ± 0.0 ^{a}	0.39 ± 0.24 ^{a*}	1.15 ± 0.08 ^{a}	0.41 ± 0.20 ^{a}	0.45 ± 0.10 ^{a*}	0.34 ± 0.13 ^{ab}	0.31 ± 0.02 ^{ab}	0.15 ± 0.09 ^{a*}	0.14 ± 0.02
	(E,Z)-2,6-nonadienal	0.98 ± 0.21 ^{a}	1.07 ± 0.14 ^{a}	0.85 ± 0.13 ^{a}	0.91 ± 0.01 ^{a}	1.20 ± 0.16 ^{a}	1.08 ± 0.08 ^{a}	0.40 ± 0.06 ^{a}	0.62 ± 0.09 ^{b}	0.65 ± 0.03 ^{b}	0.14 ± 0.0
	(E,E)-2,4-decadienal	4.59 ± 0.28 ^{a}	6.06 ± 0.57 ^{b}	4.94 ± 0.35 ^{ab}	6.28 ± 1.19 ^{a}	6.25 ± 0.70 ^{a}	6.76 ± 0.42 ^{a*}	11.5 ± 0.46 ^{a}	10.3 ± 0.18 ^{a}	14.1 ± 0.54 ^{b}	6.80 ± 0.21
	2,4-nonadienal	0.67 ± 0.04 ^{a}	1.03 ± 0.14 ^{a}	1.02 ± 0.13 ^{a}	2.09 ± 0.16 ^{a}	0.93 ± 0.13 ^{b}	0.96 ± 0.13 ^{b}	6.53 ± 0.58 ^{a}	6.59 ± 0.49 ^{a}	4.77 ± 0.02 ^{b}	0.26 ± 0.05
Alcohols	1-penten-3-ol	0.08 ± 0.0 ^{a}	0.05 ± 0.01 ^{ab}	0.01 ± 0.01 ^{b*}	11.17 ± 0.20 ^{a}	2.29 ± 1.31 ^{b}	1.03 ± 0.0 ^{b}	0.65 ± 0.01 ^{a}	0.37 ± 0.02 ^{b}	0.07 ± 0.0 ^{c}	0.02 ± 0.0
	4-methylpenten-2-ol	2.66 ± 0.07 ^{a}	1.42 ± 0.17 ^{b}	2.15 ± 0.57 ^{a}	1.14 ± 0.03 ^{a}	1.08 ± 0.57 ^{a}	1.46 ± 0.0 ^{a*}	0.57 ± 0.03 ^{a}	1.55 ± 0.10 ^{b}	1.91 ± 0.10 ^{c}	1.14 ± 0.03
	Hexanol	0.08 ± 0.01 ^{a}	0.03 ± 0.01 ^{b}	0.05 ± 0.03 ^{b*}	0.06 ± 0.0 ^{a}	0.03 ± 0.01 ^{a}	0.04 ± 0.0 ^{a*}	0.06 ± 0.0 ^{a}	0.02 ± 0.0 ^{b}	0.03 ± 0.0 ^{c}	0.06 ± 0.01
	E-2-hexen-1-ol	0.08 ± 0.0 ^{a}	0.06 ± 0.04 ^{ab}	0.11 ± 0.03 ^{a}	0.01 ± 0.01 ^{a}	0.13 ± 0.09 ^{a}	0.23 ± 0.02 ^{a}	0.04 ± 0.0 ^{a}	0.12 ± 0.01 ^{b}	0.23 ± 0.02 ^{c}	n.d.
	Z-3-hexen-1-ol	0.05 ± 0.01 ^{ab}	0.04 ± 0.01 ^{ab}	0.03 ± 0.0 ^{a}	0.05 ± 0.01 ^{a}	0.20 ± 0.14 ^{a}	0.06 ± 0.0 ^{a*}	0.01 ± 0.01 ^{a}	0.06 ± 0.0 ^{b}	0.02 ± 0.0 ^{a}	0.11 ± 0.01
Hydrocarbons	Dodecane	3.85 ± 0.58 ^{a}	4.03 ± 0.11 ^{a}	3.50 ± 0.55 ^{a}	3.22 ± 0.15 ^{a}	4.41 ± 0.59 ^{a}	3.23 ± 0.74 ^{a}	1.17 ± 0.11 ^{a}	1.79 ± 0.59 ^{a}	1.39 ± 0.08 ^{a}	0.76 ± 0.02
	Tetradecane	1.13 ± 0.22 ^{a}	1.19 ± 0.26 ^{a}	0.71 ± 0.41 ^{a*}	0.85 ± 0.01 ^{a}	0.60 ± 0.07 ^{b}	1.09 ± 0.10 ^{c}	1.18 ± 0.06 ^{a}	1.00 ± 0.06 ^{a}	1.09 ± 0.15 ^{a}	0.51 ± 0.01
	Tetradecene	1.22 ± 0.02 ^{a}	1.17 ± 0.21 ^{a}	1.09 ± 0.15 ^{a}	1.32 ± 0.19 ^{a}	1.18 ± 0.08 ^{a}	1.02 ± 0.10 ^{a}	2.66 ± 0.16 ^{a}	2.49 ± 0.37 ^{a}	2.31 ± 0.07 ^{a}	8.62 ± 0.52
	2,4-heptadienal +pentadecan	174 ± 22.6 ^{a}	208 ± 27.5 ^{b}	160 ± 19.6 ^{a}	146 ± 11.5 ^{a}	164 ± 10.5 ^{a}	172 ± 9.43 ^{a}	36.0 ± 4.65 ^{a}	51.4±8.07 ^{a}	86.5 ± 0.52 ^{b}	11.0 ± 0.11

[a–c] Different subscript letters define statistically significant difference ($p < 0.05$) among different stages of the refining process for each oil; * Concentration of volatiles in deodorized oils marked with * do not differ statistically ($p < 0.05$) from control sample; Deodorized = refined; n.d.—not detected; $n = 12$.

Chakraborty and Joseph [14] reported that sardine fish oil distillate obtained after 60 min of steam distillation under vacuum contained two prominent aldehydes, namely, 2,4-heptadienal and 2,4-decadienal. The concentrations of these compounds were also high in our study suggesting that improvement of the distillation method is necessary.

The aroma components of fish have been widely studied, however volatile compound profiles in crude fish by-products oils and in oils undergoing the refining process have rarely been reported. In general, volatile compounds of fish oils are only identified [14,33,40], without dealing with the quantification of those components (concentrations reported in mg/kg instead of in % of peak area). The volatile components in fish oils are usually a result of microbiological spoilage or oxidation processes of lipids, amino acids and proteins and the knowledge of their chemical characterization and changes during treatments is useful for feed and aquatic industry as it opens new usage possibilities of different processing by-products [14,33,41].

The changes of volatile profiles of fish oil, from tuna and anchovy by-products in chemical refining process have been previously reported by Song et al. [33]. Authors identified 63 volatile compounds, with hexanal, nonanal, undecanal, 2-nonanone, and 2-undecanone being the key volatile components of the fish oils. The study demonstrated that compounds which are most responsible for the unfavorable odour of the fish oil could be effectively removed by the refining process which directly enhances the oil quality. Oliveira et al. [42] studied the effects of chemical refining and deodorization on fatty acid profiles and sensory characteristics of the tuna (*Thunnus albacares*) by-product oil obtained by enzymatic hydrolysis. The oil was extracted from the heads and was found rich in PUFAs. In comparison to this study, authors found higher content of MUFAs in refined oil (36.78%) and lower content of PUFA (33.18%) and recommended deodorization conditions at 160 °C for 1 h and 200 °C for 1 h for PUFA rich oils.

4. Conclusions

The chemical and compositional quality of the characterization of oils from tuna by-products, tuna liver, seabass, and gilthead seabream by-products during the four stage refining process suggests that by-products are suitable and valuable raw material for PUFA-rich oil production. Crude oils showed good characteristics; and the four-stage refining process was effective in reducing oil impurities resulting in lower FFA, PV, *p*-AV, TOTOX, and TBARS values of studied oils. Refined oils also showed better oxidative stability. A beneficial compound, α-tocopherol, which might improve the oil quality was lowered by the described refining process in all oils. Volatile compounds responsible for the sensory profile of the oils were formed and removed from the oils during different refining steps without clear relation to FFA and TBARS values. In order to maintain high levels of long-chain fatty acids, such as EPA and DHA, the described refining procedure was effective, but for effective removal of volatile components from fish oil, improvement of the deodorization step is needed possibly at temperatures higher than 100 °C for a short period of time. During the search of an alternative source of raw material for fish oil production, the results of this paper have been found to contribute to a more efficient utilization of natural marine resources, clearly indicating that by-products may offer a solution that will improve waste management, an ecological aspect of fish processing, thereby adding value to "waste".

Author Contributions: Conceptualization, V.Š., J.V. and I.G.M.; methodology, V.Š., J.V., D.S., I.L.; formal analysis, J.V., D.S., B.S., I.L.; investigation, V.Š., J.V., D.S., B.S.; writing—original draft preparation, V.Š. and J.V.; writing—review and editing, I.G.M. and D.S.; visualization, V.Š.

Acknowledgments: The authors would like to thank Sardina d.o.o. (Postira, Croatia) for raw material support, technical and facilities support of this research. We thank Heidi-Christine Santoro for the language editing.

References

1. FAO. *The State of World Fisheries and Aquaculture 2018—Meeting the Sustainable Development Goals*; FAO: Rome, Italy, 2018; p. 227.
2. Constantinos, C.M.; De La Gándara, F.; Corriero, A.; Belmonte Ríos, A. Atlantic bluefin tuna (*Thunnus Thynnus*) farming and fattening in the Mediterranean Sea. *Rev. Fish. Sci.* **2010**, *18*, 266–280. [CrossRef]
3. Rustad, T. Utilization of marine by-product. *EJEAFChe* **2003**, *2*, 458–463.
4. Ivanovs, K.; Blumberga, D. Extraction of fish oil using green extraction methods: A short review. *Energy Procedia* **2017**, *128*, 477–483. [CrossRef]
5. Arason, S.; Karlsdottir, M.; Valsdottir, T.; Slizyte, R.; Rustad, T.; Falch, E.; Eysturskard, J.; Jakobsen, G. *Maximum Resource Utilisation—Value Added Fish By-Products*; Nordic Innovation Centre: Oslo, Norway, 2009; p. 108. Available online: http://nordicinnovation.org/Global/_Publications/Reports/2010/Maximum%20resource%20utilisation%20-%20Value%20added%20fish%20by-products.pdf (accessed on 24 January 2019).
6. Stevens, J.R.; Newton, R.W.; Tlusty, M.; Little, D.C. The rise of aquaculture by-products: Increasing food production, value, and sustainability through strategic utilisation. *Mar. Policy* **2018**, *90*, 115–124. [CrossRef]
7. Kara, K.; Ouanji, F.; El Lotfia, M.; El Mahia, M.; Kacimi, M.; Ziyad, M. Biodiesel production from waste fish oil with high free fatty acid content from Moroccan fish-processing industries. *Egypt. J. Pet.* **2017**, *27*, 249–255. [CrossRef]
8. Rustad, T.; Storro, I.; Slizyte, R. Possibilities for the utilisation of marine by-products. *Int. J. Food Sci. Technol.* **2011**, *46*, 2001–2014. [CrossRef]
9. Menegazzo, M.L.; Petenuci, M.E.; Fonseca, G.G. Production and characterization of crude and refined oils obtained from the co-products of Nile tilapia and hybrid sorubim processing. *Food Chem.* **2014**, *157*, 100–104. [CrossRef] [PubMed]
10. Huang, J.; Sathivel, S. Purifying salmon oil using adsorption, neutralization, and a combined neutralization and adsorption process. *J. Food Eng.* **2010**, *96*, 51–58. [CrossRef]
11. Ferdosh, S.; Sarker, Z.I.; Norulaini, N.; Oliviera, A.; Yunus, K.; Choedury, A.J.; Arkanda, J.; Omar, M. Quality of tuna fish oils extracted from processing the by- products of three species of neritic tuna using supercritical carbon dioxide. *J. Food Process Preserv.* **2015**, *39*, 432–441. [CrossRef]
12. Kuo, C.H.; Liao, H.Z.; Wang, Y.H.; Wang, H.M.D.; Shieh, C.J.; Tseng, C.Y. Highly efficient extraction of EPA/DHA-enriched oil from cobia liver using homogenization plus sonication. *Eur. J. Lipid Sci. Technol.* **2017**, *119*, 1600466. [CrossRef]
13. Nazir, N.; Diana, A.; Sayuti, K. Physicochemical and fatty acid profile of fish oil from head of tuna (Thunnus albacares) extracted from various extraction method. *IJASEIT* **2017**, *7*, 709–715. [CrossRef]
14. Chakraborty, K.; Joseph, D. Production and characterization of refined oils obtained from Indian oil sardine (*Sardinella longiceps*). *J. Agric. Food Chem.* **2015**, *63*, 998–1009. [CrossRef]
15. Šimat, V.; Vlahović, J.; Soldo, B.; Generalić Mekinić, I.; Čagalj, M.; Hamed, I.; Skroza, D. The quality of crude marine oils from seafood processing by-products: Production and characterization. *Food Biosci.* **2019**, in press.
16. AOCS. *The Official Methods and Recommended Practices of the American Oil Chemists' Society*; The American Oil Chemists' Society: Champaign, IL, USA, 1994.
17. Ke, P.; Woyewoda, A. Microdetermination of thiobarbituric acid values in marine lipids by a direct spectrophotometric method with a monophasic reaction system. *Anal. Chim. Acta* **1979**, *106*, 279–284. [CrossRef]
18. Šimat, V.; Ficović, M.; Čagalj, M.; Skroza, D.; Ljubenkov, I.; Generalić Mekinić, I. Preventive effect of herb extracts on lipid oxidation in fish oil. *Croat. J. Food Technol. Biotechnol. Nutr.* **2017**, *12*, 30–36.
19. Soldo, B.; Šimat, V.; Vlahović, J.; Skroza, D.; Ljubenkov, I.; Generalić Mekinić, I. Sardine by-products as an alternative to whole sardines in oil production: Chemical composition and quality parameters during refining process. *Eur. J. Lipid Sci. Technol.* **2019**, in press.
20. Bligh, E.G.; Dyer, W.J. A rapid method of total lipid extraction and purification. *Can. J. Biochem. Physiol.* **1959**, *37*, 911–917. [PubMed]
21. Šimat, V.; Vlahović, J. University Department of Marine Studies, University of Split, Split, Croatia. Unpublished work, 2016.

22. Honold, P.J.; Nouard, M.-L.; Jacobsen, C. Fish oil extracted from fish-fillet by-products is weakly linked to the extraction temperature but strongly linked to the omega-3 content of the raw material. *Eur. J. Lipid Sci. Technol.* **2016**, *118*, 874–884. [CrossRef]
23. Ceriani, R.; Paiva, F.R.; Goncalves, C.B.; Batista, E.A.C.; Meirelles, A.J.A. Densities and viscosities of vegetable oils of nutritional value. *Chem. Eng. Data* **2008**, *53*, 1846–1853.
24. Bimbo, A.P. Guidelines for characterization food-grade fish oil. *Inform* **1998**, *9*, 473–483.
25. Özyurt, G.; Şimşek, A.; Etyemez, M.; Polat, A. Fatty acid composition and oxidative stability of fish oil products in Turkish retail market. *J. Aquat. Food Prod. Technol.* **2013**, *22*, 322–329. [CrossRef]
26. Vaisali, C.; Charanyaa, S.; Belur, P.D.; Regupathi, I. Refining of edible oils: A critical appraisal of current and potential technologies. *Int. J. Food Sci. Technol.* **2015**, *50*, 13–23. [CrossRef]
27. Bako, T.; Victor, U.I.; Awulu, O. Criteria for the extraction of fish oil. *Agric. Eng. Int. CIGR J.* **2017**, *19*, 120–132.
28. FAO/WHO. Proposed draft standard for fish oils. In Proceedings of the 23rd Session Codex Committee on Fats and Oils, Langkawi, Malaysia, 25 February–1 March 2013.
29. Codex Alimentarius Commision. *Standards for Fish Oils*; CXS 329-2017 1–6; Codex Alimentarius Commision: Rome, Italy, 2017.
30. Crexi, V.T.; Monte, M.L.; Soares, L.A.S.; Pinto, L.A.A. Production and refinement of oil from carp (*Cyprinus carpio*) viscera. *Food Chem.* **2010**, *119*, 945–950. [CrossRef]
31. Deepika, D.; Vegneshwaran, V.R.; Julia, P.; Sukhinder, K.C.; Sheila, T.; Heather, M.; Wade, M. Investigation on oil extraction methods and its influence on omega-3 content from cultured salmon. *J. Food Process Technol.* **2014**, *5*, 12. [CrossRef]
32. Sabliov, C.M.; Fronczek, C.; Astete, C.E.; Khachaturyan, M.; Khachatryan, L.; Leonardi, C. Effects of temperature and UV light on degradation of α-tocopherol in free and dissolved form. *J. Am. Oil Chem. Soc.* **2009**, *86*, 895–902. [CrossRef]
33. Song, G.; Dai, Z.; Shen, Q.; Peng, X.; Zhang, M. Analysis of the changes in volatile compound and fatty acid profiles of fish oil in chemical refining process. *Eur. J. Lipid Sci. Technol.* **2017**, *120*, 1700219. [CrossRef]
34. FAO. *Fats and Fatty Acids in Human Nutrition: Report of an Expert Consultation*; FAO: Rome, Italy, 2010; p. 166.
35. Šimat, V.; Bogdanović, T.; Poljak, V.; Petričević, S. Changes in fatty acid composition, atherogenic and thrombogenic health lipid indices and lipid stability of bogue (*Boops boops* Linnaeus, 1758) during storage on ice: Effect of fish farming activities. *J. Food Comp. Anal.* **2015**, *40*, 120–125. [CrossRef]
36. Cameron-Smith, D.; Albert, B.B.; Cutfield, W.S. Fishing for answers: Is oxidation of fish oil supplements a problem? *J. Nutr. Sci.* **2015**, *4*, e36. [CrossRef]
37. Chung, H.; Choi, A.; Cho, I.H.; Kim, Y.-S. Changes in fatty acids and volatile components in mackerel by broiling. *Eur. J. Lipid Sci. Technol.* **2011**, *113*, 1481–1490. [CrossRef]
38. Jónsdóttir, R.; Bragadóttir, M.; Arnarson, G.Ö. Oxidatively derived volatile compounds in microencapsulated fish oil monitored by solid-phase microextraction (SPME). *J. Food Sci.* **2005**, *70*, 433–440. [CrossRef]
39. Roh, H.S.; Park, J.Y.; Park, S.Y.; Chun, B.S. Isolation of off-flavours from tuna fish oil using supercritical carbon dioxide. *Biotechnol. Bioprocess Eng.* **2006**, *11*, 496–502. [CrossRef]
40. Ghaly, A.E.; Dave, D.; Budge, S.; Brooks, M.S. Fish spoilage mechanisms and preservation techniques: Review. *Am. J Appl. Sci.* **2010**, *7*, 859–877. [CrossRef]
41. Giogios, I.; Grigorakis, K.; Nengas, I.; Papasolomontos, S.; Papaioannou, N.; Alexis, M.N. Fatty acid composition and volatile compounds of selected marine oils and meals. *J Sci. Food Agric.* **2008**, *89*, 88–100. [CrossRef]
42. De Oliveira, D.; Minozzo, M.G.; Licodiedoff, S.; Waszczynskyj, N. Physicochemical and sensory characterization of refined and deodorized tuna (*Thunnus albacares*) by-product oil obtained by enzymatic hydrolysis. *Food Chem.* **2016**, *207*, 187–194. [CrossRef]

16

Identification of Rice *Koji* Extract Components that Increase *β*-Glucocerebrosidase Levels in Human Epidermal Keratinocytes

Kazuhisa Maeda [1,2,*], Yuuka Ogino [2], Ayano Nakamura [3], Keiji Nakata [3], Manabu Kitagawa [3] and Seiki Ito [3]

1 Bionics Program, Tokyo University of Technology Graduate School, 1404-1 Katakuramachi, Hachioji City, Tokyo 192-0982, Japan
2 School of Bioscience and Biotechnology, Tokyo University of Technology, 1404-1 Katakuramachi, Hachioji City, Tokyo 192-0982, Japan; yk.lax6054@gmail.com
3 MARUKOME Co., Ltd., 883 Amori, Nagano-shi, Nagano 380-0943, Japan; ayano_nakamura@marukome.co.jp (A.N.); keiji_nakata@marukome.co.jp (K.N.); manabu_kitagawa@marukome.co.jp (M.K.); seiki_itou@marukome.co.jp (S.I.)
* Correspondence: kmaeda@stf.teu.ac.jp

Abstract: Rice miso contains many ingredients derived from rice *koji* and has been a valuable source of nutrition since ancient times. We found that the consumption of rice miso led to improvements in the moisture content of cheek stratum corneum, skin viscoelasticity, and skin texture. Further, rice miso extract was found to increase the mRNA expression and activity of β-glucocerebrosidase (β-GCase), an enzyme involved in ceramide synthesis in the stratum corneum, in cultures. In this study, we identified the lipid-derived components of rice *koji* that increase the β-GCase activity in cultured human epidermal keratinocytes. The methanol fraction of rice *koji* extract induced an increase in the mRNA expression and activity of β-GCase in keratinocytes. The active fraction of rice *koji* was found to contain phosphatidic acid (PA) and lysophosphatidic acid (LPA). The total PA concentration in rice *koji* was 973.9 ng/mg dry weight, which was 17.5 times higher than that in steamed rice. Among the molecular species, PA_18:2/18:2 was the most frequently found. The total LPA concentration in rice *koji* was 29.6 ng/mg dry weight, and 2-LPA_18:2 was the most frequently found LPA. Since PA and LPA increase the mRNA expression and activity of β-GCase in keratinocytes, they are thought to be the active ingredients in rice *koji* that increase the β-GCase levels in human epidermal keratinocytes.

Keywords: *Aspergillus oryzae*; rice *koji*; phosphatidic acid; lysophosphatidic acid; β-glucocerebrosidase

1. Introduction

Rice *koji*, which is a solid-state culture of *koji* molds (*Aspergilus oryzae*) in rice, is used as a raw material for rice miso. Rice miso contains many ingredients derived from rice *koji* and has been a valuable source of nutrition since ancient times. We found that ingesting rice miso improved the moisture content in cheek stratum corneum, skin viscoelasticity, and texture [1]. Furthermore, the effect of miso extract on ceramide synthesis in epidermal keratinocytes was examined in cultured cells, and the mRNA expression and activity of glucocerebrosidase (β-GCase) in these cells increased when the cells were treated with miso extract [1]. From these results, it was hypothesized that the moisture level of the skin improves by everyday consumption of miso soup made from rice miso and that this may occur via increasing the ceramide content of the stratum corneum [1]. *A. oryzae* produces and secretes many types of enzymes, including α-amylase, which degrades starch; glucoamylase;

transglucosidase; acid protease, which degrades protein; and acidic carboxypeptidase [2,3], as it grows. In addition, rice *koji* contains various nutrients and supplies the necessary nutrients for yeast and lactic acid bacteria. These nutrients are especially rich in vitamins of the B group and include molybdenum; biotin; vitamins B1, B2, and B6; folic acid; pantothenic acid; and niacin [4]. Furthermore, mono- and diacylglycerol are converted to free fatty acids by the lipid-decomposing enzymes of rice *koji* [5], and other studies have suggested that the free fatty acid content in miso contributes to its antimutagenic activities [6]. The main constituent fatty acids of *A. oryzae* are lignoceric acid and, particularly, 2-oxy lignoceric acid and 2,3-dioxyl lignoceric acid, with phytosphingosine reported as the major long-chain constituent [7]. Rice bran malt contains a bifidobacterial growth-promoting substance and glucosylceramide, which improve intestinal bacterial flora in mice [8,9]. It has also been reported that *A. oryzae* exhibits antioxidant activity [10] and produces multiple cathepsin B-inhibiting components [11]. Rice *koji* is used for most Japanese fermented foods, including miso, soy sauce, amazake, Japanese sake, and malt vinegar. Rice *koji* and sake lees have also been used as cosmetics and skin moisturizing agents for many years. In this paper, we report on the lipid-derived components of rice *koji* that increase β-GCase levels in cultured human epidermal keratinocytes.

2. Materials and Methods

2.1. Materials

Human epidermal keratinocytes used for a three-dimensional epidermis model were purchased from the Japan Tissue Engineering Co. Ltd. (Tokyo, Japan). Rice *koji*, which is a solid-state culture of *koji* molds (*A. oryzae*) in rice, was obtained from Marukome Co., Ltd. (Nagano, Japan). Reagents not described in the text were obtained from Wako Pure Chemical Industries, Ltd. (Osaka, Japan).

2.2. Preparation of Rice Koji Extract

Five hundred grams of fermented rice *koji* produced by an *A. oryzae* addition to steamed rice was extracted using 3 L of chloroform/methanol (2:1). The extract was filtered and concentrated under reduced pressure on a rotary evaporator. The concentrated extract was fractionated sequentially with 3 L of chloroform, 3 L of acetone, and 3 L of methanol using a silica gel column (5 cm × 35 cm), and the fractionated solution was recovered. After concentrating this solution under reduced pressure with an evaporator, the weight of the sample was measured, and each sample was adjusted to a 5 mg/mL concentration by the addition of ethanol.

2.3. Effects of Fractions of Rice Koji Extracts on Cell Proliferation and β-GCase Activity in Cultured Human Keratinocytes

Human epidermal keratinocytes were seeded in a 96-well plate at a density of 1×10^4 cells/well, cultured in Dulbecco's modified Eagle's medium containing 10% fetal bovine serum (FBS-DMEM) for 24 h and exchanged into 99 μL of 2% FBS-DMEM. Subsequently, 1 μL each of the chloroform fraction, acetone fraction, and methanol fraction of the chloroform/methanol (2:1) extract of rice *koji* was added (n = 4). Then, the cells were cultured in a CO_2 incubator for three days. After culturing, 10 μL of Cell Counting Kit-8 solution (Dojindo Laboratories, Inc., Kumamoto, Japan) was added to each well, and after 2 h, the absorbance (at 450 nm) was measured with a microplate reader (Multi-Detection Microplate Powerscan HT; BioTek, Winooski, VT, USA) to obtain the number of cells. In this method, the tetrazolium salt WST-8 (2-(2-methoxy-4-nitrophenyl)-3-(4-nitrophenyl)-5-(2,4-disulfophenyl)-2H-tetrazolium, monosodium salt) is reduced by intracellular dehydrogenases, and the absorbance at 450 nm of the generated water-soluble formazan is measured to determine the number of living cells. The number of cells and the amount of formazan produced are linearly proportional.

β-GCase activity was determined using 4-methylumbelliferyl β-D-glucopyranoside [1]. Human keratinocytes cultured for three days in the 96-well plate were washed twice with PBS, and

30 μL of 0.01 mol/L acetate buffer (pH = 5.0) and 40 μL of a 5 mmol/L 4-methylumbelliferyl β-D-glucopyranoside solution were added. After a 1 h reaction in an incubator, 50 μL of a 0.1 mol/L glycine sodium hydrate buffer solution (pH = 10.7) was added to determine the fluorescence using the microplate reader. The measurement was performed at an excitation wavelength of 360 nm and an emission wavelength of 460 nm.

2.4. Effects of Fractions from Silica Gel Column Re-Fractionated Rice Koji Extracts on Cell Proliferation and β-GCase Activity in Cultured Human Keratinocytes

Methanol fractions ①–⑦ of rice *koji* extract were separately dried and then dissolved in 6 mL of chloroform. The entire volume of dissolved lipid solution was added to 1 g of silica gel in a column (Strata SI-1, Phenomenex Inc., Torrance, CA, USA) equilibrated with chloroform and then eluted with 40 mL of chloroform/methanol (2:1). Subsequently, phospholipids other than lysophospholipids were eluted with 40 mL of chloroform/methanol (1:1). Each fraction was weighed after being dried under reduced pressure. Then, lysophospholipids were obtained with 40 mL of methanol. Each phospholipid or lysophospholipid fraction was separated and weighed after being dried under reduced pressure. Their concentrations were adjusted to 5 mg/mL. Human keratinocytes with these fractions at a concentration of 50 μg/mL were cultured in 2% FBS-DMEM for three days, and the number of cells and β-GCase activity were measured in the same manner as in Section 2.3.

2.5. TLC Analysis of Components in Rice Koji That Affect β-GCase Activity

Methanol fractions ②–⑥ (chloroform/methanol 1:1 fractionation, 10 mg/mL); methanol fractions ④–⑥ (methanol re-fractionation, 10 mg/mL); 1,2-di-(cis-9-octadecenoyl)-*sn*-glycerin 3-phosphate sodium salt (PA_C18:1/C18:1, Sigma-Aldrich Corp., St. Louis, MO, USA; 10 mg/mL), as a standard of phosphatidic acid (PA); and oleoyl-L-α-lysophosphatidic acid sodium salt (1-LPA_C18:1, Sigma-Aldrich Corp., St. Louis, MO, USA; 10 mg/mL), as a standard of lysophosphatidic acid (LPA), were spotted on a thin-layer chromatography (TLC) plate (silica gel 60 TLC aluminum plates, Merck KGaA, Darmstadt, Germany). The plate was developed with chloroform/methanol/water/triethylamine (30:35:7:35 (*v*/*v*)). The developed plate was sprayed with molybdenum blue reagent and left at room temperature till turning a blue color. Phospholipids in the sample were estimated from the Rf value of the obtained spots. The spot density was analyzed by ImageJ. The method of preparing the molybdenum blue reagent (coloring reagent) was as follows. Solution A was prepared by adding 4.01 g of molybdenum trioxide (MoO_3) to 100 mL of 25 mol/L H_2SO_4, which was then boiled gently until the solid dissolved. Solution B was prepared by adding 0.18 g of powdered molybdenum (Mo) to 50 mL of solution A, which was then boiled gently for 15 min and allowed to cool. Equal amounts of the supernatants were mixed. After diluting three times with water, an equal volume of ethanol was added, and the solution was placed in a nebulizer.

2.6. Effects of PA_C18:1/C18:1, PA_C16:0/C18:1, and 1-LPA_C18:1 on Cell Proliferation and β-GCase Activity in Cultured Human Keratinocytes

PA_C18:1/C18:1,1-palmitoyl-2-oleoyl-*sn*-glycero-3-phosphatidic acid (PA_C16:0/C18:1) from the Cayman Chemical Company, Ann Arbor, MI, USA, and 1-LPA_C18:1 were used. Their concentrations were adjusted to 10 mg/mL, 1 mg/mL, 0.1 mg/mL, and 0.01 mg/mL with ethanol, respectively. The effect of PA_C18:1/C18:1, PA_C16:0/C18:1, and 1-LPA_C18:1 on the number of cells and β-GCase activity in cultured human keratinocytes was examined as described in Section 2.3.

2.7. Effects of the PA and LPA Fractions of Rice Koji on TEWL on a Three-Dimensional Human Epidermis Model

An agar plate was placed on a warmer set at 32 °C in a room with a temperature of 22 °C and a humidity of 40%, and a three-dimensional human epidermis model, which had been cultured for four days in the presence or absence of the PA fraction ⑤ or LPA fraction ⑤ of rice *koji* (10 μg/mL,

100 μg/mL in a solvent of ethanol:water (1:99)), was placed on the agar plate inlay. The transepidermal water loss (TEWL) was measured with a Tewameter TM 210 (Courage and Khazaka Electronic GmbH, Köln, Germany) using a probe for 24-well culture inserts.

2.8. *Effects of PA and LPA on TEWL in a Three-Dimensional Human Epidermis Model*

An agar plate was placed on a warmer set at 32 °C in a room with a temperature of 22 °C and a humidity of 40%, and a three-dimensional human epidermis model, which had been cultured for four days in the presence or absence of PA_C18:1/C18:1, PA_C16:0/C18:1, or 1-LPA_C18:1 (10 μ/mL, 100 μg/mL in a solvent of ethanol:water (1:99)), was placed on the agar plate inlay. The TEWL was measured with the Tewameter TM210 using the probe for 24-well culture inserts [12].

2.9. *Effects of the PA and LPA Fractions of Rice Koji, PA_C18:1/C18:1, PA_C16:0/C18:1, and 1-LPA_C18:1 on the Amount of β-GCase mRNA in the Three-Dimensional Human Epidermis Model*

We investigated the amount of β-GCase mRNA involved in ceramide synthesis using a human epidermal model cultured for four days in the absence or presence of the PA fraction of rice *koji*, the LPA fraction, PA_C18:1/C18:1, PA_C16:0/C18:1, or 1-LPA_C18:1 (10 μg/mL, 100 μg/mL in a solvent of ethanol:water (1:99)). RNA extraction was performed using the RNeasy Protect Mini Kit (RNeasy Mini kit, Qiagen GmbH, Hilden, Germany) according to the manufacturer's instructions. cDNA conversion from the extracted RNA was performed using the One Step SYBR® Prime Script™ RT-PCR Kit II (Takara Bio Inc., Shiga, Japan) according to the package insert. The expression level of mRNA was measured using real-time PCR (Applied Biosystems 7900HT, Thermo Fisher Scientific Inc., Waltham, MA, USA). GAPDH was used as a reference gene for normalization. Primers were purchased from Qiagen. Each experiment was performed thrice. In the analysis, a threshold cycle Ct was obtained, the difference between the Ct value of the housekeeping gene and the Ct value of the target gene (ΔCt: (target gene Ct) − (housekeeping gene Ct)) was obtained, and the ratio of gene expression was calculated from the difference in ΔCt between samples (ΔΔCt).

2.10. *Measurement of the PA and LPA Contents in Steamed Rice and Rice Koji*

Five hundred microliters of methanol and 500 μL of chloroform were added to 20 mg of lyophilized powder of steamed rice and rice *koji*, and after shaking and centrifugation, 100 μL of supernatant was collected. Then, 100 μL of a methanol solution of a PA measurement internal standard (PA_16:0 D 31/18: 1 (500 ng/mL)) was added to this supernatant sample to yield an analytical sample for PA measurement. In addition, 300 μL of the supernatant was taken, and 150 μL of the methanol solution of internal standard 1-LPA_17:0, 2-LPA_17:0 (50 ng/mL) was added to prepare an analytical sample for LPA measurement. Liquid chromatography (LC) and mass spectrometry (MS) conditions are shown below.

LC conditions	
Device	UltiMate 3000 BioRS (Thermo Fisher Scientific Inc.)
Column	L-column 2 ODS metal-free column (2 mm ID × 150 mm, 3 μm, Chemicals Evaluation and Research Institute, Tokyo, Japan)
Flow rate	0.2 mL/min
Column temperature	40 °C
Sampler temperature	5 °C
Injection volume	3 μL
MS conditions	
Device	3200 QTRAP (AB Sciex Pte Ltd. Framingham, MA, USA)
Ionization method	Electrospray ionization
Measurement mode	SRM (negative)

The analysis software Analyst 1.6.1 (AB Sciex) was used for peak detection. The detection limit was set to a signal noise ratio (S/N) of 3. The area value of the detected peak was divided by the peak area value of the internal standard (PA_16:0 D 31/18:1) to calculate the ratio. The approximate concentration of each molecular species in the sample was calculated using the obtained peak area ratio. The coefficient of variation (C.V. %) for five measurements of the peak area ratio (analysis sample/internal standard) of each molecular species was 6.9 ± 2.5 (mean $\pm$ standard deviation).

2.11. Measurement of the Relative LPA Contents in Steamed Rice and Rice Koji

To prepare the lysophospholipid fraction, 15 mL of chloroform/methanol (2:1) was added to 5 g of each of the three types of steamed rice and rice *koji*, and the mixtures were stirred and extracted at room temperature for 1 h. They were divided into soluble and solid components by filtration, and distilled water was added while stirring to make a chloroform/methanol/water solution (8:4:3 volume ratio). The sample was left undisturbed, and the lower layer (chloroform layer, total lipid fraction) was collected. The total amount of collected lipids was added to a silica gel column (Strata SI-1 100 mg (Phenomenex Inc.), gel volume 1 mL) equilibrated with chloroform; neutral lipids were then eluted using 10 mL of chloroform, and glycolipids were eluted using 40 mL of acetone. Finally, a total phospholipid fraction was obtained with 10 mL of methanol. Total phospholipids were dried and then dissolved in 1 mL of chloroform. The dissolved phospholipid solution was added in its entirety to a silica gel column (Strata SI-1 100 mg, Phenomenex Inc.) equilibrated with chloroform, and phospholipids other than lysophospholipids were eluted with 10 mL of chloroform/methanol (1:1). Subsequently, a lysophospholipid fraction was obtained with 10 mL of methanol. This fraction was dried under reduced pressure and dissolved in 100 μL of 10% Triton X-100-isopropanol. For a determination of LPA concentration, the lysophospholipid fraction was methyl-esterified using a fatty acid methyl esterification kit (Nacalai Tesque, Inc., Kyoto, Japan), and the products were analyzed by GC-flame ionization detection (FID) (TC-WAX, GL Sciences Inc., Tokyo, Japan). 1-LPA_C18:1 (Tocris Bioscience, Bristol, UK) was used as a standard. The peak area ratio of each molecular species with a C.V. below 15% for three measurements was adopted.

2.12. Statistical Analysis

Statistical analysis was performed using t-tests run with MS Excel. Differences with a p value less than 5% were statistically significant (* $p < 0.05$, ** $p < 0.01$, *** $p < 0.001$), and there was no significant difference (ns) above 5%. In addition, when the ratio was greater than 5% but less than 10%, it was considered to be exhibiting a tendency ($^{+}$ $p < 0.1$).

3. Results

3.1. Effects of Rice Koji Extract Fractions on Cell Proliferation and β-GCase Activity in Cultured Human Keratinocytes

Figure 1 shows the effects of the chloroform, acetone, and methanol fractions of rice *koji* extract on the number of cells and β-GCase activity in cultured human keratinocytes. Significantly more cells were observed in treatments with methanol fractions ②–⑦ of the rice *koji* extract than in the control (Figure 1a). In addition, a significant enhancement in β-GCase activity was confirmed in cells treated with methanol fractions ⑤ and ⑥ of the rice *koji* extract (Figure 1b). The chloroform and acetone fractions of rice *koji* extract had no such effect.

(a)

(b)

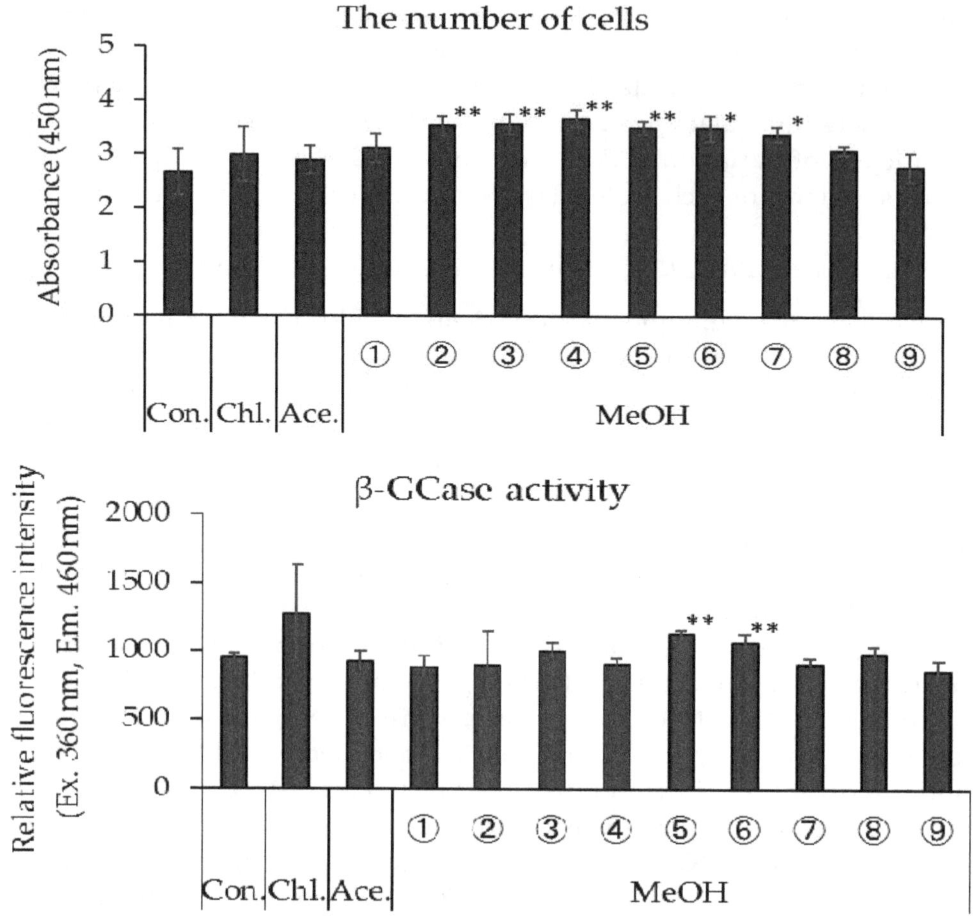

Figure 1. Effects of fractions of rice *koji* extracts on cell proliferation and β-GCase activity in cultured human keratinocytes. (**a**) The number of cells, (**b**) β-GCase activity, $n = 4$, mean ± standard deviation (S.D.), $^{+}$ $p < 0.1$ vs. control, * $p < 0.05$ vs. control, and ** $p < 0.01$ vs. control.

3.2. *Effects of Fractions from Silica Gel Column Re-Fractionated Rice Koji Extracts on Cell Proliferation and β-GCase Activity in Cultured Human Keratinocytes*

Figure 2 shows the effect of silica gel column re-fractionated rice *koji* extracts on the number of cells and β-GCase activity in cultured human keratinocytes. A significant increase in the number of cells was confirmed in treatments with silica column fractions ②, ③, and ⑤ (chloroform/methanol 1:1 re-fractionation) of the methanol fractions of rice *koji* extract, and a tendency to promote cell proliferation was observed in fraction ① (Figure 2a). In addition, a significant increase in the number of cells was observed in treatments with silica gel column fraction ① (methanol re-fractionation) of the methanol fractions of rice *koji* extract (Figure 2a). A significant increase in β-GCase activity was observed in cells treated with fractions ②–⑦ of the silica gel column fractionations (chloroform/methanol 1:1 re-fractionation) from the methanol fractions of rice *koji* extract (Figure 2b). In addition, a significant enhancement in β-GCase activity was confirmed in cells treated with silica gel column fractions ②–⑥ (methanol re-fractionation) of the methanol fractions of rice *koji* extract, and a tendency to promote β-GCase activity was observed in fraction ⑦ (Figure 2b).

(a)

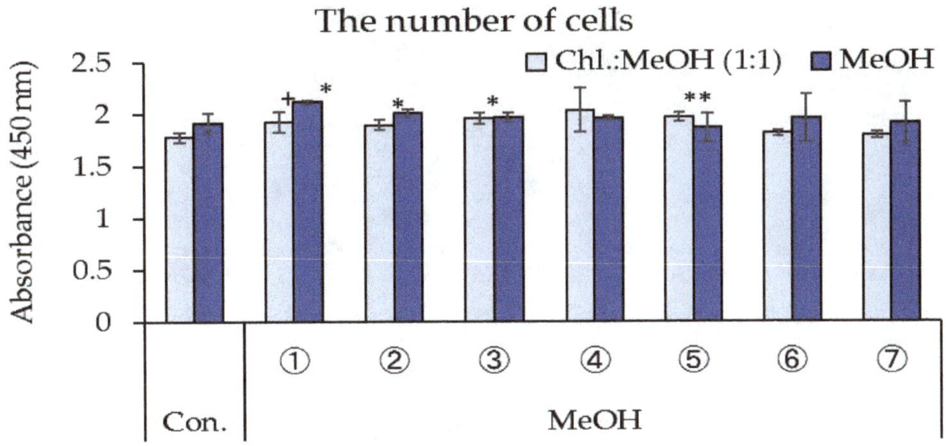

(b)

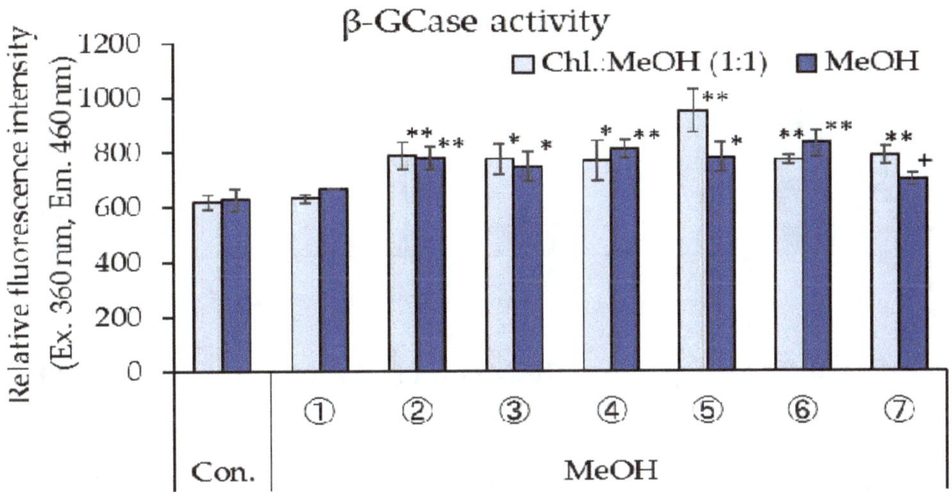

Figure 2. Effects of fractions from silica gel column re-fractionated rice *koji* extract on cell proliferation and β-GCase activity in cultured human keratinocytes. (**a**) The number of cells, (**b**) β-GCase activity, $n = 4$, mean ± S.D., + $p < 0.1$ vs. control, * $p < 0.05$ vs. control, and ** $p < 0.01$ vs. control.

3.3. TLC Analysis of Components of Rice Koji Extract That Induce β-GCase Activity

In Figure 3a, the TLC images of the chloroform and acetone extracts, methanol fractions ②–⑦ (chloroform/methanol 1:1 re-fractionation of rice *koji* extract) and methanol fractions ②–⑦ (methanol re-fractionation of rice *koji* extract) are shown. The presence of PA in methanol fractions ②–⑥ (chloroform/methanol 1:1 re-fractionation of rice *koji* extract) and LPA in methanol fractions ④–⑥ (methanol re-fractionation of rice *koji* extract) was confirmed. As a result of the analysis of spot density with ImageJ, the presence of PA in methanol fraction ⑤ (chloroform/methanol 1:1 re-fractionation of rice *koji* extract) and of LPA in methanol fractions ④ and ⑤ (methanol refraction of rice *koji* extract) was confirmed in a majority of cases (Figure 3b).

(a)

(b)

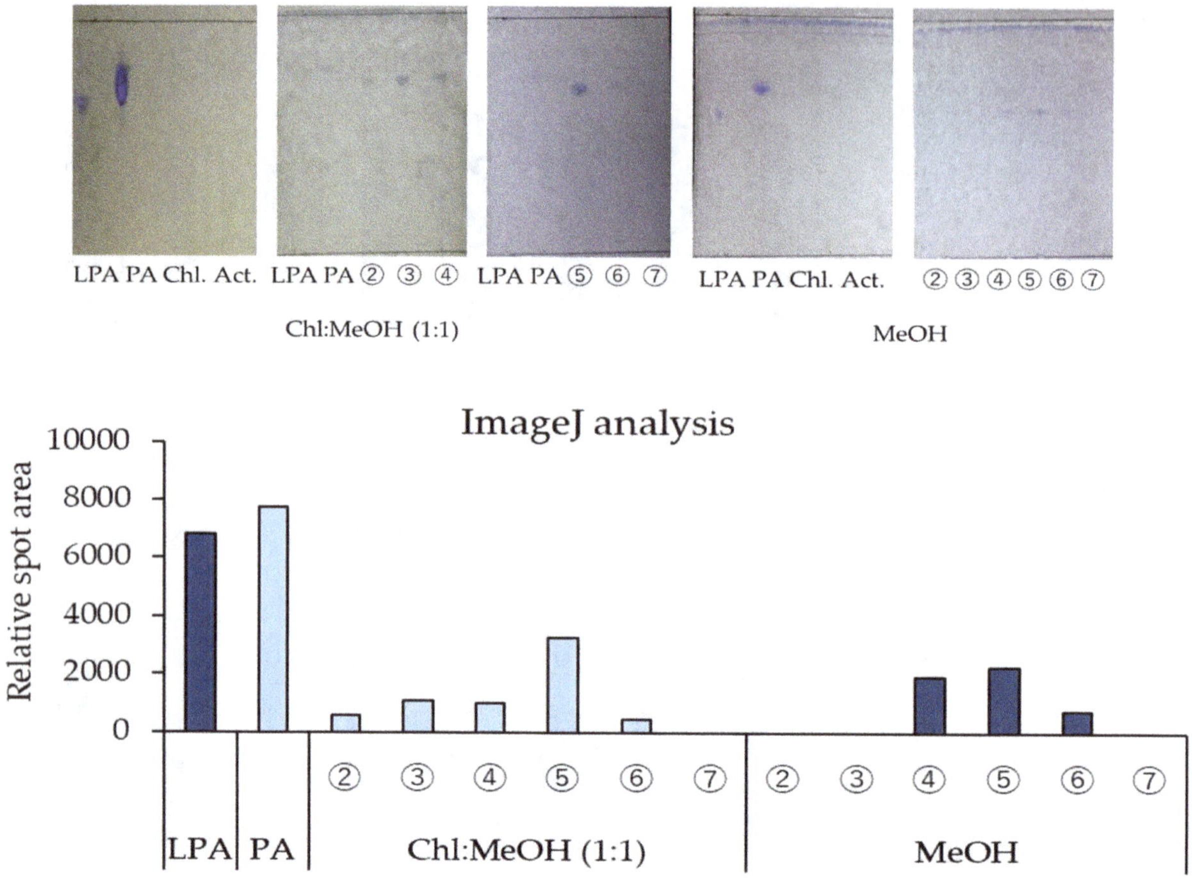

Figure 3. TLC (thin-layer chromatography) analysis of components in rice *koji* extract that increase β-GCase activity. (**a**) TLC image, (**b**) analysis of spot density with ImageJ. LPA: 1-LPA_C18:1, LA: PA_C18:1/C18:1.

3.4. Effects of PA_C18:1/C18:1 and 1-LPA_C18:1 on Cell Proliferation and β-GCase Activity in Cultured Human Keratinocytes

Figure 4 shows the effects of PA_C18:1/C18:1 and 1-LPA_C18:1 on the number of cells and β-GCase activity in cultured human keratinocytes. Treatment with PA_C18:1/C18:1 (10 μg/mL, 100 μg/mL) and 1-LPA_C18:1 (100 μg/mL) resulted in a significant increase in the number of cells (Figure 4a). In addition, a significant enhancement in β-GCase activity was observed in cells treated with either PA_C18:1/C18:1 (10 μg/mL, 100 μg/mL) or 1-LPA_C18:1 (10 μg/mL, 100 μg/mL). Treatment with PA_C18:1/C18:1 (1 μg/mL) also demonstrated a tendency towards increased β-GCase activity (Figure 4b).

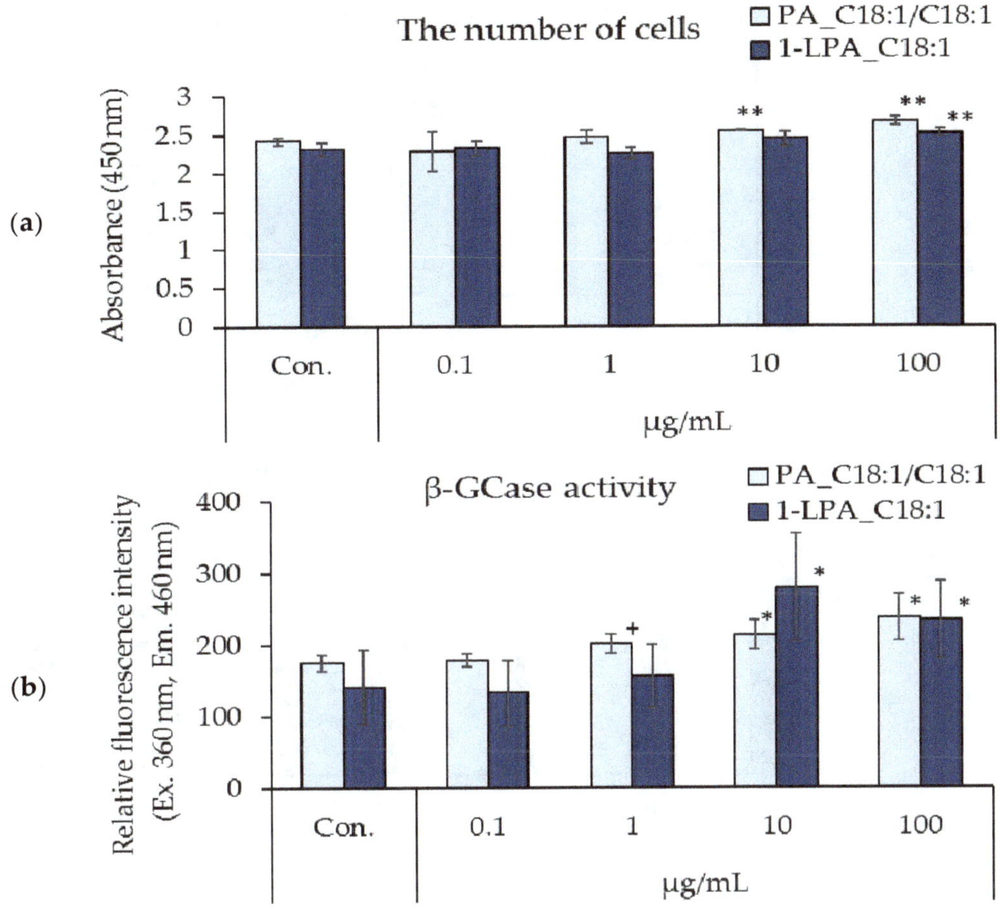

Figure 4. Effects of PA_C18:1/C18:1 and 1-LPA_C18:1 on cell proliferation and β-GCase activity in cultured human keratinocytes. (**a**) Number of cells, (**b**) β-GCase activity; $n = 4$, mean ± S.D., $^{+}$ $p < 0.1$ vs. control, * $p < 0.05$ vs. control, and ** $p < 0.01$ vs. control.

3.5. Effects of the PA and LPA Fractions of Rice Koji Extract, PA_C18:1/C18:1, PA_C16:0/C18:1, and 1-LPA_C18:1 on the TEWL in the Three-Dimensional Human Epidermal Model

Figure 5a shows the TEWL, which is the amount of moisture that transpired from the stratum corneum in the three-dimensional human epidermal model cultured for four days in the presence or absence of the PA and LPA fractions of rice *koji* extract. The TEWL from human epidermal models cultured in the presence of methanol fraction ⑤ (chloroform/methanol 1:1 re-fractionation, 10 μg/mL, 100 μg/mL) as the PA fraction and in the presence of methanol fraction ⑤ (methanol re-fractionation, 100 μg/mL) as the LPA fraction was significantly lower than that in the absence of these fractions (control). In addition, the TEWL from human epidermal models cultured in the presence of the LPA fraction (10 μg/mL) had a tendency to be lower than that in the control (Figure 5a).

Furthermore, Figure 5b shows the TEWL from human epidermal models cultured for four days in the presence or absence of either PA or LPA. The TEWL from human epidermal models cultured in the presence of PA_C18:1/C18:1 (10 μg/mL, 100 μg/mL), PA_C16:0/C18:1 (10 μg/mL, 100 μg/mL), and 1-LPA_C18:1 (100 μg/mL) was significantly lower than that in the absence of these fractions (control), and the TEWL in the epidermis model cultured for four days in the presence of 1-LPA_C18:1 (10 μg/mL) showed a tendency to be lower than the TEWL in the control (Figure 5b).

The transpiration of moisture from the stratum corneum was significantly suppressed by PA and LPA.

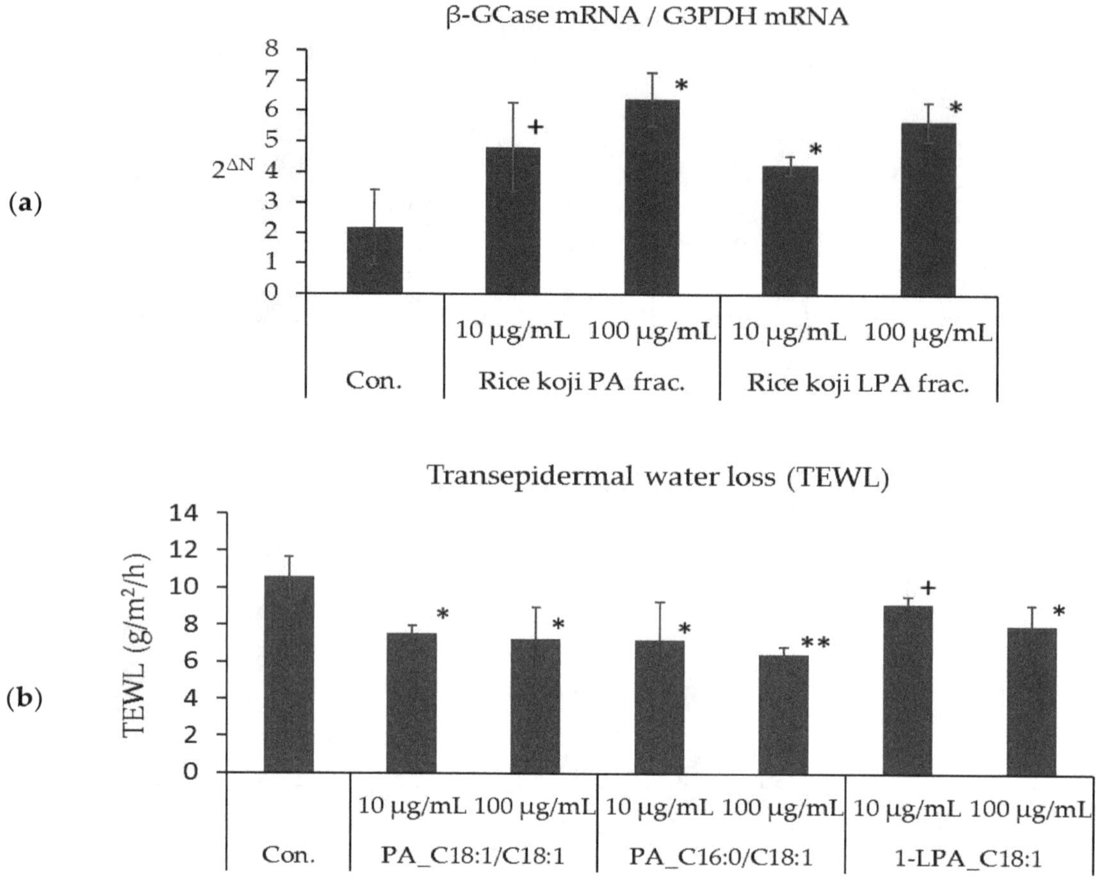

Figure 5. Effects of the PA and LPA fractions of rice *koji* extract, PA_C18:1/C18:1, PA_C16:0/C18:1, and 1-LPA_C18:1 on the TEWL from the three-dimensional epidermal model. (**a**) Effects of the PA and LPA fractions of rice *koji* extract on the TEWL, (**b**) effects of PA_C18:1/C18:1, PA_C16:0/C18:1, and 1-LPA_C18:1 on the TEWL; $n = 3$, mean ± S.D., $^{+}$ $p < 0.1$ vs. control, * $p < 0.05$ vs. control, and ** $p < 0.01$ vs. control.

3.6. Effects of the PA and LPA Fractions of Rice Koji Extract, PA_C18:1/C18:1, PA_C16:0/C18:1, and 1-LPA_C18:1 on the Expression Level of β-GCase mRNA in the Three-Dimensional Human Epidermis Model

The level of β-GCase mRNA in the three-dimensional human epidermis models cultured for four days in the presence of either rice *koji* methanol fraction ⑤ (chloroform/methanol 1:1 re-fractionation, PA fraction 100 μg/mL) or methanol fraction ⑤ (methanol re-fractionation, LPA fraction 10 μg/mL, 100 μg/mL) was significantly higher than that in the control (Figure 6a). The mRNA level of β-GCase in the epidermal model cultured for four days in the presence of methanol fraction ⑤ (chloroform/methanol 1:1 re-fractionation, PA fraction 10 μg/mL) tended to be higher than the mRNA level of β-GCase in the control (Figure 6a). Furthermore, the level of β-GCase mRNA in the epidermal models cultured for four days in the presence of PA_C18:1/C18:1 (100 μg/mL), PA_C16:0/C18:1 (100 μg/mL), or 1-LPA_C18:1 (100 μg/mL) was significantly higher than that found in the control epidermal model (Figure 6b). The level of β-GCase mRNA in the models cultured for four days in the presence of PA_C18:1/C18:1 (10 μg/mL), PA_C16:0/C18:1 (10 μg/mL), or 1-LPA_C18:1 (10 μg/mL) tended to be higher than that of the control model (Figure 6b).

(a)

(b)

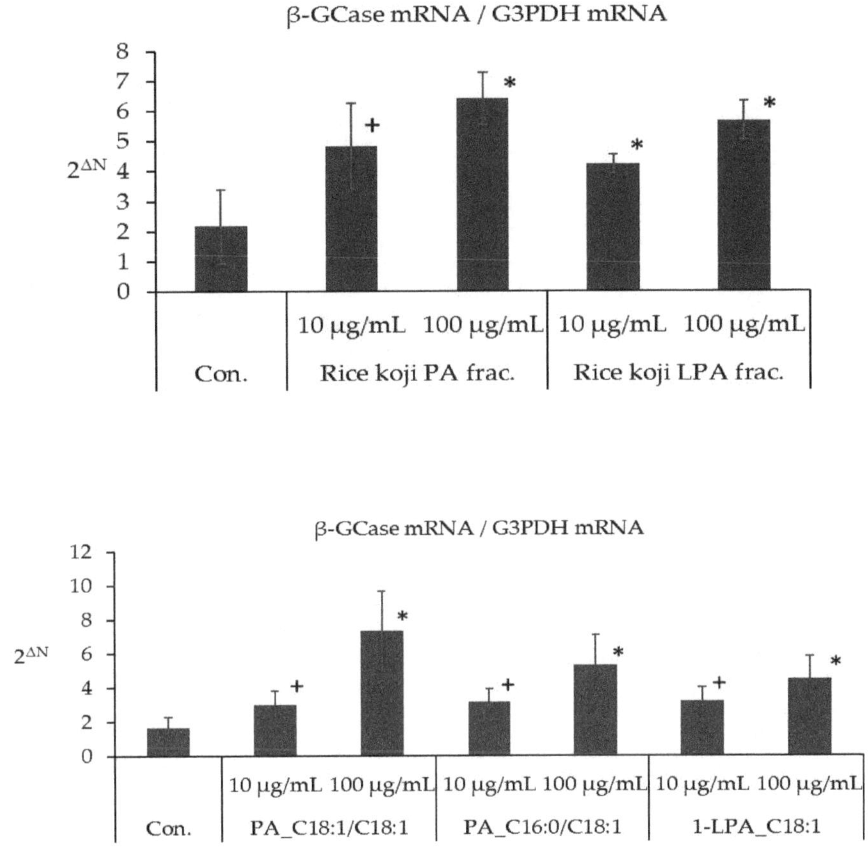

Figure 6. Effects of the PA and LPA fractions of rice *koji* extract, PA_C18:1/C18:1, PA_C16:0/C18:1, and 1-LPA_C18:1 on β-GCase mRNA expression in cultured human keratinocytes. (**a**) Effects of the PA and LPA fractions of rice *koji* extract on the level of β-GCase mRNA, (**b**) effects of PA_C18:1/C18:1, PA_C16:0/C18:1, and 1-LPA_C18:1 on the level of β-GCase mRNA; $n = 3$, mean ± S.D., $^{+}$ $p < 0.1$ vs. control, * $p < 0.05$ vs. control, and ** $p < 0.01$ vs. control.

3.7. Measurement of the PA and LPA Contents in Steamed Rice and Rice Koji

The content of PA in each molecular species of steamed rice and rice *koji* was measured, and the results are shown in Figure 7a. The total PA in rice *koji* was 973.9 ng/mg dry weight, which was 17.5 times higher than the total PA in steamed rice (55.5 ng/mg of dry weight). PA_18:2/18:2 is the most common molecular species, followed by, in decreasing order, PA_16:0/18:2, PA_18: 1/18:2, and PA _16:0/18:1 (Figure 7a). The LPA contents of steamed rice and rice *koji* are shown in Figure 7b. LPA was not detected in steamed rice, but LPA at a concentration of 29.6 ng/mg dry weight was confirmed in rice *koji*. In addition, the 2-LPA content in rice *koji* was 14 times that of 1-LPA. The 2 -LPA_18:2 species was the most frequently found 2-LPA, followed by 2-LPA_18:1. Little 1-LPA was found.

(a)

(b)

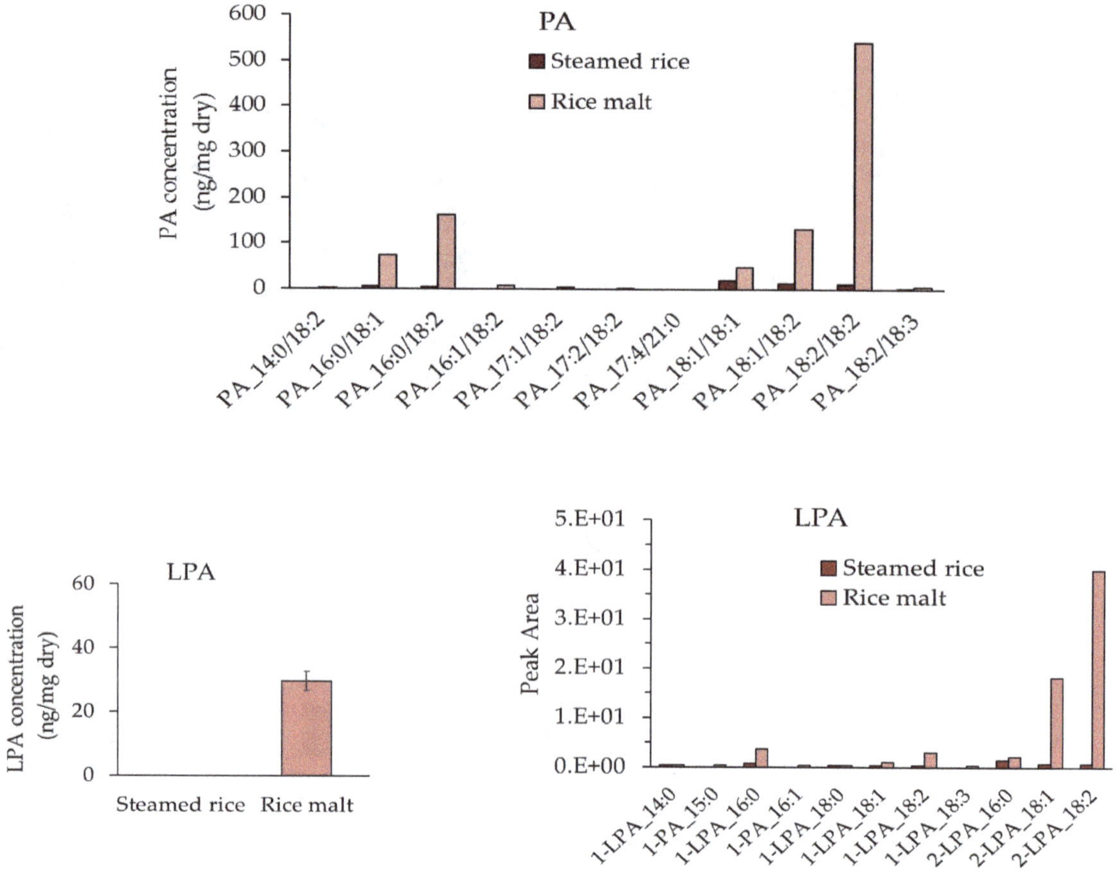

Figure 7. PA and LPA contents in steamed rice and rice *koji*. (**a**) Molecular species content of PA in steamed rice and rice *koji*, (**b**) LPA contents in steamed rice and rice *koji* (left), and molecular species content of LPA in rice *koji* relative to that in steamed rice (right).

3.8. Measurement of the PC and LPC Contents in Steamed Rice and Rice Koji

The contents of phosphatidylcholine (PC) and lysophosphatidylcholine (LPC) in steamed rice and rice *koji* are shown in Figure 8. Although PC was hardly detected in steamed rice, PC_18:2/18:2 was the most abundant PC in rice *koji*, followed by PC_18:1/18:2 and PC_16:0/18:2 (Figure 8a). Two types of 1-LPC were present in steamed rice: 1-LPC_16:0 and 1–LPC_18:2. Meanwhile, 1-LPC was also present in rice *koji*, and 1-LPC_16:0 and 1-LPC_18:2 were abundant. Both 2-LPC_16:0 and 2-LPC_18:2 were less abundant in rice *koji* than the other types of LPC (Figure 8b).

(a)

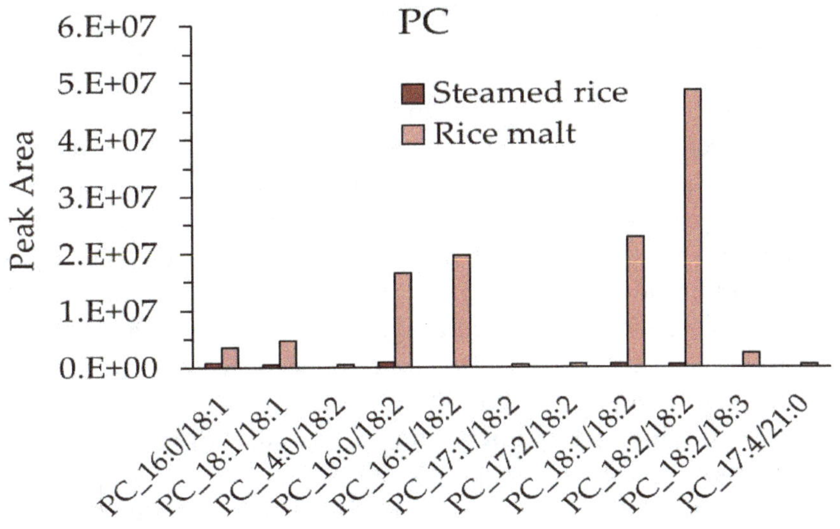

(b)

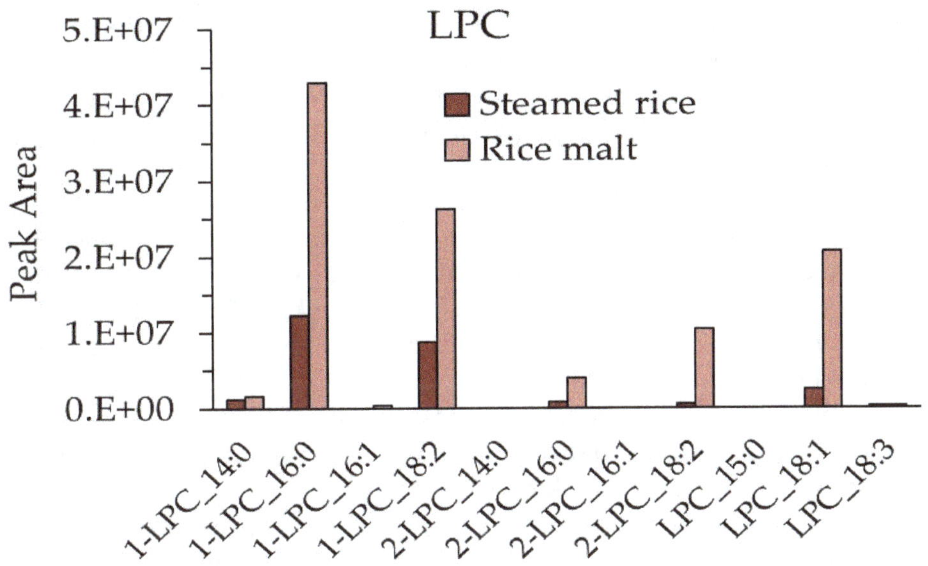

Figure 8. PC and LPC contents in steamed rice and rice *koji*. (**a**) Relative molecular species content of PC in steamed rice and rice *koji* and (**b**) relative molecular species content of LPC in steamed rice and rice *koji*.

4. Discussion

The stratum corneum intercellular lipids, which extend into the intercellular space of the stratum corneum (extracellular stratum corneum lipids), act as a barrier between the epidermis and the air of the outside world and are critical to preventing the transpiration of moisture from inside the body and moisture ingression from outside the body. When this barrier is damaged, excessive evaporation occurs, and the stratum corneum becomes dehydrated, while further deterioration causes allergic reactions in the skin, such as rough skin and atopic dermatitis [13–15]. The intercellular lipids consist of ceramides (37%), cholesterols (32%), long-chain fatty acids (16%), and cholesterol esters (15%) and form a multilayered lamellar lipid structure [16]. Among these components, ceramides are particularly important in the stratum corneum and are present in amounts 30 times or greater in the stratum corneum than in other organs. The stratum corneum ceramides are characterized not only by their large quantity, but also by the presence of various kinds of molecules [17,18]. Acylceramide, which is important for skin barrier function, is produced by β-GCase from acylglucosylceramide [19,20]. In addition, some ceramides are produced from both glucosylceramide and sphingomyelin [21,22].

We showed that the mRNA expression and activity of β-GCase, which is an enzyme involved in ceramide synthesis in the stratum corneum, increases with exposure to rice miso extract [1]. The levels of phytosphingosine- and sphingosine-type ceramides increase after such exposure [1]. During the fermentation of miso, various functional substances are produced by the enzymatic action of various fermenting microorganisms. For example, miso contains functional substances, such as essential fatty acids (linoleic acid and linolenic acid), and acylphosphatidic acid is produced by *Rhizopus oryzae* [23]. In this study, to investigate whether ceramide synthesis is involved in the skin improvement effects of rice *koji*, we examined the effects of the lipid component of rice *koji* on the mRNA level and activity of β-GCase in cultured keratinocytes. We found that both the mRNA level and activity of β-GCase were increased in cells treated with a methanol fraction of rice *koji* extract and with PA and LPA. In addition, when a methanol fraction of rice *koji* extract, PA, and LPA were allowed to act on the three-dimensional human epidermal skin model, a decrease in TEWL and increases in β-GCase activity and β-GCase mRNA expression occurred. On the other hand, the chloroform and acetone fractions of rice *koji* extract had no such effect. Rice (*Oryza sativa* L.) contains phospholipase A1 and phospholipase A2 [24], and rice bran oil contains phospholipase D [25,26]. Since steamed rice is used for the production of rice *koji*, these enzymes are thought to be inactivated. On the other hand, *A. oryzae* produces phospholipase A1 [27,28]. Rice bran oil contains phospholipids [29], and rice contains many PCs, which are phospholipids, and LPC_16:0 (3.0 to 4.7 μg/mL) and LPC_18:2 (0.8 to 2.2 μg/mL), which are both lysophospholipids [30].

In our study, PA and LPA were included in rice *koji*, and since their concentrations were higher in rice *koji* than in steamed rice, the source of phospholipids was thought to be the rice. The abundance of 2-LPA was 14 times greater than that of 1-LPA in rice *koji*. The 2-LPA_18:2 species was the most frequently found, followed by 2-LPA_18:1, and the 1-LPA level was low in rice *koji*. From these results, PA was considered to be produced from PC by phospholipase D of *A. oryzae*, and 2-LPA was produced from PA by phospholipase A1. Furthermore, these results indicated that the activity of phospholipase A1 of *A. oryzae* was higher than that of phospholipase A2. However, since the PA content in rice *koji* was 10 times greater than the LPA content, the phospholipase A1 activity of *A. oryzae* was not thought to be high. In addition, 2-LPA may be produced by phospholipase D of *A. oryzae* from the 2-LC produced by phospholipase A1 of *A. oryzae*, but the pathway by which 1-LPA is produced from 1-LC via phospholipase D of *A. oryzae* contributes less. The activity of phospholipase D of orthologous genes has not been verified in *A. oryzae* [31], and further investigating the variations in phospholipase D for each *A. oryzae* strain is necessary.

5. Conclusions

The methanol fraction of rice *koji* extract contains PA and LPA, both of which increase the mRNA expression and activity of β-GCase in cultured human epidermal keratinocytes. Therefore, PA and LPA are thought to be among the active ingredients in rice *koji* that increase the β-GCase levels in human epidermal keratinocytes. The total PA in rice *koji* was 973.9 ng/mg dry weight, which was 17.5 times higher than that in the steamed rice used as the source of rice *koji*, and contained several molecular species, of which PA_18:2/18:2 was the most abundant. The total LPA in rice *koji* was 29.6 ng/mg dry weight, and 2-LPA_18:2 was the most abundant. Based on these findings, foods containing rice *koji* (which includes high levels of PA and LPA) can presumably function in improving the moisture content, viscoelasticity, and texture of human skin.

Author Contributions: K.M. conceived and designed the experiments; Y.O. performed the experiments; K.M. and Y.O. analyzed the data; K.N., A.N., M.K., and S.I. were engaged in the manufacture of the rice *koji;* and K.M. wrote the paper.

Acknowledgments: The study was supported by a grant from the Nagano Prefecture General Industrial Technology Center. Measurements of the PA and LPA contents in steamed rice and rice *koji* were performed by the Kansai Research Institute, Inc., Japan and the Chemicals Evaluation and Research Institute, Japan.

References

1. Maeda, K.; Nakata, K.; Nakamura, A.; Kitagawa, M.; Ito, S. Improvement in skin conditions by consumption of traditional Japanese miso soup and its mechanism. *J. Nutr. Food Sci.* **2018**, *8*, 1. [CrossRef]
2. Kitamoto, K. *Bunshi Kojikin Gaku*; Revised Version; The Brewing Society of Japan: Tokyo, Japan, 2012. (In Japanese)
3. Iwano, K. Seisyu shuzou to kouso. *J. Brew. Soc. Jpn.* **1974**, *74*, 206–212. (In Japanese)
4. Ministry of Education, Culture, Sports, Science and Technology, Japan. Standard Tables of Food Composition in Japan (Seventh Revised Version). 2015. Available online: http://www.mext.go.jp/en/policy/science_technology/policy/title01/detail01/1374030.htm (accessed on 14 April 2018).
5. Ohnishi, K.; Yoshida, Y.; Toita, J.; Sekiguchi, J. Purification and characterization of a novel lipolytic enzyme from *Aspergillus oryzae*. *J. Ferment. Bioeng.* **1994**, *78*, 413–419. [CrossRef]
6. Watanabe, T.; Owari, K.; Hori, K.; Takahashi, K. Selection of *koji* mold strain for making functional miso as rich antimutagenic activity. *Nippon Shokuhin Kagaku Kogaku Kaishi* **2004**, *51*, 698–702. (In Japanese) [CrossRef]
7. Ohnishi, M.; Fujino, Y. Molecular species of free ceramides in *Aspergillus oryzae*. *Agric. Biol. Chem.* **1976**, *40*, 1419–1426. [CrossRef]
8. Hosoyama, H.; Oisawa, M.; Hamano, M. Bifidobacterium growth promoting substance in rice bran *koji* extract. *Nippon Shokuhin Kogyo Gakkaishi* **1991**, *38*, 940–944. [CrossRef]
9. Hamajima, H.; Matsunaga, H.; Fujikawa, A.; Sato, T.; Mitsutake, S.; Yanagita, T.; Nagao, K.; Nakayama, J.; Kitagaki, H. Japanese traditional dietary fungus *koji Aspergillus oryzae* functions as a prebiotic for *Blautia coccoides* through glycosylceramide: Japanese dietary fungus *koji* is a new prebiotic. *Springerplus* **2016**, *5*, 1321. [CrossRef] [PubMed]
10. Kawasumi, T.; Sato, M.; Tsuriya, Y.; Ueno, S. Antioxidant activity of a medicine based on *Aspergillus oryzae* NK *koji* measured by a modified t-butyl peroxyl radical scavenging assay. *Biosci. Biotechnol. Biochem.* **1999**, *63*, 581–584. [CrossRef] [PubMed]
11. Yamada, T.; Hiratake, J.; Aikawa, M.; Suizu, T.; Saito, Y.; Kawato, A.; Suginami, K.; Oda, J. Cysteine protease inhibitors produced by the industrial *koji* mold, *Aspergillus oryzae* O-1018. *Biosci. Biotechnol. Biochem.* **1998**, *62*, 907–914. [CrossRef] [PubMed]
12. Morimoto, H.; Gu, L.; Zeng, H.; Maeda, K. Amino carbonylation of epidermal basement membrane inhibits epidermal cell function and is suppressed by methylparaben. *Cosmetics* **2017**, *4*, 38. [CrossRef]
13. Feingold, K.R.; Elias, P.M. Role of lipids in the formation and maintenance of the cutaneous permeability barrier. *Biochim. Biophys. Acta.* **2014**, *1841*, 280–294. [CrossRef] [PubMed]
14. Groen, D.; Poole, D.S.; Gooris, G.S.; Bouwstra, J.A. Investigating the barrier function of skin lipid models with varying compositions. *Eur. J. Pharm. Biopharm.* **2011**, *79*, 334–342. [CrossRef] [PubMed]
15. Elias, P.M.; Menon, G.K. Structural and lipid biochemical correlates of the epidermal permeability barrier. *Adv. Lipid Res.* **1991**, *24*, 1–26. [PubMed]
16. Norlén, L.; Nicander, I.; Lundh Rozell, B.; Ollmar, S.; Forslind, B. Inter- and intra- individual differences in human stratum corneum lipid content related to physical parameters of skin barrier function *in vivo*. *J. Invest. Dermatol.* **1999**, *112*, 72–77. [CrossRef] [PubMed]
17. Hamanaka, S.; Hara, M.; Nishio, H.; Otsuka, F.; Suzuki, A.; Uchida, Y. Human epidermal glucosylceramides are major precursors of stratum corneum ceramides. *J. Invest. Dermatol.* **2002**, *119*, 416–423. [CrossRef] [PubMed]
18. Van Smeden, J.; Hoppel, L.; van der Heijden, R.; Hankemeier, T.; Vreeken, R.J.; Bouwstra, J.A. LC/MS analysis of stratum corneum lipids: Ceramide profiling and discovery. *J. Lipid Res.* **2011**, *52*, 1211–1221. [CrossRef] [PubMed]
19. Holleran, W.M.; Takagi, Y.; Menon, G.K.; Jackson, S.M.; Lee, J.M.; Feingold, K.R.; Elias, P.M. Permeability barrier requirements regulate epidermal beta-glucocerebrosidase. *J. Lipid Res.* **1994**, *35*, 905–912. [PubMed]
20. Hanley, K.; Jiang, Y.; Holleran, W.M.; Elias, P.M.; Williams, M.L.; Feingold, K.R. Glucosylceramide metabolism is regulated during normal and hormonally stimulated epidermal barrier development in the rat. *J. Lipid Res.* **1997**, *38*, 576–584. [PubMed]

21. Uchida, Y.; Hara, M.; Nishio, H.; Sidransky, E.; Inoue, S.; Otsuka, F.; Suzuki, A.; Elias, P.M.; Holleran, W.M.; Hamanaka, S. Epidermal sphingomyelins are precursors for selected stratum corneum ceramides. *J. Lipid Res.* **2000**, *41*, 2071–2082. [PubMed]
22. Jensen, J.M.; Fölster-Holst, R.; Baranowsky, A.; Schunck, M.; Winoto-Morbach, S.; Neumann, C.; Schütze, S.; Proksch, E. Impaired sphingomyelinase activity and epidermal differentiation in atopic dermatitis. *J. Invest. Dermatol.* **2004**, *122*, 1423–1431. [CrossRef] [PubMed]
23. Oliveira Mdos, S.; Feddern, V.; Kupski, L.; Cipolatti, E.P.; Badiale-Furlong, E.; de Souza-Soares, L.A. Changes in lipid, fatty acids and phospholipids composition of whole rice bran after solid-state fungal fermentation. *Bioresour. Technol.* **2011**, *102*, 8335–8338. [CrossRef] [PubMed]
24. Singh, A.; Baranwal, V.; Shankar, A.; Kanwar, P.; Ranjan, R.; Yadav, S.; Pandey, A.; Kapoor, S.; Pandey, G.K. Rice phospholipase A superfamily: Organization, phylogenetic and expression analysis during abiotic stresses and development. *PLoS ONE* **2012**, *7*, e30947. [CrossRef] [PubMed]
25. Lee, M.H. Phospholipase D of rice bran. I. Purification and characterization. *Plant Sci.* **1989**, *59*, 25–33. [CrossRef]
26. Ueki, J.; Morioka, S.; Komari, T.; Kumashiro, T. Purification and characterization of phospholipase D (PLD) from rice (*Oryza sativa* L.) and cloning of cDNA for PLD from rice and maize (*Zea mays* L.). *Plant Cell Physiol.* **1995**, *36*, 903–914. [CrossRef] [PubMed]
27. Watanabe, I.; Koishi, R.; Yao, Y.; Tsuji, T.; Serizawa, N. Molecular cloning and expression of the gene encoding a phospholipase A1 from *Aspergillus oryzae*. *Biosci. Biotechnol. Biochem.* **1999**, *63*, 820–826. [CrossRef] [PubMed]
28. Shiba, Y.; Ono, C.; Fukui, F.; Watanabe, I.; Serizawa, N.; Gomi, K.; Yoshikawa, H. High-level secretory production of phospholipaseA1 by *Saccharomyces cerevisiae* and *Aspergillus oryzae*. *Biosci. Biotechnol. Biochem.* **2001**, *65*, 94–101.
29. Liu, L.; Waters, D.L.; Rose, T.J.; Bao, J.; King, G.J. Phospholipids in rice: significance in grain quality and health benefits: A review. *Food Chem.* **2013**, *139*, 1133–1145. [CrossRef] [PubMed]
30. Tong, C.; Liu, L.; Waters, D.L.; Rose, T.J.; Bao, J.; King, G.J. Genotypic variation in lysophospholipids of milled rice. *J. Agric. Food Chem.* **2014**, *62*, 9353–9361. [CrossRef] [PubMed]
31. AspGD. *A. oryzae* AO090005000433 Summary. The Board of Trustees, Leland Stanford Junior University. Available online: http://www.aspergillusgenome.org/cgi-bin/locus.pl?locus=AO090005000433#citations (accessed on 14 April 2018).

17

Fatty Acid Profiles of In Vitro Digested Processed Milk

Michael H. Tunick [1] **and Diane L. Van Hekken** [2,*]

1 Center for Food and Hospitality Management, Drexel University, 101 North 33rd Street, Philadelphia, PA 19104, USA; mht39@drexel.edu
2 Dairy and Functional Foods Research Unit, Eastern Regional Research Center, Agricultural Research Service, United States Department of Agriculture (USDA), 600 East Mermaid Lane, Wyndmoor, PA 19038, USA
* Correspondence: Diane.VanHekken@ars.usda.gov

Abstract: Digestion of milkfat releases some long-chain (18-carbon) fatty acids (FAs) that can provide health benefits to the consumer, yet because they are found in small amounts and can be difficult to identify, there is limited information on the effects that common fluid milk processing may have on the digestibility of these FAs. This study provides FA profiles for raw and combinations of homogenized and/or heat-treated (high and ultra-high temperature pasteurization) milk, before and after in vitro digestion, in order to determine the effects of processing on the digestibility of these healthy fatty acids. Use of a highly sensitive separation column resulted in improved FA profiles that showed that, when milk was subjected to both pasteurization and homogenization, the release of the 18-carbon FAs, oleic acid, linoleic acid (an omega-6 FA), rumenic acid (a conjugated linoleic acid, CLA), and linolenic acid (an omega-3 FA) tended to be higher than with either pasteurization or homogenization, or with no treatment. Milk is noted for containing the omega-3 FAs and CLAs, which are associated with positive health benefits. Determining how processing factors may impact the components in milk will aid in understanding the release of healthy FAs when milk and dairy foods are consumed.

Keywords: milk; fatty acids; digestion; pasteurization; homogenization; omega-3 fatty acids; conjugated linoleic acid

1. Introduction

Milk is an important part of the diet of many people. Digestion of milk fat, 98% in the form of triacylglycerides (TAG), releases bioactive fatty acids that are absorbed by the small intestine providing a multitude of health benefits. The 18-carbon polyunsaturated fatty acids (PUFAs), making up about 2.3% of the FAs in milk, have been linked to improving mental health, reducing inflammation, inhibiting some cancers, and preventing many chronic illnesses such as cardiovascular disease, diabetes, and obesity [1–5]. The major 'healthy' FAs are the omega-3 FAs and conjugated linoleic acids (CLA). The primary omega-3 FA in milk is α-linolenic acid (*cis*-9, *cis*-12, *cis*-15 18:3). The CLAs are isomers of linoleic acid (*cis*-9, *cis*-12 18:2) with rumenic acid (*cis*-9, *trans*-11 18:2), one of the most bioactive of the CLAs, comprising 92% of the total CLAs in milk [3].

Overall, milk is considered to be a highly digestible food. Yet there are many processing factors, such as homogenization and high heat treatments, which are known to alter the stability and structure of components in milk [6] that may influence digestibility [7]. Homogenization at pressures of 10–25 MPa ruptures the protective milk fat globular membrane (MFGM) from the fat droplet and reduces it to smaller droplets (1–3 μm) [8]. High heat treatments are used to eliminate pathogens and reduce spoilage bacteria in order to extend the shelf life of milk. Common methods include high temperature, short time (HTST) pasteurization at 72 °C for 15 s or ultra-high temperature (UHT) pasteurization at 135 °C for 2 s.

Although attempts to study the effects of processing on milkfat digestion have been made, it is difficult to compare results because of the variety of methods employed. One in vivo study used fasting rats fed raw, pasteurized, or pasteurized/homogenized cream. Results showed that pasteurized cream under gastric conditions had the lowest levels of long-chain (≥14-carbons) FAs. Pasteurized/homogenized cream under intestinal conditions had the lowest levels of medium- and long-chain (≥8-carbons) FAs [9]. Another approach used human gastric juices containing pepsin and lipases as well as porcine pancreatin and bile salts in the in vitro digestion of milk samples with different-sized lipid droplets. Results showed that the small native lipid droplets released more FAs under gastric and intestinal conditions than larger native or smaller homogenized droplets. The size of the droplet also influenced the FAs released, which suggested that the size of the droplet may alter the positioning of the FAs at the droplet surface (enzyme access interface) [10].

Previous research in our laboratory used yet another approach based on the simulated fasting human gastro-intestinal model, which uses porcine pepsin and pancreatin and bovine bile extract [11] to study the digestibility of raw and processed milk [12]. Although free fatty acids (FFAs) were not released during gastric digestion, raw and homogenized samples released more FFAs than the pasteurized samples during intestinal digestion. However, the rate of FA release began to slow 30 min after lipase addition, and flattened after 90 min because of product inhibition. Comparison of FA profiles prior to digestion and after 3 h of gastro-intestinal digestion showed that stearic acid (18:0) and oleic acid (18:1) were released faster than the other FAs. All processing treatments showed similar trends in digestion for the same FA, but linoleic acid (*cis*-9, *cis*-12 18:2), its CLA isomers, and α-linolenic acid (*cis*-9, *cis*-12, *cis*-15 18:3) were not reported. Similar digestion trends were found in a follow up study that compared the quantity of FFAs released during in vitro gastro-intestinal digestion of raw and processed milk from grazing organic and confined conventional cows [13]. In that study, over half of the FFAs released in the intestinal phase were generated in the first 15 min after lipase addition. Milk from confined conventional herds, which had higher levels of palmitic (16:0) and stearic (18:0) acids, released more FFAs compared to the grazing organic herd. These FAs are typically located on the sn-1 and sn-3 TAG positions that are preferred by pancreatic lipase.

The diversity of the approaches used to study the digestion of milk offers unique opportunities to understand different aspects of the digestion process. It is imperative that the FA profiles include the healthy C18 FAs, not only to provide baselines for future research, but to aid in understanding the release of bioactive FAs in dairy foods. This work, stemming from our organic milk study [13], (1) provides complete and accurate FA profiles for milk and digested samples using a more sensitive column and (2) uses the FA profiles to evaluate the effect of homogenization and/or heat pasteurization on the gastro-intestinal digestion of milkfat.

2. Materials and Methods

2.1. Processing of Milk

Three shipments of raw milk (38 L) were obtained from an actively grazing certified organic herd located in Berks County, PA between mid-July and early September and processed that afternoon as described by Van Hekken et al. [13] in our dairy pilot plant facilities. Briefly, milk was standardized to 3.25% fat and divided into five portions. One portion remained unheated raw (R) milk control. Another portion was high temperature, short time (HTST) pasteurized (P) at 72 °C for 15 s using a Universal Pilot Plant (UPP, Waukesha Cherry-Burrell, Philadelphia, PA, USA). A third portion was HTST pasteurized and homogenized (HP) using the two-stage homogenizer (17.2/10.3 MPa) attached to the UPP. Another portion of the raw milk was warmed to 60 °C to liquefy the fat before being homogenized (H) in the off-line UPP homogenizer. The last portion was ultra-high temperature pasteurized at 135 °C for 2 s using a FT 74 P/T HTST/UHT Processing System (Armfield, Denison, IA, USA) and homogenized (HU) in the off-line UPP homogenizer. Milk samples were stored at 4 °C until digested and aliquots of milk for FA analysis were frozen at −35 °C until analyzed.

2.2. Digestion of Milk

Digestion of milk was based on the in vitro human fasting model by Gallier et al. [14] as modified by Tunick et al. [12] and described by Van Hekken et al. [13]. Raw milk samples were digested the next day and all treatments were digested within 3 days after processing; digestions were conducted once. Briefly, 50 mL of warmed (37 °C) simulated gastric fluid [11] consisting of 0.2% NaCl and 0.32% pepsin (P7000 from porcine gastric mucosa, Sigma-Aldrich, St. Louis, MO, USA), pH 1.2, was added to 100 mL of warmed (37 °C) milk, and adjusted to pH 1.5 with 6 M HCl (Fisher Scientific, Fair Lawn, NJ, USA). The mixture was constantly shaken in a water bath at 37 °C for 60 min to produce a gastric digest. A mixture of 1:1 gastric digest: simulated intestinal fluid (SIF) [11] containing 0.68% KPO_4 (Fisher) was adjusted to pH 7.0 with 0.2 N NaOH (Fisher). Bile salts (B8631 porcine bile extract, Sigma-Aldrich, St. Louis, MO, USA) were added to a concentration of 5 mg/mL SIF, along with porcine pancreatin (P1750, Sigma-Aldrich) to a concentration of 1.6 mg/mL SIF. The pH was not adjusted during digestion. Aliquots of the intestinal digests were taken after 120 min and centrifuged at 5000× g for 30 min at 10 °C (Avanti J-301; Beckman Coulter, Inc., Brea, CA, USA) to obtain the lipid portion, which was immediately frozen at −35 °C (REVCO ™ DxF; Thermo Scientific, Inc., Waltham, MA, USA) until analyzed.

2.3. Fatty Acid Profiles

Profiles of the FAs still bound to the TAG in each processed milk and digested samples were obtained based on a modified version of the procedure described by Tunick et al. [12]. Briefly, the FAs were converted to methyl esters (FAME) by reacting with sodium methoxide (Sigma-Aldrich) (free FAs were not detected by this method) and 0.5 μL samples were injected into a Trace 1300 gas chromatograph equipped with a flame ionization detector set at 270 °C (Thermo Scientific, Waltham, MA, USA) and a CP-Sil 88 column (100 m × 0.25 mm; Agilent Technologies, Wilmington, DE, USA). Helium flow was 1.0 mL/min and the injector was 20 mL/min split flow with the inlet temperature at 250 °C. The initial oven temperature was 80 °C and was increased at 4 °C/min to 220 °C and held for 5 min; the oven temperature was then increased at 4 °C/min to 240 °C and held for the remaining 10 min: The instrument's software was used to calculate percentages of FA. The internal standard added before esterification was glyceryl trinonanoate (Sigma-Aldrich), and reference standards consisted of 4–24-carbon methyl esters and conjugated methyl linoleate (Nu-Chek-Prep, Elysian, MN, USA). Data collection started with caprylic acid (8:0).

2.4. Statistical Analysis

FA profile means for each shipment were used to determine the effect of milk processing, digestion, and the processing-digestion interaction on the FAs present in the samples. Statistical software was used to conduct analysis of variance (ANOVA) using the PROC MIXED statements and the Bonferroni LSD test to determine significant differences ($p < 0.05$) (Statistical Analysis System (SAS) for Windows, version 9.4; SAS Institute Inc., Cary, NC, USA). The repeatability of the digestion method was determined using the PROC GLM (SAS) to obtain the coefficient of variance (CV) and standard deviation (SD) for the undigested ($n = 15$) and digested milk ($n = 11$) samples.

3. Results and Discussion

3.1. GC System

Use of the longer (100 m) fused silica column coated with the highly polar cyanoalkyl polysiloxane stationary phase, CP Sil 88, resulted in finer resolution of peaks and identification of more monounsaturated FAs (MUFAs) and odd-numbered FAs. In total, 8 saturated FAs (SFA), 6 MUFAs, and 3 of the healthy PUFAs (Table 1) were quantified, which is an improvement over our previous GC system that used a 60 m fused silica column with a stationary phase of biscyanopropyl/cyanopropylphenyl siloxane [12]. The major CLA in milk, rumenic acid (*cis*-9, *trans*-11 18:2), was quantified, whereas the other CLA isomers were not detected. Although 400 different FAs that have been identified in milk, only 20 FAs make up 90% of the FAs found in milk [15]. The FAs present in trace amounts, such as the other CLAs, will be difficult to isolate and identify. Further modification of the FA analysis protocol, both in sample preparation and the GC method program, may resolve overlapping peaks to identify even more FAs, including other CLAs and omega-3 FAs.

Table 1. Fatty acid concentrations (g/100 g) for differently processed milk before and after a 3 h gastro-intestinal digestion.

Fatty Acid	Common Name	R	H	P	HP	HU	SE
Undigested milk							
8:0	Caprylic acid	1.20 [a]	1.38 [a]	1.17 [a]	1.58 [a]	1.56 [a]	0.201
10:0	Capric acid	2.95 [abc]	3.57 [ab]	3.07 [abc]	2.63 [abc]	3.72 [a]	0.289
12:0	Lauric acid	3.39 [a]	4.15 [a]	3.67 [a]	3.67 [a]	4.32 [a]	0.274
14:0	Myristic acid	11.25 [c]	13.35 [c]	11.89 [c]	12.28 [c]	12.57 [c]	0.477
14:1	Myristoleic acid	1.22 [a]	1.52 [a]	1.13 [a]	1.30 [a]	1.07 [a]	0.352
15:0		1.19 [a]	1.42 [a]	1.32 [a]	1.31 [a]	1.28 [a]	0.284
15:1		0.19 [c]	0.21 [bc]	0.22 [bc]	0.22 [bc]	0.24 [bc]	0.030
16:0	Palmitic acid	29.10 [b]	30.57 [b]	29.69 [b]	28.52 [b]	28.46 [b]	1.038
16:1	Palmitoleic acid	1.30 [a]	1.53 [a]	2.31 [a]	1.79 [a]	2.69 [a]	0.312
17:0	Margaric acid	0.72 [a]	0.69 [a]	0.79 [a]	0.74 [a]	0.74 [a]	0.128
17:1		0.30 [a]	0.31 [a]	0.30 [a]	0.30 [a]	0.29 [a]	0.180
18:0	Stearic acid	13.85 [a]	11.27 [a]	11.94 [a]	12.68 [a]	10.59 [a]	1.292
cis-9 18:1	Oleic acid	23.89 [a]	21.14 [a]	23.54 [a]	24.15 [a]	24.23 [a]	1.034
trans-11 18:1	Vaccenic acid	3.85 [a]	3.39 [ab]	3.50 [ab]	3.65 [ab]	3.47 [ab]	0.172
cis-9, *cis*-12 18:2	Linoleic acid	3.74 [a]	3.72 [a]	3.64 [a]	3.52 [a]	3.36 [a]	0.203
cis-9, *trans*-11 18:2	Rumenic acid	0.97 [a]	0.97 [a]	0.93 [ab]	0.92 [ab]	0.81 [ab]	0.056
cis-9, *cis*-12, *cis*-15 18:3	α-Linolenic acid	0.77 [a]	0.78 [a]	0.67 [ab]	0.69 [ab]	0.63 [abc]	0.044
Digested milk							
8:0	Caprylic acid	1.47 [a]	0.92 [a]	0.98 [a]	0.55 [a]	0.76 [a]	0.201
10:0	Capric acid	2.16 [abc]	3.79 [ab]	2.16 [a]	1.94 [bc]	1.50 [c]	0.289
12:0	Lauric acid	4.24 [a]	4.64 [a]	3.67 [abc]	4.11 [a]	3.75 [a]	0.274
14:0	Myristic acid	18.13 [ab]	17.50 [b]	17.48 [a]	20.67 [a]	19.62 [ab]	0.477
14:1	Myristoleic acid	2.20 [a]	2.58 [a]	2.31 [b]	2.00 [a]	2.15 [a]	0.352
15:0		1.40 [a]	1.88 [a]	2.09 [a]	1.99 [a]	2.12 [a]	0.284
15:1		0.22 [bc]	0.22 [bc]	0.49 [a]	0.37 [ab]	0.31 [abc]	0.030
16:0	Palmitic acid	37.60 [a]	38.50 [a]	39.82 [a]	41.59 [a]	43.77 [a]	1.038
16:1	Palmitoleic acid	2.58 [a]	2.05 [a]	2.33 [a]	2.21 [a]	1.74 [a]	0.312
17:0	Margaric acid	1.11 [a]	1.22 [a]	0.88 [a]	0.94 [a]	1.00 [a]	0.128
17:1		0.81 [a]	0.33 [a]	0.45 [a]	0.75 [a]	0.81 [a]	0.180
18:0	Stearic acid	7.59 [a]	6.97 [a]	8.06 [a]	7.76 [a]	8.19 [a]	1.292
cis-9 18:1	Oleic acid	13.21 [b]	13.47 [b]	12.54 [b]	9.70 [b]	8.82 [b]	1.034
trans-11 18:1	Vaccenic acid	3.36 [abc]	2.22 [c]	2.86 [abc]	2.82 [bc]	2.90 [abc]	0.172
cis-9, *cis*-12 18:2	Linoleic acid	2.89 [ab]	2.76 [ab]	2.81 [ab]	1.99 [b]	1.97 [b]	0.203
cis-9, *trans*-11 18:2	Rumenic acid	0.60 [bc]	0.59 [bc]	0.57 [bc]	0.33 [c]	0.33 [c]	0.056
cis-9, *cis*-12, *cis*-15 18:3	α-Linolenic acid	0.42[bcd]	0.38 [cd]	0.41 [bcd]	0.28 [d]	0.27 [d]	0.044

Processing treatments included: raw, R; homogenized, H; pasteurized, P; homogenized and pasteurized, PU; and homogenized and UHT pasteurized, HU. [a–d] Means for the same fatty acid not sharing the same letter are significantly different ($p < 0.05$). Standard error, SE.

3.2. FA Profiles

Table 1 shows the types and levels of FAs in the milk and digested samples. The FA profiles of the milk prior to digestion were similar to those of previously published studies of milk from actively grazing cows in the USA [16–18]. All of the profiles were dominated by palmitic (16:0) and oleic (18:1) acids, comprising over 50% of the FAs. The myristic (14:0) and stearic (18:0) acids comprised about 20% of the FAs.

Rumenic acid (*cis*-9, *trans*-11 18:2) was present at nearly 1%, and none of the other 20 isomers reported in the milk [19] were detected. Statistical analysis of the milk and digested milk data resulted in coefficient of variance of 10.9 $\pm$ 0.44 and 13.6 $\pm$ 0.52, respectively, for the overall repeatability of the experiment.

The digestion system we used did not add lipase until the intestinal phase [14], and we did not detected any FFAs in the digest until then. Other studies that used the in vivo rat model [9] or human gastric juices in an in vitro model [10] reported the release of FFAs during the gastric phase. It has been suggested that gastric lipolysis enhances the efficiency of pancreatic lipase [4,10].

The profiles changed markedly with simulated intestinal digestion, due to the lipolytic activity of the added pancreatic lipases supported by the bile salts. The concentrations of many of the 18-carbon FAs decreased significantly ($p < 0.05$), which indicated the release of FFAs into the digest (Table 1). The amounts of myristic (14:0) and palmitic (16:0) acids in the digested samples appeared to increase (Table 1), although they were being released but at a slower rate than the other FAs. The slower release rate resulted in their higher concentration in the recovered digested fat sample. In bovine milk, 45–65% of myristic (14:0) and palmitic (16:0) acids are located in the sn-2 (center) position of the triacylglyceride molecule [20], partially protecting it from lipolysis. In contrast, the 18-carbon FAs (18:0, 18:1, 18:2 and 18:3) are situated in the sn-1 and sn-3 (outer) positions [20], allowing them to be readily released.

The reductions in 18-carbon FAs may be more easily visualized by noting their ratios to myristic acid before and after digestion (Table 2). The ratios for 18:1, 18:2 and 18:3 substantially decreased ($p < 0.05$) with digestion. Homogenized heat treated (HP and HU) samples tended to have lower ratios for oleic (18:1), linoleic (*cis*-9, *cis*-12 18:2), rumenic (*cis*-9, *cis*-11 18:2), and α-linolenic (*cis*-9, *cis*-12, *cis*-15 18:3) acids. These levels were reduced by more than half when the HP and HU samples were digested, and their ratios to myristic acid (14:0) were significantly lower than the corresponding ratios of the raw, homogenized and pasteurized samples. Homogenization or HTST pasteurization alone did not produce these effects, suggesting that the combination of two treatments may increase digestibility of these four FAs and will require further bench and clinical research to elucidate.

Table 2. Ratios of 18-carbon fatty acids to myristic acid (14:0) for differently processed milk before and after a 3 h gastro-intestinal digestion.

Fatty Acid	Common Name	R	H	P	HP	HU	SE
Undigested milk							
18:0	Stearic acid	1.23 [a]	0.85 [ab]	1.02 [ab]	1.03 [ab]	0.85 [ab]	0.116
trans-11 18:1	Vaccenic acid	0.34 [a]	0.26 [abc]	0.30 [a]	0.30 [a]	0.28 [ab]	0.015
cis-9 18:1	Oleic acid	2.12 [a]	1.59 [a]	1.98 [a]	1.98 [a]	1.93 [a]	0.104
cis-9, cis-12 18:2	Linoleic acid	0.33 [a]	0.28 [ab]	0.31 [a]	0.29 [a]	0.27 [abc]	0.018
cis-9, trans-11 18:2	Rumenic acid	0.086 [a]	0.073 [a]	0.078 [a]	0.075 [a]	0.065[ab]	0.005
cis-9, cis-12, cis-15 18:3	α-Linolenic acid	0.069 [a]	0.058 [a]	0.056 [a]	0.056 [a]	0.050 [a]	0.003
Digested milk							
18:0	Stearic acid	0.42 [b]	0.40 [b]	0.47 [ab]	0.38 [b]	0.42 [b]	0.116
trans-11 18:1	Vaccenic acid	0.19 [bcd]	0.13 [d]	0.16 [cd]	0.14 [d]	0.15 [d]	0.015
cis-9 18:1	Oleic acid	0.73 [b]	0.77 [b]	0.72 [b]	0.47 [b]	0.44 [b]	0.104
cis-9, cis-12 18:2	Linoleic acid	0.16 [bcd]	0.16 [cd]	0.16 [bcd]	0.10 [d]	0.10 [d]	0.018
cis-9, trans-11 18:2	Rumenic acid	0.034[bc]	0.035[bc]	0.034[bc]	0.016 [c]	0.017 [c]	0.005
cis-9, cis-12, cis-15 18:3	α-Linolenic acid	0.024 [b]	0.021 [b]	0.024 [b]	0.013 [b]	0.014 [b]	0.003

Processing treatments included: raw, R; homogenized, H; pasteurized, P; homogenized and pasteurized, PU; and homogenized and UHT pasteurized, HU. [a–d] Means for the same fatty acid not sharing the same letter are significantly different ($p < 0.05$). Standard error, SE.

Overall, our results are similar to findings from other digestion studies [9,12]. The in vivo rat study also reported that pasteurized/homogenized cream released the most FAs containing ten or more carbons, but only reported the 18-carbon FAs stearic (18:0), oleic (18:1), and linoleic (*cis*-9, *cis*-12 18:2) acids [9]. An earlier in vitro study from our lab reported greater release of stearic (18:0) and oleic (18:1) acids from homogenized and heat processed milk [12], but did not report results for the PUFAs.

Unlike our study, in vitro studies using human enzymes showed higher levels of digestion from smaller fat droplets, but found homogenization and UHT heat treatment did not enhance milk digestion [10]. They reported that the size of the lipid droplet and its surface (covered with the MFGM or casein/whey proteins) were key to lipid digestion. They also suggested that pancreatic lipases had a lower affinity to the casein coating that forms around the smaller homogenized fat droplets, thereby limiting the release of FAs.

4. Conclusions

Findings from this study showed that the use of the longer, highly polar GC column improved the resolution, identification, and quantification of the FAs present in milk and the in vitro digested milk samples. Release of the FAs was easily tracked by comparing the FA profiles before and after digestion. The 18-carbon FAs were rapidly released during intestinal digestion, although care must be taken when interpreting all FA release results to take into account the distribution of the FAs in the diminishing quantity of fat at the end of digestion. While our results suggest that pasteurizing and homogenizing milk may lead to better digestibility of healthy FAs, more research is needed using animal and human models to further investigate this phenomenon.

The diversity of the systems that have been used to digest milk offers unique opportunities to understand certain aspects of the digestion process, which, when combined, will improve our understanding of the effects that processing may have on the human health benefits from consuming milk-based foods.

Acknowledgments: The authors thank Daxi Ren, Zhejiang University, China for carrying out the digestion experiments and Anthony Bucci, Agricultural Research Service, Dairy & Functional Foods Research Unit for his contribution in preparing this manuscript and Bryan Vinyard, Agricultural Research Service, Northeast Area Statistics Group, for his statistical advise. Mention of commercial products in this publication is solely for the purpose of providing specific information and does not imply recommendation or endorsement by the USDA. USDA is an equal opportunity provider and employer.

Author Contributions: M.H. Tunick contributed to the experimental design and generation of samples, prepared the fatty acid methyl esters, conducted GC-FID analysis of lipid samples, and prepared the initial manuscript. D.L. Van Hekken contributed to the experimental design and generation of the processed milk samples, extracted lipids from the frozen samples, conducted the statistical analysis of data, and prepared the final version of the manuscript for submission.

References

1. El-Badry, A.M.; Graf, R.; Clavien, P.A. Omega 3–Omega 6: What is right for the liver? *J. Hepatol.* **2007**, *47*, 718–725. [CrossRef] [PubMed]
2. Riediger, N.D.; Othman, R.A.; Suh, M.; Moghadasian, M.H. A systemic review of the roles of n-3 fatty acids in health and disease. *J. Am. Diet. Assoc.* **2009**, *109*, 668–679. [CrossRef] [PubMed]
3. Koba, K.; Yanagita, T. Health benefits of conjugated linoleic acid (CLA). *Obs. Res. Clin. Pract.* **2014**, *8*, e525–e532. [CrossRef] [PubMed]
4. Pereira, P.C. Milk nutritional composition and its role in human health. *Nutrition* **2014**, *30*, 619–627. [CrossRef] [PubMed]
5. Simopoulos, A.P. An increase in the omega-6/omega-3 fatty acid ratio increases the risk for obesity. *Nutrients* **2016**, *8*, 128. [CrossRef] [PubMed]
6. Michalski, M.C.; Januel, C. Does homogenization affect the human health properties of cow's milk? *Trends Food Sci. Technol.* **2006**, *17*, 423–437. [CrossRef]
7. Singh, H.; Ye, A.; Horne, D. Structuring food emulsions in the gastrointestinal tract to modify lipid digestion. *Progress Lipid Res.* **2009**, *48*, 92–100. [CrossRef] [PubMed]
8. Tetra Pak. *Dairy Processing Handbook*, 3rd ed.; Tetra Pak Processing Systems AB: Lund, Sweden, 2015; pp. 131–138. ISBN 87-104227-232.
9. Gallier, S.; Zhu, X.Q.; Rutherfurd, S.M.; Ye, A.; Moughan, P.J.; Singh, H. In vivo digestion of bovine milk fat globules: Effect of processing and interfacial structural changes. II. Upper digestive tract digestion. *Food Chem.* **2013**, *141*, 3215–3223. [CrossRef] [PubMed]

10. Garcia, C.; Antona, C.; Robert, B.; Lopez, C.; Armand, M. The size and interfacial composition of milk fat globules are key factors controlling triglycerides bioavailability in simulated human gastro-duodenal digestion. *Food Hydrocoll.* **2014**, *35*, 494–504. [CrossRef]
11. US Pharmacopeia. *The National Formulary 30*; US Pharmacopeia Board of Trustees: Rockville, MD, USA, 2012; Volume 1, p. 5778.
12. Tunick, M.H.; Ren, D.X.; Van Hekken, D.L.; Bonnaillie, L.; Paul, M.; Kwoczak, R.; Tomasula, P.M. Effect of heat and homogenization on in vitro digestion of milk. *J. Dairy Sci.* **2016**, *99*, 4124–4139. [CrossRef] [PubMed]
13. Van Hekken, D.L.; Tunick, M.H.; Ren, D.X.; Tomasula, P.M. Comparing the effect of homogenization and heat processing of the properties and in vitro digestion of milk from organic and conventional dairy herds. *J. Dairy Sci.* **2017**, *100*, 6042–6052. [CrossRef] [PubMed]
14. Gallier, S.; Singh, H. Behavior of almond oil bodies during in vitro gastric and intestinal digestion. *Food Funct.* **2012**, *3*, 547–554. [CrossRef] [PubMed]
15. Masson, H.L. Fatty acids in bovine milk fat. *Food Nutr. Res.* **2008**, *52*, 1821–1823. [CrossRef]
16. Lock, A.L.; Bauman, D.E. Modifying Milk Fat Composition of Dairy Cows to Enhance Fatty Acids beneficial to human health. *Lipids* **2004**, *39*, 1197–1206. [CrossRef] [PubMed]
17. Benbrook, C.M.; Butler, G.; Latif, M.A.; Leifert, C.; Davis, D.R. Organic production enhances milk nutritional quality by shifting fatty acid composition: A United States-wide, 18-month study. *PLoS ONE* **2013**, *9*, e82429–e82435. [CrossRef] [PubMed]
18. Tunick, M.H.; Paul, M.; Ingham, E.R.; Karreman, H.J.; Van Hekken, D.L. Differences in milk characteristics between a cow herd transitioning to organic versus milk from a conventional dairy herd. *Int. J. Dairy Technol.* **2015**, *68*, 511–518. [CrossRef]
19. Kraft, J.; Collomb, M.; Möckel, P.; Sieber, R.; Jahreis, G. Differences in CLA isomer distribution of cow's milk lipids. *Lipids* **2003**, *38*, 657–664. [CrossRef] [PubMed]
20. Jensen, R.G. The composition of bovine milk lipids: January 1995 to December 2000. *J. Dairy Sci.* **2002**, *85*, 295–350. [CrossRef]

18

Accumulation γ-Aminobutyric Acid and Biogenic Amines in a Traditional Raw Milk Ewe's Cheese

Rosanna Tofalo *, Giorgia Perpetuini, Noemi Battistelli, Alessia Pepe, Andrea Ianni, Giuseppe Martino and Giovanna Suzzi

Faculty of BioScience and Technology for Food, Agriculture and Environment, University of Teramo, 64100 Teramo, Italy

* Correspondence: rtofalo@unite.it

Abstract: The influence of calf (R1), kid (R2) and pig (R3) rennets on microbiota, biogenic amines (BAs) and γ-aminobutyric acid (GABA) accumulation in raw milk ewe's cheeses was evaluated. Cheeses were investigated at different ripening times for their microbial composition, free amino acids (FAAs), BAs and GABA content. Moreover, the expression of tyrosine (*tdc*) and histidine (*hdc*) decarboxylases genes was evaluated by quantitative Real Time–Polymerase Chain Reaction (qRT-PCR). Microbial counts showed similar values in all samples. Pig rennet were cheeses were characterized by higher proteolysis and the highest values of BAs. The BAs detected were putrescine, cadaverine and tyramine, while histamine was absent. qRT-PCR confirmed this data, in fact *hdc* gene was not upregulated, while *tdc* gene expression increased over time in agreement with the increasing content of tyramine and the highest fold changes were detected in R3 cheeses. GABA showed the highest concentration in R2 cheeses reaching a value of 672 mg/kg. These results showed that the accumulation of BAs and GABA in Pecorino di Farindola is influenced by ripening time and type of coagulant. Further studies are required to develop starter cultures to reduce BAs content and improve health characteristics of raw milk ewe's cheeses.

Keywords: γ-aminobutyric acid; biogenic amines; raw milk ewe's cheese; Pecorino di Farindola; histidine decarboxylase (*hdc*) gene; tyrosine decarboxylase (*tdc*) gene

---

1. Introduction

Pecorino di Farindola is an artisanal cheese of the Abruzzo region (Italy) produced following traditional practices. Farindola is a town located in National Park of Gran Sasso, Italy, at an altitude of 530 m (1740 ft). This cheese is produced only in this geographical area and has a soft texture with a thin yellow rind or can appear with a harder texture and intense/piquant flavour as the ripening time increases. It is exclusively produced with raw ewes' milk and pig rennet without the use of natural or commercial starter cultures [1–3].

Lamb and kid rennet are the main coagulants used in Mediterranean countries for the production of Protected Denomination Origin (PDO) ovine and goat cheeses, like Pecorino Romano, Fiore Sardo and Canestrato Pugliese in Italy and Feta cheese in Greece [4,5]. Di Giacomo et al. [6] reported that pig rennet was already used by the ancient Romans to produce a "cheese of Vestini" (an ancient tribe of Abruzzo). Pig rennet is obtained from stomach mucus membrane and after an incubation of 2–3 days in salt, it is mixed with white vinegar, white wine and chili pepper and stored for 3–4 months. Finally, it is filtered for 5–6 days and only at this point it is ready to use [7–9]. Pig pepsin is unstable above pH 6.0 [9]. Its clotting activity strongly depends on pH, in fact coagulation does not occur above pH 6.7 [10]. Previous studies evaluated the influence of pig rennet in the manufacture of Pecorino di Farindola in terms of physico chemical properties, microbiota, proteolysis, volatile molecule profiles and other characteristics [3,9]. The studies showed that the use of pig makes it possible to distinguish the traditional variant from cheeses made with other coagulants.

Pecorino di Farindola cheese production is not standardized and autochthonous lactic acid bacteria (LAB) are the main responsible of the definition of final product characteristics [1]. On the other hand, non-starter lactic acid bacteria (LAB) deriving from raw milk or from the dairy environment play an important action during ripening in terms of sensory characteristics and safety issues, such as biogenic amines (BAs) accumulation [11]. Type of cheese, ripening time, manufacturing process and microorganisms highly influence the BAs content [12] and for this it can be extremely variable. BAs were found in Pecorino di Farindola cheeses examined by Schirone et al., [1]. Their total content ranged from 209.0 to 2393.0 mg/kg cheese and tyramine was the main BA detected.

BAs, mainly histamine, can lead to intoxications and adverse reactions to human health, especially after the ingestion of food products rich in BAs content [13,14]. The "cheese syndrome" caused by tyramine is rather a side effect of monoamino oxidase (MAO) drugs than a food safety issue. The consumption of cheese containing tyramine is unlikely to cause health problems in healthy individuals. EFSA report showed the absence of negative effects on health for healthy individuals after the exposure to following BA levels in food: (a) 50 mg histamine; (b) 600 mg tyramine for individuals not taking monoamino oxidase inhibitor (MAOI) drugs, but 50 mg for those using third generation MAOI drugs or 6 mg for those taking classical MAOI drugs. For putrescine and cadaverine not enough information is available [15].The intoxications related to BAs consumption can get worse in association with alcohol, other amines and monoamine and diamine oxidase-inhibiting drugs, resulting in serious problems for human health [14]. Diamine oxidase inhibitor (DAOI) drugs can also be responsible of histamine related symptomatology. Monoamine oxidase (MAO), diamine oxidase (DAO) and polyamine oxidase (PAO) are enzymes naturally present in the organism and responsible of BAs detoxification through acetylation and oxidation [16,17].

Moreover, in cheeses, there are also substances present without a defined nutritional function which could have a beneficial impact on human health and, among these compounds, γ-aminobutyric acid (GABA) has been reported with numerous positive effects on animal and human metabolic disorders [18]. This compound is synthesized by glutamate decarboxylase (GAD) catalysing the decarboxylation of L-glutamate to GABA [19]. Some studies revealed the ability of this to decrease arterial pressure and to reduce blood pressure in hypertensive patients [20–22]. Therefore, several GABA-enriched food products have been manufactured, such as GABA-enriched green tea [23], rice germ [24], tempeh and fermented beverages [25]. Dairy products fermented with GABA-producing LAB have also been studied and found to have physiological effects [26,27]. In fact, native caseins contain a high proportion of L-glutamate that can be released during milk fermentation and proteolysis.

Because of its positive impact on health, it gained the attention of the food and pharmaceutical industries. GABA is a non-protein amino acid with multiple physiological functions produced by some yeasts and bacteria. Recently, the development of functional GABA-enriched foods, such as cheese, have been reported [26,27]. In this study the role of pig rennet in the safety hazards and bioactive compounds production in Pecorino di Farindola was evaluated. In particular, cheeses were produced with three different coagulants (pig, lamb and kid) and obtained cheeses were compared in terms of microbiota, BAs and GABA.

2. Materials and Methods

2.1. Cheese Manufacture

Cheese samples were made with raw ewe's milk according to the traditional protocol [23]. Calf (R1), kid (R2) (Colombo s.r.l., Sirtori, Italy) and pig (R3) rennets (Azienda Agricola Martinelli Pietropaolo, Farindola, Italy), were used to coagulate three different milk batches obtained during the milking day, as reported by Tofalo et al. [9]. Three experimental batches consisting of 24 cheeses were carried out. After pressing and dry salting, the cheeses (~2.8 kg each) were placed in a ripening chamber at 14–15 °C. Analysis were performed after 7, 15, 30, 60, 90, 180 and 270 days of ripening.

2.2. Microbial Analysis

For the microbiological analysis, serial dilutions in sodium citrate (2% *w/v*) were prepared starting from 10 g of each cheese The following microorganisms were investigated: aerobic mesophilic bacteria (AMB) on Plate Count Agar (PCA; Oxoid, Milan, Italy) at 30 °C for 2 days; mesophilic lactobacilli on MRS agar (Oxoid, Basingstoke, UK), acidified to pH 5.4 with acetic acid, at 30 °C for 2 days in anaerobic conditions using the Gas-Pack anaerobic system (AnaeroGen; Oxoid, Basingstoke, UK); lactococci on M17 (Oxoid, Basingstoke, UK), containing 1% (*w/v*) lactose (Fluka Chimica, Milan, Italy), at 30 °C for 2 days in anaerobic conditions; enterococci on Slanetz-Bartley agar (Oxoid, Basingstoke, UK) at 37 °C for 48 h; *Enterobacteriaceae* on Violet Red Bile Glucose Agar (VRBGA; Oxoid, Basingstoke, UK) at 37 °C for 24 h. Cell counts were performed in duplicate.

2.3. qPCR Analysis

Tyrosine decarboxylase (*tdc*) and histidine decarboxylase (*hdc*) genes were detected as described by Nadkarni et al. [28], Torriani et al. [29] and Fernández et al. [30]. Primer pairs and qPCR conditions are reported in Table 1. Total RNA was extracted using a MO BIO RNA Power Soil Kit (QIAgen, Milan, Italy), according to the manufacturer's instructions. The possible presence of contaminating DNA was checked by PCR and eventually the DNase treatment was repeated. One µg of total RNA was retrotranscribed using the iScript™ cDNA Synthesis Kit (Bio-Rad, Milan, Italy), according to the manufacturer's instructions. Real-time analysis was performed using an iCycler IQ realtime PCR Detection System (Bio-Rad, Milan, Italy). A reaction mixture of 25 µL containing 12.5 µL 2XIQ SYBR Green PCR Supermix™ (Bio-Rad, Milan, Italy), 0.2 µmol/L of each primer (Life Technologies-Invitrogen, Milan, Italy) was prepared. Fold changes were determined as previously described [31]. 16S rRNA was used as reference genes. Its relative stability was evaluated using NormFinder program [32]. After real-time PCR, a melting-curve analysis was performed by measuring fluorescence during heating from 50 to 95 °C at a transition rate of 0.2 °C/s to verify the presence of unspecific products or primer dimers. A single peak was obtained highlighting the specificity of the amplification. All analyses were performed in triplicate.

Table 1. Primer sequences and PCR conditions used in this study.

Primer	Sequence (5′-3′)	qPCR Conditions	References
16SF *16SR*	TCCTACGGGAGGCAGCAGT GGACTACCAGGGTATCTAATCCTGTT	95 °C for 10 min, 40 cycles at 95 °C for 15 s, 60 °C for 1 min, 72 °C for 45 s	[28]
Tyr3 *Tyr4*	CGTACACATTCAGTTGCATGGCAT ATGTCCTACTTCTTCTTCCATTTG	94 °C for 5 min, 35 cycles at 94 °C for 20 s, 58 °C for 30 s, 72 °C for 45 s	[29]
Hdc1 *Hdc2*	TTGACCGTATCTCAGTGAGTCCAT ACGGTCATACGAAACAATACCATC	95 °C for 10 min, 40 cycles at 95 °C for 15 s, 58 °C for 1 min, 72 °C for 45 s	[30]

2.4. Free amino Acids (FAAs)

Free amino acids (FAAs, expressed as mg leucine/g) were evaluated at 507 nm after reaction with Cd-ninhydrin according to Folkertsma and Fox [33]. Analyses were performed in triplicate on each sample.

2.5. Biogenic Amines Determination

Determination of BAs was performed by acid extraction and derivatization according to Eerola, et al. (1993) [34], and Moret and Conte [35], as reported by Tittarelli et al. [17]. The presence of putrescine, cadaverine, tyramine, histamine, spermidine and spermine was determined homogenizing

2 g of cheese in 20 mL of 0.1 M HCl containing 100 mg/L of 1,7-diaminoheptane (Fluka, Milano, Italy) used as internal standard. A Waters Alliance High Performance Liquid Cromatography (HPLC) system (Waters SpA, Vimodrone, Italy), equipped with a Waters 2695 separation module connected to a Waters 2996 photodiode array detector was used. Analytes were separated using a Waters Spherisorb C18 S3ODS-2 column (3 μm particle size, 150 mm × 4.6 mm I.D.). Acetonitrile (A) and ultrapure water (B) were used for the separation of BAs. The following elution gradient was applied: 57% A for 5 min; concentration was increased up to 80% linearly in 4 min, 90% A for 5 min. The flow rate was 0.8 mL/min and the column temperature was set at 30 °C ± 0.1 °C. The peaks were detected at 254 nm. The system was controlled by Waters Empower personal computer software. Identification of the BAs was based on their retention times.

2.6. GABA Determination

GABA was determined according to Kőrös, et al. [36] and Ianni et al. [37]. Analyses were performed using the High Pressure chromatographic system (Perkin-Elmer, Monza, Italy) equipped with an autosampler and a UV-VIS detector set at 210 nm with an ion-exchange column (Phenomenex Gemini C18, dimensions: 250 × 4.6 mm, particle size: 5 μm, pore size: 110 Å) (Phenomenex, Bologna, Italy). GABA was derivatized with phthaldialdehyde Reagent (Sigma-Aldrich, Milan, Italy) and injected into the HPLC system.

3. Results and Discussion

Due to the increasing awareness towards the impact of diet on human health, issues relating to food safety and quality, have a crucial role on the consumers' behaviour. Therefore, dairy industries are developing foods with improved nutritional quality. Cheese is one of the most important fermented food product. Despite it is rich in positive compounds for human health (e.g., GABA) [38], it is also associated to BAs intoxication [13]. For this reason, the European Food Safety Authority (EFSA) Panel on Biological Hazards (BIOHAZ) has put forth an opinion on risk assessment related to BAs pointing out that the actual knowledge of their toxicity is still limited, and that further research is needed [15]. In this study, the influence of different animal rennets on microbiota, BAs and GABA accumulation in Pecorino di Farindola cheese during ripening was evaluated.

3.1. Microbial Analysis

The evolution of microbial populations at different days of ripening is reported in Figure 1. In general, no significant differences were observed. After 90 days of ripening a decrease of cell counts was detected for all microbial groups, with *Enterobacteriaceae* disappearing. The highest values of *Enterobacteriaceae* were detected in R2 cheeses with cell counts of 3.69 Log CFU/g at 90 days.

Enterobacteriaceae are an indicator of the hygienic conditions in milk and cheese production. Their occurrence has been reported in some raw milk cheeses of the Mediterranean basin after 30 days of ripening [39,40]. Moreover, some studies highlighted that this microbial group can influence taste, aroma and texture, of some artisanal cheeses [41,42]. Enterococci were present with cell counts of about 6 Log CFU/mL in all samples until 90 days of ripening, while after this time a decrease of about 3 Log was observed. Their occurrence has been reported in other Pecorino cheeses [9,43]. Their presence can be due to milk contamination and to their ability to face the conditions of cheese manufacture and ripening since they are able to develop at different temperatures and are tolerant to heat and salt [44]. Moreover, they have a crucial role in cheese ripening and aging influencing aroma and flavour thanks to their proteolytic and lipolytic activities as a result of citrate metabolism [44]. On the other hand, enterococci have often been associated with clinical infections and BAs production, such as tyramine and histamine [45].

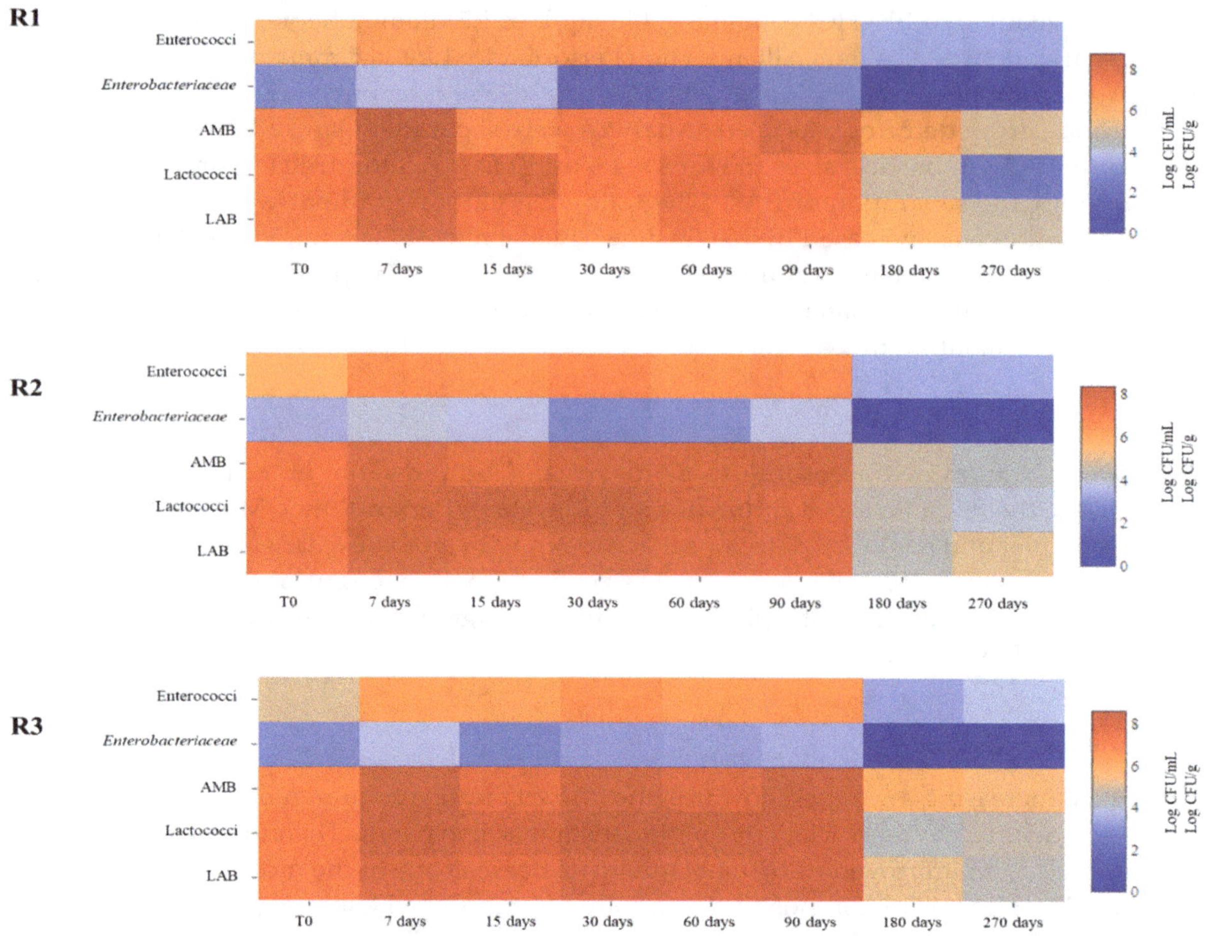

Figure 1. Heat maps depicting abundance of microbial groups characterizing the cheeses obtained with different rennets throughout ripening. Calf (**R1**), kid (**R2**) and pig (**R3**) rennets. Aerobic Mesophilic Bacteria (AMB); Lactic Acid Bacteria (LAB).

Lactococci were present in lower concentration at the end of ripening, about 4 Log CFU/mL in R2 and R3 cheeses and about 2 Log CFU/mL in R1 cheese. LAB counts throughout the ripening were similar to those observed for AMB suggesting that they were the predominant microorganisms. Similar results have been reported by Renes et al. [46]. Their counts increased during the first days of ripening reaching values of about 8 Log CFU/g in R2 and R3 cheeses after 90 days of ripening, while in R1 cheeses cell counts of about 7 Log CFU/mL were observed. LAB are the main components of the autochthonous cheese and are known to participate to the fermentation process and maturation of cheeses, producing a number of desirable substances that can improve the flavour, texture, nutritional value, shelf-life, and safety of foods [46–48]. However, some LAB species have been shown to include strains producing high amounts of BAs such as histamine and tyramine [46,49–54].

3.2. Biogenic Amines

BAs accumulation in cheese depends on several factors including ripening time, the manufacturing process, presence of decarboxylase positive microorganisms and precursors availability [14,46]. In general, during cheese ripening secondary proteolysis occurs with the accumulation of FAAs which can be decarboxylated to BAs by the microbiota [46]. Therefore, the level of protein degradation was firstly evaluated.

Figure 2 shows the evolution of FAAs during the ripening period. Obtained data revealed a certain variability of FAAs content among samples. The FAAs content increased significantly during ripening in all samples, reaching values of 233.74, 252.54 and 296.84 mg leucine/g in R1, R2 and R3 cheeses respectively after 270 days of ripening. This increase is in agreement with previous observations in Caciocavallo Pugliese, in Picante cheese, in Kashkaval cheese and in other Pecorino cheeses [9,55–58]. The greater proteolytic activity in R3 cheeses was in agreement with Tofalo et al., (2015) [9] who observed a higher proteolytic activity for pig rennet than for calf and kid ones. R3 cheeses contained the highest total concentrations of BAs (1293 mg/kg) (Figure 3). However, all the studied cheeses accumulated high total BAs contents even if with quantitative differences. It could be assumed that milk quality produced by the sheep in the Gran Sasso area is a relevant factor influencing the high BAs content of Pecorino di Farindola, probably also depending on the autochthonous microbiota [59,60].

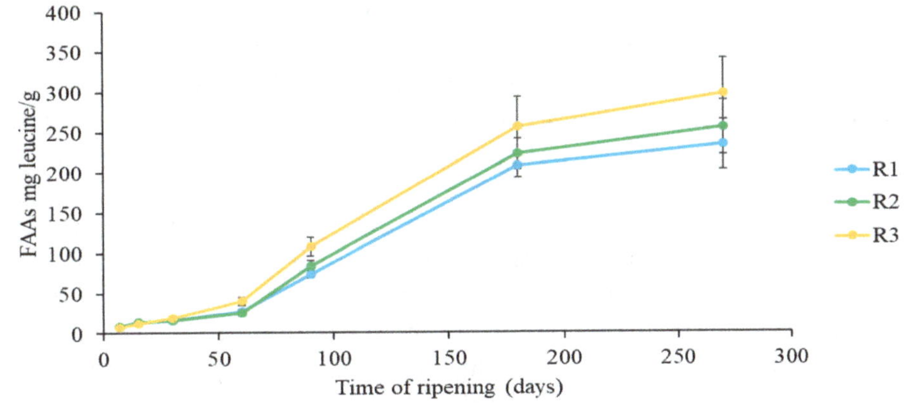

Figure 2. Evolution of free amino acids throughout ripening in Pecorino di Farindola produced with with different rennets. calf (R1), kid (R2) and pig (R3).

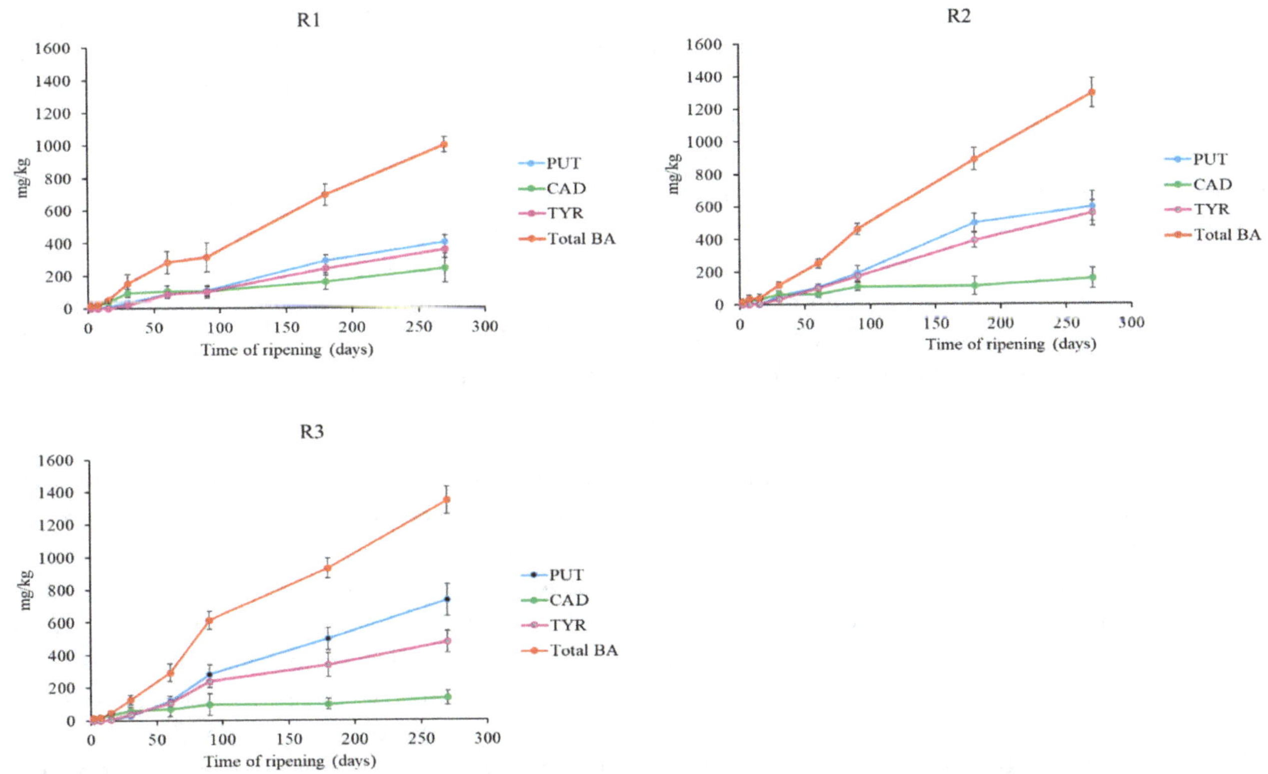

Figure 3. Biogenic amines evolution in Pecorino di Farindola manufactured with the three different rennets: calf (R1), 216 kid (R2) and pig (R3). Putrescine (PUT); Cadaverine (CAD); Tyramine (TYR); Biogenic Amine (BA).

The main BAs detected were putrescine, cadaverine and tyramine, while histamine was not detected. Putrescine showed the highest concentration with values of 400 mg/kg, 598 mg/kg and 732 mg/kg in R1, R2 and R3 cheeses, respectively after 270 days. Cadaverine presented values ranging from 241 mg/kg (R1) to 154 mg/kg (R2) at the end of ripening. These BAs are considered indicators contamination and markers of the hygiene standards of the production process. Their production mainly relies on Gram-negative bacteria, especially belonging to the families *Enterobacteriaceae* and *Pseudomonadaceae*, generally associated with spoilage [61]. LAB and staphylococci have also been reported [62]. Tyramine was present in all samples and its concentration increased over time. To our knowledge, Enterococci play a predominant role in the formation of tyramine [63]. The high BAs content detected in cheeses could be related to the productions practices associated to Pecorino di Farindola. In fact, it is produced starting from raw milk from sheep fed in a limited mountain area (Gran Sasso) and pig rennet as coagulant. The combination of these two factors could be a cause of high BAs content in the cheese. In fact, it has been already proved that there is a relationship between alpine pastures and milk quality during grazing [64].

Tyramine presents several negative effects on human health such as headaches, migraine, neurological disorders, nausea, vomiting, respiratory disorders, hypertension [13,65]. However, even though histamine was considered as the most toxic BA for a long time, recently Linares et al. [66] revealed that tyramine is even more toxic than histamine reporting the cytotoxicity threshold detected for histamine (441 mg/kg) and for tyramine (302 mg/kg). Amino acid decarboxylase activity is strain dependent rather than species specific, thus suggesting the occurrence of horizontal gene transfer events as part of a mechanism of survival and adaptation to specific environments [67]. Wüthrich et al. [68] sequenced the histamine positive strain FAM21731 of *L. parabuchneri* showing that *hdc* gene cluster was located in a genomic island, transferred within this species. This species has been frequently reported in dairy products and is responsible for the accumulation of histamine in many types of cheeses [49–51]. Its occurrence in milk is probably related to a contamination focus at farm level, because its capacity to adhere to stainless steel [50,52,53]. Moreover, *L. parabuchneri* strains are able to develop and to produce histamine also at refrigeration temperatures, suggesting that when *L. parabuchneri* is present, refrigeration can only delay but not prevent the accumulation of histamine in cheese [54]. For this reason, aminogenic strains may be found within the contaminant species but also as part of the spontaneous fermentative microbiota. Therefore, the expression of *tdc* and *hdc* genes was checked by qRT-PCR. In all samples *hdc* gene was not upregulated confirming the absence of histamine in cheeses, whereas *tdc* expression increased over time in agreement with the increasing content of tyramine (Figure 4). The strongest increase in *tdc* expression was found in R3 cheese after 270 days of ripening (a 93-fold increase), whereas the other cheeses showed 61- (R1) and 82- (R2) fold increases of the *tdc* gene.

This development was expected, because in LAB, BAs formation provides metabolic energy and/or acid resistance during a long ripening [69,70]. In general, a positive correlation between *tdc* expression and tyramine production was observed (Figure 4). This evidence is in agreement with other studies and suggests that the expression of this gene can be used to predict tyramine accumulation [13,17,43]. The high content of tyramine could be related with the high content of putrescine. In fact, agmatine deiminase pathway genes, involved in putrescine production, are linked to the tyrosine decarboxylation operon in LAB [71]. The agmatine deiminase and the tyrosine decarboxylase pathways, appear to be widespread throughout several species of LAB and are often simultaneously present [72]. Moreover, the formation of the different BAs could be also influenced by the microbial contamination in the processed milk.

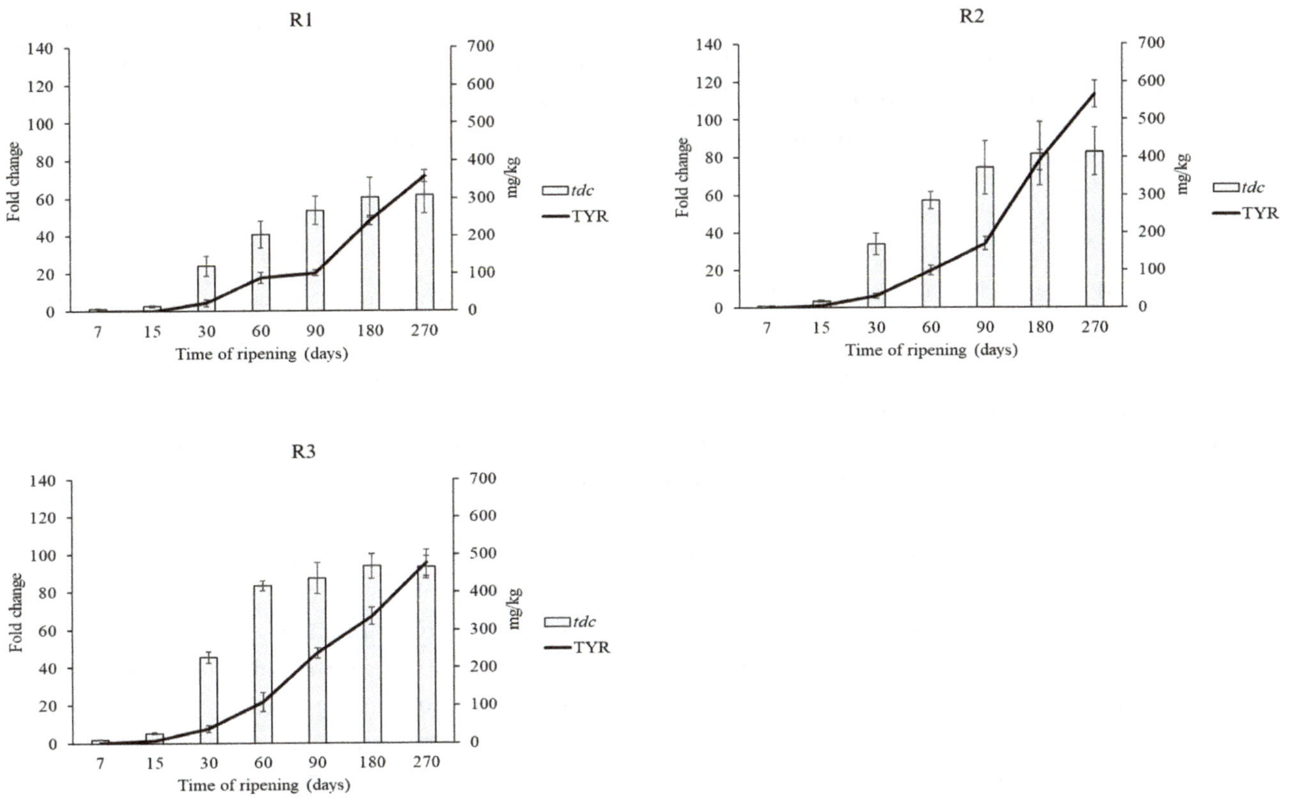

Figure 4. Tyramine content and relative transcript levels of *tdc* gene during ripening. Transcript levels are expressed as x-fold increase in comparison with the expression at T0. Three biological replicates were performed. Calf (R1), kid (R2) and pig (R3).

3.3. γ-Aminobutyric Acid

The GABA content determined in this study is reported in Figure 5. The highest concentrations of GABA were found in R2 and R3 cheeses, with values of 672 and 554 mg/kg, respectively.

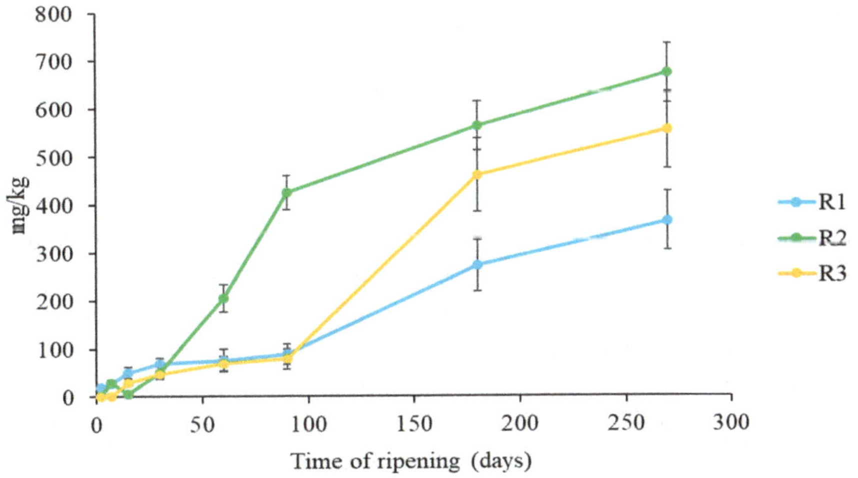

Figure 5. Evolution of GABA content in Pecorino di Farindola made with the three different rennets: calf (R1), kid (R2) and pig (R3).

These results are in agreement with the proteolysis outcome, in fact in R1 cheeses a slower proteolysis was observed. In general, GABA production is associated to different LAB species in a strain dependent way [73]. Siragusa et al. [73] studied 22 Italian cheese varieties for their GABA concentrations that varied from 0.26 to 391 mg/kg. The highest values of GABA were found in five varieties of Pecorino cheeses, but especially in Pecorino di Filiano (391 mg/kg). Moreover, Nomura et al. [74] analysed seven commercial cheeses (Camembert, Gouda, Blue, Cream, Cheddar, Edam and Emmental) and reported GABA concentration lower that those obtained in this study. In general ewe's milk quality and coagulant seem to have some influence on GABA accumulation in cheese.

4. Conclusions

Traditional cheeses like Pecorino di Farindola, maintain high diversity in cheese-making practices as well as in autochthonous cheese microbial communities. The combination of hygienic quality of raw ewe's milk, the different handling and cheesemaking processes and pig rennet could be a cause of its high BAs content. However, it is expected to see a total BAs content rise in cheese as a consequence of many BAs precursors released by coagulants from a raw milk with a high proteins content. Pig rennet imparts specific features to Pecorino di Farindola cheese, probably through its specific proteolytic patterns resulting from the unique enzymatic composition of this coagulant. However, this study confirms a greater BAs formation and proteolytic activity, as suggested by FAA values, in cheese made by pig rennet than those made by calf and kid rennet. It is difficult to modify the process without denaturing the organoleptic and sensorial characteristics of this traditional cheese. A possibility could be the pasteurization of raw milk, but this procedure denatures milk enzymes and reduces the levels of milk natural microbiota. Moreover, the pasteurized cheeses are negatively perceived by consumers compared with the sensory characteristics of cheese made with raw milk. A possible strategy for reducing BAs accumulation, increasing the safety and maintaining the sensorial characteristics of traditional cheese could be the selection of autochthonous amine-negative and amine-oxidizing LAB. These strains could be used as a starter or an adjunct/attenuated starter. In addition, Pecorino di Farindola contains high amounts of GABA which can be correlated with the use of ewe's milk, time of ripening and type of coagulant. This cheese together with other Italian "Pecorino" cheeses could be a source of microorganisms able to synthesize GABA for the production of dairy products with functional and probiotic properties.

Author Contributions: Conceptualization, R.T. and G.S.; Data curation, G.P. and N.B.; Formal analysis, N.B. and A.P.; Funding acquisition, G.M.; Methodology, G.P.; Supervision, R.T.; Writing—review & editing, R.T. and A.I.

Acknowledgments: The authors are grateful to "Azienda Agricola Martinelli Pietropaolo" for kind cooperation.

References

1. Schirone, M.; Tofalo, R.; Mazzone, G.; Corsetti, A.; Suzzi, G. Biogenic amine content and microbiological profile of Pecorino di Farindola cheese. *Food Microbiol.* **2011**, *28*, 128–136. [CrossRef] [PubMed]
2. Di Giacomo, F.; Casolani, N.; Signore, A. Cheese making using pig rennet and calf rennet: Microorganisms and volatile compounds in Farindola ewe cheese. *Ital. J. Food Sci.* **2014**, *26*, 2.
3. Suzzi, G.; Sacchetti, G.; Patrignani, F.; Corsetti, A.; Tofalo, R.; Schirone, M.; Fasoli, G.; Gardini, F.; Perpetuini, G.; Lanciotti, R. Influence of pig rennet on fatty acid composition, volatile molecule profile, texture and sensory properties of Pecorino di Farindola cheese. *J. Sci. Food Agric.* **2015**, *95*, 2252–2263. [CrossRef] [PubMed]
4. Addis, M.; Piredda, G.; Pirisi, A. The use of lamb rennet paste in traditional sheep milk cheese production. *Small Rumin. Res.* **2008**, *79*, 2–10. [CrossRef]
5. Addis, M.; Pirisi, A.; Di Salvo, R.; Podda, F.; Piredda, G. The influence of the enzymatic composition of lamb rennet paste on some properties of experimentally produced PDO Fiore Sardo cheese. *Int. Dairy J.* **2005**, *15*, 1271–1278. [CrossRef]
6. Di Giacomo, F.; Del Signore, A.; Giaccio, M. Pig rennet in making Farindola ewe cheese. *Prog. Nutr.* **2013**, *15*, 226–238.

7. Awad, S.; Lüthi-Peng, Q.-Q.; Puhan, Z. Proteolytic activities of chymosin and porcine pepsin on buffalo, cow, and goat whole and β-casein fractions. *J. Agric. Food Chem.* **1998**, *46*, 4997–5007. [CrossRef]
8. Boudjellab, N.; Grosclaude, J.; Zhao, X.; Collin, J.C. Development of an inhibition enzyme-linked immunosorbent assay for the detection of residual porcine pepsin in a soft cheese sample. *J. Agric. Food Chem.* **1998**, *46*, 4030–4033. [CrossRef]
9. Tofalo, R.; Schirone, M.; Fasoli, G.; Perpetuini, G.; Patrignani, F.; Manetta, A.C.; Lanciotti, R.; Corsetti, A.; Martino, G.; Suzzi, G. Influence of pig rennet on proteolysis, organic acids content and microbiota of Pecorino di Farindola, a traditional Italian ewe's raw milk cheese. *Food Chem.* **2015**, *175*, 121–127. [CrossRef]
10. Dalgleish, D.G. The enzymatic coagulation of milk. In *Cheese: Chem, Phys and Microbiol*; Springer: Boston, MA, USA, 1993; pp. 69–100.
11. Barbieri, F.; Montanari, C.; Gardini, F.; Tabanelli, G. Biogenic amine production by lactic acid bacteria: A Review. *Foods* **2019**, *8*, 17. [CrossRef]
12. Ordoñez, A.I.; Ibanez, F.C.; Torre, P.; Barcina, Y. Characterization of the casein hydrolysis of Idiazábal cheese manufactured from ovine milk. *J. Dairy Sci.* **1998**, *81*, 2089–2095. [CrossRef]
13. Ladero, V.; Martinez, N.; Martín, M.C.; Fernández, M.; Alvarez, M.A. qPCR for quantitative detection of tyramine-producing bacteria in dairy products. *Food Res. Int.* **2010**, *43*, 289–295. [CrossRef]
14. Tofalo, R.; Perpetuini, G.; Schirone, M.; Suzzi, G. Biogenic Amines: toxicology and health effect. *Encyclopedia Food Health* **2016**, 424–429. [CrossRef]
15. EFSA Panel on Biological Hazards (BIOHAZ). Scientific opinion on risk based control of biogenic amine formation in fermented foods. *EFSA J.* **2011**, *9*, 2393. [CrossRef]
16. Ruiz-Capillas, C. Biogenic amine content in Spanish retail market meat products treated with protective atmosphere and high pressure. *Eur. Food Res. Technol.* **2004**, *218*, 237–241. [CrossRef]
17. Tittarelli, F.; Perpetuini, G.; Di Gianvito, P.; Tofalo, R. Biogenic amines producing and degrading bacteria: A snapshot from raw ewes' cheese. *LWT* **2019**, *101*, 1–9. [CrossRef]
18. Diana, M.; Quilez, J.; Rafecas, M. Gamma-aminobutyric acid as a bioactive compound in foods: A review. *J. Funct. Foods* **2014**, *10*, 407–420. [CrossRef]
19. Tajabadi, N.; Baradaran, A.; Ebrahimpour, A.; Rahim, R.A.; Bakar, F.A.; Manap, M.Y.A.; Mohammed, A.S.; Saari, N. Overexpression and optimization of glutamate decarboxylase in *Lactobacillus plantarum* Taj-Apis362 for high gamma-aminobutyric acid production. *Microb. Biotechnol.* **2015**, *8*, 623–632. [CrossRef]
20. Hayakawa, K.; Kimura, M.; Kasaha, K.; Matsumoto, K.; Sansawa, H.; Yamori, Y. Effect of a γ-aminobutyric acid-enriched dairy product on the blood pressure of spontaneously hypertensive and normotensive Wistar–Kyoto rats. *Br. J. Nutr.* **2004**, *92*, 411–417. [CrossRef]
21. Kajimoto, O.; Hirata, H.; Nakagawa, S.; Kajimoto, Y.; Hayakawa, K.; Kimura, M. Hypotensive Effect of Fermented milk containing gamma-aminobutyric acid (GABA) in subjects with high normal blood pressure. *Nippon. Shokuhin Kagaku Kogaku Kaishi* **2004**, *51*, 79–86. [CrossRef]
22. Inoue, K.; Shirai, T.; Ochiai, H.; Kasao, M.; Hayakawa, K.; Kimura, M.; Sansawa, H. Blood-pressure-lowering effect of a novel fermented milk containing γ-aminobutyric acid (GABA) in mild hypertensives. *Eur. J. Clin. Nutr.* **2003**, *57*, 490–495. [CrossRef] [PubMed]
23. Ohmori, M. Effect of anaerobically treated tea on blood pressure of spontaneous hypertensive rats. *Nippon Nogeik. Kaishi* **1987**, *61*, 1449–1451. [CrossRef]
24. Leenhouts, K.; Burghoorn, J.; Brands, J.R.; Sanders, J.W.; Venema, G.; Kok, J. A chloride-inducible acid resistance mechanism in Lactococcus lactis and its regulation. *Mol. Microbiol.* **1998**, *27*, 299–310.
25. Aoki, H.; Furuya, Y.; Endo, Y.; Fujimoto, K. Effect of γ-Aminobutyric acid-enriched Tempeh-like fermented soybean (GABA-Tempeh) on the blood pressure of spontaneously hypertensive rats. *Biosci. Biotechnol. Biochem.* **2003**, *67*, 1806–1808. [CrossRef] [PubMed]
26. Park, K.-B.; Oh, S.-H. Production of yogurt with enhanced levels of gamma-aminobutyric acid and valuable nutrients using lactic acid bacteria and germinated soybean extract. *Bioresour. Technol.* **2007**, *98*, 1675–1679. [CrossRef] [PubMed]
27. Sun, T.; Zhao, S.; Wang, H.; Cai, C.; Chen, Y.; Zhang, H. ACE-inhibitory activity and gamma-aminobutyric acid content of fermented skim milk by *Lactobacillus helveticus* isolated from Xinjiang koumiss in China. *Eur. Food Res. Technol.* **2009**, *228*, 607–612. [CrossRef]
28. Nadkarni, M.A.; Hunter, N.; Jacques, N.A.; Martin, F.E. Determination of bacterial load by real-time PCR using a broad-range (universal) probe and primers set. *Microbiology* **2002**, *148*, 257–266. [CrossRef]

29. Torriani, S.; Gatto, V.; Sembeni, S.; Tofalo, R.; Suzzi, G.; Belletti, N.; Gardini, F.; Bover-Cid, S. Rapid detection and quantification of tyrosine decarboxylase gene (*tdc*) and its expression in gram-positive bacteria associated with fermented foods using PCR-based methods. *J. Food Prot.* **2008**, *71*, 93–101. [CrossRef]
30. Fernández, M.; Del Río, B.; Linares, D.; Martín, M.; Alvarez, M. Real-Time polymerase chain reaction for quantitative detection of histamine-producing bacteria: Use in cheese production. *J. Dairy Sci.* **2006**, *89*, 3763–3769. [CrossRef]
31. Livak, K.J.; Schmittgen, T.D. Analysis of relative gene expression data using real-time quantitative PCR and the $2^{-\Delta\Delta CT}$ Method. *Methods* **2001**, *25*, 402–408. [CrossRef]
32. Andersen, C.L.; Jensen, J.L.; Ørntoft, T.F. Normalization of real-time quantitative reverse transcription-PCR Data: A model-based variance estimation approach to identify genes suited for normalization, applied to bladder and colon cancer data sets. *Cancer Res.* **2004**, *64*, 5245–5250. [CrossRef] [PubMed]
33. Folkertsma, B.; Fox, P.F. Use of the Cd-ninhydrin reagent to assess proteolysis in cheese during ripening. *J. Dairy Res.* **1992**, *59*, 217–224. [CrossRef]
34. Eerola, S.; Hinkkanen, R.; Lindfors, E.; Hirvi, T. Liquid chromatographic determination of biogenic amines in dry sausages. *J. AOAC Int.* **1993**, *76*, 575–577. [PubMed]
35. Morea, M.; Matarante, A.; Di Cagno, R.; Baruzzi, F.; Minervini, F. Contribution of autochthonous non-starter lactobacilli to proteolysis in Caciocavallo Pugliese cheese. *Int. Dairy J.* **2007**, *17*, 525–534. [CrossRef]
36. Moret, S.; Conte, L.S. High-performance liquid chromatographic evaluation of biogenic amines in foods an analysis of different methods of sample preparation in relation to food characteristics. *J. Chromatogr. A* **1996**, *729*, 363–369. [CrossRef]
37. Kőrös, A.; Varga, Z.; Molnár-Perl, I. Simultaneous analysis of amino acids and amines as their o-phthalaldehyde-ethanethiol-9-fluorenylmethyl chloroformate derivatives in cheese by high-performance liquid chromatography. *J. Chromatogr. A* **2008**, *1203*, 146–152. [CrossRef] [PubMed]
38. Ianni, A.; Di Maio, G.; Pittia, P.; Grotta, L.; Perpetuini, G.; Tofalo, R.; Cichelli, A.; Martino, G. Chemical–nutritional quality and oxidative stability of milk and dairy products obtained from Friesian cows fed with a dietary supplementation of dried grape pomace. *J. Sci. Food Agric.* **2019**, *99*, 3635–3643. [CrossRef]
39. Diana, M.; Rafecas, M.; Arco, C.; Quilez, J. Free amino acid profile of Spanish artisanal cheeses: Importance of gamma-aminobutyric acid (GABA) and ornithine content. *J. Food Compos. Anal.* **2014**, *35*, 94–100. [CrossRef]
40. Montel, M.-C.; Buchin, S.; Mallet, A.; Delbès-Paus, C.; Vuitton, D.A.; Desmasures, N.; Berthier, F. Traditional cheeses: Rich and diverse microbiota with associated benefits. *Int. J. Food Microbiol.* **2014**, *177*, 136–154. [CrossRef]
41. Coton, M.; Delbès-Paus, C.; Irlinger, F.; Desmasures, N.; Le Flèche, A.; Stahl, V.; Montel, M.-C.; Coton, E. Diversity and assessment of potential risk factors of Gram-negative isolates associated with French cheeses. *Food Microbiol.* **2012**, *29*, 88–98. [CrossRef]
42. Dahl, S.; Tavaria, F.K.; Malcata, F.X.; Malcata, F. Relationships between flavour and microbiological profiles in Serra da Estrela cheese throughout ripening. *Int. Dairy J.* **2000**, *10*, 255–262. [CrossRef]
43. Schirone, M.; Tofalo, R.; Fasoli, G.; Perpetuini, G.; Corsetti, A.; Manetta, A.C.; Ciarrocchi, A.; Suzzi, G. High content of biogenic amines in Pecorino cheeses. *Food Microbiol.* **2013**, *34*, 137–144. [CrossRef] [PubMed]
44. Morales, P.; Feliu, I.; Fernández-García, E.; Nuñez, M. Volatile compounds produced in cheese by Enterobacteriaceae strains of dairy origin. *J. Food Prot.* **2004**, *67*, 567–573. [CrossRef] [PubMed]
45. Giraffa, G. Functionality of enterococci in dairy products. *Int. J. Food Microbiol.* **2003**, *88*, 215–222. [CrossRef]
46. Suzzi, G.; Caruso, M.; Gardini, F.; Lombardi, A.; Vannini, L.; Guerzoni, M.E.; Andrighetto, C.; Lanorte, M.T. A survey of the enterococci isolated from an artisanal Italian goat's cheese (semicotto caprino). *J. Appl. Microbiol.* **2000**, *89*, 267–274. [CrossRef]
47. Renes, E.; Ladero, V.; Tornadijo, M.; Fresno, J. Production of sheep milk cheese with high γ-aminobutyric acid and ornithine concentration and with reduced biogenic amines level using autochthonous lactic acid bacteria strains. *Food Microbiol.* **2019**, *78*, 1–10. [CrossRef]
48. Rodgers, S. Novel applications of live bacteria in food services: probiotics and protective cultures. *Trends Food Sci. Technol.* **2008**, *19*, 188–197. [CrossRef]
49. Settanni, L.; Moschetti, G. Non-starter lactic acid bacteria used to improve cheese quality and provide health benefits. *Food Microbiol.* **2010**, *27*, 691–697. [CrossRef]

50. Diaz, M.; Ladero, V.; Redruello, B.; Sanchez-Llana, E.; Del Rio, B.; Fernandez, M.; Martin, M.C.; Alvarez, M.A. A PCR-DGGE method for the identification of histamine-producing bacteria in cheese. *Food Control.* **2016**, *63*, 216–223. [CrossRef]
51. Ascone, P.; Maurer, J.; Haldemann, J.; Irmler, S.; Berthoud, H.; Portmann, R.; Fröhlich-Wyder, M.-T.; Wechsler, D. Prevalence and diversity of histamine-forming *Lactobacillus parabuchneri* strains in raw milk and cheese—A case study. *Int. Dairy J.* **2017**, *70*, 26–33. [CrossRef]
52. Berthoud, H.; Wüthrich, D.; Bruggmann, R.; Wechsler, D.; Fröhlich-Wyder, M.-T.; Irmler, S. Development of new methods for the quantitative detection and typing of *Lactobacillus parabuchneri* in dairy products. *Int. Dairy J.* **2017**, *70*, 65–71. [CrossRef]
53. Diaz, M.; Del Rio, B.; Sanchez-Llana, E.; Ladero, V.; Redruello, B.; Fernández, M.; Martín, M.C.; Alvarez, M.A. Histamine-producing Lactobacillus parabuchneri strains isolated from grated cheese can form biofilms on stainless steel. *Food Microbiol.* **2016**, *59*, 85–91. [CrossRef] [PubMed]
54. Diaz, M.; Ladero, V.; Del Rio, B.; Redruello, B.; Fernández, M.; Martín, M.C.; Alvarez, M.A. Biofilm-forming capacity in biogenic amine-producing bacteria isolated from dairy products. *Front. Microbiol.* **2016**, *7*, 357. [CrossRef] [PubMed]
55. Diaz, M.; Del Rio, B.; Sanchez-Llana, E.; Ladero, V.; Redruello, B.; Fernandez, M.; Martín, M.C.; Alvarez, M.A. Lactobacillus parabuchneri produces histamine in refrigerated cheese at a temperature-dependent rate. *Int. J. Food Sci. Technol.* **2018**, *53*, 2342–2348. [CrossRef]
56. Freitas, A.; Pintado, A.E.; Pintado, M.E.; Malcata, F.; Pintado, M.M.; Malcata, F. Role of dominant microflora of Picante cheese on proteolysis and lipolysis. *Int. Dairy J.* **1999**, *9*, 593–603. [CrossRef]
57. Sulejmani, E.; Hayaloglu, A.A. Influence of curd heating on proteolysis and volatiles of Kashkaval cheese. *Food Chem.* **2016**, *211*, 160–170. [CrossRef]
58. Schirone, M.; Tofalo, R.; Perpetuini, G.; Manetta, A.C.; Di Gianvito, P.; Tittarelli, F.; Battistelli, N.; Corsetti, A.; Suzzi, G.; Martino, G. Influence of iodine feeding on microbiological and physico-chemical characteristics and biogenic amines content in a raw ewes' milk cheese. *Foods* **2018**, *7*, 108. [CrossRef]
59. Curtin, A.; McSweeney, P. Catabolism of amino acids in cheese during ripening. *Cheese Chem. Phys. Microbiol.* **2004**, *1*, 435–454.
60. Hong-Xin, J.; Mi-Ya, S.; Guang-Yu, G. Influence of *Lactobacillus casei* LC2W on the proteolysis and aroma compounds of Cheddar cheese during ripening period. *CyTA J. Food* **2015**, *13*, 1–8. [CrossRef]
61. López-Caballero, M.; Sánchez-Fernández, J.; Moral, A. Growth and metabolic activity of Shewanella putrefaciens maintained under different CO2 and O2 concentrations. *Int. J. Food Microbiol.* **2001**, *64*, 277–287. [CrossRef]
62. Arena, M.; De Nadra, M.M. Biogenic amine production by *Lactobacillus*. *J. Appl. Microbiol.* **2001**, *90*, 158–162. [CrossRef] [PubMed]
63. Pircher, A.; Bauer, F.; Paulsen, P. Formation of cadaverine, histamine, putrescine and tyramine by bacteria isolated from meat, fermented sausages and cheeses. *Eur. Food Res. Technol.* **2007**, *226*, 225–231. [CrossRef]
64. Gorlier, A.; Lonati, M.; Renna, M.; Lussiana, C.; Lombardi, G.; Battaglini, L.M. Changes in pasture and cow milk compositions during a summer transhumance in the western Ital. Alps. *J. Appl. Botany Food Qual.* **2013**, *85*, 216–223.
65. Tofalo, R.; Cocchi, S.; Suzzi, G. Polyamines and gut microbiota. *Front. Nutr.* **2019**, *6*, 16. [CrossRef] [PubMed]
66. Linares, D.M.; Del Rio, B.; Redruello, B.; Ladero, V.; Martin, M.C.; Fernandez, M.; Ruas-Madiedo, P.; Alvarez, M.A. Comparative analysis of the in vitro cytotoxicity of the dietary biogenic amines tyramine and histamine. *Food Chem.* **2016**, *197*, 658–663. [CrossRef] [PubMed]
67. Coton, E.; Coton, M. Evidence of horizontal transfer as origin of strain to strain variation of the tyramine production trait in *Lactobacillus brevis*. *Food Microbiol.* **2009**, *26*, 52–57. [CrossRef]
68. Wüthrich, D.; Berthoud, H.; Wechsler, D.; Eugster, E.; Irmler, S.; Bruggmann, R. The histidine decarboxylase gene cluster of *Lactobacillus parabuchneri* was gained by horizontal gene transfer and is mobile within the species. *Front. Microbiol.* **2017**, *8*, 218. [CrossRef] [PubMed]
69. Molenaar, D.; Bosscher, J.S.; Driessen, A.J.; Konings, W.N.; Brink, B.T. Generation of a proton motive force by histidine decarboxylation and electrogenic histidine/histamine antiport in *Lactobacillus buchneri*. *J. Bacteriol.* **1993**, *175*, 2864–2870. [CrossRef]
70. Fernández, M.; Zuñiga, M. Amino Acid Catabolic Pathways of Lactic Acid Bacteria. *Crit. Rev. Microbiol.* **2006**, *32*, 155–183. [CrossRef]

71. Lucas, P.M.; Blancato, V.S.; Claisse, O.; Magni, C.; Lolkema, J.S.; Lonvaud-Funel, A.; Blancato, V. Agmatine deiminase pathway genes in *Lactobacillus brevis* are linked to the tyrosine decarboxylation operon in a putative acid resistance locus. *Microbiology* **2007**, *153*, 2221–2230. [CrossRef]
72. Arena, M.P.; Russo, P.; Capozzi, V.; Beneduce, L.; Spano, G. Effect of abiotic stress conditions on expression of the Lactobacillus brevis IOEB 9809 tyrosine decarboxylase and agmatine deiminase genes. *Ann. Microbiol.* **2011**, *61*, 179–183. [CrossRef]
73. Siragusa, S.; De Angelis, M.; Di Cagno, R.; Rizzello, C.G.; Coda, R.; Gobbetti, M. Synthesis of γ-aminobutyric acid by lactic acid bacteria isolated from a variety of Italian cheese. *Appl. Environ. Microbiol.* **2007**, *73*, 7283–7290. [CrossRef] [PubMed]
74. Nomura, M.; Kimoto, H.; Someya, Y.; Furukawa, S.; Suzuki, I. Production of γ-aminobutyric acid by cheese starters during cheese ripening. *J. Dairy Sci.* **1998**, *81*, 1486–1491. [CrossRef]

19

Phenolic Profiling and Antioxidant Capacity of *Eugenia uniflora* L. (Pitanga) Samples Collected in Different Uruguayan Locations

Ignacio Migues [1], Nieves Baenas [2], Amadeo Gironés-Vilaplana [2], María Verónica Cesio [1], Horacio Heinzen [1] and Diego A. Moreno [2,*]

[1] Facultad de Química, UdelaR, Av. Gral. Flores 2124, 11800 Montevideo, Uruguay; imigues@fq.edu.uy (I.M.); cs@fq.edu.uy (M.V.C.); heinzen@fq.edu.uy (H.H.)

[2] CEBAS-CSIC, Food Science and Technology Department, Phytochemistry and Healthy Foods Laboratory, Campus Universitario Espinardo-25, E-30100 Espinardo, Murcia, Spain; nbaenas@cebas.csic.es (N.B.); amadeo.girones@elpozo.com (A.G.-V.)

* Correspondence: dmoreno@cebas.csic.es

Abstract: The use of nutrient-rich foods to enhance the wellness, health and lifestyle habits of consumers is globally encouraged. Native fruits are of great interest as they are grown and consumed locally and take part of the ethnobotanic knowledge of the population. Pitanga is an example of a native fruit from Uruguay, consumed as a jelly or an alcoholic beverage. Pitanga has a red-violet pigmentation, which is a common trait for foods that are a good source of antioxidants. Hence, fruits from different Uruguayan regions were analyzed via miniaturized sample preparation method, HPLC-DAD-ESI/MS^n and RP-HPLC-DAD techniques to identify and quantify phenolic compounds, respectively. The antioxidant capacity was evaluated via DPPH and ORAC (Oxygen Radical Absorbance Capacity) assays. A multivariate linear regression was applied to correlate the observed antioxidant capacity with the phenolic content. Furthermore, Principal Components Analysis was performed to highlight characteristics between the various samples studied. The main results indicated differences between northern and southern Uruguayan samples. Delphinidin-3-hexoside was present in southern samples (mean of 293.16 μmol/100 g dry weight (DW)) and absent in the sample collected in the north (sample 3). All the samples contain high levels of cyanidin-3-hexoside, but a noticeable difference was found between the northern sample (150.45 μmol/100 g DW) and the southern sample (1121.98 μmol/100 g DW). The antioxidant capacity (mean ORAC of 56370 μmol Trolox®/100 g DW) were high in all the samples compared to the Food and Drug Administration (FDA) database of similar berry-fruits. The results of this study highlight the nutraceutical value of a native fruit that has not been exploited until now.

Keywords: *Eugenia uniflora* L.; nutraceuticals; antioxidant activity; polyphenols

---

1. Introduction

Eugenia uniflora L. belongs to Myrtaceae family and grows naturally in subtropical Latin-American zones [1]. Its cultivation has extended to other regions outside the American continent with similar climatic conditions. It grows mainly in Brazil, which is why it is known as "Brazilian Cherry", but it is also grown in Argentina, Paraguay and Uruguay [2]. Its fruits have a high carbohydrates content (around 38%) where maltose, lactose and fructose are the main identified compounds [3,4]. It has a high content of vitamin C, vitamin A, riboflavin (B12) and niacin (B3) [4]. Immature fruits show a high content of polyphenols that decreases with maturation [5]. On the other hand, carotenoid content increases with maturation evidenced by an increase in a reddish-orange coloration [6].

Pitanga leaves are often used in Brazilian traditional medicine due to its diuretic, antirheumatic, antifebrile, anti-inflammatory and hypocholesterolemic properties [7–10]. However, there is little information regarding the medicinal use of the fruit. The fruit has an acidic and sweet flavor and can be consumed fresh, in compotes, jams or juices [6]. Purple fleshed Pitanga fruit in its latest maturation stage has an edible portion (pulp and skin) of 61.76%, a vitamin C content of 38.35 mg/100 g and total anthocyanin content of 29.60 mg/100 g [11]. Additionally, a high content of total phenols (799.80 mg of gallic acid/100 g) and total carotenoids (5.86 μg of β-carotene/g) [4]. Recently, Pitanga juice showed an anti-inflammatory effect on oral gum epithelial cells; these results could be associated to the presence of cyanidin-3-glucoside and oxidoselina-1,3,7(11)-trien-8-one [12,13]. Hence, Pitanga's beneficial properties could be exploited in the nutraceutical industry.

According to DeFelice a nutraceutical can be defined as "a food or part of it, that has some health benefit, including the prevention and/or treatment of a disease" [14]. Therefore, research has driven evaluation/re-evaluation of foods and their beneficial properties. Antioxidant rich foods have received a lot of interest; promoting their consumption to decrease oxidative stress caused by stress, lack of sleep, poor diet, metabolic problems, etc.

Currently, a large number of different approaches to determine antioxidant activity have been established [15–17]. All tests differ in substrates, probes, reaction conditions, instrumentation, and quantification methods. Hence, it is difficult to compare the results obtained by one method or another. Based on the reactions involved, the tests can be further classified into two groups: HAT (Hydrogen Atom Transfer) and SET (Single Electron Transfer) [18]. In the HAT group, antioxidants must donate a hydrogen atom to stabilize the generated free radicals (a synthetic free radical generator and an oxidizable molecular probe are used to evaluate the kinetics of the reaction). SET-type assays involve a redox reaction where the antioxidant must donate an electron to the generated free radical. In both methods the "competition" with the oxidant radical is measured instead of the antioxidant capacity [18].

The ORAC (Oxygen Radical Absorbance Capacity) assay measures the overall antioxidant activity or capacity of a sample's ability to "quench or neutralize" peroxyl radicals. The peroxyl radicals are reactive species comparable to those ROS (Reactive Oxygen Species) biologically generated in the organism. In the ORAC assay, the peroxyl radicals, generated from the azo-compound AAPH (2,2′-azobis-(2-methylpropionamidine)dihydrochloride) react with fluorescein as a substrate. The fluorescence of the latter compound decreases over time, forming an area under the curve (fluorescence vs. time). In the presence of antioxidant compounds, the area under the curve increases linearly and proportionally to the concentration of antioxidants.

The ORAC assay quantifies via the HAT mechanism and measures the antioxidant activity of polyphenol and non-polyphenolic compounds present in each sample. It is important to note that the antioxidant activity does not have a direct correlation to the polyphenol nature of a sample [19]. The ORAC test reflects the overall capacity or antioxidant activity of a sample, due to the individual components and their additive, synergistic interactions. The ORAC value is usually expressed as micromoles of Trolox® equivalents/100 g of sample. Trolox® is an analogue of vitamin E and is often used as a comparative standard due to its solubility in water [18,20].

The DPPH method name stems from the reactant used (2,2-diphenyl-1-picrylhidracyl) to evaluate the ability of a sample's antioxidants to "quench or neutralize" a free radical. The DPPH assay utilizes molecules that differ completely from any free radical or reactive species generated by our organism as a source of free radicals. Although the reactant is easy to use, it places this method as a distant analytical approximation of the high reactivity that typically characterizes the ROS generated in biological systems [21]. This method is classified in the SET group. However, can be classified as a HAT-type assay according to the antioxidant present in the sample [13]. In this test the sample is incubated for 35 min and the decay of the absorbance is measured at 515 nm.

Based on previous reports of bioactivity [22] of South-Brazilian Pitanga fruit, the objective of the present work was to extract, identify and quantify the phenolic compounds in mature fruits of *Eugenia uniflora* L. The antioxidant capacity was evaluated via ORAC and DPPH; and the phenolic profiles of *E. uniflora* from different Uruguayan locations were compared. Pitanga is considered a South American native fruit and its consumption is not among the most common in the region. However, its ethnobotanical characteristics, traditional uses and its antioxidant properties highlights its potential to improve the quality of life of those who consume it [23]. Hence, this study seeks to explore and further promote the value of the Uruguayan native Pitanga fruit that has not been exploited until now.

2. Materials and Methods

2.1. Chemicals

2,2-Diphenyl-1-picrylhidracyl (DPPH), fluorescein, 2,2′-azobis-(2-methylpropionamidine) dihydrochloride (AAPH), monobasic sodium phosphate and dibasic sodium phosphate were obtained from Sigma-Aldrich (Steinheim, Germany). 6-hydroxy-2,5,7,8-tetramethylchroman-2-carboxilic acid (Trolox®) was purchased from Fluka Chemika (Neu-Ulm, Germany). Cyanidin-3-*O*-glucoside and rutin were obtained from Polyphenols Laboratories AS (Sandnes, Norway). Ultrapure water was produced using a Millipore Milli-Q® Ultrapure Water Solutions Type 1. All solvents used were HPLC grade from Sigma-Aldrich (Steinheim, Germany).

2.2. Samples

The fruits (purple fleshed Pitanga breeding lines) were collected in different Uruguayan locations (described below), they were identified and kept at the Jose Arechavaleta Herbarium in the Faculty of Chemistry, UdelaR, Uruguay (Voucher number MVFQ 4427). Samples 1, 5, 6 & 7 were collected in the north of Montevideo Department (−34.804951, −56.230206) in December 2014, November 2015, December 2015 and April 2016, respectively. Sample 2 was collected in the south of Montevideo Department (−34.884536, −56.073039), sample 3 in Paysandú Department (−32.322604, −58.088243) and sample 4 in Ciudad de la Costa, Canelones Department (−34.799105, −55.908381); samples 2, 3 & 4 were collected in December 2014. All samples were freeze-dried, and the water content calculated by weight before and after lyophilization.

2.3. Extraction

Each lyophilized grinded sample (100 mg) was mixed with 1 mL of methanol/water/formic acid (70:29:1, $v/v/v$) in a 2 mL conical polypropylene tube (Eppendorf, Madrid, Spain). Then, the samples were vortexed and subjected to indirect sonication in an ultrasound cleaning bath for 60 min (BRANSONIC® Ultrasonic cleaner mod. 5510E-MTH, Ultrasonic frequency: 135 W or 42 KHz + 6%). The samples were kept overnight at 4 °C and sonicated again for 60 min. The supernatant was separated from the solid residue after centrifugation (9500× g, 15 min), filtered using a 0.45 µm PVDF filter (Millex HV13, Millipore, Bedford, MA, USA) and stored at 4 °C until they were analyzed.

2.4. Identification of Phenolic Compounds Via HPLC-DAD-ESI/MS^n and Quantification Via RP-HPLC-DAD

The identification analyses were carried out using an Agilent HPLC 1100 series model equipped with a photodiode array detector and a mass detector in series (Agilent Technologies, Waldbronn, Germany). It consisted of a binary pump (model G1312A), a degasser (model G1322A), an autosampler (model G1313A), and a photodiode array detector (model G1315B). The HPLC system was controlled by ChemStation for LC 3D Systems software Rev. B.01.03-SR2 (204) (Agilent Technologies Spain S.L., Madrid, Spain). The mass detector was an ion trap spectrometer (model G2445A) equipped with an electrospray ionization interface and was controlled by LC/MS software (Esquire Control Ver. 6.1. Build No. 534.1., Bruker Daltoniks GmbH, Bremen, Germany). The ionization conditions were 350 °C capillary temperature and 4 kV voltage, the nebulizer pressure was 65.0 psi and the nitrogen flow rate was 11 L/min. Full-Scan mass covered the range of m/z from 100 to 1200. Collision-induced fragmentation experiments were performed in the ion trap using helium as the collision gas, with voltage ramping cycles from 0.3 to 2 V. The mass spectrometry data were acquired in the positive ionization mode for anthocyanins and in the negative ionization mode for other flavonoids. The MS^n was carried out in the automatic mode on the more abundant fragment ion in $MS^{(n-1)}$. A Luna C_{18} column (250 × 4.6 mm, 5 μm particle diameter; Phenomenex, Macclesfield, UK) was used. Mobile phase A: water/formic acid (99:1, *v*/*v*), mobile phase B: acetonitrile, initial conditions: 8% solvent B, reaching 15% solvent B at 25 min, 22% at 55 min, and 40% at 60 min, which was maintained isocratic until 70 min. The flow rate was 0.8 mL/min during the whole run, all gradients were linear, and the injection volume was 7 μL. Chromatograms were recorded at 280, 320, 360 and 520 nm.

For quantification experiments the same conditions were applied, except for the injection volume was set to 20 μL and the flow rate was 0.9 mL/min. Anthocyanins were quantified as cyanidin 3-*O*-glucoside at 520 nm and flavonols as rutin at 360 nm.

2.5. DPPH Antioxidant Activity Measurements

Experiments were carried out using 96-well micro plates (Nunc, Roskilde, Denmark) and an Infinite® M200 micro plate reader (Tecan, Grödig, Austria). The antioxidant activity was evaluated measuring the change of the absorbance at 515 nm after 35 min of reaction with the radical DPPH· (2 μL of the sample + 250 μL of DPPH· solution). The results were expressed as μmol of Trolox®/100 g dry weight.

2.6. ORAC Antioxidant Activity Measurements

The antioxidant assay was performed using black-walled 96-well plates (Nunc, Roskilde, Denmark) and an Infinite® M200 micro plate reader (Tecan, Grödig, Austria). Each well with a final volume of 200 μL. 10 mM phosphate buffer (pH 7.4) was used to prepare 1 μM fluorescein and 250 mM AAPH solutions. Each well received 150 μL of fluorescein solution and 25 μL of phosphate buffer, Trolox® solutions or sample solution to measure the blank, the curve or the samples respectively. The plate was placed into the microplate reader and after 30 min of incubation at 37 °C, 25 μL AAPH solution were added to each well and fluorescence was recorded every 5 min for 120 min using an excitation wavelength of 485 nm and an emission wavelength of 520 nm. ORAC values were calculated using the difference in Areas Under the Fluorescein Decay Curve (AUC) between the blank and a sample. The results were expressed as μmol of Trolox®/100 g dry weight.

2.7. Statistical Analysis

Data shown are mean values (n = 3), subjected to Analysis of Variance (ANOVA) and multiple range test (Tukey's test), using RStudio software (Version 1.1.383, RStudio, Boston, MA, USA) and InfoStat (Version 2017, Universidad Nacional de Córdoba, Córdoba, Argentina) [24].

3. Results and Discussion

3.1. Water Content

The results of the water content of the samples are shown in Table 1.

Table 1. Water content calculated by weighing the samples before and after lyophilization.

Sample	Location/Sampling Date	% Water (% *w*/*w*) [1]
1	North of Montevideo/December 2014	$68.1^{c,d} \pm 0.9$
2	South of Montevideo/December 2014	$63.6^{b,c} \pm 1.7$
3	Paysandú/December 2014	$66.1^{b,c,d} \pm 0.9$
4	Canelones/December 2014	$46.4^{a} \pm 6.4$
5	North of Montevideo/November 2015	$66.5^{b,c,d} \pm 4.1$
6	North of Montevideo/December 2015	$58.3^{b} \pm 0.6$
7	North of Montevideo/April 2016	$73.0^{d} \pm 2.7$

[1] Means (n = 3) followed by different letters are significantly different at $p < 0.05$ according to Tukey's test.

The stress generated by the lack of precipitations, is associated to the increased concentration of sugar and phenolic compounds in grapes [25]. For grapes this enhances fermentation and wine quality. However, in a study where water availability and photosynthetic efficiency of Pitanga plants was evaluated the main influencing factor that determined the quality of the fruits was not water availability, but light exposure [26].

During 2014, Uruguay suffered from excess precipitations, especially in the south of the country (60% above the regular precipitation rate) [27]. However, sample 4 showed a smaller water %, which could be due to its location near the beach, where water availability was less due to the sandy ground. During 2015, Uruguay suffered from slight droughts and higher temperatures at the end of the year, which could be the cause of the decreased water content in sample 6. The first two months of 2016 experienced a lot of rain and consequently, the water content of sample 7 was much higher in comparison to the other studied samples.

3.2. *Identification and Quantification of Phenolic Compounds*

As expected, all samples resulted in similar phenolic profiles. Hence, the different climate situations had no influence, see Table 2. Two anthocyanins were identified, delphinidin-3-hexoside and cyanidin-3-hexoside, the latter was the main anthyocyanin present in all samples. The results are in agreement with previously obtained values by Einbond in 2004 [28]. Thirteen flavonols were identified and myricetin-rhamnoside was the most abundant in all samples. Samples collected from northern Montevideo showed variable levels of total flavonol content (TFC) that ranged from 120 to 860 μmol/100 g dry weight, but the Paysandú sample showed a much higher level of TFC (1050 μmol/100 g dry weight), see Table 3.

The total anthocyanin content (TAC), total quercetin derivatives content (TQC), total myricetin derivatives content (TMC), total flavonol content (TFC), total catechol derivatives content (TCC), total pyrogallol derivatives content (TPC) and total polyphenol content (TPPC) were calculated for each sample and the results are shown in Table 3.

3.3. *Antioxidant Activity*

The results of the antioxidant assays (ORAC and DPPH) are shown in Table 4, the results for both assays are expressed as (μmol Trolox®/100 g dry weight).

In general, samples collected in the north of Montevideo showed greater level of ORAC scavenging activity, but similar levels of DPPH activity compared to the other samples. The direct correlation between ORAC-TAC, ORAC-TFC, DPPH-TAC, and DPPH-TFC was not statistically significant ($R^2 < 0.3$ in all cases). However, the ORAC and DPPH activity of all Pitanga samples were higher compared to other Latin-American berries [29].

All the samples collected in southern Uruguay contained delphinidin together with cyanidin. This is a clear difference with the findings of Celli [5] that described cyanidin as the only occurring anthocyanin in Brazilian Pitanga samples. Northern Uruguay is naturally connected with southern Brazil but the continuity towards southern Uruguay is broken by the Negro river, these results could point out a region related chemo-diversity. Furthermore, three other myricetin derivatives were not identified in the Brazilian samples.

Studying the linear correlation (Figure 1) between the identified compounds grouped as it is shown in Table 3, we can see that when the concentration of anthocyanins increased, the flavonol content decreased, that is a negative correlation (shown in red spots, bigger spots represents a stronger correlation). A strong positive correlation between quercetin and myricetin derivatives, and a negative correlation of both flavonol groups to the anthocyanins concentration is shown. When the biosynthesis of anthocyanins is favored, there is less biosynthesis of flavonols as expected from their common biosynthetic pathway, similarly described for bilberries [30].

Table 2. Phenolic compounds identified and quantified (μmol/100 g dry weight) in different samples [1].

Compound [2]	Rt	$[M-H]^+$	MS^n	Sample 1	Sample 2	Sample 3	Sample 4	Sample 5	Sample 6	Sample 7
C1	29.8	465	303	19.99 ^{a} ± 3.34	373.24 ^{c} ± 3.98	ND ^{3,a}	381.38 ^{c} ± 31.81	282.99 ^{b} ± 24.49	215.53 ^{b} ± 19.42	485.81 ^{d} ± 26.25
C2	33.8	449	287	115.01 ^{a} ± 8.56	1757.29 ^{d} ± 18.34	150.45 ^{a} ± 0.25	987.77 ^{c} ± 49.63	916.35 ^{b,c} ± 85.15	706.78 ^{b} ± 68.87	2248.68 ^{e} ± 98.76
		$[M-H]^-$								
C3	48.4	631	479, 317, 271	8.07 ^{d} ± 1.15	14.18 ^{f} ± 0.34	10.67 ^{e} ± 0.34	ND ^{3,a}	3.63 ^{b,c} ± 0.08	2.41 ^{b} ± 0.57	4.94 ^{c} ± 0.36
C4	53.6	479	317, 271	34.33 ^{c} ± 1.28	46.41 ^{d} ± 0.43	56.53 ^{e} ± 1.11	6.11 ^{a} ± 0.18	12.97 ^{b} ± 1.52	8.77 ^{a} ± 0.86	17.05 ^{b} ± 2.14
C5	54.7	479	317, 271	32.37 ^{d} ± 2.52	35.82 ^{d} ± 0.34	22.59 ^{c} ± 1.49	6.53 ^{a,b} ± 0.50	4.85 ^{a} ± 1.76	7.57 ^{a,b} ± 0.78	10.25 ^{b} ± 2.45
C6	56.8	449	317, 271, 179	23.44 ^{d} ± 0.26	6.79 ^{b,c} ± 0.51	9.39 ^{c} ± 4.91	1.22 ^{a} ± 1.46	2.15 ^{a,b} ± 0.24	1.52 ^{a} ± 0.18	3.33 ^{a,b} ± 0.35
C7	58.0	615	463, 301, 271	8.45 ^{c} ± 0.09	11.10 ^{d} ± 0.64	16.87 ^{e} ± 0.43	0.92 ^{a} ± 0.81	7.61 ^{b,c} ± 0.65	5.27 ^{b} ± 0.75	11.59 ^{d} ± 1.19
C8	61.0	449	317, 271, 179	49.91 ^{d} ± 3.46	4.57 ^{a,b} ± 0.94	26.30 ^{c} ± 0.85	2.09 ^{a} ± 0.20	5.33 ^{a,b} ± 1.10	3.96 ^{a} ± 0.78	8.34 ^{b} ± 1.11
C9	61.9	463	317, 271, 179	378.69 ^{f} ± 10.72	138.43 ^{d} ± 3.37	243.25 ^{e} ± 1.20	16.81 ^{a} ± 1.04	41.63 ^{b} ± 3.49	29.16 ^{a,b} ± 3.76	56.62 ^{c} ± 3.33
C10	62.9	463	301	29.25 ^{c} ± 2.13	64.65 ^{d} ± 2.39	167.25 ^{e} ± 0.00	4.11 ^{a} ± 1.50	14.97 ^{b} ± 0.59	8.17 ^{a} ± 0.66	18.48 ^{b} ± 1.05
C11	63.5	463	301	38.30 ^{b} ± 2.65	71.26 ^{c} ± 4.27	101.54 ^{d} ± 3.59	13.11 ^{a} ± 3.81	8.22 ^{a} ± 0.80	8.32 ^{a} ± 1.02	10.61 ^{a} ± 0.20
C12	64.5	433	301	8.97 ^{c} ± 1.24	10.59 ^{c} ± 0.04	19.64 ^{d} ± 0.30	2.57 ^{a,b} ± 0.14	2.41 ^{a,b} ± 0.48	1.75 ^{a} ± 0.42	4.17 ^{b} ± 1.35
C13	64.9	433	301	28.44 ^{d} ± 1.75	8.71 ^{c} ± 2.43	55.81 ^{e} ± 0.38	6.55 ^{a} ± 1.35	11.36 ^{a,b} ± 2.30	6.79 ^{a} ± 0.96	16.48 ^{b,c} ± 1.55
C14	65.4	433	301	36.12 ^{d} ± 0.43	36.21 ^{d} ± 0.13	92.95 ^{e} ± 0.17	3.37 ^{a} ± 0.51	15.12 ^{b} ± 2.32	9.98 ^{b} ± 2.93	22.92 ^{c} ± 2.90
C15	65.7	447	301	80.74 ^{d} ± 0.13	93.13 ^{e} ± 1.54	224.17 ^{f} ± 0.04	15.21 ^{a} ± 0.33	34.62 ^{b} ± 3.82	26.44 ^{b} ± 4.27	53.22 ^{c} ± 3.34

[1] Means (n = 3) in the same rows followed by different letters are significantly different at $p < 0.05$ according to Tukey's test. [2] Compounds: anthocyanins quantified at 520 nm: **C1**: delphinidin-3-hexoside, **C2**: cyanidin-3-hexoside. Flavonols quantified at 360 nm: **C3**: myricetin-galloyl-hexoside, **C4**: myricetin-hexoside 1, **C5**: myricetin-hexoside 2, **C6**: myricetin-pentoside 1, **C7**: quercetin galloyl hexoside, **C8**: myricetin-pentoside 2, **C9**: myricetin-rhamnoside, **C10**: quercetin hexoside 1, **C11**: quercetin hexoside 2, **C12**: quercetin pentoside 1, **C13**: quercetin pentoside 2, **C14**: quercetin pentoside 3 and **C15**: quercetin rhamnoside. [3] ND = not detected.

Table 3. Total anthocyanin content (TAC), total quercetin derivatives content (TQC), total myricetin derivatives content (TMC), total flavonol content (TFC), total catechol derivatives content (TCC), total pyrogallol derivatives content (TPC) and total polyphenol content (TPPC) results expressed as μmol/100 g dry weight.

	Sample 1	Sample 2	Sample 3	Sample 4	Sample 5	Sample 6	Sample 7
TAC	134.98 ^{a} ± 11.90	2130.53 ^{d} ± 14.35	150.45 ^{a} ± 0.24	1369.15 ^{c} ± 79.26	1199.35 ^{b,c} ± 109.47	922.32 ^{b} ± 87.78	2734.50 ^{e} ± 125.00
TQC	230.26 ^{d} ± 1.61	308.45 ^{e} ± 8.03	678.25 ^{f} ± 4.14	45.84 ^{a} ± 2.98	94.33 ^{b} ± 8.56	66.70 ^{a} ± 7.42	137.44 ^{c} ± 11.21
TMC	526.83 ^{f} ± 17.08	246.20 ^{d} ± 3.43	368.79 ^{e} ± 6.24	32.76 ^{a} ± 1.65	70.54 ^{b} ± 8.14	53.39 ^{a,b} ± 6.56	100.50 ^{c} ± 9.57
TFC	757.09 ^{f} ± 18.69	554.65 ^{e} ± 11.47	1047.04 ^{g} ± 10.38	78.60 ^{a} ± 2.50	164.87 ^{c} ± 14.57	120.08 ^{b} ± 7.39	237.94 ^{d} ± 17.48
TCC	345.25 ^{a} ± 10.18	2065.75 ^{d} ± 10.30	828.70 ^{b,c} ± 4.38	1033.62 ^{c} ± 49.24	1010.68 ^{c} ± 92.65	773.48 ^{b} ± 65.14	2386.12 ^{e} ± 100.13
TPC	546.82 ^{c} ± 20.42	619.43 ^{c} ± 7.42	368.79 ^{b} ± 6.28	414.13 ^{b} ± 31.28	353.54 ^{a,b} ± 32.23	268.92 ^{a} ± 25.93	586.32 ^{c} ± 35.30
TPPC	892.07 ^{a} ± 30.59	2685.18 ^{d} ± 2.89	1197.49 ^{b,c} ± 10.62	1447.75 ^{c} ± 77.27	1364.21 ^{c} ± 124.02	1042.40 ^{a,b} ± 90.94	2972.43 ^{d} ± 135.41

Means (n = 3) in the same rows followed by different letters are significantly different at $p < 0.05$ according to Tukey's test.

Table 4. Oxygen Radical Absorbance Capacity (ORAC) and 2,2-diphenyl-1-picrylhidracyl (DPPH) antioxidant activity results for each sample.

Assay	Sample 1	Sample 2	Sample 3	Sample 4	Sample 5	Sample 6	Sample 7
ORAC	57,440 ^{b,c} ± 1090	44,510 ^{a,b} ± 460	22,800 ^{a} ± 300	57,560 ^{b,c} ± 10,040	57,400 ^{b,c} ± 16,380	82,340 ^{c} ± 9070	72,550 ^{c} ± 15,280
DPPH	44,170 ^{b} ± 4480	11,940 ^{a} ± 2200	10,070 ^{a} ± 1200	12,200 ^{a} ± 650	15,430 ^{a} ± 70	12,960 ^{a} ± 1250	13,950 ^{a} ± 560

Means (n = 3) in the same rows followed by different letters are significantly different at $p < 0.05$ according to Tukey's test.

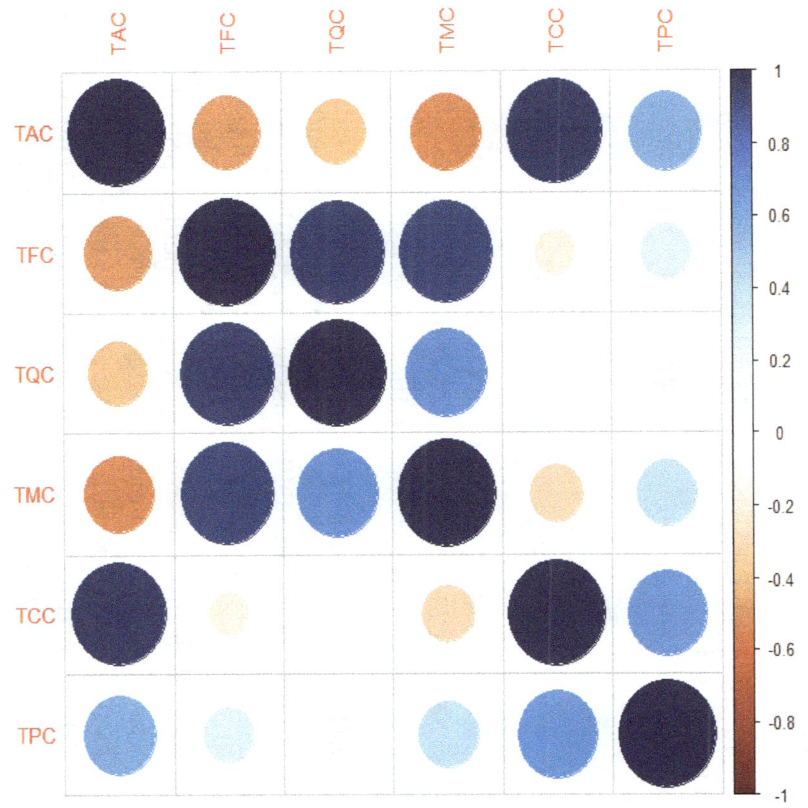

Figure 1. Correlation boxplot between identified and quantified compounds.

A PCA was performed using the phenolic content to identify the compounds that weighted the most when classifying the samples. Figure 2a shows that all the samples are grouped together according mainly to PC1 (69.62% of the variance), except for the sample collected in Paysandú (sample 3). Sample 7 is located closer to the anthocyanins than the rest of the samples, mainly because of PC2 (15.68% of the variance).

When we analyze the samples collected in 2014, sample 4 (Canelones) and 2 (south of Montevideo) correlate with a high anthocyanin content, which is coherent with the TAC of the samples. On the other hand, Sample 1 (north of Montevideo) correlated with the myricetin glycosides (C6, C8 and C9), while sample 3 had a stronger correlation to the quercetin derivatives. This PCA diagram explains 88.11% of the total variance (PC1 = 68.58% and PC2 = 19.53%).

Samples 1, 4, 5, 6 and 7 were labeled as high ORAC samples (H), while samples 2 and 3 were labeled as low ORAC samples (L). The compounds that classified the H samples were the anthocyanins while the flavonols classified the L samples, see Figure 3.

In order to predict the ORAC and DPPH values of a new sample based on the concentration of the identified compounds, we performed a stepwise multivariate linear regression analysis, the equations described below were obtained:

$$\begin{gathered}\mathrm{ORAC} = 69825.66 - 552.22[\mathrm{C11}] + 378.91[\mathrm{C5}] \\ (R^2 = 0.7345,\ p\text{-value} = 1.876 \times 10^{-5},\ \mathrm{RSE} = 9050 \text{ on 15 Degrees of Freedom})\end{gathered} \tag{1}$$

$$\begin{gathered}\mathrm{DPPH} = 14108.99 - 97.55[\mathrm{C11}] + 168.64[\mathrm{C9}] - 246.19[\mathrm{C15}] + 421.48[\mathrm{C14}] - 260.30[\mathrm{C5}] - \\ 367.10[\mathrm{C8}] - 80.43[\mathrm{C10}] + 287.09[\mathrm{C4}] - 527.05[\mathrm{C3}] - 80.35[\mathrm{C6}] \\ (R^2 = 0.9995,\ p\text{-value} = 8.487 \times 10^{-12},\ \mathrm{RSE} = 238.3 \text{ on 7 Degrees of Freedom})\end{gathered} \tag{2}$$

An increased number of reports have shown the non-additivity of the antioxidant properties of polyphenols, in the ORAC and DPPH assays. Particularly, they can act negatively on the overall value of the measurement, depending on the certain mixture of polyphenols and the point they enter in the reaction chain cycle, either as oxidants or reductants. The anthocyanins, due to their positive formal charge, are kinetically more reactive than the neutral polyphenols when reacting with DPPH. The reaction chain thus triggered could foster negative contributions of the quercetin derivatives, but positive ones from the myricetin ones, based on the positive or negative contributions shown in Equation (2). These mixture effects were "partly explained by regeneration mechanisms between antioxidants, depending on the chemical structure of molecules and on the possible formation of stable intermolecular complexes" [31]. Further work is required to understand the global behavior of complex mixtures of different classes of polyphenols in these widely used bench-top bioassays.

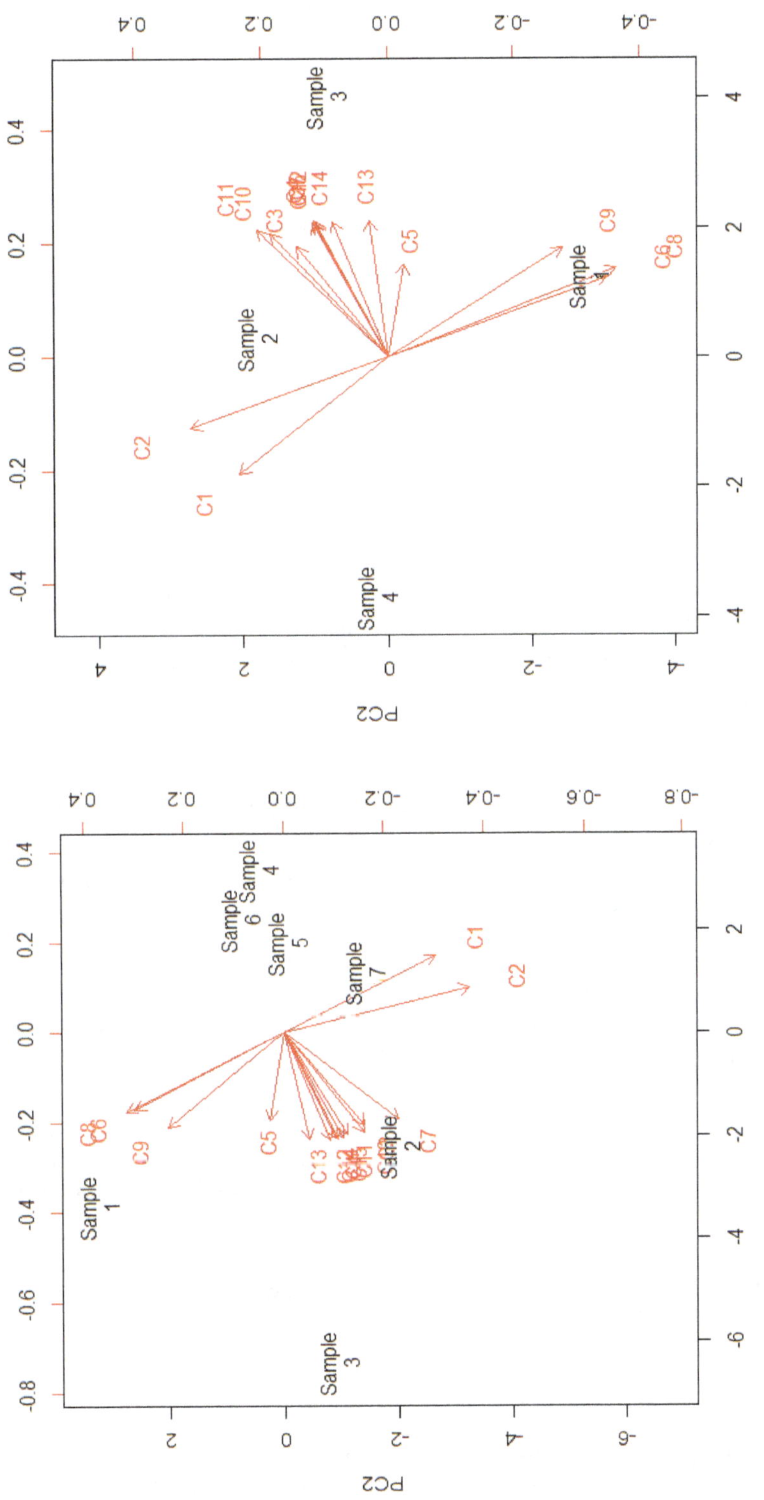

Figure 2. Phenolic content PCA of: (**a**) all samples, and (**b**) samples collected in December 2014.

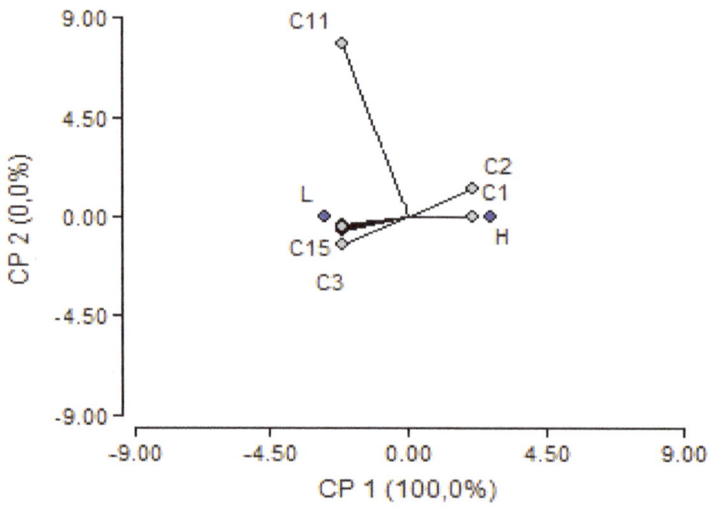

Figure 3. PCA where all identified compounds are classified according to low (L) and high (H) ORAC results.

4. Conclusions

The samples from different Uruguayan locations were very similar on their composition but presented different levels of antioxidant activity. The sample collected in 2014 in the north of Montevideo showed the highest ORAC and DPPH values. Several samples were collected until April 2016 and the evaluated. There is no clear relationship between the TAC and TFC values and the bioactivity studied; due to the presence of secondary metabolites with antioxidant activity in Pitanga fruit, for example carotenoids [6]. However, we could identify the phenolic compounds responsible for the separation between samples using PCA diagrams. Furthermore, the different location samples were characterized by specific types of phenolic compounds.

The sample collected in April 2016 (sample 7) showed a TPC three times higher than the sample collected in December 2015 (sample 6) probably because of the ripening during summer season where light exposure enhances the quality of the fruits.

In contrast to the results obtained by Celli et al. [5], the main compounds identified amongst all flavonols were myricetin derivatives and not quercetin derivatives, these results can be used as a characteristic of Uruguayan Pitanga fruits, with high antioxidant capacity.

Author Contributions: D.A.M. conceived and designed the experiments; I.M., A.G.-V. and N.B. performed the experiments; I.M., A.G.-V. and N.B. analyzed the data; D.A.M. contributed reagents/materials/analysis tools; I.M., M.V.C. and H.H. gathered the samples and wrote the drafts as well as the final version and the corrections of the paper.

Acknowledgments: The authors gratefully acknowledge the CYTED program for the support of the international collaboration through the Thematic Network AGL 112RT0460 CORNUCOPIA.

References

1. Bicas, J.L.; Molina, G.; Dionísio, A.P.; Barros, F.F.C.; Wagner, R.; Maróstica, M.R.; Pastore, G.M. Volatile constituents of exotic fruits from Brazil. *Food Res. Int.* **2011**, *44*, 1843–1855. [CrossRef]
2. Consolini, A.E.; Sarubbio, M.G. Pharmacological effects of Eugenia uniflora (Myrtaceae) aqueous crude extract on rat's heart. *J. Ethnopharmacol.* **2002**, *81*, 57–63. [CrossRef]
3. Amoo, A.; Adebayo, O.; Oyeleye, A. Chemical evaluation of winged beans (*Psophocarpus Tetragonolobus*), Pitanga cherries (*Eugenia uniflora*) and orchid fruit (*Orchid fruit myristica*). *Afr. J. Food Agric. Nutr. Dev.* **2006**, *6*, 3–12.

4. Vasconcelos Costa, A.G.; Garcia-Diaz, D.F.; Jimenez, P.; Ibrahim Silva, P. Bioactive compounds and health benefits of exotic tropical red–blackberries. *J. Funct. Foods* **2013**, *5*, 539–549. [CrossRef]
5. Celli, G.B.; Pereira-Netto, A.B.; Beta, T. Comparative analysis of total phenolic content, antioxidant activity, and flavonoids profile of fruits from two varieties of Brazilian cherry (*Eugenia uniflora* L.) throughout the fruit developmental stages. *Food Res. Int.* **2011**, *44*, 2442–2451. [CrossRef]
6. Galvão de Lima, V.L.; Almeida Mélo, E.; da Silva Lima, D.E. Fenólicos e carotenóides totais em pitanga. *Sci. Agric.* **2002**, *59*, 447–450. [CrossRef]
7. Corrêa, P. *Dicionário das Plantas Uteis do Brasil e das Exóticas Cultivadas*; Imprensa National-Ministerio da Agricultural: Rio de Janeiro, Brazil, 1984; Volume 5.
8. Rücker, G.; Brasil e Silva, G.A.A.; Bauer, L.; Schikarski, M. Neu Inhaltstoffe von *Stenoealyx michelii* (New constituents of Stenoealyx michelii). *Planta Med.* **1977**, *31*, 322–327. [CrossRef]
9. Ferro, E.; Schinini, A.; Maldonado, M.; Rosner, J.; Schmeda-Hirschmann, G. *Eugenia unliflora* leaf extract and lipid metabolism in Cebus apella monkeys. *J. Ethnopharmacol.* **1988**, *24*, 321–325. [CrossRef]
10. Schapoval, E.E.S.; Silveira, S.M.; Miranda, M.L.; Alice, C.B.; Henriques, A.T. Evaluation of some pharmacological activities of *Eugenia uniflora* L. *J. Ethnopharmacol.* **1994**, *44*, 137–142. [CrossRef]
11. Vizzotto, M.; Cabral, L.; Santos Lopes, S. Pitanga (*Eugenia uniflora* L.). In *Postharvest Biology and Technology of Tropical and Subtropical Fruits. Mangosteen to White Sapote*; Yahia, E., Ed.; Woodhead Publishing: Cambridge, UK, 2011; Volume 4, pp. 272–286.
12. Soares, D.J.; Walker, J.; Pignitter, M.; Walker, J.M.; Imboeck, J.M.; Ehrnhoefer-Ressler, M.M.; Montenegro Brasil, I.; Veronika, S. Pitanga (*Eugenia uniflora* L.) fruit juice and two major constituents thereof exhibit anti-inflammatory properties in human gingival and oral gum epithelial cells. *Food Funct.* **2014**, *5*, 2981–2988. [CrossRef] [PubMed]
13. Soares, D.J.; Pignitter, M.; Ehrnhöfer-Ressler, M.M.; Walker, J.; Montenegro, I.; Somoza, V. Identification and Quantification of Oxidoselina-1,3,7-Trien-8-One and Cyanidin-3-Glucoside as One of the Major Volatile and Non-Volatile Low-Molecular- Weight Constituents in Pitanga Pulp. *PLoS ONE* **2015**, *10*, e0138809. [CrossRef]
14. DeFelice, S.L. The nutraceutical revolution: Its impact on food industry R&D. *Trends Food Sci. Technol.* **1995**, *6*, 59–61.
15. Tai, A.; Sawano, T.; Yazama, F.; Ito, H. Evaluation of antioxidant activity of vanillin by using multiple antioxidant assays. *Biochim. Biophys. Acta Gen. Subj.* **2011**, *1810*, 170–177. [CrossRef] [PubMed]
16. Jones, A.; Acquaviva, A.; Dennis, G.R.; Shalliker, R.A.; Soliven, A. High throughput screening of phenolic constituents in a complex sample matrix using post-column derivatisations employing reaction flow HPLC columns. *Microchem. J.* **2018**. [CrossRef]
17. Acquaviva, A.; Jones, A.; Dennis, G.R.; Shalliker, R.A.; Soliven, A. Phenolic profiling of complex tea samples via simultaneous multiplexed detection employing reaction flow HPLC columns and colorimetric post column derivatisation. *Microchem. J.* **2018**, *138*, 533–539. [CrossRef]
18. Huang, D.; Ou, B.; Prior, R.L. The Chemistry behind Antioxidant Capacity Assays. *J. Agric. Food Chem.* **2005**, *53*, 1841–1856. [CrossRef] [PubMed]
19. Acquaviva, A.; Jones, A.; Dennis, G.R.; Shalliker, R.A.; Soliven, A. Detection selectivity in the analysis of "reactive" chemical compounds derived from natural samples via reaction flow chromatography. *Microchem. J.* **2018**, *139*, 315–321. [CrossRef]
20. Prior, R.L.; Wu, X.; Schaich, K. Standardized Methods for the Determination of Antioxidant Capacity and Phenolics in Foods and Dietary Supplements. *J. Agric. Food Chem.* **2005**, *53*, 4290–4302. [CrossRef] [PubMed]
21. Xie, J.; Schaich, K.M. Re-evaluation of the 2,2-diphenyl-1-picrylhydrazyl Free Radical (DPPH) Assay for Antioxidant Activity. *J. Agric. Food Chem.* **2014**, *62*, 4251–4260. [CrossRef] [PubMed]
22. Bagetti, M.; Facco, E.M.P.; Piccolo, J.; Hirsch, G.E.; Rodriguez-Amaya, D.; Kobori, C.N.; Vizzotto, M.; Emanuelli, T. Physicochemical characterization and antioxidant capacity of pitanga fruits (*Eugenia uniflora* L.). *Ciênc. Tecnol. Aliment.* **2011**, *31*, 147–154. [CrossRef]
23. Lim, T.K. *Edible Medicinal and Non-Medicinal Plants*; Springer: Dordrecht, The Netherlands, 2012; pp. 620–630, ISBN 978-94-007-1764-0.
24. Di Rienzo, J.; Casanoves, F.; Balzarini, M.G.; Gonzalez, L.; Tablada, M.; Robledo, C.W. *InfoStat Versión 2017*; InfoStat: Córdoba, Argentina, 2017.

25. Romero, P.; Gil-Muñoz, R.; del Amor, F.M.; Valdés, E.; Fernández, J.I.; Martinez-Cutillas, A. Regulated Deficit Irrigation based upon optimum water status improves phenolic composition in Monastrell grapes and wines. *Agric. Water Manag.* **2013**, *121*, 85–101. [CrossRef]
26. Mielke, M.S.; Schaffer, B. Photosynthetic and growth responses of *Eugenia uniflora* L. seedlings to soil flooding and light intensity. *Environ. Exp. Bot.* **2010**, *68*, 113–121. [CrossRef]
27. INUMET ANOMALIAS CLIMATICAS Durante 2014 en Uruguay. Available online: http://www.meteorologia.com.uy/reportes/noticias/docs/pdf/rrpp/168_53868.pdf (accessed on 15 October 2016).
28. Einbond, L.S.; Reynertson, K.A.; Luo, X.-D.; Basile, M.J.; Kennelly, E.J. Anthocyanin antioxidants from edible fruits. *Food Chem.* **2004**, *84*, 23–28. [CrossRef]
29. Gironés-Vilaplana, A.; Baenas, N.; Villaño, D.; Speisky, H.; García-Viguera, C.; Moreno, D.A. Evaluation of Latin-American fruits rich in phytochemicals with biological effects. *J. Funct. Foods* **2014**, *7*, 599–608. [CrossRef]
30. Jaakola, L.; Määttä, K.; Pirttilä, A.M.; Törrönen, R.; Kärenlampi, S.; Hohtola, A. Expression of Genes Involved in Anthocyanin Biosynthesis in Relation to Anthocyanin, Proanthocyanidin, and Flavonol Levels during Bilberry Fruit Development. *Plant Physiol.* **2002**, *130*, 729–739. [CrossRef] [PubMed]
31. Peyrat-Maillard, M.N.; Cuvelier, M.E.; Berset, C. Antioxidant activity of phenolic compounds in 2,2′-azobis (2-amidinopropane) dihydrochloride (AAPH)-induced oxidation: Synergistic and antagonistic effects. *J. Am. Oil Chem. Soc.* **2003**, *80*, 1007–1012. [CrossRef]

PERMISSIONS

All chapters in this book were first published by MDPI; hereby published with permission under the Creative Commons Attribution License or equivalent. Every chapter published in this book has been scrutinized by our experts. Their significance has been extensively debated. The topics covered herein carry significant findings which will fuel the growth of the discipline. They may even be implemented as practical applications or may be referred to as a beginning point for another development.

The contributors of this book come from diverse backgrounds, making this book a truly international effort. This book will bring forth new frontiers with its revolutionizing research information and detailed analysis of the nascent developments around the world.

We would like to thank all the contributing authors for lending their expertise to make the book truly unique. They have played a crucial role in the development of this book. Without their invaluable contributions this book wouldn't have been possible. They have made vital efforts to compile up to date information on the varied aspects of this subject to make this book a valuable addition to the collection of many professionals and students.

This book was conceptualized with the vision of imparting up-to-date information and advanced data in this field. To ensure the same, a matchless editorial board was set up. Every individual on the board went through rigorous rounds of assessment to prove their worth. After which they invested a large part of their time researching and compiling the most relevant data for our readers.

The editorial board has been involved in producing this book since its inception. They have spent rigorous hours researching and exploring the diverse topics which have resulted in the successful publishing of this book. They have passed on their knowledge of decades through this book. To expedite this challenging task, the publisher supported the team at every step. A small team of assistant editors was also appointed to further simplify the editing procedure and attain best results for the readers.

Apart from the editorial board, the designing team has also invested a significant amount of their time in understanding the subject and creating the most relevant covers. They scrutinized every image to scout for the most suitable representation of the subject and create an appropriate cover for the book.

The publishing team has been an ardent support to the editorial, designing and production team. Their endless efforts to recruit the best for this project, has resulted in the accomplishment of this book. They are a veteran in the field of academics and their pool of knowledge is as vast as their experience in printing. Their expertise and guidance has proved useful at every step. Their uncompromising quality standards have made this book an exceptional effort. Their encouragement from time to time has been an inspiration for everyone.

The publisher and the editorial board hope that this book will prove to be a valuable piece of knowledge for researchers, students, practitioners and scholars across the globe.

LIST OF CONTRIBUTORS

Daniela Fracassetti, Ileana Vigentini, Roberto Foschino and Antonio Tirelli
Department of Food, Environmental and Nutritional Sciences, Università degli Studi di Milano, Via G. Celoria 2, 20133 Milan, Italy

Alfredo Fabrizio Francesco Lo Faro and Marica Orioli
Department of Biomedical, Surgical and Dental Sciences, Università degli Studi di Milano, Via Mangiagalli 37, 20133 Milan, Italy

Patrizia De Nisi and Marcello Iriti
Department of Agricultural and Environmental Sciences - Production, Landscape, Agroenergy, Università degli Studi di Milano, Via G. Celoria 2, 20133 Milan, Italy

Julien Stanisiere, Pierre-Yves Mousset and Sophie Lafay
GYNOV SAS, 5 rue Salneuve, 75017 Paris, France

Caroline Orfila, Melvin Holmes and Lisa J. Marshall
School of Food Science and Nutrition, University of Leeds, Leeds LS2 9JT, UK

Benjapor Phongnarisorn
School of Food Science and Nutrition, University of Leeds, Leeds LS2 9JT, UK
Faculty of Agricultural Technology, Phuket Rajabhat University, Phuket 83000, Thailand

Ronan Lordan, Eoin O'Keeffe, Alexandros Tsoupras and Ioannis Zabetakis
Department of Biological Sciences, University of Limerick, Limerick V94 T9PX, Ireland

Duy Tien Doan, Duc Phuong Luu and Thanh Duong Nguyen
Institute of Chemistry, Vietnam Academy of Science and Technology, 18 Hoang Quoc Viet St., Cau Giay Dist., Hanoi 10072, Vietnam

Bich Hoang Thi
Institute of Natural Products Chemistry, Vietnam Academy of Science and Technology, 18 Hoang Quoc Viet St., Cau Giay Dist., Hanoi 10072, Vietnam

Hong Minh Pham Thi, Huu Nghi Do, Minh Quan Pham and Quoc Toan Tran
Institute of Natural Products Chemistry, Vietnam Academy of Science and Technology, 18 Hoang Quoc Viet St., Cau Giay Dist., Hanoi 10072, Vietnam
Graduate University of Science and Technology, Vietnam Academy of Science and Technology, Hanoi 10072, Vietnam

Van Huyen Luu
Hanoi University of Natural Resources and Environment, Hanoi 10072, Vietnam

The Dan Pham
Institute of Natural Products Chemistry, Vietnam Academy of Science and Technology, 18 Hoang Quoc Viet St., Cau Giay Dist., Hanoi 10072, Vietnam
Vietnam Academy of Science and Technology, University of Science and Technology of Hanoi, Hanoi 10072, Vietnam

Van Thai Than
NTT Institute of High Technology, Nguyen Tat Thanh University, Ho Chi Minh City 700000, Vietnam

Hai Ha Pham Thi
Faculty of Biotechnology, Nguyen Tat Thanh University, Ho Chi Minh City 700000, Vietnam

Jay Udani, Ollie Tan and Jhanna Molina
Medical Private Practice, Agoura Hills, CA 91301, USA

Takuya Yamane
Center for Research and Development Bioresources, Organization for Research Promotion, Osaka Prefecture University, Sakai, Osaka 599-8570, Japan
Department of Applied Life Sciences, Graduate School of Life and Environmental Sciences, Osaka Prefecture University, Sakai, Osaka 599-8531, Japan
Institute of Food Sciences, Nakagaki Consulting Engineer and Co., Ltd., Nishi-ku, Sakai 593-8328, Japan

Tatsuji Sakamoto and Yoshihisa Nakano
Center for Research and Development Bioresources, Organization for Research Promotion, Osaka Prefecture University, Sakai, Osaka 599-8570, Japan
Department of Applied Life Sciences, Graduate School of Life and Environmental Sciences, Osaka Prefecture University, Sakai, Osaka 599-8531, Japan

Takenori Nakagaki
Institute of Food Sciences, Nakagaki Consulting Engineer and Co., Ltd., Nishi-ku, Sakai 593-8328, Japan

Sumanto Haldar, Joseph Lim, Siok Ching Chia and Shalini Ponnalagu
Clinical Nutrition Research Centre (CNRC), Singapore Institute for Clinical Sciences (SICS), Agency for Science Technology and Research (A*STAR), 30 Medical Drive, Singapore 117609, Singapore

Christiani Jeyakumar Henry
Clinical Nutrition Research Centre (CNRC), Singapore Institute for Clinical Sciences (SICS), Agency for Science Technology and Research (A*STAR), 30 Medical Drive, Singapore 117609, Singapore
Department of Biochemistry, National University of Singapore, Singapore 119077, Singapore

Michela Verni and Carlo Giuseppe Rizzello
Department of Soil, Plant and Food Science, University of Bari Aldo Moro, 70126 Bari, Italy

Vito Verardo
Department of Nutrition and Food Science, University of Granada, Campus Universitario de Cartuja, E-18071 Granada, Spain
Institute of Nutrition and Food Technology 'José Mataix', Biomedical Research Centre, University of Granada, Avenida del Conocimiento s/n, E-18071 Granada, Spain

Ayse Sevgili and Osman Erkmen
Department of Food Engineering, Faculty of Engineering, University of Gaziantep, 27310 Gaziantep, Turkey

Rattanamanee Chomchan and Bandhita Saibandith
Interdisciplinary Graduate School of Nutraceutical and Functional Food, Prince of Songkla University, Hat-Yai, Songkhla 90112, Thailand

Sunisa Siripongvutikorn
Department of Food Technology, Faculty of Agro-Industry, Prince of Songkla University, Hat-Yai, Songkhla 90112, Thailand

Pattaravan Maliyam
Department of Pharmacognosy and Pharmaceutical Botany, Faculty of Pharmaceutical Sciences, Prince of Songkla University, Hat-Yai, Songkhla 90112, Thailand

Panupong Puttarak
Department of Pharmacognosy and Pharmaceutical Botany, Faculty of Pharmaceutical Sciences, Prince of Songkla University, Hat-Yai, Songkhla 90112, Thailand
Phytomedicine and Pharmaceutical Biotechnology Excellence Center (PPBEC), Prince of Songkla University, Hat-Yai, Songkhla 90112, Thailand

Bojana Filipčev, Jovana Kojić, Jelena Krulj, Marija Bodroža-Solarov and Nebojša Ilić
Institute of Food Technology, University of Novi Sad, 21000 Novi Sad, Serbia

Manuel Venturi and Simona Guerrini
FoodMicroTeam s.r.l., Via di Santo Spirito, 14, 50125 Florence, Italy

Viola Galli, Niccolò Pini and Lisa Granchi
Department of Agriculture, Food, Environment and Forestry (DAGRI), University of Florence, Piazzale delle Cascine, 18, 50144 Florence, Italy

MCarment Martínez-Ballesta
Department of Plant Nutrition, Centro de Edafología y Biología Aplicada del Segura-Spanish Council for Scientific Research (CEBAS-CSIC), Campus de Espinardo 25, 30100 Espinardo, Murcia, Spain

Ángel Gil-Izquierdo, Cristina García-Viguera and Raúl Domínguez-Perles
Research Group on Quality, Safety and Bioactivity of Plant Foods, Department of Food Science and Technology, Centro de Edafología y Biología Aplicada del Segura-Spanish Council for Scientific Research (CEBAS-CSIC), Campus de Espinardo 25, 30100 Espinardo, Murcia, Spain

Vida Šimat
Department of Marine Studies, University of Split, Ruđera Boškovi´ca 37, HR-21000 Split, Croatia

Jelena Vlahović
Department of Marine Studies, University of Split, Ruđera Boškovi´ca 37, HR-21000 Split, Croatia
Sardina d.o.o., Ratac 1, HR-21410 Postira, Croatia

Barbara Soldo and Ivica Ljubenkov
Department of Chemistry, Faculty of Science, University of Split, Ruđera Boškovi´ca 33, HR-21000 Split, Croatia

Ivana Generalić Mekinić and Danijela Skroza
Department of Food Technology and Biotechnology, Faculty of Chemistry and Technology, University of Split, Ruđera Boškovi´ca 35, HR-21000 Split, Croatia

Kazuhisa Maeda
Bionics Program, Tokyo University of Technology Graduate School, 1404-1 Katakuramachi, Hachioji City, Tokyo 192-0982, Japan
School of Bioscience and Biotechnology, Tokyo University of Technology, 1404-1 Katakuramachi, Hachioji City, Tokyo 192-0982, Japan

Yuuka Ogino
School of Bioscience and Biotechnology, Tokyo University of Technology, 1404-1 Katakuramachi, Hachioji City, Tokyo 192-0982, Japan

Ayano Nakamura, Keiji Nakata, Manabu Kitagawa and Seiki Ito
MARUKOME Co., Ltd., 883 Amori, Nagano-shi, Nagano 380-0943, Japan

Michael H. Tunick
Center for Food and Hospitality Management, Drexel University, 101 North 33rd Street, Philadelphia, PA 19104, USA

Diane L. Van Hekken
Dairy and Functional Foods Research Unit, Eastern Regional Research Center, Agricultural Research Service, United States Department of Agriculture (USDA), 600 East Mermaid Lane, Wyndmoor, PA 19038, USA

Rosanna Tofalo, Giorgia Perpetuini, Noemi Battistelli, Alessia Pepe, Andrea Ianni, Giuseppe Martino and Giovanna Suzzi
Faculty of BioScience and Technology for Food, Agriculture and Environment, University of Teramo, 64100 Teramo, Italy

Ignacio Migues, María Verónica Cesio and Horacio Heinzen
Facultad de Química, UdelaR, Av. Gral. Flores 2124, 11800 Montevideo, Uruguay

Nieves Baenas, Amadeo Gironés-Vilaplana and Diego A. Moreno
CEBAS-CSIC, Food Science and Technology Department, Phytochemistry and Healthy Foods Laboratory, Campus Universitario Espinardo-25, E-30100 Espinardo, Murcia, Spain

Index

www.ingramcontent.com/pod-product-compliance
Lightning Source LLC
LaVergne TN
LVHW081413160926
848178LV00067B/96